ACSM's
Guidelines for Exercise Testing and Prescription

TENTH EDITION

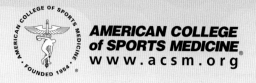

**AMERICAN COLLEGE
of SPORTS MEDICINE**
w w w . a c s m . o r g

ACSM's
Guidelines for Exercise Testing and Prescription

TENTH EDITION

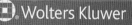

Philadelphia · Baltimore · New York · London
Buenos Aires · Hong Kong · Sydney · Tokyo

Executive Editor: Michael Nobel
Senior Product Development Editor: Amy Millholen
Marketing Manager: Shauna Kelley
Production Product Manager: David Orzechowski
Design Coordinator: Stephen Druding
Art Director: Jennifer Clements
Manufacturing Coordinator: Margie Orzech
Compositor: Absolute Service, Inc.
ACSM Committee on Certification and Registry Boards Chair: William Simpson, PhD, FACSM
ACSM Publications Committee Chair: Jeffrey Potteiger, PhD, FACSM
ACSM Group Publisher: Katie Feltman

Tenth Edition

Copyright 2018 American College of Sports Medicine

9 8 7 6 5 4 3 2 1

Printed in China

Library of Congress Cataloging-in-Publication Data

Names: American College of Sports Medicine, author, issuing body. | Riebe,
    Deborah, editor. | Ehrman, Jonathan K., 1962- editor. | Liguori, Gary,
    1965- editor. | Magal, Meir, editor.
Title: ACSM's guidelines for exercise testing and prescription / senior
    editor, Deborah Riebe ; associate editors, Jonathan K. Ehrman, Gary
    Liguori, Meir Magal.
Other titles: American College of Sports Medicine's guidelines for exercise
    testing and prescription | Guidelines for exercise testing and prescription
Description: Tenth edition. | Philadelphia, PA : Wolters Kluwer Health,
    [2018] | Includes bibliographical references and index.
Identifiers: LCCN 2016042823 | ISBN 9781496339065
Subjects: | MESH: Motor Activity | Exercise Test—standards | Exercise
    Therapy—standards | Physical Exertion | Guideline
Classification: LCC RC684.E9 | NLM WE 103 | DDC 615.8/2—dc23 LC record available at
https://lccn.loc.gov/2016042823

DISCLAIMER

Care has been taken to confirm the accuracy of the information present and to describe generally accepted practices. However, the authors, editors, and publisher are not responsible for errors or omissions or for any consequences from application of the information in this publication and make no warranty, expressed or implied, with respect to the currency, completeness, or accuracy of the contents of the publication. Application of this information in a particular situation remains the professional responsibility of the practitioner; the clinical treatments described and recommended may not be considered absolute and universal recommendations.

The authors, editors, and publisher have exerted every effort to ensure that drug selection and dosage set forth in this text are in accordance with the current recommendations and practice at the time of publication. However, in view of ongoing research, changes in government regulations, and the constant flow of information relating to drug therapy and drug reactions, the reader is urged to check the package insert for each drug for any change in indications and dosage and for added warnings and precautions. This is particularly important when the recommended agent is a new or infrequently employed drug.

Some drugs and medical devices presented in this publication have Food and Drug Administration (FDA) clearance for limited use in restricted research settings. It is the responsibility of the health care provider to ascertain the FDA status of each drug or device planned for use in their clinical practice.

This book is dedicated to the hundreds of volunteer professionals who have, since 1975, contributed thousands of hours developing these internationally adopted Guidelines. Now in its 10th edition, it is the most widely circulated set of guidelines established for exercise professionals. This edition is dedicated to the editors, the writing teams, and the reviewers of this and previous editions who have not only provided their collective expertise but also sacrificed precious time with their colleagues, friends, and families to make sure that these Guidelines meet the highest standards in both science and practice.

The American College of Sports Medicine (ACSM) *Guidelines* origins are within the ACSM Committee on Certification and Registry Boards (CCRB, formerly known as the Certification and Education Committee and the Preventive and Rehabilitative Exercise Committee). Today, the *Guidelines* remain under the auspices of the CCRB and have become the primary resource for anyone conducting exercise testing or exercise programs. The *Guidelines* provide the foundation of content for its supporting companion texts produced by ACSM, which include the fifth edition of *ACSM's Certification Review*, fifth edition of *ACSM's Resources for the Personal Trainer*, second edition of *ACSM's Resources for the Exercise Physiologist*, fifth edition of *ACSM's Health-Related Physical Fitness Assessment Manual*, and several other key ACSM titles.

The first edition of the *Guidelines* was published in 1975, with updated editions published approximately every 4 to 6 years. The outstanding scientists and clinicians who have served in leadership positions as chairs and editors of the *Guidelines* since 1975 are:

First Edition, 1975
Karl G. Stoedefalke, PhD, FACSM, Cochair
John A. Faulkner, PhD, FACSM, Cochair

Second Edition, 1980
Anne R. Abbott, PhD, FACSM, Chair

Third Edition, 1986
Steven N. Blair, PED, FACSM, Chair

Fourth Edition, 1991
Russell R. Pate, PhD, FACSM, Chair

Fifth Edition, 1995
W. Larry Kenney, PhD, FACSM, Senior Editor
Reed H. Humphrey, PhD, PT, FACSM, Associate
  Editor Clinical
Cedric X. Bryant, PhD, FACSM, Associate
  Editor Fitness

Sixth Edition, 2000
Barry A. Franklin, PhD, FACSM, Senior Editor
Mitchell H. Whaley, PhD, FACSM, Associate
  Editor Clinical
Edward T. Howley, PhD, FACSM, Associate
  Editor Fitness

Seventh Edition, 2005
Mitchell H. Whaley, PhD, FACSM, Senior
  Editor

Peter H. Brubaker, PhD, FACSM, Associate
  Editor Clinical
Robert M. Otto, PhD, FACSM, Associate Editor
  Fitness

Eighth Edition, 2009
Walter R. Thompson, PhD, FACSM, Senior
  Editor
Neil F. Gordon, MD, PhD, FACSM, Associate
  Editor
Linda S. Pescatello, PhD, FACSM, Associate
  Editor

Ninth Edition, 2013
Linda S. Pescatello, PhD, FACSM, Senior Editor
Ross Arena, PT, PhD, FAHA, Associate Editor
Deborah Riebe, PhD, FACSM, Associate Editor
Paul D. Thompson, MD, FACSM, FACC,
  Associate Editor

Tenth Edition, 2016
Deborah Riebe, PhD, FACSM, Senior Editor
Jonathan K. Ehrman, PhD, FACSM, FAACVPR,
  Associate Editor
Gary Liguori, PhD, FACSM, Associate Editor
Meir Magal, PhD, FACSM, Associate Editor

Preface

The 10th edition of *ACSM's Guidelines for Exercise Testing and Prescription* will continue the efforts of the editors and contributing authors of the eighth and ninth editions to make it a true *guidelines* book rather than a sole and inclusive *resource*. It was the original intent of the *Guidelines* to be user-friendly, easily accessible, and a current primary resource for exercise and other health professionals who conduct exercise testing and exercise programs. To this effect, in this edition, text descriptions have been minimized; more tables, boxes, and figures have been included; and key Web sites conclude each chapter.

The reader of this edition of *ACSM's Guidelines for Exercise Testing and Prescription* will notice several innovations. The 10th edition of the *Guidelines* presents ACSM's new recommendations for the preparticipation health screening process, which represents a significant change from previous versions. Recommendations for the Frequency, Intensity, Time, and Type (FITT) principle of exercise prescription are presented using a new succinct format for quick reference. Some of the book content has been reorganized to make it easier to locate information quickly. Finally, there was a substantial increase in the number of external reviewers. In lieu of chapter reviewers, the 10th edition used content expert reviewers for specific sections within chapters. This included the development of an expert panel which met several times to develop the new preparticipation health screening process. We have integrated the most recent guidelines and recommendations available from ACSM position stands and other relevant professional organizations' scientific statements so that the *Guidelines* are the most current, primary resource for exercise testing and prescription. It is important for the readership to know that new themes and innovations included in the 10th edition were developed with input from the ACSM membership prior to the initiation of this project via an electronic survey and focus groups conducted at the 2014 ACSM Annual Meeting that asked respondents and participants, respectively, for their suggestions regarding the content.

Any updates made in this edition of the *Guidelines* after their publication and prior to the publication of the next edition of the *Guidelines* can be accessed from the ACSM Certification link (http://certification.acsm.org/updates). Furthermore, the reader is referred to the ACSM Get Certified link for a listing of ACSM Certifications at www.acsmcertification.org/get-certified) and to http://certification.acsm .org/outlines for detailed exam content outlines..

ACKNOWLEDGMENTS

It is in this preface that the editors of the 10th edition have the opportunity to thank the many people who helped to see this project to completion. First and foremost, we thank our families and friends for their understanding of the extensive time commitment we made to this project that encompassed over three years.

We are in great debt to the contributing authors of the 10th edition of the *Guidelines* for volunteering their expertise and valuable time to ensure the *Guidelines* meet the highest standards in exercise science and practice. The 10th edition contributing authors are listed in the following section.

The *Guidelines* review process was extensive, undergoing many layers of expert scrutiny to ensure the highest quality of content. We thank the external and ACSM Committee on Certification and Registry Boards (CCRB) reviewers of the 10th edition for their careful reviews. These reviewers are listed later in this front matter.

This book could not have been completed without the patience, expertise, and guidance of Katie Feltman, ACSM Director of Publishing. We thank Richard T. Cotton, ACSM National Director of Certification; Traci Sue Rush, ACSM Assistant Director of Certification Programs; Kela Webster, ACSM Certification Coordinator; Robin Ashman and Dru Romanini, ACSM Certification Department Assistants; Angela Chastain, ACSM Editorial Services Office; Jeffrey Potteiger, ACSM Publications Committee Chair; and the extraordinarily hardworking Publications Committee.

We thank our publisher, and in particular Michael Nobel, Executive Editor; Amy Millholen, Senior Product Development Editor; and Shauna Kelley, Marketing Manager.

We thank the ACSM CCRB for their valuable insights into the content of this edition of the *Guidelines* and council on administrative issues related to seeing this project to completion. The ACSM CCRB tirelessly reviewed manuscript drafts to ensure the content of this edition of the *Guidelines* meets the highest standards in exercise science and practice.

On a more personal note, I thank my three associate editors — Dr. Jonathan Ehrman, Dr. Gary Liguori, and Dr. Meir Magal — who selflessly devoted their valuable time and expertise to the 10th edition of the *Guidelines*. Their strong sense of commitment to the *Guidelines* emanated from an underlying belief held by the editorial team of the profound importance the *Guidelines* have in informing and directing the work we do in exercise science and practice. Words cannot express the extent of my gratitude to the three of you for your tireless efforts to see this project to completion.

Deborah Riebe, PhD, FACSM
Senior Editor

ADDITIONAL RESOURCES

ACSM's Guidelines for Exercise Testing and Prescription, Tenth Edition, includes additional resources for instructors that are available on the book's companion Web site at http://thepoint.lww.com/.

Instructors

Approved adopting instructors will be given access to the following additional resources:

- Brownstone test generator
- PowerPoint presentations
- Image bank
- Angel/Blackboard/Moodle ready cartridges

Nota Bene

The views and information contained in the 10th edition of *ACSM's Guidelines for Exercise Testing and Prescription* are provided as guidelines — as opposed to *standards of practice*. This distinction is an important one because specific legal connotations may be attached to standards of practice that are not attached to guidelines. This distinction is critical inasmuch as it gives the professional in exercise testing and programmatic settings the freedom to deviate from these guidelines when necessary and appropriate in the course of using independent and prudent judgment. *ACSM's Guidelines for Exercise Testing and Prescription* presents a framework whereby the professional may certainly — and in some cases has the obligation to — tailor to individual client or patient needs while balancing institutional or legal requirements.

Contributing Authors to the Tenth Edition*

Stamatis Agiovlasitis, PhD, FACSM, ACSM-CEP

Mississippi State University
Mississippi State, Mississippi
Chapter 11: Exercise Testing and Prescription for Populations with Other Chronic Diseases and Health Conditions

Meghan Baruth, PhD

Saginaw Valley State University
University Center, Michigan
Chapter 12: Behavioral Theories and Strategies for Promoting Exercise

Tracy Baynard, PhD, FACSM

University of Illinois at Chicago
Chicago, Illinois
Chapter 11: Exercise Testing and Prescription for Populations with Other Chronic Diseases and Health Conditions

Darren T. Beck, PhD

Edward Via College of Osteopathic Medicine—Auburn Campus
Auburn, Alabama
Appendix A: Common Medications
Appendix C: Electrocardiogram Interpretation

Clinton A. Brawner, PhD, FACSM, ACSM-RCEP, ACSM-CEP

Henry Ford Hospital
Detroit, Michigan
Chapter 5: Clinical Exercise Testing and Interpretation

Monthaporn S. Bryant, PT, PhD

Michael E DeBakey VA Medical Center
Houston, Texas
Chapter 11: Exercise Testing and Prescription for Populations with Other Chronic Diseases and Health Conditions

John W. Castellani, PhD

United States Army Research Institute of Environmental Medicine
Natick, Massachusetts
Chapter 8: Environmental Considerations for Exercise Prescription

Linda H. Chung, PhD

UCAM Research Center for High Performance Sport; Universidad Católica de Murcia
Guadalupe, Murcia, Spain
Chapter 11: Exercise Testing and Prescription for Populations with Other Chronic Diseases and Health Conditions

Sheri R. Colberg-Ochs, PhD, FACSM

Old Dominion University
Norfolk, Virginia
Chapter 10: Exercise Prescription for Individuals with Metabolic Disease and Cardiovascular Disease Risk Factors

Marisa Colston, PhD, ATC

The University of Tennessee at Chattanooga
Chattanooga, Tennessee
Chapter 7: Exercise Prescription for Healthy Populations with Special Considerations

*See Appendix F for a list of contributors for the previous two editions.

Michael R. Deschenes, PhD, FACSM
College of William & Mary in Virginia
Williamsburg, Virginia
Chapter 6: General Principles of Exercise
  Prescription

Charles L. Dumke, PhD, FACSM
University of Montana
Missoula, Montana
Chapter 4: Health-Related Physical
  Fitness Testing and Interpretation

**Jonathan K. Ehrman, PhD, FACSM,
FAACVPR, ACSM-CEP, ACSM-PD**
Henry Ford Hospital
Detroit, Michigan
Chapter 5: Clinical Exercise Testing and
  Interpretation
Chapter 9: Exercise Prescription for
  Patients with Cardiac, Peripheral,
  Cerebrovascular, and Pulmonary
  Disease
Chapter 10: Exercise Prescription for
  Individuals with Metabolic Disease and
  Cardiovascular Disease Risk Factors
Chapter 11: Exercise Testing and
  Prescription for Populations with
  Other Chronic Diseases and Health
  Conditions

Stephen F. Figoni, PhD, FACSM
VA Long Beach Healthcare System
Long Beach, California
Chapter 11: Exercise Testing and
  Prescription for Populations with
  Other Chronic Diseases and Health
  Conditions

Charles J. Fountaine, PhD
University of Minnesota Duluth
Duluth, Minnesota
Chapter 7: Exercise Prescription for
  Healthy Populations with Special
  Considerations

**Barry A. Franklin, PhD, FACSM,
ACSM-PD, ACSM-CEP**
William Beaumont Hospital
Royal Oak, Michigan
Chapter 2: Exercise Preparticipation
  Health Screening

**Carol Ewing Garber, PhD, FACSM,
ACSM-ETT, ACSM-RCEP, ACSM-HFS,
ACSM-PD**
Teachers College, Columbia University
New York, New York
Chapter 6: General Principles of Exercise
  Prescription

Gregory A. Hand, PhD, MPH, FACSM
West Virginia University
Morgantown, West Virginia
Chapter 11: Exercise Testing and
  Prescription for Populations with
  Other Chronic Diseases and Health
  Conditions

**Samuel A. Headley, PhD, FACSM,
ACSM-RCEP, ACSM-CEP, ACSM-ETT**
Springfield College
Springfield, Massachusetts
Chapter 3: Preexercise Evaluation
Chapter 11: Exercise Testing and
  Prescription for Populations with
  Other Chronic Diseases and Health
  Conditions

Jason R. Jaggers, PhD
University of Louisville
Louisville, Kentucky
Chapter 11: Exercise Testing and
  Prescription for Populations with
  Other Chronic Diseases and Health
  Conditions

Josh Johann, MS, EIM
University of Tennessee at Chattanooga
Chattanooga, Tennessee
Chapter 10: Exercise Prescription for
  Individuals with Metabolic Disease and
  Cardiovascular Disease Risk Factors

Robert W. Kenefick, PhD, FACSM
United States Army Research Institute of
  Environmental Medicine
Natick, Massachusetts
Chapter 8: Environmental Considerations
  for Exercise Prescription

Steven J. Keteyian, PhD, ACSM-RCEP
Henry Ford Hospital
Detroit, Michigan
Chapter 9: Exercise Prescription for
  Patients with Cardiac, Peripheral,
  Cerebrovascular, and Pulmonary
  Disease

Peter Kokkinos, PhD
Veterans Affairs Medical Center
Washington, District of Columbia
Chapter 10: Exercise Prescription for
  Individuals with Metabolic Disease and
  Cardiovascular Disease Risk Factors

Kathy Lemley, PT, PhD
Concordia University Wisconsin
Mequon, Wisconsin
Chapter 11: Exercise Testing and
  Prescription for Populations with
  Other Chronic Diseases and Health
  Conditions

Andrew Lemmey, PhD
Bangor University
Bangor Gwynedd, Wales, United
  Kingdom
Chapter 11: Exercise Testing and
  Prescription for Populations with
  Other Chronic Diseases and Health
  Conditions

**Gary Liguori, PhD, FACSM,
ACSM-CEP**
University of Rhode Island
Kingston, Rhode Island
Chapter 10: Exercise Prescription for
  Individuals with Metabolic Disease and
  Cardiovascular Disease Risk Factors

Meir Magal, PhD, FACSM, ACSM-CEP
North Carolina Wesleyan College
Rocky Mount, North Carolina
Chapter 1: Benefits and Risks Associated
  with Physical Activity

Kyle J. McInnis, ScD, FACSM
Merrimack College
North Andover, Massachusetts
Appendix B: Emergency Risk Management

Miriam C. Morey, PhD, FACSM
Durham VA Medical Center
Durham, North Carolina
Chapter 7: Exercise Prescription for
  Healthy Populations with Special
  Considerations

Stephen R. Muza, PhD, FACSM
United States Army Research Institute of
  Environmental Medicine
Natick, Massachusetts
Chapter 8: Environmental Considerations
  for Exercise Prescription

David L. Nichols, PhD, FACSM
Texas Woman's University
Denton, Texas
Chapter 11: Exercise Testing and
  Prescription for Populations with
  Other Chronic Diseases and Health
  Conditions

Jennifer R. O'Neill, PhD, MPH
University of South Carolina
Columbia, South Carolina
Chapter 7: Exercise Prescription for
  Healthy Populations with Special
  Considerations

Quinn R. Pack, MD, MSc
Baystate Medical Center
Springfield, Massachusetts
Chapter 10: Exercise Prescription for
  Individuals with Metabolic Disease and
  Cardiovascular Disease Risk Factors

Russell R. Pate, PhD, FACSM
University of South Carolina
Columbia, South Carolina
Chapter 7: Exercise Prescription for
  Healthy Populations with Special
  Considerations

Ken Pitteti, PhD
Wichita State University
Wichita, Kansas
Chapter 11: Exercise Testing and
  Prescription for Populations with
  Other Chronic Diseases and Health
  Conditions

Elizabeth J. Protas, PhD, FACSM

University of Texas Medical Branch
Galveston, Texas
Chapter 11: Exercise Testing and
    Prescription for Populations with
    Other Chronic Diseases and Health
    Conditions

Amy E. Rauworth, MS

National Center on Health, Physical
    Activity and Disability
Birmingham, Alabama
Chapter 11: Exercise Testing and
    Prescription for Populations with
    Other Chronic Diseases and Health
    Conditions

**Deborah Riebe, PhD, FACSM,
ACSM EP-C**

University of Rhode Island
Kingston, Rhode Island
Appendix D: American College of Sports
    Medicine Certifications
Appendix E: Accreditation of Exercise
    Science Programs

Mickey Scheinowitz, PhD, FACSM

Tel-Aviv University and Neufeld Cardiac
    Research Institute at Sheba Medical
    Center Ramat-Aviv
Tel-Hashomer, Israel
Chapter 1: Benefits and Risks Associated
    with Physical Activity

**Kathryn H. Schmitz, PhD, MPH,
FACSM**

University of Pennsylvania
Philadelphia, Pennsylvania
Chapter 11: Exercise Testing and
    Prescription for Populations with
    Other Chronic Diseases and Health
    Conditions

Thomas W. Storer, PhD

Brigham and Women's Hospital, Harvard
    Medical School
Boston, Massachusetts
Chapter 9: Exercise Prescription for
    Patients with Cardiac, Peripheral,
    Cerebrovascular, and Pulmonary
    Disease

Cooker Storm, PhD

Pepperdine University
Malibu, California
Chapter 7: Exercise Prescription for
    Healthy Populations with Special
    Considerations

Dennis A. Tighe, MD

University of Massachusetts Medical
    School
Worcester, Massachusetts
Chapter 3: Preexercise Evaluation

Jared M. Tucker, PhD

Helen DeVos Children's Hospital
Grand Rapids, Michigan
Chapter 7: Exercise Prescription for
    Healthy Populations with Special
    Considerations

Sara Wilcox, PhD, FACSM

University of South Carolina
Columbia, South Carolina
Chapter 12: Behavioral Theories and
    Strategies for Promoting Exercise

Reviewers for Tenth Edition*

Robert S. Axtell, PhD, FACSM, ACSM-ETT
Southern Connecticut State University
New Haven, Connecticut

Marie Hoeger Bement, MPT, PhD
Marquette University
Milwaukee, Wisconsin

Robert Berry, MS, ACSM-RCEP, ACSM-CEP, EIM 3
Henry Ford Medical Group
Detroit, Michigan

Susan Bloomfield, PhD, FACSM
Texas A&M University
College Station, Texas

*Andrew M. Bosak, PhD, ACSM EP-C
Liberty University
Lynchburg, Virginia

Douglas Casa, PhD, ATC, FACSM
University of Connecticut
Storrs, Connecticut

James Churilla, PhD, MPH, FACSM, ACSM-PD, ACSM-RCEP, ACSM-CEP, ACSM EP-C
University of North Florida
Jacksonville, Florida

*Robert J. Confessore, PhD, FACSM, ACSM-RCEP, ACSM-CEP, ACSM EP-C, EIM 3
Kalispell Regional Medical Center
Kalispell, Montana

*Richard T. Cotton, MA, ACSM-PD, ACSM-CEP
American College of Sports Medicine
Indianapolis, Indiana

Matthew Delmonico, PhD
University of Rhode Island
Kingston, Rhode Island

Devon Dobrosielski, PhD, ACSM-CEP
Towson University
Towson, Maryland

David R. Dolbow, PhD, DPT, RKT
University of Southern Mississippi
Hattiesburg, Mississippi

J. Larry Durstine, PhD, FACSM
University of South Carolina
Columbia, South Carolina

Gregory Dwyer, PhD, FACSM, ACSM-PD, ACSM-RCEP, ACSM-CEP, ACSM-ETT, EIM 3
East Stroudsburg University
East Stroudsburg, Pennsylvania

*Michael R. Esco, PhD, ACSM-RCEP, ACSM EP-C, EIM 2
The University of Alabama
Tuscaloosa, Alabama

Nicholas H. Evans, MHS, ACSM-CEP
Shepherd Center
Atlanta, Georgia

Kelly Evenson, PhD, FACSM
The University of North Carolina at Chapel Hill
Chapel Hill, North Carolina

*Yuri Feito, PhD, MPH, FACSM, ACSM-RCEP, ACSM-CEP, EIM 3
Kennesaw State University
Kennesaw, Georgia

Carl Foster, PhD, FACSM
University of Wisconsin—La Crosse
La Crosse, Wisconsin

Charles Fountaine, PhD
University of Minnesota Duluth
Duluth, Minnesota

*Janet T. Peterson, DrPH, FACSM, ACSM-RCEP, ACSM EP-C

Linfield College
McMinnville, Oregon

*Peter J. Ronai, MS, FACSM, ACSM-PD, ACSM-RCEP, ACSM-CEP, ACSM EP-C, ACSM-ETT, EIM 3

Sacred Heart University
Fairfield, Connecticut

*Brad A. Roy, PhD, FACSM, ACSM-CEP, EIM 3

Kalispell Regional Medical Center
Kalispell, Montana

John M. Schuna Jr, PhD

Oregon State University
Corvallis, Oregon

JoAnn Eickhoff-Shemek, PhD, PACSM, FAWHP, ACSM-HFD, ACSM EP-C, ACSM-ETT

University of South Florida
Tampa, Florida

Ronald J. Sigal, MD, MPH, FRCPC

University of Calgary
Alberta, Canada

Barbara Smith, PhD, RN, FACSM, ACSM-PD

Michigan State University
East Lansing, Michigan

Erin M. Snook, PhD

Datalys Center for Sports Injury Research and Prevention
Indianapolis, Indiana

Bradford Strand, PhD

North Dakota State University
Fargo, North Dakota

*Amy Jo Sutterluety, PhD, FACSM, ACSM-CES, EIM 3

Baldwin Wallace University
Berea, Ohio

*Ann M. Swank, PhD

University of Louisville
Louisville, Kentucky

*Benjamin C. Thompson, PhD, FACSM, ACSM EP-C, EIM 2

Metropolitan State University of Denver
Denver, Colorado

Dennis A. Tighe, MD

University of Massachusetts Medical School
Worcester, Massachusetts

David Verrill, MS, ACSM-PD, ACSM-RCEP, ACSM-CEP

The University of North Carolina at Charlotte
Charlotte, North Carolina

Sean Walsh, PhD, FACSM

Central Connecticut State University
New Britain, Connecticut

*Christie Ward-Ritacco, PhD, ACSM EP-C, EIM 2

University of Rhode Island
Kingston, Rhode Island

*Michael Webster, PhD, FACSM, ACSM-CEP

Valdosta State University
Valdosta, Georgia

*M. Allison Williams, PhD, FACSM, ACSM EP-C

Queens College
Queens, New York

*Denotes reviewers who were also members of the ACSM Committee on Certification and Registry Boards.

Contents

Abbreviations

AACVPR	American Association of Cardiovascular and Pulmonary Rehabilitation		BIA	bioelectrical impedance analysis
ABI	ankle/brachial pressure index		BLS	basic life support
ACC	American College of Cardiology		BMD	bone mineral density
			BMI	body mass index
ACE-I	angiotensin-converting enzyme inhibitors		BMT	bone marrow transplantation
ACLS	advanced cardiac life support		BP	blood pressure
ACS	Acute coronary syndrome		BUN	blood urea nitrogen
ACSM	American College of Sports Medicine		CAAHEP	Commission on Accreditation of Allied Health Education Programs
ADL	activities of daily living		CABG(S)	coronary artery bypass graft (surgery)
ADT	androgen deprivation therapy		CAC	coronary artery calcium
AEDs	automated external defibrillators		CAD	coronary artery disease
			CCB	calcium channel blockers
AHA	American Heart Association		CDC	Centers for Disease Control and Prevention
AHFS	American Hospital Formulary Service		CEP	ACSM Certified Clinical Exercise Physiologist®
AIDS	acquired immunodeficiency syndrome		CHF	congestive heart failure
			CKD	chronic kidney disease
ALT	alanine transaminase		CM	cardiomyopathy
AMI	acute myocardial infarction		CNS	central nervous system
AMS	acute mountain sickness		CoAES	Committee on Accreditation for the Exercise Sciences
ARBs	angiotensin II receptor blockers		COPD	chronic obstructive pulmonary disease
ART	antiretroviral therapy		CP	cerebral palsy
AS	ankylosing spondylitis		CPET	cardiopulmonary exercise test
ASH	American Society of Hypertension		CPISRA	Cerebral Palsy International Sport and Recreation Association
AST	aspartate aminotransferase			
ATP III	Adult Treatment Panel III		CPR	cardiopulmonary resuscitation
ATS	American Thoracic Society			
AV	atrioventricular		CPT	ACSM Certified Personal Trainer^SM
AVD	atherosclerotic vascular disease			

CR	cardiac rehabilitation
CRF	cardiorespiratory fitness
CVD	cardiovascular disease
CWR	constant work rate
DASH	Dietary Approaches to Stop Hypertension
Db	body density
DBP	diastolic blood pressure
DBS	deep brain stimulation
DEXA	dual-energy X-ray absorptiometry
DM	diabetes mellitus
DMARD	disease-modifying antirheumatic drug
DOMS	delayed onset muscle soreness
DRI	direct renin inhibitor
DS	Down syndrome
DVR	dynamic variable resistance
EAS	European Atherosclerosis Society
ECG	electrocardiogram (electrocardiographic)
EDSS	Kurtzke Expanded Disability Status Scale
EE	energy expenditure
EI	energy intake
EIB	exercise-induced bronchoconstriction
EIM	Exercise is Medicine
EMS	emergency medical service
EP-C	ACSM Certified Exercise Physiologist[SM]
ERS	European Respiratory Society
ESC	European Society of Cardiology
ESRD	end-stage renal disease
ETT	exercise tolerance testing
Ex R_x	exercise prescription
FES-LCE	functional electrical stimulation-leg cycle ergometry
$FEV_{1.0}$	forced expiratory volume in one second
FFBd	fat-free body density
FFM	fat-free mass
FITT-VP	Frequency, Intensity, Time, Type, Volume, and Progression
FM	fat mass
FN	false negative
FP	false positive
FPG	fasting plasma glucose
FRAX	Fracture Risk Algorithm
FRIEND	Fitness Registry and the Importance of Exercise National Database
FVC	forced vital capacity
GEI	ACSM Certified Group Exercise Instructor[SM]
GFR	glomerular filtration rate
GLP-1	glucagon-like peptide 1
GOLD	Global Initiative for Chronic Obstructive Lung Disease
GXT	graded exercise test
HACE	high-altitude cerebral edema
HAPE	high-altitude pulmonary edema
HbA1C	glycolated hemoglobin
HBM	health belief model
HCTZ	hydrochlorothiazide
HDL-C	high-density lipoprotein cholesterol
HFpEF	heart failure with preserved ejection fraction
HFrEF	heart failure with reduced ejection fraction
HIIT	high intensity interval training
HIPAA	Health Insurance Portability and Accountability Act
HIV	human immunodeficiency virus
HMG-CoA	hydroxymethylglutaryl-CoA
HR	heart rate
HR_{max}	maximal heart rate
HR_{peak}	peak heart rate
HRR	heart rate reserve

HR_{rest}	resting heart rate		MVV	maximal voluntary ventilation
hs-CRP	high-sensitivity C-reactive protein		6MWT	6-min walk test
HSCT	hematopoietic stem cell transplantation		NCCA	National Commission for Certifying Agencies
HTN	hypertension		NCEP	National Cholesterol Education Program
ICD	implantable cardioverter defibrillator		NFCI	nonfreezing cold injuries
ID	intellectual disability		NHANES	National Health and Nutrition Examination Survey
IDF	International Diabetes Federation		NHLBI	National Heart, Lung, and Blood Institute
IDL	intermediate-density lipoprotein		NOTF	National Obesity Task Force
IFG	impaired fasting glucose		NSAIDs	nonsteroidal anti-inflammatory drugs
IGT	impaired glucose tolerance		NSTE	non–ST-segment elevation
IHD	ischemic heart disease		NSTEMI	non–ST-segment elevation myocardial infarction
IMT	inspiratory muscle training			
ISH	International Society of Hypertension		NYHA	New York Heart Association
IVC	inspiration vital capacity		OA	osteoarthritis
IVCD	intraventricular conduction delay		OGTT	oral glucose tolerance test
			OSHA	Occupational Safety and Health Administration
JTA	job task analysis			
KSs	knowledge and skills		OUES	oxygen uptake efficiency slope
LABS	Longitudinal Assessment of Bariatric Surgery		PA	physical activity
LBP	low back pain		PAD	peripheral artery disease
LDL-C	low-density lipoprotein cholesterol		$PaCO_2$	partial pressure of carbon dioxide
L-G-L	Lown-Ganong-Levine		PAH	pulmonary arterial hypertension
LLN	lower limit of normal			
LVAD	left ventricular assist device		P_aO_2	partial pressure of arterial oxygen
LVEF	left ventricular ejection fraction			
LVH	left ventricular hypertrophy		PAR-Q+	Physical Activity Readiness Questionnaire+
MAP	mean arterial pressure		PCI	percutaneous coronary intervention
MET	metabolic equivalent			
Metsyn	metabolic syndrome		PD	Parkinson disease
MI	myocardial infarction		PEF	peak expiratory flow
MR	mitral regurgitation		PG	plasma glucose
MS	multiple sclerosis		PKU	phenylketonuria
MSI	musculoskeletal injury		PNF	proprioceptive neuromuscular facilitation
MVC	maximal voluntary contraction			

PPMS	primary progressive multiple sclerosis
PR	pulmonary rehabilitation
PRMS	progressive relapsing multiple sclerosis
PTCA	percutaneous transluminal coronary angioplasty
PVC	premature ventricular contraction
$\dot{Q}$	cardiac output
QTc	QT corrected for heart rate
RA	rheumatoid arthritis
RCEP	ACSM Registered Clinical Exercise Physiologist®
RER	respiratory exchange ratio
RHR	resting heart rate
1-RM	one repetition maximum
ROM	range of motion
RPE	rating of perceived exertion
RRMS	relapsing-remitting multiple sclerosis
RVH	right ventricular hypertrophy
SaO_2	percent saturation of arterial oxygen
SBP	systolic blood pressure
SCA	sudden cardiac arrest
SCD	sudden cardiac death
SCI	spinal cord injury
SCT	social cognitive theory
SD	standard deviation
SDT	self-determination theory
SEE	standard error of the estimate
SET	social ecological theory
SIT	sprint interval training
SpO_2	percent saturation of arterial oxygen
SPPB	Short Physical Performance Battery
SRT	shuttle run test
T1DM	Type 1 diabetes mellitus

T2DM	Type 2 diabetes mellitus
TAVR	transcatheter aortic valve replacement
TG	triglycerides
THR	target heart rate
TLC	total lung capacity
TN	true negative
TOBEC	total body electrical conductivity
TP	true positive
TPB	theory of planned behavior
TTM	transtheoretical model
VAT	ventilatory-derived anaerobic threshold
VC	vital capacity
$\dot{V}CO_2$	volume of carbon dioxide per minute
$\dot{V}E$	expired ventilation per minute
VF	ventricular fibrillation
VHD	valvular heart disease
VLDL	very low-density lipoprotein
$\dot{V}O_2$	volume of oxygen consumed per minute
$\dot{V}O_{2max}$	maximal volume of oxygen consumed per minute (maximal oxygen uptake, maximal oxygen consumption)
$\dot{V}O_{2peak}$	peak oxygen uptake
$\dot{V}O_2R$	oxygen uptake reserve
%$\dot{V}O_2R$	percentage of oxygen uptake reserve
VT	ventilatory threshold
WBGT	wet-bulb globe temperature
WCT	Wind Chill Temperature Index
WHR	waist-to-hip ratio
W-P-W	Wolff-Parkinson-White

CHAPTER 1

Benefits and Risks Associated with Physical Activity

INTRODUCTION

The purpose of this chapter is to provide current information on the benefits and risks of physical activity (PA) and/or exercise. For clarification purposes, key terms used throughout the *Guidelines* related to PA and fitness are defined in this chapter. Additional information specific to a disease, disability, or health condition are explained within the context of the chapter in which they are discussed in the *Guidelines*. PA continues to take on an increasingly important role in the prevention and treatment of multiple chronic diseases, health conditions, and their associated risk factors. Therefore, *Chapter 1* focuses on the public health perspective that forms the basis for the current PA recommendations (5,26,34,70,93). *Chapter 1* concludes with recommendations for reducing the incidence and severity of exercise-related complications for primary and secondary prevention programs.

PHYSICAL ACTIVITY AND FITNESS TERMINOLOGY

PA and exercise are often used interchangeably, but these terms are not synonymous. *PA* is defined as any bodily movement produced by the contraction of skeletal muscles that results in a substantial increase in caloric requirements over resting energy expenditure (14,78). *Exercise* is a type of PA consisting of planned, structured, and repetitive bodily movement done to improve and/or maintain one or more components of physical fitness (14). *Physical fitness* has been defined in several ways, but the generally accepted definition is the ability to carry out daily tasks with vigor and alertness, without undue fatigue, and with ample energy to enjoy leisure-time pursuits and meet unforeseen emergencies (76). Physical fitness is composed of various elements that can be further grouped into health-related and skill-related components which are defined in *Box 1.1*.

In addition to defining PA, exercise, and physical fitness, it is important to clearly define the wide range of intensities associated with PA (see *Table 6.1*). Methods for quantifying the relative intensity of PA include specifying a percentage

Box 1.1	Health-Related and Skill-Related Components of Physical Fitness

Health-Related Physical Fitness Components

- Cardiorespiratory endurance: the ability of the circulatory and respiratory system to supply oxygen during sustained physical activity
- Body composition: the relative amounts of muscle, fat, bone, and other vital parts of the body
- Muscular strength: the ability of muscle to exert force
- Muscular endurance: the ability of muscle to continue to perform without fatigue
- Flexibility: the range of motion available at a joint

Skill-Related Physical Fitness Components

- Agility: the ability to change the position of the body in space with speed and accuracy
- Coordination: the ability to use the senses, such as sight and hearing, together with body parts in performing tasks smoothly and accurately
- Balance: the maintenance of equilibrium while stationary or moving
- Power: the ability or rate at which one can perform work
- Reaction time: the time elapsed between stimulation and the beginning of the reaction to it
- Speed: the ability to perform a movement within a short period of time

Adapted from (96). Available from http://www.fitness.gov/digest_mar2000.htm

of oxygen uptake reserve ($\dot{V}O_2R$), heart rate reserve (HRR), oxygen consumption ($\dot{V}O_2$), heart rate (HR), or metabolic equivalents (METs) (see *Box 6.2*). Each of these methods for describing the intensity of PA has strengths and limitations. Although determining the most appropriate method is left to the exercise professional, *Chapter 6* provides the methodology and guidelines for selecting a suitable method.

METs are a useful, convenient, and standardized way to describe the absolute intensity of a variety of physical activities. Light intensity PA is defined as requiring 2.0–2.9 METs, moderate as 3.0–5.9 METs, and vigorous as ≥6.0 METs (26). *Table 1.1* gives specific examples of activities in METs for each of the intensity ranges. A complete list of physical activities and their associated estimates of energy expenditure can be found elsewhere (2).

Maximal aerobic capacity usually declines with age (26). For this reason, when older and younger individuals work at the same MET level, the relative exercise intensity (*e.g.*, %$\dot{V}O_{2max}$) will usually be different (see *Chapter 6*). In other words, the older individual will be working at a greater relative percentage of maximal oxygen consumption ($\dot{V}O_{2max}$) than their younger counterparts. Nonetheless, physically active older adults may have aerobic capacities comparable to or greater than those of physically inactive younger adults.

TABLE 1.1

Metabolic Equivalents (METs) Values of Common Physical Activities Classified as Light, Moderate, or Vigorous Intensity

Very Light/Light (<3.0 METs)	Moderate (3.0–5.9 METs)	Vigorous (≥6.0 METs)
Walking	**Walking**	**Walking, jogging, and running**
Walking slowly around home, store, or office = 2.0[a]	Walking 3.0 mi · h^{-1} = 3.0[a] Walking at very brisk pace (4 mi · h^{-1}) = 5.0[a]	Walking at very, very brisk pace (4.5 mi · h^{-1}) = 6.3[a] Walking/hiking at moderate pace and grade with no or light pack (<10 lb) = 7.0
Household and occupation	**Household and occupation**	Hiking at steep grades and pack 10–42 lb = 7.5–9.0
Standing performing light work, such as making bed, washing dishes, ironing, preparing food, or store clerk = 2.0–2.5	Cleaning, heavy — washing windows, car, clean garage = 3.0 Sweeping floors or carpet, vacuuming, mopping = 3.0–3.5	Jogging at 5 mi · h^{-1} = 8.0[a] Jogging at 6 mi · h^{-1} = 10.0[a] Running at 7 mi · h^{-1} = 11.5[a]
Leisure time and sports	Carpentry — general = 3.6 Carrying and stacking wood = 5.5	**Household and occupation**
Arts and crafts, playing cards = 1.5 Billiards = 2.5 Boating — power = 2.5 Croquet = 2.5 Darts = 2.5 Fishing — sitting = 2.5 Playing most musical instruments = 2.0–2.5	Mowing lawn — walk power mower = 5.5 **Leisure time and sports** Badminton — recreational = 4.5 Basketball — shooting around = 4.5 Dancing — ballroom slow = 3.0; ballroom fast = 4.5 Fishing from riverbank and walking = 4.0 Golf — walking, pulling clubs = 4.3 Sailing boat, wind surfing = 3.0 Table tennis = 4.0 Tennis doubles = 5.0 Volleyball — noncompetitive = 3.0–4.0	Shoveling sand, coal, etc. = 7.0 Carrying heavy loads, such as bricks = 7.5 Heavy farming, such as bailing hay = 8.0 Shoveling, digging ditches = 8.5 **Leisure time and sports** Bicycling on flat — light effort (10–12 mi · h^{-1}) = 6.0 Basketball game = 8.0 Bicycling on flat — moderate effort (12–14 mi · h^{-1}) = 8.0; fast (14–16 mi · h^{-1}) = 10.0 Skiing cross-country — slow (2.5 mi · h^{-1}) = 7.0; fast (5.0–7.9 mi · h^{-1}) = 9.0 Soccer — casual = 7.0; competitive = 10.0 Swimming leisurely = 6.0[b]; swimming — moderate/hard = 8.0–11.0[b] Tennis singles = 8.0 Volleyball — competitive at gym or beach = 8.0

[a]On flat, hard surface.
[b]MET values can vary substantially from individual to individual during swimming as a result of different strokes and skill levels.
Adapted from (2).

PUBLIC HEALTH PERSPECTIVE FOR CURRENT RECOMMENDATIONS

Over 20 yr ago, the American College of Sports Medicine (ACSM) in conjunction with the Centers for Disease Control and Prevention (CDC) (73), the U.S. Surgeon General (93), and the National Institutes of Health (75) issued landmark publications on PA and health. An important goal of these reports was to clarify for exercise professionals and the public the amount and intensity of PA needed to improve health, lower susceptibility to disease (morbidity), and decrease premature mortality (73,75,93). In addition, these reports documented the dose-response relationship between PA and health (*i.e.*, some activity is better than none, and more activity, up to a point, is better than less).

In 1995, the CDC and ACSM recommended that "every U.S. adult should accumulate 30 min or more of moderate PA on most, preferably all, days of the week" (73). The intent of this statement was to increase public awareness of the importance of the health-related benefits of moderate intensity PA. As a result of an increasing awareness of the adverse health effects of physical inactivity and because of some confusion and misinterpretation of the original PA recommendations, the ACSM and American Heart Association (AHA) issued updated recommendations for PA and health in 2007 (*Box 1.2*) (34).

More recently, the federal government convened an expert panel, the 2008 Physical Activity Guidelines Advisory Committee, to review the scientific evidence on PA and health published since the 1996 U.S. Surgeon General's Report (76). This committee found compelling evidence regarding the benefits of PA for health as well as the presence of a dose-response relationship for many diseases and health conditions. Two important conclusions from the *Physical Activity*

| Box 1.2 | The ACSM-AHA Primary Physical Activity (PA) Recommendations (33) |

- All healthy adults aged 18–65 yr should participate in moderate intensity aerobic PA for a minimum of 30 min on 5 d · wk^{-1} or vigorous intensity aerobic activity for a minimum of 20 min on 3 d · wk^{-1}.
- Combinations of moderate and vigorous intensity exercise can be performed to meet this recommendation.
- Moderate intensity aerobic activity can be accumulated to total the 30 min minimum by performing bouts each lasting ≥10 min.
- Every adult should perform activities that maintain or increase muscular strength and endurance for a minimum of 2 d · wk^{-1}.
- Because of the dose-response relationship between PA and health, individuals who wish to further improve their fitness, reduce their risk for chronic diseases and disabilities, and/or prevent unhealthy weight gain may benefit by exceeding the minimum recommended amounts of PA.

ACSM, American College of Sports Medicine; AHA, American Heart Association.

Guidelines Advisory Committee Report that influenced the development of the PA recommendations are the following:

- Important health benefits can be obtained by performing a moderate amount of PA on most, if not all, days of the week.
- Additional health benefits result from greater amounts of PA. Individuals who maintain a regular program of PA that is longer in duration, of greater intensity, or both are likely to derive greater benefit than those who engage in lesser amounts.

Similar recommendations have been made in the 2008 federal PA guidelines (http://www.health.gov/PAguidelines) (93) based on the *2008 Physical Activity Guidelines Advisory Committee Report* (76) (*Box 1.3*).

Since the release of the *U.S. Surgeon General's Report* in 1996 (93), several reports have advocated PA levels above the minimum CDC-ACSM PA recommendations (22,26,80,92). These guidelines and recommendations primarily refer to the volume of PA required to prevent weight gain and/or obesity and should not be viewed as contradictory. In other words, PA that is sufficient to reduce the risk of developing chronic diseases and delaying mortality may be insufficient to prevent or reverse weight gain and/or obesity given the typical American lifestyle. PA beyond the minimum recommendations combined with proper nutrition is likely needed in many individuals to manage and/or prevent weight gain and obesity (22,42).

Several large-scale epidemiology studies have been performed that document the dose-response relationship between PA and cardiovascular disease (CVD) and premature mortality (52,57,72,79,88,107). Williams (104) performed a meta-analysis of 23 sex-specific cohorts reporting varying levels of PA or cardiorespiratory fitness (CRF) representing 1,325,004 individual-years of follow-up and showed a dose-response relationship between PA or CRF and the risks of coronary artery disease (CAD) and CVD (*Figure 1.1*). It is clear that greater amounts of PA or increased CRF levels provide additional health benefits. *Table 1.2* provides the

Box 1.3	**The Primary Physical Activity Recommendations from the 2008 *Physical Activity Guidelines Advisory Committee Report* (93)**

- All Americans should participate in an amount of energy expenditure equivalent to 150 min $\cdot$ wk^{-1} of moderate intensity aerobic activity, 75 min $\cdot$ wk^{-1} of vigorous intensity aerobic activity, or a combination of both that generates energy equivalency to either regimen for substantial health benefits.
- These guidelines further specify a dose-response relationship, indicating additional health benefits are obtained with 300 min $\cdot$ wk^{-1} or more of moderate intensity aerobic activity, 150 min $\cdot$ wk^{-1} or more of vigorous intensity aerobic activity, or an equivalent combination of moderate and vigorous intensity aerobic activity.
- Adults should do muscle strengthening activities that are moderate or high intensity and involve all major muscle groups in $\geq$2 d $\cdot$ wk^{-1} because these activities provide additional health benefits.

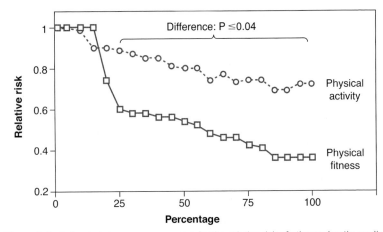

Figure 1.1 Estimated dose-response curve for the relative risk of atherosclerotic cardio-vascular disease by sample percentages of fitness and physical activity. Studies weighted by individual-years of experience. Used with permission from (104).

strength of evidence for the dose-response relationships among PA and numerous health outcomes.

The ACSM and AHA have also released two publications examining the relationship between PA and public health in older adults (5,70). In general, these publications offered some recommendations that are similar to the updated guidelines for adults (26,34), but the recommended intensity of aerobic activity reflected in these guidelines is related to the older adult's CRF level. In addition, age-specific recommendations are made concerning the importance of flexibility, neuromotor, and muscle strengthening activities. The *2008 Physical Activity Guidelines for Americans* made age-specific recommendations targeted at adults (18–64 yr) and older adults (≥65 yr) as well as children and adolescents (6–17 yr) (http://www.health.gov/PAguidelines) (93) that are similar to recommendations by the ACSM and AHA.

Despite the well-known health benefits, physical inactivity is a global pandemic that has been identified as one of the four leading contributors to premature mortality (30,50). Globally, 31.1% of adults are physically inactive (30). In the United States, 51.6% of adults meet aerobic activity guidelines, 29.3% meet muscle strengthening guidelines, and 20.6% meet both the aerobic and muscle strengthening guidelines (15).

SEDENTARY BEHAVIOR AND HEALTH

Prolonged periods of sitting or sedentary behavior are associated with deleterious health consequences (see *Chapter 6*) (35,36,44,47) independent of PA levels (8,51, 63,82). This is concerning from a public health perspective because population-based studies have demonstrated that more than 50% of an average person's waking day involves activities associated with prolonged sitting such as television viewing and computer use (62). A recent meta-analysis demonstrated that after statistical adjustment

TABLE 1.2		
Evidence for Dose-Response Relationship between Physical Activity and Health Outcome		
Variable	**Evidence for Inverse Dose-Response Relationship**	**Strength of Evidence**[a]
All-cause mortality	Yes	Strong
Cardiorespiratory health	Yes	Strong
Metabolic health	Yes	Moderate
Energy balance:		
Weight maintenance	Insufficient data	Weak
Weight loss	Yes	Strong
Weight maintenance following weight loss	Yes	Moderate
Abdominal obesity	Yes	Moderate
Musculoskeletal health:		
Bone	Yes	Moderate
Joint	Yes	Strong
Muscular	Yes	Strong
Functional health	Yes	Moderate
Colon and breast cancers	Yes	Moderate
Mental health:		
Depression and distress	Yes	Moderate
Well-being:		
Anxiety, cognitive health, and sleep	Insufficient data	Weak

[a]Strength of the evidence was classified as follows:
"Strong" — Strong, consistent across studies and populations
"Moderate" — Moderate or reasonable, reasonably consistent
"Weak" — Weak or limited, inconsistent across studies and populations
Adapted from (76).

for PA, sedentary time was independently associated with a greater risk for all-cause mortality, CVD incidence or mortality, cancer incidence or mortality (breast, colon, colorectal, endometrial, and epithelial ovarian), and Type 2 diabetes mellitus (T2DM) in adults (8). However, sedentary time was associated with a 30% lower relative risk for all-cause mortality among those with high levels of PA as compared with those with low levels of PA, suggesting that the adverse outcomes associated with sedentary time decrease in magnitude among persons who are more physically active (8).

HEALTH BENEFITS OF REGULAR PHYSICAL ACTIVITY AND EXERCISE

Evidence to support the inverse relationship between regular PA and/or exercise and premature mortality, CVD/CAD, hypertension, stroke, osteoporosis, T2DM, metabolic syndrome (Metsyn), obesity, 13 cancers (breast, bladder, rectal, head and neck, colon, myeloma, myeloid leukemia, endometrial, gastric cardia, kidney, lung, liver, esophageal adenocarcinoma), depression, functional health, falls, and cognitive function continues to accumulate (26,67,76). For many of these diseases and health conditions, there is also strong evidence of a dose-response relationship with PA (see *Table 1.2*). This evidence has resulted from clinical intervention studies as well as large-scale, population-based, observational studies (26,34,37,45,54,69,94,100,103).

Several large-scale epidemiology studies have clearly documented a dose-response relationship between PA and risk of CVD and premature mortality in men and women and in ethnically diverse participants (52,57,69,71,76,88,107). It is also important to note that aerobic capacity (*i.e.*, CRF) has an inverse relationship with risk of premature death from all causes and specifically from CVD, and higher levels of CRF are associated with higher levels of habitual PA, which in turn are associated with many health benefits (10,11,26,49,84,99,103). *Box 1.4* summarizes the benefits of regular PA and/or exercise.

HEALTH BENEFITS OF IMPROVING MUSCULAR FITNESS

The health benefits of enhancing muscular fitness (*i.e.*, the functional parameters of muscle strength, endurance, and power) are well established (26,93,102). Higher levels of muscular strength are associated with a significantly better cardiometabolic risk factor profile, lower risk of all-cause mortality, fewer CVD events, lower risk of developing physical function limitations, and lower risk for nonfatal disease (26). There is an impressive array of changes in health-related biomarkers that can be derived from regular participation in resistance training including improvements in body composition, blood glucose levels, insulin sensitivity, and blood pressure in individuals with mild or moderate hypertension (17,26,74). Recent evidence suggests that resistance training is as effective as aerobic training in the management and treatment of T2DM (106) and in improving the blood lipid profiles of individuals who are overweight/obese (83). Resistance training positively affects walking distance and velocity in those with peripheral artery disease (PAD) (6,106). Further health benefits attributed to resistance training were confirmed by a recent meta-analysis of published reports which revealed that regimens featuring mild-to-moderate intensity isometric muscle actions were more effective in reducing blood pressure in both normotensive and hypertensive people than aerobic training or dynamic resistance training (13). Accordingly, resistance training may be effective for preventing and treating the dangerous constellation of conditions referred to as Metsyn (26) (see *Chapter 10*).

Exercise that enhances muscle strength and mass also increases bone mass (*i.e.*, bone mineral density and content) and bone strength of the specific bones stressed and may serve as a valuable measure to prevent, slow, or reverse the loss of bone mass in individuals with osteoporosis (5,26,93) (see *Chapter 11*). Resistance training can reduce pain and disability in individuals with osteoarthritis (26,65) and has been shown to be effective in the treatment of chronic back pain (57,97).

Box 1.4	Benefits of Regular Physical Activity and/or Exercise

Improvement in Cardiovascular and Respiratory Function

- Increased maximal oxygen uptake resulting from both central and peripheral adaptations
- Decreased minute ventilation at a given absolute submaximal intensity
- Decreased myocardial oxygen cost for a given absolute submaximal intensity
- Decreased heart rate and blood pressure at a given submaximal intensity
- Increased capillary density in skeletal muscle
- Increased exercise threshold for the accumulation of lactate in the blood
- Increased exercise threshold for the onset of disease signs or symptoms (*e.g.*, angina pectoris, ischemic ST-segment depression, claudication)

Reduction in Cardiovascular Disease Risk Factors

- Reduced resting systolic/diastolic pressure
- Increased serum high-density lipoprotein cholesterol and decreased serum triglycerides
- Reduced total body fat, reduced intra-abdominal fat
- Reduced insulin needs, improved glucose tolerance
- Reduced blood platelet adhesiveness and aggregation
- Reduced inflammation

Decreased Morbidity and Mortality

- Primary prevention (*i.e.*, interventions to prevent the initial occurrence)
  - Higher activity and/or fitness levels are associated with lower death rates from CAD
  - Higher activity and/or fitness levels are associated with lower incidence rates for CVD, CAD, stroke, Type 2 diabetes mellitus, metabolic syndrome, osteoporotic fractures, cancer of the colon and breast, and gallbladder disease
- Secondary prevention (*i.e.*, interventions after a cardiac event to prevent another)
  - Based on meta-analyses (*i.e.*, pooled data across studies), cardiovascular and all-cause mortality are reduced in patients with post-myocardial infarction (MI) who participate in cardiac rehabilitation exercise training, especially as a component of multifactorial risk factor reduction (Note: randomized controlled trials of cardiac rehabilitation exercise training involving patients with post-MI do not support a reduction in the rate of nonfatal reinfarction).

Other Benefits

- Decreased anxiety and depression
- Improved cognitive function
- Enhanced physical function and independent living in older individuals
- Enhanced feelings of well-being
- Enhanced performance of work, recreational, and sport activities
- Reduced risk of falls and injuries from falls in older individuals
- Prevention or mitigation of functional limitations in older adults
- Effective therapy for many chronic diseases in older adults

CAD, coronary artery disease; CVD, cardiovascular disease.

Adapted from (45,70,94).

Preliminary work suggests that resistance exercise may prevent and improve depression and anxiety, increase vigor, and reduce fatigue (26,86).

RISKS ASSOCIATED WITH PHYSICAL ACTIVITY AND EXERCISE

Although the benefits of regular PA are well established, participation in exercise is associated with an increased risk for musculoskeletal injury (MSI) and cardiovascular complications (26). MSI is the most common exercise-related complication and is often associated with exercise intensity, the nature of the activity, preexisting conditions, and musculoskeletal anomalies. Adverse cardiovascular events such as sudden cardiac death (SCD) and acute myocardial infarction (AMI) are usually associated with vigorous intensity exercise (3,66,93). SCD and AMI are much less common than MSI but may lead to long-term morbidity and mortality (4).

Exercise-Related Musculoskeletal Injury

Participation in exercise and PA increases the risk of MSI (68,76). The intensity and type of exercise may be the most important factors related to the incidence of injury (26). Walking and moderate intensity physical activities are associated with a very low risk of MSI, whereas jogging, running, and competitive sports are associated with an increased risk of injury (26,39,40). The risk of MSI is higher in activities where there is direct contact between participants or with the ground (e.g., football, wrestling) versus activities where the contact between participants or with the ground is minimal or nonexistent (i.e., baseball, running, walking) (38,76). In 2012, over 6 million Americans received medical attention for sport-related injuries, with the highest rates found in children between the ages of 12 and 17 yr (91.34 injury episodes per 1,000 population) and children younger than the age of 12 yr (20.03 injury episodes per 1,000 population) (1). The most common anatomical sites for MSI are the lower extremities with higher rates in the knees followed by the foot and ankle (39,40).

The literature on injury consequences of PA participation often focuses on men from nonrepresentative populations (e.g., military personnel, athletes) (43). A prospective study of community-dwelling women found that meeting the national guidelines of ≥ 150 min $\cdot$ wk^{-1} of moderate-to-vigorous intensity PA resulted in a modest increase in PA-related MSI compared to women not meeting the PA guidelines (68). However, the risk for developing MSI is inversely related to physical fitness level (76). For any given dose of PA, individuals who are physically inactive are more likely to experience MSI when compared to their more active counterparts (76).

Commonly used methods to reduce MSI (e.g., stretching, warm-up, cool-down, and gradual progression of exercise intensity and volume) may be helpful in some situations; however, there is a lack of controlled studies confirming the effectiveness of these methods (26). A comprehensive list of strategies that may prevent MSI can be found elsewhere (12,28).

SUDDEN CARDIAC DEATH AMONG YOUNG INDIVIDUALS

The cardiovascular causes of exercise-related sudden death in young athletes are shown in *Table 1.3* (4). It is clear from these data that the most common causes of SCD in young individuals are congenital and hereditary abnormalities including

TABLE 1.3			
Cardiovascular Causes of Exercise-Related Sudden Death in Young Athletes[a]			
	Van Camp et al. ($n = 100$)[b] (95)	Maron et al. ($n = 134$) (60)	Corrado et al. ($n = 55$)[c] (18)
Hypertrophic CM	51	36	1
Probable hypertrophic CM	5	10	0
Coronary anomalies	18	23	9
Valvular and subvalvular aortic stenosis	8	4	0
Possible myocarditis	7	3	5
Dilated and nonspecific CM	7	3	1
Atherosclerotic CVD	3	2	10
Aortic dissection/rupture	2	5	1
Arrhythmogenic right ventricular CM	1	3	11
Myocardial scarring	0	3	0
Mitral valve prolapse	1	2	6
Other congenital abnormalities	0	1.5	0
Long QT syndrome	0	0.5	0
Wolff-Parkinson-White syndrome	1	0	1
Cardiac conduction disease	0	0	3
Cardiac sarcoidosis	0	0.5	0
Coronary artery aneurysm	1	0	0
Normal heart at necropsy	7	2	1
Pulmonary thromboembolism	0	0	1

[a]Ages ranged from 13 to 24 yr (95), 12 to 40 yr (60), and 12 to 35 yr (18). References (95) and (60) used the same database and include many of the same athletes. All (95), 90% (60), and 89% (18) had symptom onset during or within an hour of training or competition.
[b]Total exceeds 100% because several athletes had multiple abnormalities.
[c]Includes some athletes whose deaths were not associated with recent exertion. Includes aberrant artery origin and course, tunneled arteries, and other abnormalities.
CM, cardiomyopathy; CVD, cardiovascular disease.

Used with permission from (4).

hypertrophic cardiomyopathy, coronary artery abnormalities, and aortic stenosis. The absolute annual risk of exercise-related death among high school and college athletes is 1 per 133,000 men and 769,000 women (95). It should be noted that these rates, although low, include all sports-related nontraumatic deaths. Of the 136 total identifiable causes of death, 100 were caused by CVD. A more recent estimate places the annual incidence of cardiovascular deaths among young competitive athletes in the United States as 1 death per 185,000 men and 1.5 million women. (58). Some experts, however, believe the incidence of exercise-related sudden death in young sports participants is higher, ranging between 1 per 40,000 and 1 per 80,000 athletes per year (32). Furthermore, death rates seem to be higher in African American male athletes and basketball players (32,59). Experts debate on why estimates of the incidence of exercise-related sudden deaths vary among studies. These variances are likely due to differences in (a) the populations studied, (b) estimation of the number of sport participants, and (c) subject and/or incident case assignment. In an effort to reduce the risk of SCD incidence in young individuals, well-recognized organizations such as the International Olympic Committee and AHA have endorsed the practice of preparticipation cardiovascular screening (19,53,61). The recent position stand by the American Medical Society for Sports Medicine presents the latest evidence based research on cardiovascular preparticipation screening in athletes (23).

EXERCISE-RELATED CARDIAC EVENTS IN ADULTS

In general, exercise does not provoke cardiovascular events in healthy individuals with normal cardiovascular systems. The risk of SCD and AMI is very low in apparently healthy individuals performing moderate intensity PA (76,101). There is an acute and transient increase in the risk of SCD and AMI in individuals performing vigorous intensity exercise, particularly in sedentary men and women with diagnosed or occult CVD (3,4,29,66,85,90,105). However, this risk decreases with increasing volumes of regular exercise (89). *Chapter 2* includes an exercise preparticipation health screening algorithm to help identify individuals who may be at risk for exercise-related cardiovascular events.

It is well established that the transient risks of SCD and AMI are substantially higher during acute vigorous physical exertion as compared with rest (29,66,85,91,105). A recent meta-analysis reported a fivefold increased risk of SCD and 3.5-fold increased risk of AMI during or shortly after vigorous intensity PA (20). The risk of SCD or AMI is higher in middle-aged and older adults than in younger individuals due to the higher prevalence of CVD in the older population. The rates of SCD and AMI are disproportionately higher in the most sedentary individuals when they perform unaccustomed or infrequent exercise (4). For example, the Onset Study (65) showed that the risk of AMI during or immediately following vigorous intensity exercise was 50 times higher for the habitually sedentary compared to individuals who exercised vigorously for 1-h sessions ≥ 5 d $\cdot$ wk^{-1} (*Figure 1.2*).

Although the *relative* risks of SCD and AMI are higher during sudden vigorous physical exertion versus rest, the *absolute* risk of these events is very low.

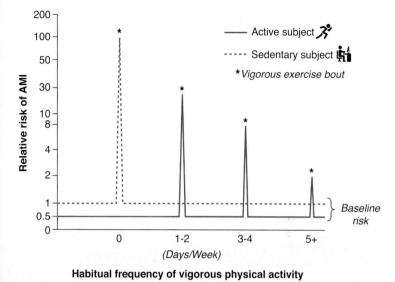

Figure 1.2 The relationship between habitual frequency of vigorous physical activity and the relative risk of acute myocardial infarction (AMI). Used with permission from (24).

Prospective evidence from the Physicians' Health Study and Nurses' Health Study suggests that SCD occurs every 1.5 million episodes of vigorous physical exertion in men (3) and every 36.5 million h of moderate-to-vigorous exertion in women (101). Retrospective analyses also support the rarity of these events. Thompson et al. (90) reported 1 death per 396,000 h of jogging. An analysis of exercise-related cardiovascular events among participants at YMCA sports centers found 1 death per 2,897,057 person-hours, although exercise intensity was not documented (55). Kim et al. (46) studied over 10 million marathon and half-marathon runners and identified an overall cardiac arrest incidence rate of 1 per 184,000 runners and an SCD incidence rate of 1 per 256,000 runners, which translates to 0.20 cardiac arrests and 0.14 SCDs per 100,000 estimated runner-hours.

Although the risk is extremely low, vigorous intensity exercise has a small but measurable acute risk of CVD complications; therefore, mitigating this risk in susceptible individuals is important (see *Chapter 2*). The exact mechanism of SCD during vigorous intensity exercise with asymptomatic adults is not completely understood. However, evidence exists that the increased frequency of cardiac contraction and excursion of the coronary arteries produces bending and flexing of the coronary arteries may be the underlying cause. This response may cause cracking of the atherosclerotic plaque with resulting platelet aggregation and possible acute thrombosis and has been documented angiographically in individuals with exercise-induced cardiac events (9,16,31).

EXERCISE TESTING AND THE RISK OF CARDIAC EVENTS

As with vigorous intensity exercise, the risk of cardiac events during exercise testing varies directly with the prevalence of diagnosed or occult CVD in the study population. Several studies have documented these risks during exercise testing (7,27,41,48,64,78,87). *Table 1.4* summarizes the risks of various cardiac events including AMI, ventricular fibrillation, hospitalization, and death. These data indicate in a mixed population the risk of exercise testing is low with approximately six cardiac events per 10,000 tests. One of these studies includes data for which the exercise testing was supervised by nonphysicians (48). In addition, the majority of these studies used symptom-limited maximal exercise tests. Therefore, it would be expected that the risk of submaximal testing in a similar population would be lower.

TABLE **1.4**								
Cardiac Complications during Exercise Testing[a]								
Reference	Year	Site	No. of Tests	MI	VF	Death	Hospitalization	Comment
Rochmis and Blackburn (78)	1971	73 U.S. centers	170,000	NA	NA	1	3	34% of tests were symptom limited; 50% of deaths in 8 h; 50% over the next 4 d
Irving et al. (41)	1977	15 Seattle facilities	10,700	NA	4.67	0	NR	
McHenry (64)	1977	Hospital	12,000	0	0	0	0	
Atterhög et al. (7)	1979	20 Swedish centers	50,000	0.8	0.8	6.4	5.2	
Stuart and Ellestad (87)	1980	1,375 U.S. centers	518,448	3.58	4.78	0.5	NR	VF includes other dysrhythmias requiring treatment.
Gibbons et al. (27)	1989	Cooper Clinic	71,914	0.56	0.29	0	NR	Only 4% of men and 2% of women had CVD.
Knight et al. (48)	1995	Geisinger Cardiology Service	28,133	1.42	1.77	0	NR	25% were inpatient tests supervised by non-MDs.

[a]Events are per 10,000 tests.
CVD, cardiovascular disease; MD, medical doctor; MI, myocardial infarction; NA, not applicable; NR, not reported; VF, ventricular fibrillation.

TABLE 1.5

Summary of Contemporary Exercise-Based Cardiac Rehabilitation Program Complication Rates

Investigator	Year	Patient Exercise Hours	Cardiac Arrest	Myocardial Infarction	Fatal Events	Major Complications[a]
Van Camp and Peterson (96)	1980–1984	2,351,916	1/111,996[b]	1/293,990	1/783,972	1/81,101
Digenio et al. (21)	1982–1988	480,000	1/120,000[c]		1/160,000	1/120,000
Vongvanich et al. (98)	1986–1995	268,503	1/89,501[d]	1/268,503[d]	0/268,503	1/67,126
Franklin et al. (25)	1982–1998	292,254	1/146,127[d]	1/97,418[d]	0/292,254	1/58,451
Average			1/116,906	1/219,970	1/752,365	1/81,670

[a]Myocardial infarction and cardiac arrest.
[b]Fatal 14%.
[c]Fatal 75%.
[d]Fatal 0%.

Used with permission from (4).

RISKS OF CARDIAC EVENTS DURING CARDIAC REHABILITATION

The highest risk of cardiovascular events occurs in those individuals with diagnosed CAD. In one survey, there was one nonfatal complication per 34,673 h and one fatal cardiovascular complication per 116,402 h of cardiac rehabilitation (33). Other studies have found a lower rate: one cardiac arrest per 116,906 patient-hours, one AMI per 219,970 patient-hours, one fatality per 752,365 patient-hours, and one major complication per 81,670 patient-hours (21,25,96,98). These studies are presented in *Table 1.5* (4). A more recent study demonstrated an even lower rate of cardiovascular complications during cardiac rehabilitation with one cardiac arrest per 169,344 patient-hours, no AMI per 338,638 patient-hours, and one fatality per 338,638 patient-hours (81). Although these complication rates are low, it should be noted that patients were screened and exercised in medically supervised settings equipped to handle cardiac emergencies. The mortality rate appears to be six times higher when patients exercised in facilities without the ability to successfully manage cardiac arrest (4,21,25,96,98). Interestingly, however, a review of home-based cardiac rehabilitation programs found no increase in cardiovascular complications versus formal center-based exercise programs (100).

PREVENTION OF EXERCISE-RELATED CARDIAC EVENTS

Because of the low incidence of cardiac events related to vigorous intensity exercise, it is very difficult to test the effectiveness of strategies to reduce the occurrence of these events. According to a recent statement by the ACSM and AHA (4), "Physicians should not overestimate the risks of exercise because the benefits of habitual physical activity substantially outweigh the risks." This report also recommends several strategies to reduce these cardiac events during vigorous intensity exercise (4):

- Health care professionals should know the pathologic conditions associated with exercise-related events so that physically active children and adults can be appropriately evaluated.
- Physically active individuals should know the nature of cardiac prodromal symptoms (*e.g.*, excessive, unusual fatigue and pain in the chest and/or upper back) and seek prompt medical care if such symptoms develop (see *Table 2.1*).
- High school and college athletes should undergo preparticipation screening by qualified professionals.
- Athletes with known cardiac conditions or a family history should be evaluated prior to competition using established guidelines.
- Health care facilities should ensure their staff is trained in managing cardiac emergencies and have a specified plan and appropriate resuscitation equipment (see *Appendix B*).
- Physically active individuals should modify their exercise program in response to variations in their exercise capacity, habitual activity level, and the environment (see *Chapters 6* and *8*).

Although strategies for reducing the number of cardiovascular events during vigorous intensity exercise have not been systematically studied, it is incumbent on the exercise professional to take reasonable precautions when working with individuals who wish to become more physically active/fit and/or increase their PA/fitness levels. These precautions are particularly true when the exercise program will be of vigorous intensity. Although many sedentary individuals can safely begin a light-to-moderate intensity exercise program, all individuals should participate in the exercise preparticipation screening process to determine the need for medical clearance (see *Chapter 2*).

Exercise professionals who supervise exercise and fitness programs should have current training in basic and/or advanced cardiac life support and emergency procedures. These emergency procedures should be reviewed and practiced at regular intervals (see *Appendix B*). Finally, individuals should be educated on the signs and symptoms of CVD and should be referred to a physician for further evaluation should these symptoms occur.

ONLINE RESOURCES

American College of Sports Medicine Position Stand on the Quantity and
  Quality of Exercise:
  http://www.acsm.org
2008 Physical Activity Guidelines for Americans:
  http://www.health.gov/PAguidelines

REFERENCES

1. Adams PF, Kirzinger WK, Martinez M. Summary health statistics for the U.S. population: National Health Interview Survey, 2012. *Vital Health Stat*. 2013;10(259):1–95.
2. Ainsworth BE, Haskell WL, Whitt MC, et al. Compendium of physical activities: an update of activity codes and MET intensities. *Med Sci Sports Exerc*. 2000;32(Suppl 9):S498–504.
3. Albert CM, Mittleman MA, Chae CU, Lee IM, Hennekens CH, Manson JE. Triggering of sudden death from cardiac causes by vigorous exertion. *N Engl J Med*. 2000;343(19):1355–61.
4. American College of Sports Medicine, American Heart Association. Exercise and acute cardiovascular events: placing the risks into perspective. *Med Sci Sports Exerc*. 2007;39(5):886–97.
5. American College of Sports Medicine, Chodzko-Zajko WJ, Proctor DN, et al. American College of Sports Medicine Position Stand. Exercise and physical activity for older adults. *Med Sci Sports Exerc*. 2009;41(7):1510–30.
6. Askew CD, Parmenter B, Leicht AS, Walker PJ, Golledge J. Exercise & Sports Science Australia (ESSA) position statement on exercise prescription for patients with peripheral arterial disease and intermittent claudication. *J Sci Med Sport*. 2014;17(6):623–9.
7. Atterhög JH, Jonsson B, Samuelsson R. Exercise testing: a prospective study of complication rates. *Am Heart J*. 1979;98(5):572–9.
8. Biswas A, Oh PI, Faulkner GE, et al. Sedentary time and its association with risk for disease incidence, mortality, and hospitalization in adults: a systematic review and meta-analysis. *Ann Intern Med*. 2015;162(2):123–32.
9. Black A, Black MM, Gensini G. Exertion and acute coronary artery injury. *Angiology*. 1975;26(11):759–83.
10. Blair SN, Kohl HW III, Barlow CE, Paffenbarger RS Jr, Gibbons LW, Macera CA. Changes in physical fitness and all-cause mortality. A prospective study of healthy and unhealthy men. *JAMA*. 1995;273(14):1093–8.
11. Blair SN, Kohl HW III, Paffenbarger RS Jr, Clark DG, Cooper KH, Gibbons LW. Physical fitness and all-cause mortality. A prospective study of healthy men and women. *JAMA*. 1989;262(17): 2395–401.
12. Bullock SH, Jones BH, Gilchrist J, Marshall SW. Prevention of physical training-related injuries recommendations for the military and other active populations based on expedited systematic reviews. *Am J Prev Med*. 2010;38:S156–181.
13. Carlson DJ, Dieberg G, Hess NC, Millar PJ, Smart NA. Isometric exercise training for blood pressure management: a systematic review and meta-analysis. *Mayo Clin Proc*. 2014;89(3):327–34.
14. Caspersen CJ, Powell KE, Christenson GM. Physical activity, exercise, and physical fitness: definitions and distinctions for health-related research. *Public Health Rep*. 1985;100(2):126–31.
15. Centers for Disease Control and Prevention. Adult participation in aerobic and muscle-strengthening activities — United States, 2011. *MMWR Morb Mortal Wkly Rep*. 2013;62(17):326–30.
16. Ciampricotti R, Deckers JW, Taverne R, el Gamal M, Relik-van Wely L, Pool J. Characteristics of conditioned and sedentary men with acute coronary syndromes. *Am J Cardiol*. 1994;73(4):219–22.
17. Colberg SR, Sigal RJ, Fernhall B, et al. Exercise and type 2 diabetes: the American College of Sports Medicine and the American Diabetes Association: joint position statement. *Diabetes Care*. 2010;33(12):e147–67.
18. Corrado D, Basso C, Rizzoli G, Schiavon M, Thiene G. Does sports activity enhance the risk of sudden death in adolescents and young adults? *J Am Coll Cardiol*. 2003;42(11):1959–63.
19. Corrado D, Pelliccia A, Bjørnstad HH, et al. Cardiovascular pre-participation screening of young competitive athletes for prevention of sudden death: proposal for a common European protocol. Consensus Statement of the Study Group of Sport Cardiology of the Working Group of Cardiac Rehabilitation and Exercise Physiology and the Working Group of Myocardial and Pericardial Diseases of the European Society of Cardiology. *Eur Heart J*. 2005;26(5):516–24.
20. Dahabreh IJ, Paulus J. Association of episodic physical and sexual activity with triggering of acute cardiac events: systematic review and meta-analysis. *JAMA*. 2011;305(12):1225–33.
21. Digenio AG, Sim JG, Dowdeswell RJ, Morris R. Exercise-related cardiac arrest in cardiac rehabilitation. The Johannesburg experience. *S Afr Med J*. 1991;79(4):188–91.

22. Donnelly JE, Blair SN, Jakicic JM, et al. American College of Sports Medicine Position Stand. Appropriate physical activity intervention strategies for weight loss and prevention of weight regain for adults. *Med Sci Sports Exerc.* 2009;41(2):459–71.

23. Drezner JA, O'Connor FG, Harmon KG, et al. AMSSM position statement on cardiovascular preparticipation screening in athletes: current evidence, knowledge gaps, recommendations and future directions. *Curr Sports Med Rep.* 2016;15(5):359–75.

24. Franklin BA. Preventing exercise-related cardiovascular events: is a medical examination more urgent for physical activity or inactivity? *Circulation.* 2014;129(10):1081–4.

25. Franklin BA, Bonzheim K, Gordon S, Timmis GC. Safety of medically supervised outpatient cardiac rehabilitation exercise therapy: a 16-year follow-up. *Chest.* 1998;114(3):902–6.

26. Garber CE, Blissmer B, Deschenes MR, et al. American College of Sports Medicine position stand. The quantity and quality of exercise for developing and maintaining cardiorespiratory, musculoskeletal, and neuromotor fitness in apparently healthy adults: guidance for prescribing exercise. *Med Sci Sports Exerc.* 2011;43(7):1334–559.

27. Gibbons L, Blair SN, Kohl HW, Cooper K. The safety of maximal exercise testing. *Circulation.* 1989;80(4):846–52.

28. Gilchrist J, Jones BH, Sleet DA, Kimsey C. Exercise-related injuries among women: strategies for prevention from civilian and military studies. *MMWR Recomm Rep.* 2000;49(RR-2):15–33.

29. Giri S, Thompson PD, Kiernan FJ, et al. Clinical and angiographic characteristics of exertion-related acute myocardial infarction. *JAMA.* 1999;282(18):1731–6.

30. Hallal PC, Andersen LB, Bull FC, et al. Global physical activity levels: surveillance progress, pitfalls, and prospects. *Lancet.* 2012;380(9838):247–57.

31. Hammoudeh AJ, Haft J. Coronary-plaque rupture in acute coronary syndromes triggered by snow shoveling. *N Engl J Med.* 1996;335(26):2001.

32. Harmon KG, Drezner JA, Wilson MG, Sharma S. Incidence of sudden cardiac death in athletes: a state-of-the-art review. *Heart.* 2014;100(16):1227–34.

33. Haskell WL. Cardiovascular complications during exercise training of cardiac patients. *Circulation.* 1978;57(5):920–4.

34. Haskell WL, Lee IM, Pate RR, et al. Physical activity and public health: updated recommendation for adults from the American College of Sports Medicine and the American Heart Association. *Med Sci Sports Exerc.* 2007;39(8):1423–34.

35. Healy GN, Dunstan DW, Salmon J, et al. Breaks in sedentary time: beneficial associations with metabolic risk. *Diabetes Care.* 2008;31(4):661–6.

36. Healy GN, Matthews CE, Dunstan DW, Winkler EA, Owen N. Sedentary time and cardio-metabolic biomarkers in US adults: NHANES 2003-06. *Eur Heart J.* 2011;32(5):590–7.

37. Hollingworth M, Harper A, Hamer M. Dose–response associations between cycling activity and risk of hypertension in regular cyclists: the UK Cycling for Health Study. *J Hum Hypertens.* 2015;29(4):219–23.

38. Hootman JM, Dick R, Agel J. Epidemiology of collegiate injuries for 15 sports: summary and recommendations for injury prevention initiatives. *J Athl Train.* 2007;42(2):311–9.

39. Hootman JM, Macera CA, Ainsworth BE, Addy CL, Martin M, Blair SN. Epidemiology of musculoskeletal injuries among sedentary and physically active adults. *Med Sci Sports Exerc.* 2002;34(5):838–44.

40. Hootman JM, Macera CA, Ainsworth BE, Martin M, Addy CL, Blair SN. Association among physical activity level, cardiorespiratory fitness, and risk of musculoskeletal injury. *Am J Epidemiol.* 2001;154(3):251–8.

41. Irving JB, Bruce RA, DeRouen TA. Variations in and significance of systolic pressure during maximal exercise (treadmill) testing. *Am J Cardiol.* 1977;39(6):841–8.

42. Jensen MD, Ryan DH, Apovian CM, et al. 2013 AHA/ACC/TOS guideline for the management of overweight and obesity in adults: a report of the American College of Cardiology/American Heart Association Task Force on Practice Guidelines and The Obesity Society. *J Am Coll Cardiol.* 2014;63(25):2985–3023.

43. Kaplan RM, Hermann AK, Morrison JT, DeFina LF, Morrow JR Jr. Costs associated with women's physical activity musculoskeletal injuries: the women's injury study. *J Phys Act Health.* 2014;11(6):1149–55.

44. Katzmarzyk PT, Church TS, Craig CL, Bouchard C. Sitting time and mortality from all causes, cardiovascular disease, and cancer. *Med Sci Sports Exerc*. 2009;41(5):998–1005.

45. Kesaniemi YK, Danforth E Jr, Jensen MD, Kopelman PG, Lefèbvre P, Reeder BA. Dose-response issues concerning physical activity and health: an evidence-based symposium. *Med Sci Sports Exerc*. 2001;33(Suppl 6):S351–8.

46. Kim JH, Malhotra R, Chiampas G, et al. Cardiac arrest during long-distance running races. *N Engl J Med*. 2012;366(2):130–40.

47. Kim Y, Wilkens LR, Park SY, Goodman MT, Monroe KR, Kolonel LN. Association between various sedentary behaviours and all-cause, cardiovascular disease and cancer mortality: the Multiethnic Cohort Study. *Int J Epidemiol*. 2013;42(4):1040–56.

48. Knight JA, Laubach CA Jr, Butcher RJ, Menapace FJ. Supervision of clinical exercise testing by exercise physiologists. *Am J Cardiol*. 1995;75(5):390–1.

49. Kodama S, Saito K, Tanaka S, et al. Cardiorespiratory fitness as a quantitative predictor of all-cause mortality and cardiovascular events in healthy men and women: a meta-analysis. *JAMA*. 2009;301(19):2024–35.

50. Kohl HW III, Craig CL, Lambert EV, et al. The pandemic of physical inactivity: global action for public health. *Lancet*. 2012;380(9838):294–305.

51. Koster A, Caserotti P, Patel KV, et al. Association of sedentary time with mortality independent of moderate to vigorous physical activity. *PLoS One*. 2012;7(6):e37696.

52. Lee IM, Rexrode KM, Cook NR, Manson JE, Buring JE. Physical activity and coronary heart disease in women: is "no pain, no gain" passe? *JAMA*. 2001;285(11):1447–54.

53. Ljungqvist A, Jenoure P, Engebretsen L, et al. The International Olympic Committee (IOC) consensus statement on periodic health evaluation of elite athletes, March 2009. *Br J Sports Med*. 2009;43(9):631–43.

54. Loprinzi PD, Lee H, Cardinal BJ. Dose response association between physical activity and biological, demographic, and perceptions of health variables. *Obes Facts*. 2013;6(4):380–92.

55. Malinow M, McGarry D, Kuehl K. Is exercise testing indicated for asymptomatic active people? *J Cardiac Rehab*. 1984;4:376–9.

56. Manniche C, Lundberg E, Christensen I, Bentzen L, Hesselsøe G. Intensive dynamic back exercises for chronic low back pain: a clinical trial. *Pain*. 1997;47(1):53–63.

57. Manson JE, Greenland P, LaCroix AZ, et al. Walking compared with vigorous exercise for the prevention of cardiovascular events in women. *N Engl J Med*. 2002;347(10):716–25.

58. Maron BJ, Doerer JJ, Haas TS, Tierney DM, Mueller FO. Sudden deaths in young competitive athletes: analysis of 1866 deaths in the United States, 1980-2006. *Circulation*. 2009;119(8):1085–92.

59. Maron BJ, Haas TS, Murphy CJ, Ahluwalia A, Rutten-Ramos S. Incidence and causes of sudden death in U.S. college athletes. *J Am Coll Cardiol*. 2014;63(16):1636–43.

60. Maron BJ, Shirani J, Poliac LC, Mathenge R, Roberts WC, Mueller FO. Sudden death in young competitive athletes. Clinical, demographic, and pathological profiles. *JAMA*. 1996;276(3):199–204.

61. Maron BJ, Thompson PD, Ackerman MJ, et al. Recommendations and considerations related to preparticipation screening for cardiovascular abnormalities in competitive athletes: 2007 update: a scientific statement from the American Heart Association Council on Nutrition, Physical Activity, and Metabolism: endorsed by the American College of Cardiology Foundation. *Circulation*. 2007;115(12):1643–455.

62. Matthews CE, Chen KY, Freedson PS, et al. Amount of time spent in sedentary behaviors in the United States, 2003–2004. *Am J Epidemiol*. 2008;167(7):875–81.

63. Matthews CE, George SM, Moore SC, et al. Amount of time spent in sedentary behaviors and cause-specific mortality in US adults. *Am J Clin Nutr*. 2012;95(2):437–45.

64. McHenry PL. Risks of graded exercise testing. *Am J Cardiol*. 1977;39(6):935–7.

65. Messier SP. Obesity and osteoarthritis: disease genesis and nonpharmacologic weight management. *Med Clin North Am*. 2009;93(1):145–159.

66. Mittleman MA, Maclure M, Tofler GH, Sherwood JB, Goldberg RJ, Muller JE. Triggering of acute myocardial infarction by heavy physical exertion. Protection against triggering by regular exertion. Determinants of Myocardial Infarction Onset Study Investigators. *N Engl J Med*. 1993;329(23):1677–83.

67. Moore SC, Lee I, Weiderpass E, et al. Association of leisure-time physical activity with risk of 26 types of cancer in 1.44 million adults. *JAMA Intern Med*. 2016;176(6):816–25. doi:10.1001/jamainternmed.2016.1548

68. Morrow JR Jr, DeFina LF, Leonard D, Trudelle-Jackson E, Custodio MA. Meeting physical activity guidelines and musculoskeletal injury: the WIN study. *Med Sci Sports Exerc*. 2012;44(10): 1986–92.

69. Naci H, Ioannidis J. Comparative effectiveness of exercise and drug interventions on mortality outcomes: metaepidemiological study. *BMJ*. 2013;347:f5577.

70. Nelson ME, Rejeski WJ, Blair SN, et al. Physical activity and public health in older adults: recommendation from the American College of Sports Medicine and the American Heart Association. *Med Sci Sports Exerc*. 2007;39(8):1435–45.

71. Paffenbarger RS Jr, Hyde RT, Wing AL, Lee IM, Jung DL, Kampert JB. The association of changes in physical-activity level and other lifestyle characteristics with mortality among men. *N Engl J Med*. 1993;328(8):538–45.

72. Paffenbarger RS Jr, Lee IM. Smoking, physical activity, and active life expectancy. *Clin J Sport Med*. 1999;9(4):244.

73. Pate RR, Pratt M, Blair SN, et al. Physical activity and public health. A recommendation from the Centers for Disease Control and Prevention and the American College of Sports Medicine. *JAMA*. 1995;273(5):402–7.

74. Pescatello LS, Franklin BA, Fagard R, et al. American College of Sports Medicine position stand. Exercise and hypertension. *Med Sci Sports Exerc*. 2004;36(3):533–53.

75. Physical activity and cardiovascular health. NIH Consensus Development Panel on Physical Activity and Cardiovascular Health. *JAMA*. 1996;276(3):241–6.

76. Physical Activity Guidelines Advisory Committee. *Physical Activity Guidelines Advisory Committee Report, 2008* [Internet]. Washington (DC): U.S. Department of Health and Human Services; 2008 [updated Sep 24]. 683 p. Available from: http://www.health.gov/paguidelines/Report/pdf/CommitteeReport.pdf

77. President's Council on Physical Fitness and Sports. *Definitions — Health, Fitness, and Physical Activity* [Internet]. Washington (DC): President's Council on Physical Fitness and Sports; 2000 [cited 2016 Jun 6]. Available from: http://purl.access.gpo.gov/GPO/LPS21074

78. Rochmis P, Blackburn H. Exercise tests. A survey of procedures, safety, and litigation experience in approximately 170,000 tests. *JAMA*. 1971;217(8):1061–6.

79. Rockhill B, Willett WC, Manson JE, et al. Physical activity and mortality: a prospective study among women. *Am J Public Health*. 2001;91(4):578–83.

80. Saris WH, Blair SN, van Baak MA, et al. How much physical activity is enough to prevent unhealthy weight gain? Outcome of the IASO 1st Stock Conference and consensus statement. *Obes Rev*. 2003;4(2):101–14.

81. Scheinowitz M, Harpaz D. Safety of cardiac rehabilitation in a medically supervised, community-based program. *Cardiology*. 2005;103(3):113–7.

82. Schmid D, Ricci C, Leitzmann MF. Associations of objectively assessed physical activity and sedentary time with all-cause mortality in US adults: the NHANES study. *PLoS One*. 2015;10(3):e0119591.

83. Schwingshackl L, Missbach B, Dias S, König J, Hoffmann G. Impact of different training modalities on glycaemic control and blood lipids in patients with type 2 diabetes: a systematic review and network meta-analysis. *Diabetologia*. 2014;57(9):1789–97.

84. Sesso HD, Paffenbarger RS Jr, Lee IM. Physical activity and coronary heart disease in men: the Harvard Alumni Health Study. *Circulation*. 2000;102(9):975–80.

85. Siscovick DS, Weiss NS, Fletcher RH, Lasky T. The incidence of primary cardiac arrest during vigorous exercise. *N Engl J Med*. 1984;311(14):874–7.

86. Strickland JC, Smith M. The anxiolytic effects of resistance exercise. *Front Psychol*. 2014;5:753.

87. Stuart RJ Jr, Ellestad MH. National survey of exercise stress testing facilities. *Chest*. 1980;77(1):94–7.

88. Tanasescu M, Leitzmann MF, Rimm EB, Willett WC, Stampfer MJ, Hu FB. Exercise type and intensity in relation to coronary heart disease in men. *JAMA*. 2002;288(16):1994–2000.

89. Thompson PD, Franklin BA, Balady GJ, et al. Exercise and acute cardiovascular events placing the risks into perspective: a scientific statement from the American Heart Association Council on Nutrition, Physical Activity, and Metabolism and the Council on Clinical Cardiology. *Circulation*. 2007;115(17):2358–68.

90. Thompson PD, Funk EJ, Carleton RA, Sturner WQ. Incidence of death during jogging in Rhode Island from 1975 through 1980. *JAMA*. 1982;247(18):2535–8.

91. Thompson PD, Stern MP, Williams P, Duncan K, Haskell WL, Wood PD. Death during jogging or running. A study of 18 cases. *JAMA*. 1979;242(12):1265–7.

92. U.S. Department of Agriculture, U.S. Department of Health and Human Services. *Dietary Guidelines for Americans, 2010*. 7th ed. Washington (DC): U.S. Government Printing Office; 2010. 112 p.

93. U.S. Department of Health and Human Services. *2008 Physical Activity Guidelines for Americans* [Internet]. Washington (DC): U.S. Department of Health and Human Services; 2008 [cited 2016 Jun 6]. Available from: http://health.gov/paguidelines/pdf/paguide.pdf

94. U.S. Department of Health and Human Services. *Physical Activity and Health: A Report of the Surgeon General*. Atlanta (GA): U.S. Department of Health and Human Services, Public Health Service, Centers for Disease Control and Prevention, National Center for Chronic Disease Prevention and Health Promotion; 1996. 278 p.

95. Van Camp SP, Bloor CM, Mueller FO, Cantu RC, Olson HG. Nontraumatic sports death in high school and college athletes. *Med Sci Sports Exerc*. 1995;27(5):641–7.

96. Van Camp SP, Peterson RA. Cardiovascular complications of outpatient cardiac rehabilitation programs. *JAMA*. 1986;256(9):1160–3.

97. Vincent HK, George SZ, Seay AN, Vincent KR, Hurley RW. Resistance exercise, disability, and pain catastrophizing in obese adults with back pain. *Med Sci Sports Exerc*. 2014;46(9):1693–701.

98. Vongvanich P, Paul-Labrador MJ, Merz CN. Safety of medically supervised exercise in a cardiac rehabilitation center. *Am J Cardiol*. 1996;77(15):1383–5.

99. Wang CY, Haskell WL, Farrell SW, et al. Cardiorespiratory fitness levels among US adults 20-49 years of age: findings from the 1999-2004 National Health and Nutrition Examination Survey. *Am J Epidemiol*. 2010;171(4):426–35.

100. Wenger NK, Froelicher ES, Smith LK, et al. Cardiac rehabilitation as secondary prevention. Agency for Health Care Policy and Research and National Heart, Lung, and Blood Institute. *Clin Pract Guidel Quick Ref Guide Clin*. 1995;(17):1–23.

101. Whang W, Manson JE, Hu FB, et al. Physical exertion, exercise, and sudden cardiac death in women. *JAMA*. 2006;295(12):1399–403.

102. Williams MA, Haskell WL, Ades PA, et al. Resistance exercise in individuals with and without cardiovascular disease: 2007 update: a scientific statement from the American Heart Association Council on Clinical Cardiology and Council on Nutrition, Physical Activity, and Metabolism. *Circulation*. 2007;116(5):572–84.

103. Williams PT. Dose-response relationship of physical activity to premature and total all-cause and cardiovascular disease mortality in walkers. *PLoS One*. 2013;8(11):e78777.

104. Williams PT. Physical fitness and activity as separate heart disease risk factors: a meta-analysis. *Med Sci Sports Exerc*. 2001;33(5):754–61.

105. Willich SN, Lewis M, Löwel H, Arntz HR, Schubert F, Schröder R. Physical exertion as a trigger of acute myocardial infarction. Triggers and Mechanisms of Myocardial Infarction Study Group. *N Engl J Med*. 1993;329(23):1684–90.

106. Yang Z, Scott CA, Mao C, Tang J, Farmer AJ. Resistance exercise versus aerobic exercise for type 2 diabetes: a systematic review and meta-analysis. *Sports Med*. 2014;44(4):487–99.

107. Yu S, Yarnell JW, Sweetnam PM, Murray L. What level of physical activity protects against premature cardiovascular death? The Caerphilly study. *Heart*. 2003;89(5):502–6.

Exercise Preparticipation Health Screening

INTRODUCTION

Historically, the exercise preparticipation health screening process centered on the risk classification (*i.e.*, low, moderate, high) of all individuals which was based on (a) the number of cardiovascular disease (CVD) risk factors and (b) the presence of signs or symptoms and/or known cardiovascular (CV), metabolic, and/or pulmonary disease. Recommendations for a preparticipation medical examination and exercise testing were then based on the risk classification and proposed exercise intensity. These recommendations were designed to avoid exposing habitually inactive individuals with known or occult CVD to the transiently heightened risks of unaccustomed vigorous intensity exercise, including sudden cardiac death (SCD) and acute myocardial infarction (AMI) as discussed in *Chapter 1*.

Although the overarching goal of exercise preparticipation health screening remains the same as in the previous editions of the *Guidelines*, the updated version of *Chapter 2*:

- Bases the exercise preparticipation health screening process on (a) the individual's current level of physical activity (PA); (b) the presence of signs or symptoms and/or known CV, metabolic, or renal disease; and (c) the desired exercise intensity because these three factors have been identified as important risk modulators of exercise-related CV events.
- No longer includes the CVD risk factor profile as part of the decision making for referral to a health care provider prior to the initiating a moderate-to-vigorous intensity exercise program.
- No longer recommends a low, moderate, or high risk classification scheme.
- Makes general recommendations for *medical clearance* versus specific recommendations for *medical exams* or *exercise tests*, leaving the manner of clearance to the discretion of the health care provider.
- Does not automatically refer individuals with pulmonary disease for medical clearance prior to the initiation of an exercise program.

This edition of the *Guidelines* not only continues to encourage preparticipation health screening for persons interested in initiating or progressing exercise or other PA programs but also seeks to further simplify the preparticipation health screening process that was updated in the ninth edition in order to remove unnecessary barriers to adopting a physically active lifestyle (23). This edition of the *Guidelines* also continues to recommend that exercise professionals consult with their medical colleagues when there are questions about patients with known disease or signs and symptoms suggestive of disease or any other concern about an individual's ability to safely participate in an exercise program. The new exercise preparticipation health screening recommendations are not a replacement for sound clinical judgment, and decisions about referral to a health care provider for medical clearance prior to the initiation of an exercise program should continue to be made on an individual basis.

This updated preparticipation process is based on the outcomes of a scientific roundtable sponsored by the American College of Sports Medicine (ACSM) in 2014 (25). The expert panel unanimously agreed that the relative risk of a CV event is transiently increased during vigorous intensity exercise as compared with rest but that the absolute risk of an exercise-related acute cardiac event is low in healthy asymptomatic individuals (see *Figure 1.2*) (1,15,19,20,28–30,35). Accordingly, preparticipation screening was deemed necessary, but screening recommendations needed refinement to better reflect the state of the science and reduce potential barriers to the adoption of PA. The new evidence-informed model for exercise preparticipation health screening is based on a screening algorithm with recommendations for medical clearance based on an individual's current PA level, presence of signs or symptoms and/or known CV, metabolic, or renal disease, and the anticipated or desired exercise intensity (25). These factors are included because among adults, the risk for activity-associated SCD and AMI is known to be highest among those with underlying CVD who perform unaccustomed vigorous PA (7,20,29). The relative risk of SCD and AMI during vigorous-to-near maximal intensity exercise is directly related to the presence of CVD and/or exertional symptoms (29) and is inversely related to the habitual level of PA (1,2,5,8,20,23,24). The relative and absolute risks of an adverse CV event during exercise are extremely low even during vigorous intensity exercise in asymptomatic individuals (26,28,30).

Insufficient evidence is available to suggest that the presence of CVD risk factors *without* underlying disease confers substantial risk of adverse exercise-related CV events. The high prevalence of CVD risk factors among adults (36), combined with the rarity of exercise-related SCD and AMI (28,29), suggests that the ability to predict these rare events by assessing risk factors is low, especially among otherwise healthy adults (29,31). Furthermore, recent evidence suggests that conventional CVD risk factor–based exercise preparticipation health screening may be overly conservative due to the high prevalence of risk factors and may generate excessive physician referrals, particularly in older adults (36). Although removed from preparticipation screening, this edition of the *Guidelines* affirms the importance of identifying and controlling CVD risk factors as an important objective of overall CV and metabolic disease prevention and management. Exercise professionals are encouraged to complete a CVD risk factor assessment with their patients/clients as part of the preexercise evaluation (see *Chapter 3*). Regardless of the number of risk factors, the exercise professional should use clinical judgment and make decisions about referral to a health care provider for medical clearance on an individual basis.

The decision to recommend general *medical clearance* rather than *medical examination* or *exercise testing* builds on changes introduced in the ninth edition of the *Guidelines* and is intended to better align with recent relevant evidence that exercise testing is not a uniformly recommended screening procedure. As noted in the ninth edition of the *Guidelines*, exercise testing is a poor predictor of acute cardiac events in asymptomatic individuals. Although exercise testing may detect flow-limiting coronary lesions via the provocation of ischemic ST-segment depression, angina pectoris, or both, SCD and AMI are usually triggered by the rapid progression of a previously nonobstructive lesion (29). Furthermore, lack of consensus exists regarding the extent of the medical evaluation (*i.e.*, physical exam; peak or symptom-limited exercise testing) needed as part of the preparticipation health screening process prior to initiating an exercise program, even when the program will be of vigorous intensity. The American College of Cardiology (ACC)/American Heart Association (AHA) recommend exercise testing prior to moderate or vigorous intensity exercise programs when the risk of CVD is increased but acknowledge that these recommendations are based on conflicting evidence and divergent opinions (9). The U.S. Preventive Services Task Force recommends against the use of routine diagnostic testing or exercise electrocardiography as a screening tool in asymptomatic individuals who are at low risk for CVD events and concluded that there is insufficient evidence to evaluate the benefits and harm of exercise testing before initiating a PA program. Furthermore, the U.S. Preventive Services Task Force did not make specific recommendations regarding the need for exercise testing for individuals at intermediate and high risk for CVD events (22). Similarly, others have emphasized that randomized trial data on the clinical value of exercise testing for screening purposes are absent; in other words, it is presently not known if exercise testing in asymptomatic adults reduces the risk of premature mortality or major cardiac morbidity (17). The 2008 Physical Activity Guidelines Advisory Committee Report to the Secretary of Health and Human Services (23) states that "symptomatic persons or those with cardiovascular disease, diabetes, or other active chronic conditions who want to begin engaging in *vigorous* PA and who have not already developed a PA plan with their health care provider may wish to do so" but does not mandate medical clearance. There also is evidence from decision analysis modeling that routine screening using exercise testing prior to initiating an exercise program is not warranted regardless of baseline individual risk (16). These considerations and other recent reports (10,23) further shaped the present ACSM recommendation that the inclusion of exercise testing or any other type of exam, as part of medical clearance, should be left to the clinical judgment of qualified health care providers.

In the new exercise preparticipation health screening procedures, individuals with pulmonary disease are no longer automatically referred for medical clearance because pulmonary disease does not increase the risks of nonfatal or fatal CV complications during or immediately after exercise; in fact, it is the associated inactive and sedentary lifestyle of many patients with pulmonary disease that may increase the risk of these events (13). However, chronic obstructive pulmonary disease

(COPD) and CVD are often comorbid due to the common risk factor of smoking, and the presence of COPD in current or former smokers is an independent predictor of overall CV events (6). Thus, careful attention to the presence of signs and symptoms of CV and metabolic disease is warranted in individuals with COPD during the exercise preparticipation health screening process. Nevertheless, despite this change, the presence of pulmonary or other diseases remains an important consideration for determining the safest and most effective exercise prescription (Ex R$_x$) (25).

The goals of the new ACSM exercise preparticipation health screening process are to identify individuals (a) who should receive medical clearance before initiating an exercise program or increasing the frequency, intensity, and/or volume of their current program; (b) with clinically significant disease(s) who may benefit from participating in a medically supervised exercise program; and (c) with medical conditions that may require exclusion from exercise programs until those conditions are abated or better controlled. This chapter provides guidance for using the new exercise preparticipation health screening algorithm with respect to:

- Determining current PA levels
- Identifying signs and symptoms of underlying CV, metabolic, and renal disease (*Table 2.1*)
- Identifying individuals with diagnosed CV and metabolic disease
- Using signs and symptoms, disease history, current exercise participation, and desired exercise intensity to guide recommendations for preparticipation medical clearance

By following a preparticipation screening algorithm taking into account the preceding points, exercise professionals are better able to identify participants who are at risk for exercise- or PA-related CV complications. The algorithm is designed to identify individuals who should receive medical clearance before initiating an exercise program or increasing the frequency, intensity, and/or volume of their current program and may also help to identify those with clinically significant disease(s) who may benefit from participating in a medically supervised exercise program and those with medical conditions that may require exclusion from exercise programs until those conditions are abated or better controlled (18,25).

PREPARTICIPATION HEALTH SCREENING

The following section provides guidance for preparticipation screening for exercise professionals working with the general, nonclinical population. Recommendations for those individuals who are working in a clinical or cardiac rehabilitation setting are presented separately, later in the chapter.

Preparticipation health screening before initiating PA or an exercise program is a two-stage process:

1. The need for medical clearance before initiating or progressing exercise programming is determined using the updated and revised ACSM screening algorithm (see *Figure 2.2*) and the help of a qualified exercise or health

TABLE 2.1

Major Signs or Symptoms Suggestive of Cardiovascular, Metabolic, and Renal Disease[a]

Signs or Symptoms	Clarification/Significance
Pain; discomfort (or other anginal equivalent) in the chest, neck, jaw, arms, or other areas that may result from myocardial ischemia	One of the cardinal manifestations of cardiac disease; in particular, coronary artery disease Key features *favoring an ischemic origin* include the following: ■ *Character*: constricting, squeezing, burning, "heaviness," or "heavy feeling" ■ *Location*: substernal, across midthorax, anteriorly; in one or both arms, shoulders; in neck, cheeks, teeth; in forearms, fingers in interscapular region ■ *Provoking factors*: exercise or exertion, excitement, other forms of stress, cold weather, occurrence after meals Key features *against an ischemic origin* include the following: ■ *Character*: dull ache; "knifelike," sharp, stabbing; "jabs" aggravated by respiration ■ *Location*: in left submammary area; in left hemithorax ■ *Provoking factors*: after completion of exercise, provoked by a specific body motion
Shortness of breath at rest or with mild exertion	Dyspnea (defined as an abnormally uncomfortable awareness of breathing) is one of the principal symptoms of cardiac and pulmonary disease. It commonly occurs during strenuous exertion in healthy, well-trained individuals and during moderate exertion in healthy, untrained individuals. However, it should be regarded as abnormal when it occurs at a level of exertion that is not expected to evoke this symptom in a given individual. Abnormal exertional dyspnea suggests the presence of cardiopulmonary disorders; in particular, left ventricular dysfunction or chronic obstructive pulmonary disease.
Dizziness or syncope	Syncope (defined as a loss of consciousness) is most commonly caused by a reduced perfusion of the brain. Dizziness and, in particular, syncope *during* exercise may result from cardiac disorders that prevent the normal rise (or an actual fall) in cardiac output. Such cardiac disorders are potentially life threatening and include severe coronary artery disease, hypertrophic cardiomyopathy, aortic stenosis, and malignant ventricular dysrhythmias. Although dizziness or syncope shortly *after* cessation of exercise should not be ignored, these symptoms may occur even in healthy individuals as a result of a reduction in venous return to the heart.
Orthopnea or paroxysmal nocturnal dyspnea	Orthopnea refers to dyspnea occurring at rest in the recumbent position that is relieved promptly by sitting upright or standing. Paroxysmal nocturnal dyspnea refers to dyspnea, beginning usually 2–5 h after the onset of sleep, which may be relieved by sitting on the side of the bed or getting out of bed. Both are symptoms of left ventricular dysfunction. Although nocturnal dyspnea may occur in individuals with chronic obstructive pulmonary disease, it differs in that it is usually relieved following a bowel movement rather than specifically by sitting up.

(continued)

TABLE 2.1	
Major Signs or Symptoms Suggestive of Cardiovascular, Metabolic, and Renal Disease[a] (Continued)	
Signs or Symptoms	**Clarification/Significance**
Ankle edema	Bilateral ankle edema that is most evident at night is a characteristic sign of heart failure or bilateral chronic venous insufficiency. Unilateral edema of a limb often results from venous thrombosis or lymphatic blockage in the limb. Generalized edema (known as anasarca) occurs in individuals with the nephrotic syndrome, severe heart failure, or hepatic cirrhosis.
Palpitations or tachycardia	Palpitations (defined as an unpleasant awareness of the forceful or rapid beating of the heart) may be induced by various disorders of cardiac rhythm. These include tachycardia, bradycardia of sudden onset, ectopic beats, compensatory pauses, and accentuated stroke volume resulting from valvular regurgitation. Palpitations also often result from anxiety states and high cardiac output (or hyperkinetic) states, such as anemia, fever, thyrotoxicosis, arteriovenous fistula, and the so-called idiopathic hyperkinetic heart syndrome.
Intermittent claudication	Intermittent claudication refers to the pain that occurs in the lower extremities with an inadequate blood supply (usually as a result of atherosclerosis) that is brought on by exercise. The pain does not occur with standing or sitting, is reproducible from day to day, is more severe when walking upstairs or up a hill, and is often described as a cramp, which disappears within 1–2 min after stopping exercise. Coronary artery disease is more prevalent in individuals with intermittent claudication. Patients with diabetes are at increased risk for this condition.
Known heart murmur	Although some may be innocent, heart murmurs may indicate valvular or other cardiovascular disease. From an exercise safety standpoint, it is especially important to exclude hypertrophic cardiomyopathy and aortic stenosis as underlying causes because these are among the more common causes of exertion-related sudden cardiac death.
Unusual fatigue or shortness of breath with usual activities	Although there may be benign origins for these symptoms, they also may signal the onset of or change in the status of cardiovascular disease or metabolic disease.

[a]These signs or symptoms must be interpreted within the clinical context in which they appear because they are not all specific for cardiovascular, metabolic, or renal diseases.

Modified from (12).

care professional. In the absence of professional assistance, interested individuals may use self-guided methods (discussed later).

2. If indicated during screening (see *Figure 2.2*), medical clearance should be sought from an appropriate health care provider (*e.g.*, primary care or internal medicine physician, cardiologist). The manner of clearance should be determined by the clinical judgment and discretion of the health care provider.

Preparticipation health screening before initiating an exercise program should be distinguished from a periodic medical examination (23), which should be encouraged as part of routine health maintenance.

SELF-GUIDED METHODS

Preparticipation health screening by a self-screening tool should be done for all individuals wishing to initiate an exercise program. A notable change in this section is the omission of the Physical Activity Readiness Questionnaire (PAR-Q) and AHA/ACSM Health/Fitness Facility Preparticipation Screening Questionnaire and the addition of the PAR-Q+ (3,34). The traditional AHA/ACSM questionnaire was excluded because it relies heavily on risk factor profiling which is no longer a part of the exercise preparticipation health screening process. The PAR-Q was recently updated to the PAR-Q+ (*Figure 2.1*), which now includes several additional follow-up questions to better guide preparticipation recommendations (34). The updated PAR-Q+ is evidence-based and was developed, in part, to reduce barriers for exercise and false positive screenings (14). The tool uses follow-up questions to better tailor preexercise recommendations based on relevant medical history and symptomatology. The PAR-Q+ may be used as a self-guided exercise preparticipation health screening tool or as a supplemental tool for professionals that may want additional screening resources beyond the new algorithm. Notably, the cognitive ability required to fully answer the PAR-Q+ may be higher than the original PAR-Q; thus, some individuals may need assistance completing the PAR-Q+.

AMERICAN COLLEGE OF SPORTS MEDICINE PREPARTICIPATION SCREENING ALGORITHM

The ACSM preparticipation screening algorithm (*Figure 2.2*) is a new instrument designed to identify participants at risk for CV complications during or immediately after aerobic exercise. Although resistance training is growing in popularity (32), current evidence is insufficient regarding CV complications during resistance training to warrant formal prescreening recommendations. Because there are few data regarding CV complications during resistance training, this risk cannot currently be determined but appears to be low (10,11,38).

Algorithm Components

The screening algorithm (see *Figure 2.2*) begins by classifying individuals who do or do not currently participate in regular exercise. The intent is to better identify those individuals unaccustomed to regular physical exertion for whom exercise may place disproportionate demands on the CV system and increase the risk of complications. As designated, participants classified as current exercisers should have a history of performing planned, structured PA of at least

2014 PAR-Q+

The Physical Activity Readiness Questionnaire for Everyone

The health benefits of regular physical activity are clear; more people should engage in physical activity every day of the week. Participating in physical activity is very safe for MOST people. This questionnaire will tell you whether it is necessary for you to seek further advice from your doctor OR a qualified exercise professional before becoming more physically active.

GENERAL HEALTH QUESTIONS

Please read the 7 questions below carefully and answer each one honestly: check YES or NO.	YES	NO
1) Has your doctor ever said that you have a heart condition ☐ OR high blood pressure ☐?	☐	☐
2) Do you feel pain in your chest at rest, during your daily activities of living, **OR** when you do physical activity?	☐	☐
3) Do you lose balance because of dizziness **OR** have you lost consciousness in the last 12 months? Please answer **NO** if your dizziness was associated with over-breathing (including during vigorous exercise).	☐	☐
4) Have you ever been diagnosed with another chronic medical condition (other than heart disease or high blood pressure)? **PLEASE LIST CONDITION(S) HERE:** _____	☐	☐
5) Are you currently taking prescribed medications for a chronic medical condition? **PLEASE LIST CONDITION(S) AND MEDICATIONS HERE:** _____	☐	☐
6) Do you currently have (or have had within the past 12 months) a bone, joint, or soft tissue (muscle, ligament, or tendon) problem that could be made worse by becoming more physically active? Please answer **NO** if you had a problem in the past, but it *does not limit your current ability* to be physically active. **PLEASE LIST CONDITION(S) HERE:** _____	☐	☐
7) Has your doctor ever said that you should only do medically supervised physical activity?	☐	☐

☑ **If you answered NO to all of the questions above, you are cleared for physical activity.**
Go to Page 4 to sign the PARTICIPANT DECLARATION. You do not need to complete Pages 2 and 3.

▶ Start becoming much more physically active – start slowly and build up gradually.

▶ Follow International Physical Activity Guidelines for your age (www.who.int/dietphysicalactivity/en/).

▶ You may take part in a health and fitness appraisal.

▶ If you are over the age of 45 yr and **NOT** accustomed to regular vigorous to maximal effort exercise, consult a qualified exercise professional before engaging in this intensity of exercise.

▶ If you have any further questions, contact a qualified exercise professional.

⬤ **If you answered YES to one or more of the questions above, COMPLETE PAGES 2 AND 3.**

⚠ **Delay becoming more active if:**

☑ You have a temporary illness such as a cold or fever; it is best to wait until you feel better.

☑ You are pregnant - talk to your health care practitioner, your physician, a qualified exercise professional, and/or complete the ePARmed-X+ at **www.eparmedx.com** before becoming more physically active.

☑ Your health changes - answer the questions on Pages 2 and 3 of this document and/or talk to your doctor or a qualified exercise professional before continuing with any physical activity program.

 OSHF

Figure 2.1 The Physical Activity Readiness Questionnaire + (PAR-Q+). Reprinted with permission from the PAR-Q+ Collaboration and the authors of the PAR-Q+ (3). (*continued*)

2014 PAR-Q+

FOLLOW-UP QUESTIONS ABOUT YOUR MEDICAL CONDITION(S)

1. **Do you have Arthritis, Osteoporosis, or Back Problems?**

If the above condition(s) is/are present, answer questions 1a-1c   If **NO** ☐ go to question 2

1a. Do you have difficulty controlling your condition with medications or other physician-prescribed therapies? (Answer **NO** if you are not currently taking medications or other treatments)   YES☐ NO☐

1b. Do you have joint problems causing pain, a recent fracture or fracture caused by osteoporosis or cancer, displaced vertebra (e.g., spondylolisthesis), and/or spondylolysis/pars defect (a crack in the bony ring on the back of the spinal column)?   YES☐ NO☐

1c. Have you had steroid injections or taken steroid tablets regularly for more than 3 months?   YES☐ NO☐

2. **Do you have Cancer of any kind?**

If the above condition(s) is/are present, answer questions 2a-2b   If **NO** ☐ go to question 3

2a. Does your cancer diagnosis include any of the following types: lung/bronchogenic, multiple myeloma (cancer of plasma cells), head, and neck?   YES☐ NO☐

2b. Are you currently receiving cancer therapy (such as chemotherapy or radiotherapy)?   YES☐ NO☐

3. **Do you have a Heart or Cardiovascular Condition?** *This includes Coronary Artery Disease, Heart Failure, Diagnosed Abnormality of Heart Rhythm*

If the above condition(s) is/are present, answer questions 3a-3d   If **NO** ☐ go to question 4

3a. Do you have difficulty controlling your condition with medications or other physician-prescribed therapies? (Answer **NO** if you are not currently taking medications or other treatments)   YES☐ NO☐

3b. Do you have an irregular heart beat that requires medical management? (e.g., atrial fibrillation, premature ventricular contraction)   YES☐ NO☐

3c. Do you have chronic heart failure?   YES☐ NO☐

3d. Do you have diagnosed coronary artery (cardiovascular) disease and have not participated in regular physical activity in the last 2 months?   YES☐ NO☐

4. **Do you have High Blood Pressure?**

If the above condition(s) is/are present, answer questions 4a-4b   If **NO** ☐ go to question 5

4a. Do you have difficulty controlling your condition with medications or other physician-prescribed therapies? (Answer **NO** if you are not currently taking medications or other treatments)   YES☐ NO☐

4b. Do you have a resting blood pressure equal to or greater than 160/90 mmHg with or without medication? (Answer **YES** if you do not know your resting blood pressure)   YES☐ NO☐

5. **Do you have any Metabolic Conditions?** *This includes Type 1 Diabetes, Type 2 Diabetes, Pre-Diabetes*

If the above condition(s) is/are present, answer questions 5a-5e   If **NO** ☐ go to question 6

5a. Do you often have difficulty controlling your blood sugar levels with foods, medications, or other physician-prescribed therapies?   YES☐ NO☐

5b. Do you often suffer from signs and symptoms of low blood sugar (hypoglycemia) following exercise and/or during activities of daily living? Signs of hypoglycemia may include shakiness, nervousness, unusual irritability, abnormal sweating, dizziness or light-headedness, mental confusion, difficulty speaking, weakness, or sleepiness.   YES☐ NO☐

5c. Do you have any signs or symptoms of diabetes complications such as heart or vascular disease and/or complications affecting your eyes, kidneys, **OR** the sensation in your toes and feet?   YES☐ NO☐

5d. Do you have other metabolic conditions (such as current pregnancy-related diabetes, chronic kidney disease, or liver problems)?   YES☐ NO☐

5e. Are you planning to engage in what for you is unusually high (or vigorous) intensity exercise in the near future?   YES☐ NO☐

Figure 2.1 (*Continued*)

2014 PAR-Q+

6.	**Do you have any Mental Health Problems or Learning Difficulties?** This includes Alzheimer's, Dementia, Depression, Anxiety Disorder, Eating Disorder, Psychotic Disorder, Intellectual Disability, Down Syndrome	
	If the above condition(s) is/are present, answer questions 6a-6b If **NO** ☐ go to question 7	
6a.	Do you have difficulty controlling your condition with medications or other physician-prescribed therapies? (Answer **NO** if you are not currently taking medications or other treatments)	YES☐ NO☐
6b.	Do you **ALSO** have back problems affecting nerves or muscles?	YES☐ NO☐
7.	**Do you have a Respiratory Disease?** This includes Chronic Obstructive Pulmonary Disease, Asthma, Pulmonary High Blood Pressure	
	If the above condition(s) is/are present, answer questions 7a-7d If **NO** ☐ go to question 8	
7a.	Do you have difficulty controlling your condition with medications or other physician-prescribed therapies? (Answer **NO** if you are not currently taking medications or other treatments)	YES☐ NO☐
7b.	Has your doctor ever said your blood oxygen level is low at rest or during exercise and/or that you require supplemental oxygen therapy?	YES☐ NO☐
7c.	If asthmatic, do you currently have symptoms of chest tightness, wheezing, laboured breathing, consistent cough (more than 2 days/week), or have you used your rescue medication more than twice in the last week?	YES☐ NO☐
7d.	Has your doctor ever said you have high blood pressure in the blood vessels of your lungs?	YES☐ NO☐
8.	**Do you have a Spinal Cord Injury?** This includes Tetraplegia and Paraplegia	
	If the above condition(s) is/are present, answer questions 8a-8c If **NO** ☐ go to question 9	
8a.	Do you have difficulty controlling your condition with medications or other physician-prescribed therapies? (Answer **NO** if you are not currently taking medications or other treatments)	YES☐ NO☐
8b.	Do you commonly exhibit low resting blood pressure significant enough to cause dizziness, light-headedness, and/or fainting?	YES☐ NO☐
8c.	Has your physician indicated that you exhibit sudden bouts of high blood pressure (known as Autonomic Dysreflexia)?	YES☐ NO☐
9.	**Have you had a Stroke?** This includes Transient Ischemic Attack (TIA) or Cerebrovascular Event	
	If the above condition(s) is/are present, answer questions 9a-9c If **NO** ☐ go to question 10	
9a.	Do you have difficulty controlling your condition with medications or other physician-prescribed therapies? (Answer **NO** if you are not currently taking medications or other treatments)	YES☐ NO☐
9b.	Do you have any impairment in walking or mobility?	YES☐ NO☐
9c.	Have you experienced a stroke or impairment in nerves or muscles in the past 6 months?	YES☐ NO☐
10.	**Do you have any other medical condition not listed above or do you have two or more medical conditions?**	
	If you have other medical conditions, answer questions 10a-10c If **NO** ☐ read the Page 4 recommendations	
10a.	Have you experienced a blackout, fainted, or lost consciousness as a result of a head injury within the last 12 months **OR** have you had a diagnosed concussion within the last 12 months?	YES☐ NO☐
10b.	Do you have a medical condition that is not listed (such as epilepsy, neurological conditions, kidney problems)?	YES☐ NO☐
10c.	Do you currently live with two or more medical conditions?	YES☐ NO☐
	PLEASE LIST YOUR MEDICAL CONDITION(S) AND ANY RELATED MEDICATIONS HERE: _____	

> ## GO to Page 4 for recommendations about your current medical condition(s) and sign the PARTICIPANT DECLARATION.

OSHF

Figure 2.1 (Continued)

2014 PAR-Q+

✓ **If you answered NO to all of the follow-up questions about your medical condition,
you are ready to become more physically active - sign the PARTICIPANT DECLARATION below:**

▶ It is advised that you consult a qualified exercise professional to help you develop a safe and effective physical activity plan to meet your health needs.

▶ You are encouraged to start slowly and build up gradually - 20 to 60 minutes of low to moderate intensity exercise, 3-5 days per week including aerobic and muscle strengthening exercises.

▶ As you progress, you should aim to accumulate 150 minutes or more of moderate intensity physical activity per week.

▶ If you are over the age of 45 yr and **NOT** accustomed to regular vigorous to maximal effort exercise, consult a qualified exercise professional before engaging in this intensity of exercise.

⦿ **If you answered YES to one or more of the follow-up questions** about your medical condition:
You should seek further information before becoming more physically active or engaging in a fitness appraisal. You should complete the specially designed online screening and exercise recommendations program - the **ePARmed-X+ at www.eparmedx.com** and/or visit a qualified exercise professional to work through the ePARmed-X+ and for further information.

⚠ **Delay becoming more active if:**

You have a temporary illness such as a cold or fever; it is best to wait until you feel better.

You are pregnant - talk to your health care practitioner, your physician, a qualified exercise professional, and/or complete the ePARmed-X+ **at www.eparmedx.com** before becoming more physically active.

Your health changes - talk to your doctor or qualified exercise professional before continuing with any physical activity program.

● You are encouraged to photocopy the PAR-Q+. You must use the entire questionnaire and NO changes are permitted.
● The authors, the PAR-Q+ Collaboration, partner organizations, and their agents assume no liability for persons who undertake physical activity and/or make use of the PAR-Q+ or ePARmed-X+. If in doubt after completing the questionnaire, consult your doctor prior to physical activity.

PARTICIPANT DECLARATION

● All persons who have completed the PAR-Q+ please read and sign the declaration below.

● If you are less than the legal age required for consent or require the assent of a care provider, your parent, guardian or care provider must also sign this form.

I, the undersigned, have read, understood to my full satisfaction and completed this questionnaire. I acknowledge that this physical activity clearance is valid for a maximum of 12 months from the date it is completed and becomes invalid if my condition changes. I also acknowledge that a Trustee (such as my employer, community/fitness centre, health care provider, or other designate) may retain a copy of this form for their records. In these instances, the Trustee will be required to adhere to local, national, and international guidelines regarding the storage of personal health information ensuring that the Trustee maintains the privacy of the information and does not misuse or wrongfully disclose such information.

NAME _____   DATE _____

SIGNATURE _____   WITNESS _____

SIGNATURE OF PARENT/GUARDIAN/CARE PROVIDER _____

───── **For more information, please contact** ─────
www.eparmedx.com
Email: eparmedx@gmail.com

The PAR-Q+ was created using the evidence-based AGREE process (1) by the PAR-Q+ Collaboration chaired by Dr. Darren E. R. Warburton with Dr. Norman Gledhill, Dr. Veronica Jamnik, and Dr. Donald C. McKenzie (2). Production of this document has been made possible through financial contributions from the Public Health Agency of Canada and the BC Ministry of Health Services. The views expressed herein do not necessarily represent the views of the Public Health Agency of Canada or the BC Ministry of Health Services.

Citation for PAR-Q+
Warburton DER, Jamnik VK, Bredin SSD, and Gledhill N on behalf of the PAR-Q+ Collaboration. The Physical Activity Readiness Questionnaire for Everyone (PAR-Q+) and Electronic Physical Activity Readiness Medical Examination (ePARmed-X+). Health & Fitness Journal of Canada 4(2):3-23, 2011.

Key References
1. Jamnik VK, Warburton DER, Makarski J, McKenzie DC, Shephard RJ, Stone J, and Gledhill N. Enhancing the effectiveness of clearance for physical activity participation; background and overall process. APNM 36(S1):S3-S13, 2011.
2. Warburton DER, Gledhill N, Jamnik VK, Bredin SSD, McKenzie DC, Stone J, Charlesworth S, and Shephard RJ. Evidence-based risk assessment and recommendations for physical activity clearance; Consensus Document. APNM 36(S1):S266-S298, 2011.

 OSHF

Copyright © 2014 PAR-Q+ Collaboration   4 / 4
08-01-2014

Figure 2.1 (*Continued*)

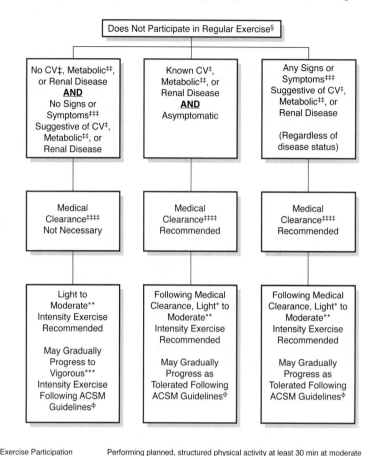

§Exercise Participation	Performing planned, structured physical activity at least 30 min at moderate intensity on at least 3 d · wk⁻¹ for at least the last 3 mo	
*Light Intensity Exercise	30%–39% HRR or V̇O₂R, 2–2.9 METs, RPE 9–11, an intensity that causes slight increases in HR and breathing	
**Moderate Intensity Exercise	40%–59% HRR or V̇O₂R, 3–5.9 METs, RPE 12–13, an intensity that causes noticeable increases in HR and breathing	
***Vigorous Intensity Exercise	≥60% HRR or V̇O₂R, ≥6 METs, RPE ≥14, an intensity that causes substantial increases in HR and breathing	
‡Cardiovascular (CV) Disease	Cardiac, peripheral vascular, or cerebrovascular disease	
‡‡Metabolic Disease	Type 1 and 2 diabetes mellitus	
‡‡‡Signs and Symptoms	At rest or during activity. Includes pain, discomfort in the chest, neck, jaw, arms, or other areas that may result from ischemia; shortness of breath at rest or with mild exertion; dizziness or syncope; orthopnea or paroxysmal nocturnal dyspnea; ankle edema; palpitations or tachycardia; intermittent claudication; known heart murmur; unusual fatigue or shortness of breath with usual activities.	
‡‡‡‡Medical Clearance	Approval from a health care professional to engage in exercise	
ΦACSM Guidelines	See *ACSM's Guidelines for Exercise Testing and Prescription*, 10th edition, 2018	

Figure 2.2 The American College of Sports Medicine preparticipation screening algorithm. ACSM, American College of Sports Medicine; HR, heart rate; HRR, heart rate reserve; METs, metabolic equivalents; RPE, rating of perceived exertion; V̇O₂R, oxygen uptake reserve. Used with permission from (25). (*continued*)

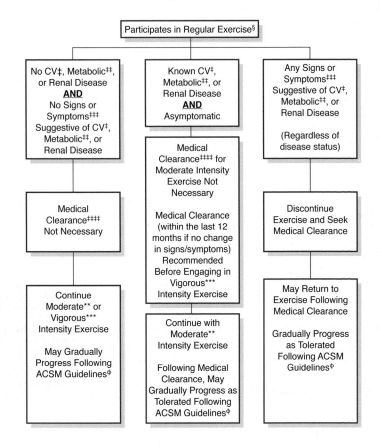

	Participates in Regular Exercise§	
No CV‡, Metabolic‡‡, or Renal Disease AND No Signs or Symptoms‡‡‡ Suggestive of CV‡, Metabolic‡‡, or Renal Disease	**Known CV‡, Metabolic‡‡, or Renal Disease AND** Asymptomatic	**Any Signs or Symptoms‡‡‡** Suggestive of CV‡, Metabolic‡‡, or Renal Disease (Regardless of disease status)
Medical Clearance‡‡‡‡ Not Necessary	Medical Clearance‡‡‡‡ for Moderate Intensity Exercise Not Necessary	Discontinue Exercise and Seek Medical Clearance
Continue Moderate** or Vigorous*** Intensity Exercise	Medical Clearance (within the last 12 months if no change in signs/symptoms) Recommended Before Engaging in Vigorous*** Intensity Exercise	May Return to Exercise Following Medical Clearance
May Gradually Progress Following ACSM Guidelinesφ	Continue with Moderate** Intensity Exercise	Gradually Progress as Tolerated Following ACSM Guidelinesφ
	Following Medical Clearance, May Gradually Progress as Tolerated Following ACSM Guidelinesφ	

§Exercise Participation	Performing planned, structured physical activity at least 30 min at moderate intensity on at least 3 d · wk⁻¹ for at least the last 3 mo
*Light Intensity Exercise	30%–39% HRR or $\dot{V}O_2R$, 2–2.9 METs, RPE 9–11, an intensity that causes slight increases in HR and breathing
**Moderate Intensity Exercise	40%–59% HRR or $\dot{V}O_2R$, 3–5.9 METs, RPE 12–13, an intensity that causes noticeable increases in HR and breathing
***Vigorous Intensity Exercise	≥60% HRR or $\dot{V}O_2R$, ≥6 METs, RPE ≥14, an intensity that causes substantial increases in HR and breathing
‡Cardiovascular (CV) Disease	Cardiac, peripheral vascular, or cerebrovascular disease
‡‡Metabolic Disease	Type 1 and 2 diabetes mellitus
‡‡‡Signs and Symptoms	At rest or during activity. Includes pain, discomfort in the chest, neck, jaw, arms, or other areas that may result from ischemia; shortness of breath at rest or with mild exertion; dizziness or syncope; orthopnea or paroxysmal nocturnal dyspnea; ankle edema; palpitations or tachycardia; intermittent claudication; known heart murmur; unusual fatigue or shortness of breath with usual activities.
‡‡‡‡Medical Clearance	Approval from a health care professional to engage in exercise
φACSM Guidelines	See *ACSM's Guidelines for Exercise Testing and Prescription, 10th edition, 2018*

Figure 2.2 (*Continued*)

moderate intensity for at least 30 min on three or more days per week during the past 3 mo.

The next level of classification involves identifying individuals with known CV, metabolic, or renal diseases or those with signs or symptoms suggestive of cardiac, peripheral vascular, or cerebrovascular disease, Types 1 and 2 diabetes mellitus (DM), and renal diseases. During the preparticipation screening process, participants should be asked if a physician or other qualified health care provider has ever diagnosed them with any of these conditions. During preparticipation health screening, hypertension should be considered a CVD risk factor and not a cardiac disease (4). Refer to *Chapter 3* for additional information on CVD risk factor appraisal.

Once an individual's disease status has been ascertained, attention should shift toward signs and symptoms suggestive of these diseases. The CV, metabolic, and renal diseases of concern for preparticipation health screening may be present but undiagnosed in exercise participants. To better identify those individuals who may have undiagnosed disease, participants should be screened for the presence or absence of signs and symptoms suggestive of these diseases, as described in *Table 2.1*. Care should be taken to interpret the signs and symptoms within the context of the participant's recent history, and additional information should be sought to clarify vague or ambiguous responses. For example, a participant may describe recent periods of noticeable breathlessness. This occurrence is a nonspecific symptom of CVD as many factors can cause shortness of breath. Pertinent follow-up questions may include "What were you doing during these periods?" or "Were you more breathless than you would have expected for this activity?" These questions may provide better clarification to better distinguish expected from potentially pathological signs and symptoms. An exercise preparticipation health screening checklist (*Figure 2.3*) is included to guide the exercise professional through the prescreening process.

Desired exercise intensity is the final component in the preparticipation screening algorithm. Because vigorous intensity exercise is more likely to trigger acute CV events, versus light-to-moderate intensity exercise, in selected individuals (20,29), identifying the intensity at which a participant intends to exercise is important. Guidance is offered in the footnotes of the algorithm on the aforementioned designations as well as what constitutes light, moderate, and vigorous intensity exercise. Additional information on exercise intensity can be found in *Table 6.1*.

Using the Algorithm

According to the preparticipation screening algorithm, participants are grouped into one of six categories. Each category is explained later, moving from left to right across *Figure 2.2*. Importantly, exercise professionals using this algorithm should monitor participants for changes that may alter their categorization and recommendations. For example, participants who initially declare no signs or symptoms of disease may develop signs or symptoms only after beginning

Exercise Preparticipation Health Screening Questionnaire for Exercise Professionals

Assess your client's health needs by marking all *true* statements.

Step 1

SYMPTOMS
Does your client experience:
____ chest discomfort with exertion
____ unreasonable breathlessness
____ dizziness, fainting, blackouts
____ ankle swelling
____ unpleasant awareness of a forceful, rapid or irregular heart rate
____ burning or cramping sensations in your lower legs when walking short distance

If you **did** mark any of these statements under the symptoms, **STOP**, your client should should seek medical clearance before engaging in or resuming exercise. Your client may need to use a facility with a **medically qualified staff**.

If you **did not** mark any symptoms, continue to steps 2 and 3.

Step 2

CURRENT ACTIVITY
Has your client performed planned, structured physical activity for at least 30 min at moderate intensity on at least 3 days per week for at least the last 3 months?

Yes ☐ No ☐

Continue to Step 3.

Step 3

MEDICAL CONDITIONS
Has your client had or do they currently have:
____ a heart attack
____ heart surgery, cardiac catheterization, or coronary angioplasty
____ pacemaker/implantable cardiac defibrillator/rhythm disturbance
____ heart valve disease
____ heart failure
____ heart transplantation
____ congenital heart disease
____ diabetes
____ renal disease

Evaluating Steps 2 and 3:

- If you **did not mark any of the statements in Step 3**, medical clearance is not necessary.
- If you marked Step 2 "**yes**" and **marked any of the statements in Step 3**, your client may continue to exercise at light to moderate intensity without medical clearance. Medical clearance is recommended before engaging in vigorous exercise.
- If you marked Step 2 "**no**" and **marked any of the statements in Step 3**, medical clearance is recommended. Your client may need to use a facility with a **medically qualified staff**.

Figure 2.3 Exercise preparticipation health screening questionnaire for exercise professionals. Used with permission from (18).

an exercise program, and this would necessitate more aggressive screening recommendations.

- Apparently, healthy participants who do not currently exercise and have no history or signs or symptoms of CV, metabolic, or renal disease can immediately, and without medical clearance, initiate an exercise program at light-to-moderate intensity. If desired, progression beyond moderate intensity should follow the principles of Ex R_x covered in *Chapter 6*.

- Participants who do not currently exercise and have (a) known CV, metabolic, or renal disease and (b) are asymptomatic should obtain medical clearance before initiating a structured exercise program of any intensity. Following medical clearance, the individual may embark on light-to-moderate intensity exercise and progress as tolerated following ACSM *Guidelines*.

- Symptomatic participants who do not currently exercise should seek medical clearance regardless of disease status. If signs or symptoms are present with activities of daily living, medical clearance may be urgent. Following medical clearance, the individual may embark on light-to-moderate intensity exercise and progress as tolerated following ACSM *Guidelines* (see *Chapter 6*).

- Participants who already exercise regularly and have no history or signs or symptoms of CV, metabolic, or renal disease may continue with their current exercise volume/intensity or progress as appropriate without medical clearance.

- Participants who already exercise regularly; have a known history of CV, metabolic, or renal disease; but have no current signs or symptoms (*i.e.*, are clinically "stable") may continue with moderate intensity exercise without medical clearance. However, if these individuals desire to progress to vigorous intensity aerobic exercise, medical clearance is recommended.

- Participants who already exercise regularly but experience signs or symptoms suggestive of CV, metabolic, or renal disease (regardless of disease status) should discontinue exercise and obtain medical clearance before continuing exercise at any intensity.

When participants are identified for whom medical clearance is warranted, they should be referred to an appropriate physician or other health care provider. Importantly, the type of medical clearance is left to the discretion and clinical judgment of the provider to whom the participant is referred because there is no single, universally recommended screening test. The type of procedures conducted during clearance may vary widely from provider to provider and may include verbal consultations, resting or stress electrocardiogram (ECG)/echocardiogram, computed tomography for the assessment of coronary artery calcium, or even nuclear medicine imaging studies or angiography. Exercise professionals may request written clearance along with special instructions or restrictions (*e.g.*, exercise intensity) for the participant in question, and continued communication between health care providers and exercise professionals is strongly encouraged. To better understand the preparticipation screening algorithm, case studies are presented in *Box 2.1*.

Box 2.1	Case Studies to Determine Need for Exercise Preparticipation Medical Clearance

CASE STUDY I

A 50-yr-old nonsmoking male was recently invited by colleagues to participate in a 10-km trail run. He reports currently walking 40 min on Monday, Wednesday, and Friday — something he has done "for years." His goal is to run the entire race without stopping, and he is seeking training services. He reports having what he describes as a "mild heart attack" at 45 yr old, completed cardiac rehabilitation, and has had no problems since. He takes a statin, an angiotensin-converting enzyme (ACE) inhibitor, and aspirin daily. During the last visit with his cardiologist, which took place 2 yr ago, the cardiologist noted no changes in his medical condition.

CASE STUDY II

A 22-yr-old recent college graduate is joining a gym. Since becoming an accountant 6 mo ago, she no longer walks across campus or plays intramural soccer and has concerns about her now sedentary lifestyle. Although her body mass index (BMI) is slightly above normal, she reports no significant medical history and no symptoms of any diseases, even when walking up three flights of stairs to her apartment. She would like to begin playing golf.

CASE STUDY III

A 45-yr-old former collegiate swimmer turned lifelong triathlete requests assistance with run training. His only significant medical history is a series of overuse injuries to his shoulders and Achilles tendon. In recent weeks, he notes his workouts are unusually difficult and reports feeling constriction in his chest with exertion — something he attributes to deficiencies in core strength. Upon further questioning, he explains that the chest constriction is improved with rest and that he often feels dizzy during recovery.

CASE STUDY IV

A 60-yr-old woman is beginning a professionally led walking program. Two years ago, she had a drug-eluting stent placed in her left anterior descending coronary artery after a routine exercise stress test revealed significant ST-segment depression. She completed a brief cardiac rehabilitation program in the 2 mo following the procedure but has been inactive since. She reports no signs or symptoms and takes a cholesterol-lowering statin and antiplatelet medications as directed by her cardiologist.

CASE STUDY V

A 35-yr-old business consultant is in town for 2 wk and seeking a temporary membership at a fitness club. She and her friends have been training for a long-distance charity bike ride for the past 16 wk; she is unable to travel with her bike and she does not want to lose her fitness. She reports no current symptoms of CV or metabolic disease and has no medical history except hyperlipidemia, for which she takes a HMG-CoA reductase inhibitor (statin) daily.

	Case Study I	Case Study II	Case Study III	Case Study IV	Case Study V
Currently participates in regular exercise?	Yes	No	Yes	No	Yes
Known CV, metabolic, or renal disease?	Yes	No	No	Yes	No
Signs or symptoms suggestive of disease?	No	No	Yes	No	No
Desired intensity?	Vigorous	Moderate	Vigorous	Moderate	Vigorous
Medical clearance needed?	Yes	No	Yes	Yes	No

RISK STRATIFICATION FOR PATIENTS IN CARDIAC REHABILITATION AND MEDICAL FITNESS FACILITIES

Previous sections in this chapter presented a preparticipation screening algorithm for the general, nonclinical public. Exercise professionals working with patients with known CVD in exercise-based cardiac rehabilitation and medical fitness settings are advised to use more in-depth risk stratification procedures (37). Risk stratification criteria from the American Association of Cardiovascular and Pulmonary Rehabilitation (AACVPR) are presented in *Box 2.2* (37).

The AACVPR guidelines provide recommendations for participant and/or patient monitoring and exercise supervision and for activity prescription and restriction. Clinical exercise professionals should recognize that the AACVPR guidelines do not consider comorbidities (*e.g.*, Type 2 DM, morbid obesity, severe pulmonary disease, debilitating neurological and orthopedic conditions) that may require modification of the recommendations for monitoring and supervision during exercise training.

SUMMARY

- The ACSM updated preparticipation health screening algorithm (see *Figure 2.2*) was developed for exercise professionals to systematically determine a participant's need for medical clearance prior to beginning an exercise program.
- The need for medical clearance prior to beginning an exercise program is based on current exercise participation; history of CV, metabolic, or renal disease; signs or symptoms suggestive of CV, metabolic, or renal disease (see *Table 2.1*); and desired exercise intensity.
- Individuals initiating exercise without assistance or outside of fitness facilities may choose to use the PAR-Q+ (see *Figure 2.1*) as a self-screening tool.

Box 2.2	**American Association of Cardiovascular and Pulmonary Rehabilitation Risk Stratification Criteria for Patients with Cardiovascular Disease**

LOWEST RISK

Characteristics of patients at lowest risk for exercise participation (all characteristics listed must be present for patients to remain at lowest risk)

- Absence of complex ventricular dysrhythmias during exercise testing and recovery
- Absence of angina or other significant symptoms (*e.g.*, unusual shortness of breath, light-headedness, or dizziness, during exercise testing and recovery)
- Presence of normal hemodynamics during exercise testing and recovery (*i.e.*, appropriate increases and decreases in heart rate and systolic blood pressure with increasing workloads and recovery)
- Functional capacity ≥ 7 metabolic equivalents (METs)

Nonexercise Testing Findings

- Resting ejection fraction $\geq 50\%$
- Uncomplicated myocardial infarction or revascularization procedure
- Absence of complicated ventricular dysrhythmias at rest
- Absence of congestive heart failure
- Absence of signs or symptoms of postevent/postprocedure myocardial ischemia
- Absence of clinical depression

MODERATE RISK

Characteristics of patients at moderate risk for exercise participation (any one or combination of these findings places a patient at moderate risk)

- Presence of angina or other significant symptoms (*e.g.*, unusual shortness of breath, light-headedness, or dizziness occurring only at high levels of exertion [≥ 7 METs])
- Mild-to-moderate level of silent ischemia during exercise testing or recovery (ST-segment depression < 2 mm from baseline)
- Functional capacity < 5 METs

Nonexercise Testing Findings

- Rest ejection fraction 40%–49%

HIGHEST RISK

Characteristics of patients at high risk for exercise participation (any one or combination of these findings places a patient at high risk)

- Presence of complex ventricular dysrhythmias during exercise testing or recovery
- Presence of angina or other significant symptoms (*e.g.*, unusual shortness of breath, light-headedness, dizziness at low levels of exertion [< 5 METs] or during recovery)
- High level of silent ischemia (ST-segment depression ≥ 2 mm from baseline) during exercise testing or recovery

(continued)

Box 2.2 *(continued)*
- Presence of abnormal hemodynamics with exercise testing (*i.e.*, chronotropic incompetence or flat or decreasing systolic blood pressure with increasing workloads) or recovery (*i.e.*, severe postexercise hypotension)

Nonexercise Testing Findings
- Rest ejection fraction <40%
- History of cardiac arrest or sudden death
- Complex dysrhythmias at rest
- Complicated myocardial infarction or revascularization procedure
- Presence of congestive heart failure
- Presence of signs or symptoms of postevent/postprocedure myocardial ischemia
- Presence of clinical depression

Reprinted from (37), with permission from Elsevier.

- The methods or procedures used for clearance are left to the discretion of the medical provider.
- Cardiac rehabilitation and medical fitness facilities are encouraged to use the AACVPR stratification presented in *Box 2.2*.

The purpose of preparticipation health screening is to identify individuals who are at risk for adverse exercise-related CV events. Overall, there is a low risk of SCD and AMI associated with participation in an exercise program and much of the risk associated with vigorous exercise is mitigated by adopting a progressive transitional phase (~2–3 mo) during which the duration and intensity of exercise are gradually increased (23,25). When previously sedentary individuals initiate an exercise program, such individuals are strongly recommended to begin with light-to-moderate intensity (*e.g.*, 2–3 metabolic equivalents [METs]) and gradually increase the intensity of exertion (*e.g.*, 3–5 METs) over time, provided that the individual remains symptom free. Such a gradual progression appears prudent because these intensities are below the vigorous intensity threshold (≥6 METs) that is commonly associated with the triggering of acute CV events in susceptible individuals (21,29). This "progressive transitional phase" will help to minimize the risk of musculoskeletal injury as well as allow sedentary individuals to improve their cardiorespiratory fitness without going through a period during which each session of vigorous exercise is associated with large spikes in relative CV risk (27).

ONLINE RESOURCES

ACSM Exe*Rx*cise is Medicine:
    http://exerciseismedicine.org
2008 Physical Activity Guidelines for Americans:
    http://www.health.gov/PAguidelines

REFERENCES

1. Albert CM, Mittleman MA, Chae CU, Lee IM, Hennekens CH, Manson JE. Triggering of sudden death from cardiac causes by vigorous exertion. *N Engl J Med*. 2000;343(19):1355–61.
2. Berlin JA, Colditz GA. A meta-analysis of physical activity in the prevention of coronary heart disease. *Am J Epidemiol*. 1990;132:612–28.
3. Bredin SS, Gledhill N, Jamnik VK, Warburton DE. PAR-Q+ and ePARmed-X+: new risk stratification and physical activity clearance strategy for physicians and patients alike. *Can Fam Physician*. 2013;59(3):273–7.
4. Contractor AS, Gordon TL, Gordon NF. Hypertension. In: Ehrman JK, Gordon PM, Visich PS, Keteyian SJ, editors. *Clinical Exercise Physiology*. Champaign (IL): Human Kinetics; 2013. p. 137–53.
5. Dahabreh IJ, Paulus JK. Association of episodic physical and sexual activity with triggering of acute cardiac events: systematic review and meta-analysis. *JAMA*. 2011;305(12):1225–33.
6. de Barros e Silva PG, Califf RM, Sun J, et al. Chronic obstructive pulmonary disease and cardiovascular risk: insights from the NAVIGATOR trial. *Int J Cardiol*. 2014;176(3):1126–8.
7. Franklin BA. Preventing exercise-related cardiovascular events: is a medical examination more urgent for physical activity or inactivity? *Circulation*. 2014;129(10):1081–4.
8. Franklin BA, McCullough P. Cardiorespiratory fitness: an independent and additive marker of risk stratification and health outcomes. *Mayo Clin Proc*. 2009;84(9):776–9.
9. Gibbons RJ, Balady GJ, Bricker JT, et al. ACC/AHA 2002 guideline update for exercise testing: summary article. A report of the American College of Cardiology/American Heart Association Task Force on Practice Guidelines (Committee to Update the 1997 Exercise Testing Guidelines). *J Am Coll Cardiol*. 2002;40(8):1531–40.
10. Goodman JM, Thomas SG, Burr J. Evidence-based risk assessment and recommendations for exercise testing and physical activity clearance in apparently healthy individuals. *Appl Physiol Nutr Metab*. 2011;36:S14–32.
11. Gordon NF, Kohl HW III, Pollock MI, Vaandrager H, Gibbons LW, Blair SN. Cardiovascular safety of maximal strength testing in healthy adults. *Am J Cardiol*. 1995;76(11):851–3.
12. Gordon SMBS. Health appraisal in the non-medical setting. In: Durstine JL, editor. *ACSM's Resource Manual for Guidelines for Exercise Testing and Prescription*. 2nd ed. Philadelphia (PA): Lea & Febiger; 1993. p. 219–28.
13. Hill K, Gardiner P, Cavalheri V, Jenkins S, Healy G. Physical activity and sedentary behavior: applying lessons to chronic obstructive pulmonary disease. *Intern Med J*. 2015;45(5):474–82.
14. Jamnik VK, Warburton DE, Makarski J, et al. Enhancing the effectiveness of clearance for physical activity participation: background and overall process. *Appl Physiol Nutr Metab*. 2011;36:S3–13.
15. Kim JH, Malhotra R, Chiampas G, et al. Cardiac arrest during long-distance running races. *N Engl J Med*. 2012;366(2):130–40.
16. Lahav D, Leshno M, Brezis M. Is an exercise tolerance test indicated before beginning regular exercise? A decision analysis. *J Gen Intern Med*. 2009;24(8):934–8.
17. Lauer M, Froelicher ES, Williams M, Kligfield P. Exercise testing in asymptomatic adults: a statement for professionals from the American Heart Association Council on Clinical Cardiology, Subcommittee on Exercise, Cardiac Rehabilitation, and Prevention. *Circulation*. 2005;112(5):771–6.
18. Magal M, Riebe D. New preparticipation health screening recommendations: what exercise professionals need to know. *ACSM Health Fitness J*. 2016;20(3):22–7.
19. Malinow M, McGarry D, Kuehl K. Is exercise testing indicated for asymptomatic active people? *J Cardiac Rehabil*. 1984;4:376–9.
20. Mittleman MA, Maclure M, Tofler GH, Sherwood JB, Goldberg RJ, Muller JE. Triggering of acute myocardial infarction by heavy physical exertion. Protection against triggering by regular exertion. Determinants of Myocardial Infarction Onset Study Investigators. *N Engl J Med*. 1993;329(23):1677–83.
21. Mittleman MA, Mostofsky E. Physical, psychological and chemical triggers of acute cardiovascular events. Prevention strategies. *Circulation*. 2011;124(3):346–54.

22. Moyer VA. Screening for coronary heart disease with electrocardiography: U.S. Preventive Services Task Force recommendation statement. *Ann Intern Med.* 2012;157(7):512–8.

23. Physical Activity Guidelines Advisory Committee. *Physical Activity Guidelines Advisory Committee Report, 2008* [Internet]. Washington (DC): U.S. Department of Health and Human Services; 2008 [updated Sep 24]. 683 p. Available from: http://www.health.gov/paguidelines/Report/pdf/CommitteeReport.pdf

24. Powell KE, Thompson PD, Caspersen CJ, Kendrick JS. Physical activity and the incidence of coronary heart disease. *Annu Rev Public Health.* 1987;8:253–87.

25. Riebe D, Franklin BA, Thompson PD, et al. Updating ACSM's recommendations for exercise preparticipation health screening. *Med Sci Sports Exerc.* 2015;47(11):2473–9.

26. Rognmo Ø, Moholdt T, Bakken H, et al. Cardiovascular risk of high- versus moderate-intensity aerobic exercise in coronary heart disease patients. *Circulation.* 2012;126(12):1436–40.

27. Sallis R, Franklin B, Joy L, Ross R, Sabgir D, Stone J. Strategies for promoting physical activity in clinical practice. *Prog Cardiovasc Dis.* 2015;57(4):375–86.

28. Siscovick DS, Weiss NS, Fletcher RH, Lasky T. The incidence of primary cardiac arrest during vigorous exercise. *N Engl J Med.* 1984;311(14):874–7.

29. Thompson PD, Franklin BA, Balady GJ, et al. Exercise and acute cardiovascular events placing the risks into perspective: a scientific statement from the American Heart Association Council on Nutrition, Physical Activity, and Metabolism and the Council on Clinical Cardiology. *Circulation.* 2007;115(17):2358–68.

30. Thompson PD, Funk EJ, Carleton RA, Sturner WQ. Incidence of death during jogging in Rhode Island from 1975 through 1980. *JAMA.* 1982;247(18):2535–8.

31. Thompson PD, Stern MP, Williams P, Duncan K, Haskell WL, Wood PD. Death during jogging or running. A study of 18 cases. *JAMA.* 1979;242(12):1265–7.

32. Thompson WR. Now trending: worldwide survey of fitness trends for 2014. *ACSM Health Fitness J.* 2013;17(6):10–20.

33. Warburton DE, Gledhill N, Jamnik VK, et al. Evidence-based risk assessment and recommendations for physical activity clearance: Consensus Document 2011. *Appl Physiol Nutr Metab.* 2011;36:S266–98.

34. Warburton DE, Jamnik VK, Bredin SS, et al. Evidence-based risk assessment and recommendations for physical activity clearance: an introduction. *Appl Physiol Nutr Metab.* 2011;36:S1–2.

35. Whang W, Manson JE, Hu FB, et al. Physical exertion, exercise, and sudden cardiac death in women. *JAMA.* 2006;295(12):1399–403.

36. Whitfield GP, Pettee Gabriel KK, Rahbar MH, Kohl HW III. Application of the American Heart Association/American College of Sports Medicine Adult Preparticipation Screening Checklist to a nationally representative sample of US adults aged ≥40 years from the National Health and Nutrition Examination Survey 2001 to 2004. *Circulation.* 2014;129(10):1113–20.

37. Williams MA. Exercise testing in cardiac rehabilitation. Exercise prescription and beyond. *Cardiol Clin.* 2001;19(3):415–31.

38. Williams MA, Haskell WL, Ades PA, et al. Resistance exercise in individuals with and without cardiovascular disease: 2007 update: a scientific statement from the American Heart Association Council on Clinical Cardiology and Council on Nutrition, Physical Activity, and Metabolism. *Circulation.* 2007;116(5):572–84.

Preexercise Evaluation

INTRODUCTION

This chapter contains information related to the preexercise evaluation and serves as a bridge among the preparticipation health screening concepts presented in *Chapter 2*, the fitness assessment in *Chapter 4*, and the clinical exercise testing concepts in *Chapter 5*. *Chapter 3* contents (*e.g.*, informed consent procedures, medical history and cardiovascular disease [CVD] risk factor assessment, physical examination and laboratory tests, participant instructions) relate to both the health/fitness and the clinical exercise settings.

If an individual is referred for medical clearance, the extent of the preexercise evaluation is based on the discretion of the health care provider (see *Chapter 2*). A preexercise evaluation that includes a physical examination, an exercise test, and/or laboratory tests may be warranted for any individual whenever the exercise professional or health care provider has concerns about an individual's health status or requires additional information to design an exercise prescription (Ex R_x) or when the exercise participant has concerns about starting an exercise program of any intensity without such a medical evaluation.

The healthier populations typically encountered in the health fitness setting generally warrant a less intensive approach to the preexercise evaluation. However, individuals with chronic disease and other health challenges may be encountered in these settings, so exercise professionals are urged to be prudent in identifying those who need medical clearance.

A comprehensive preexercise evaluation in the clinical setting generally includes a medical history and risk factor assessment, physical examination, and laboratory tests, the results of which should be documented in the client's or patient's file. The goal of *Chapter 3* is not to be totally inclusive or to supplant more specific considerations that may surround the exercise participant but rather to provide a concise set of guidelines for the various components of the preexercise evaluation.

INFORMED CONSENT

Obtaining adequate informed consent from participants before exercise testing in health/fitness or clinical settings is an important ethical and legal consideration. Although the content and extent of consent forms may vary, enough information must be present in the informed consent process to ensure that the participant knows and understands the purposes and risks associated with the test or exercise program in health/fitness or clinical settings. The consent form should be verbally explained and include a statement indicating the client or patient has been given an opportunity to ask questions about the procedure and has sufficient information to give informed consent. Note specific questions from the participant on the form along with the responses provided. The consent form must indicate the participant is free to withdraw from the procedure at any time. If the participant is a minor, a legal guardian or parent must sign the consent form. It is advisable to check with authoritative bodies (*e.g.*, hospital risk management, institutional review boards, facility legal counsel) to determine what is appropriate for an acceptable informed consent process. Also, all reasonable efforts must be made to protect the privacy of the patient's health information (*e.g.*, medical history, test results) as described in the Health Insurance Portability and Accountability Act (HIPAA) of 1996. A sample consent form for exercise testing is provided in *Figure 3.1*. No sample form should be adopted for a specific test or program unless approved by local legal counsel and/or the appropriate institutional review board.

When the exercise test is for purposes other than diagnosis or Ex R$_x$ (*i.e.*, for research purposes), this should be indicated during the consent process and reflected on the *informed consent form*, and applicable policies for the testing of human subjects must be implemented. Health care professionals and scientists should obtain approval from their institutional review board when conducting an exercise test for research purposes.

Because most consent forms include the statement "emergency procedures and equipment are available," the program must ensure available personnel are appropriately trained and authorized to carry out emergency procedures that use such equipment. Written emergency policies and procedures should be in place, and emergency drills should be practiced at least once every 3 mo or more often when there is a change in staff (28). See *Appendix B* for more information on emergency management.

MEDICAL HISTORY AND CARDIOVASCULAR DISEASE RISK FACTOR ASSESSMENT

The preexercise medical history should be thorough and include past and current information. Appropriate components of the medical history are presented in *Box 3.1*. Although no longer part of the exercise preparticipation health screening process, identifying and controlling CVD risk factors continues to be

Informed Consent for an Exercise Test

1. **Purpose and Explanation of the Test**

   You will perform an exercise test on a cycle ergometer or a motor-driven treadmill. The exercise intensity will begin at a low level and will be advanced in stages depending on your fitness level. We may stop the test at any time because of signs of fatigue or changes in your heart rate, electrocardiogram, or blood pressure, or symptoms you may experience. It is important for you to realize that you may stop when you wish because of feelings of fatigue or any other discomfort.

2. **Attendant Risks and Discomforts**

   There exists the possibility of certain changes occurring during the test. These include abnormal blood pressure; fainting; irregular, fast, or slow heart rhythm; and, in rare instances, heart attack, stroke, or death. Every effort will be made to minimize these risks by evaluation of preliminary information relating to your health and fitness and by careful observations during testing. Emergency equipment and trained personnel are available to deal with unusual situations that may arise.

3. **Responsibilities of the Participant**

   Information you possess about your health status or previous experiences of heart-related symptoms (*e.g.*, shortness of breath with low-level activity; pain; pressure; tightness; heaviness in the chest, neck, jaw, back and/or arms) with physical effort may affect the safety of your exercise test. Your prompt reporting of these and any other unusual feelings with effort during the exercise test itself is very important. You are responsible for fully disclosing your medical history as well as symptoms that may occur during the test. You are also expected to report all medications (including nonprescription) taken recently and, in particular, those taken today to the testing staff.

4. **Benefits To Be Expected**

   The results obtained from the exercise test may assist in the diagnosis of your illness, in evaluating the effect of your medications, or in evaluating what type of physical activities you might do with low risk.

5. **Inquiries**

   Any questions about the procedures used in the exercise test or the results of your test are encouraged. If you have any concerns or questions, please ask us for further explanations.

6. **Use of Medical Records**

   The information that is obtained during exercise testing will be treated as privileged and confidential as described in the Health Insurance Portability and Accountability Act of 1996. It is not to be released or revealed to any individual except your referring physician without your written consent. However, the information obtained may be used for statistical analysis or scientific purposes with your right to privacy retained.

7. **Freedom of Consent**

   I hereby consent to voluntarily engage in an exercise test to determine my exercise capacity and state of cardiovascular health. My permission to perform this exercise test is given voluntarily. I understand that I am free to stop the test at any point if I so desire.

I have read this form, and I understand the test procedures that I will perform and the attendant risks and discomforts. Knowing these risks and discomforts, and having had an opportunity to ask questions that have been answered to my satisfaction, I consent to participate in this test.

_____ Date	_____ Signature of Patient
_____ Date	_____ Signature of Witness
_____ Date	_____ Signature of Physician or Authorized Delegate

Figure 3.1 Sample of informed consent form for a symptom-limited exercise test.

Box 3.1	Components of the Medical History

Appropriate components of the medical history may include the following:

■ Medical diagnoses and history of medical procedures: cardiovascular disease risk factors including hypertension, obesity, dyslipidemia, and diabetes; cardiovascular disease including heart failure, valvular dysfunction (*e.g.*, aortic stenosis/mitral valve disease), myocardial infarction, and other acute coronary syndromes; percutaneous coronary interventions including angioplasty and coronary stent(s), coronary artery bypass surgery, and other cardiac surgeries such as valvular surgeries; cardiac transplantation; pacemaker and/or implantable cardioverter defibrillator; ablation procedures for dysrhythmias; peripheral vascular disease; pulmonary disease including asthma, emphysema, and bronchitis; cerebrovascular disease including stroke and transient ischemic attacks; anemia and other blood dyscrasias (*e.g.*, lupus erythematosus); phlebitis, deep vein thrombosis, or emboli; cancer; pregnancy; osteoporosis; musculoskeletal disorders; emotional disorders; and eating disorders

■ Previous physical examination findings: murmurs, clicks, gallop rhythms, other abnormal heart sounds, and other unusual cardiac and vascular findings; abnormal pulmonary findings (*e.g.*, wheezes, rales, crackles), high blood pressure, and edema

■ Laboratory findings: plasma glucose, HbA1C, hs-CRP, serum lipids and lipoproteins, or other significant laboratory abnormalities

■ History of symptoms: discomfort (*e.g.*, pressure, tingling sensation, pain, heaviness, burning, tightness, squeezing, numbness) in the chest, jaw, neck, back, or arms; light-headedness, dizziness, or fainting; temporary loss of visual acuity or speech; transient unilateral numbness or weakness; shortness of breath; rapid heartbeat or palpitations, especially if associated with physical activity, eating a large meal, emotional upset, or exposure to cold (or any combination of these activities)

■ Recent illness, hospitalization, new medical diagnoses, or surgical procedures

■ Orthopedic problems including arthritis, joint swelling, and any condition that would make ambulation or use of certain test modalities difficult

■ Medication use (including dietary/nutritional supplements) and drug allergies

■ Other habits including caffeine, alcohol, tobacco, or recreational (illicit) drug use

■ Exercise history: information on readiness for change and habitual level of activity: frequency, duration or time, type, and intensity or FITT of exercise

■ Work history with emphasis on current or expected physical demands, noting upper and lower extremity requirements

■ Family history of cardiac, pulmonary, or metabolic disease, stroke, or sudden death

FITT, Frequency, Intensity, Time, and Type; HbA1C, glycolated hemoglobin; hs-CRP, high-sensitivity C-reactive protein.

an important objective of overall cardiovascular and metabolic disease prevention and management (10,15). Qualified exercise or health care professionals are encouraged to complete a CVD risk factor assessment with their patients/clients to determine if the individual meets any of the criteria for CVD risk factors shown in *Table 3.1*. If the presence or absence of a CVD risk factor is not disclosed or is not available, that CVD risk factor should be counted as a risk factor. For patient/client education and lifestyle counseling, it is common practice to

TABLE **3.1**	
Atherosclerotic Cardiovascular Disease (CVD) Risk Factors and Defining Criteria (27,41)	
Risk Factors[a]	**Defining Criteria**
Age	Men ≥45 yr; women ≥55 yr (13)
Family history	Myocardial infarction, coronary revascularization, or sudden death before 55 yr in father or other male first-degree relative or before 65 yr in mother or other female first-degree relative
Cigarette smoking	Current cigarette smoker or those who quit within the previous 6 mo or exposure to environmental tobacco smoke (42)
Physical inactivity	Not participating in at least 30 min of moderate intensity physical activity (40%–59% $\dot{V}O_2R$) on at least 3 d of the week for at least 3 mo (31,40)
Obesity	Body mass index ≥30 kg · m^{-2} or waist girth >102 cm (40 in) for men and >88 cm (35 in) for women (20)
Hypertension	Systolic blood pressure ≥140 mm Hg and/or diastolic ≥90 mm Hg, confirmed by measurements on at least two separate occasions, or on antihypertensive medication (8)
Dyslipidemia	Low-density lipoprotein cholesterol ≥130 mg · dL^{-1} (3.37 mmol · L^{-1}) or high-density lipoprotein[a] cholesterol (HDL-C) <40 mg · dL^{-1} (1.04 mmol · L^{-1}) or on lipid-lowering medication. If total serum cholesterol is all that is available, use ≥200 mg · dL^{-1} (5.18 mmol · L^{-1}) (29)
Diabetes	Fasting plasma glucose ≥126 mg · dL^{-1} (7.0 mmol · L^{-1}) or 2 h plasma glucose values in oral glucose tolerance test (OGTT) ≥200 mg · dL^{-1} (11.1 mmol · L^{-1}) or HbA1C ≥6.5% (1)
Negative Risk Factors	**Defining Criteria**
HDL-C[b]	≥60 mg · dL^{-1} (1.55 mmol · L^{-1})

[a]If the presence or absence of a CVD risk factor is not disclosed or is not available, that CVD risk factor should be counted as a risk factor.
[b]High HDL-C is considered a negative risk factor. For individuals having high HDL ≥60 mg · dL^{-1} (1.55 mmol · L^{-1}), for these individuals one positive risk factor is subtracted from the sum of positive risk factors.
HbA1C, glycolated hemoglobin; $\dot{V}O_2R$, oxygen uptake reserve.

sum the number of positive risk factors. Because of the cardioprotective effect of high-density lipoprotein cholesterol (HDL-C), it is considered a negative CVD risk factor. For individuals having HDL-C $\geq$60 mg $\cdot$ dL^{-1} (1.55 mmol $\cdot$ L^{-1}), one positive CVD risk factor is subtracted from the sum of positive CVD risk factors. Please refer to the case studies in *Box 3.2* that provide a framework for conducting CVD risk factor assessment.

CVD risk factor assessment provides important information for the development of a client or patient's Ex R$_x$ as well as his or her need for lifestyle modification and is an important opportunity for patient education about CVD risk reduction.

| Box 3.2 | Case Studies to Conduct Cardiovascular Disease Risk Factor Assessment |

CASE STUDY I

Female, age 21 yr, smokes socially on weekends ($\sim$10–20 cigarettes). Drinks alcohol one or two nights a week, usually on weekends. Height = 63 in (160 cm), weight = 124 lb (56.4 kg), BMI = 22.0 kg $\cdot$ m^{-2}. RHR = 76 beats $\cdot$ min^{-1}, resting BP = 118/72 mm Hg. Total cholesterol = 178 mg $\cdot$ dL^{-1} (4.61 mmol $\cdot$ L^{-1}), LDL-C = 98 mg $\cdot$ dL^{-1} (2.54 mmol $\cdot$ L^{-1}), HDL-C = 62 mg $\cdot$ dL^{-1} (1.60 mmol $\cdot$ L^{-1}), FBG = 96 mg $\cdot$ dL^{-1} (5.33 mmol $\cdot$ L^{-1}). Currently taking oral contraceptives. Attends group exercise class two to three times a week. Both parents living and in good health.

CASE STUDY II

Man, age 45 yr, nonsmoker. Height = 72 in (182.9 cm), weight = 168 lb (76.4 kg), BMI = 22.8 kg $\cdot$ m^{-2}. RHR = 64 beats $\cdot$ min^{-1}, resting BP = 124/78 mm Hg. Total cholesterol = 187 mg $\cdot$ dL^{-1} (4.84 mmol $\cdot$ L^{-1}), LDL-C = 103 mg $\cdot$ L^{-1} (2.67 mmol $\cdot$ L^{-1}), HDL-C = 39 mg $\cdot$ dL^{-1} (1.01 mmol $\cdot$ L^{-1}), FBG = 88 mg $\cdot$ dL^{-1} (4.84 mmol $\cdot$ L^{-1}). Recreationally competitive runner, runs 4–7 d $\cdot$ wk^{-1}, completes one to two marathons and numerous other road races every year. No medications other than over-the-counter ibuprofen as needed. Father died at age 51 yr of a heart attack; mother died at age 81 yr of cancer.

CASE STUDY III

Man, age 44 yr, nonsmoker. Height = 70 in (177.8 cm), weight = 216 lb (98.2 kg), BMI = 31.0 kg $\cdot$ m^{-2}. RHR = 62 beats $\cdot$ min^{-1}, resting BP = 128/84 mm Hg. Total serum cholesterol = 184 mg $\cdot$ dL^{-1} (4.77 mmol $\cdot$ L^{-1}), LDL-C = 106 mg $\cdot$ dL^{-1} (2.75 mmol $\cdot$ L^{-1}), HDL-C = 44 mg $\cdot$ dL^{-1} (1.14 mmol $\cdot$ L^{-1}), FBG = 130 mg $\cdot$ dL^{-1} (7.22 mmol $\cdot$ L^{-1}). Reports that he does not have time to exercise. Father had Type 2 diabetes and died at age 67 yr of a heart attack; mother living, no CVD. No medications.

CASE STUDY IV

Woman, age 36 yr, nonsmoker. Height = 64 in (162.6 cm), weight = 108 lb (49.1 kg), BMI = 18.5 kg · m^{-2}. RHR = 61 beats · min^{-1}, resting BP = 142/86 mm Hg. Total cholesterol = 174 mg · dL^{-1} (4.51 mmol · L^{-1}), blood glucose normal with insulin injections. Type 1 diabetes mellitus diagnosed at age 7 yr. Teaches dance aerobic classes three times a week, walks approximately 45 min four times a week. Both parents in good health with no history of CVD.

	Case Study I	Case Study II	Case Study III	Case Study IV
CVD risk factors:				
Age?	No	Yes	No	No
Family history?	No	Yes	No	No
Cigarette smoking?	Yes	No	No	No
Physical inactivity?	No	No	Yes	No
Obesity?	No	No	Yes	No
Hypertension?	No	No	No	Yes
Dyslipidemia?	No	Yes	No	No
Diabetes?	No	No	Yes	Yes
Negative risk factor: HDL-C ≥60 mg · dL^{-1}	Yes	No	No	No
Number of CVD risk factors	Zero	Three	Three	Two

BMI, body mass index; BP, blood pressure; CVD, cardiovascular disease; FBG, fasting blood glucose; HDL-C, high-density lipoprotein cholesterol; LDL-C, low-density lipoprotein cholesterol; RHR, resting heart rate.

PHYSICAL EXAMINATION AND LABORATORY TESTS

If warranted, a preliminary physical examination should be performed by a physician or other qualified health care provider. Appropriate components of the physical examination specific to subsequent exercise testing are presented in *Box 3.3*, and the recommended laboratory tests are listed in *Box 3.4*. Although detailed descriptions of all the physical examination procedures and the recommended laboratory tests are beyond the scope of the *Guidelines*, additional basic information related to assessment of blood pressure (BP), lipids and lipoproteins, other blood chemistries, and pulmonary function are provided in the following sections. For more detailed descriptions of these assessments, the reader is referred to the work of Bickley (7).

Identification and risk stratification of individuals with CVD and those at high risk for developing CVD are facilitated by review of previous test results, if available, such as coronary angiography, myocardial perfusion imaging, echocardiography, coronary artery calcium (CAC) score studies, ankle/brachial systolic pressure

Box 3.3	Components of the Preparticipation Physical Examination

Appropriate components of the physical examination may include the following:

- Body weight; in many instances, determination of body mass index, waist girth, and/or body composition (body fat percentage) is desirable.
- Apical pulse rate and rhythm
- Resting blood pressure: seated, supine, and standing
- Auscultation of the lungs with specific attention to uniformity of breath sounds in all areas (absence of rales, wheezes, and other breathing sounds)
- Palpation of the cardiac apical impulse and point of maximal impulse
- Auscultation of the heart with specific attention to murmurs, gallops, clicks, and rubs
- Palpation and auscultation of carotid, abdominal, and femoral arteries
- Evaluation of the abdomen for bowel sounds, masses, visceromegaly, and tenderness
- Palpation and inspection of lower extremities for edema and presence of arterial pulses
- Absence or presence of tendon xanthoma and skin xanthelasma
- Follow-up examination related to orthopedic or other medical conditions that would limit exercise testing
- Tests of neurologic function including reflexes and cognition (as indicated)
- Inspection of the skin, especially of the lower extremities in known patients with diabetes mellitus

Adapted from (7).

index, or high-sensitivity C-reactive protein (hs-CRP) determination (15,17). Additional testing may include ambulatory electrocardiogram (ECG) or Holter monitor ECG and pharmacologic stress testing to further clarify the need for and extent of intervention, assess response to treatment such as medical therapies and revascularization procedures, or determine the need for additional assessment. As outlined in *Box 3.4*, other laboratory tests may be warranted based on the clinical status of the patient, especially for those with diabetes mellitus (DM). These laboratory tests may include, but are not limited to, serum chemistries, complete blood count, serum lipids and lipoproteins, inflammatory markers, fasting plasma glucose, glucose tolerance test, glycolated hemoglobin (HbA1C), and pulmonary function.

For asymptomatic adults aged 40–79 yr without established coronary artery disease (CAD) or risk equivalents (*i.e.,* peripheral arterial disease, symptomatic carotid artery disease, or abdominal aortic aneurysm) and with low-density lipoprotein cholesterol (LDL-C) <190 mg $\cdot$ dL^{-1}, assessment of demographic factors, lipoprotein analysis, presence or absence of DM, smoking status, and BP level and treatment status can be used to provide sex- and race-specific estimates of an individual's 10-yr risk for suffering a first CVD event using a risk calculator such as the

Box 3.4 Recommended Laboratory Tests

All Individuals

- Fasting serum total cholesterol, LDL cholesterol, HDL cholesterol, and triglycerides
- Fasting plasma glucose. For all patients, particularly those who are overweight or obese (BMI $\geq$25 kg · m^{-2} or $\geq$23 kg · m^{-2} in Asian Americans), testing should begin at age 45 yr. Testing should be considered in all adults regardless of age who are overweight or obese and have one or more additional risk factors for Type 2 diabetes mellitus: a first-degree relative with diabetes, member of a high-risk ethnic population (*e.g.*, African American, Latino, Native American, Asian American, Pacific Islander), delivered a baby weighing >9 lb (4.08 kg) or history of gestational diabetes, hypertension (BP $\geq$140/90 mm Hg in adults) or on therapy for hypertension, HDL cholesterol <35 mg · dL^{-1} (<0.90 mmol · L^{-1}) and/or triglycerides $\geq$250 mg · dL^{-1} ($\geq$2.82 mmol · L^{-1}), polycystic ovary disease, previously identified impaired glucose tolerance or impaired fasting glucose (fasting glucose $\geq$100 mg · dL^{-1}; $\geq$5.55 mmol · L^{-1}) or HbA1C $\geq$5.7%, habitual physical inactivity, other clinical conditions associated with insulin resistance (*e.g.*, severe obesity, acanthosis nigricans), and history of atherosclerotic vascular disease (1).

Individuals with Signs/Symptoms or Known Cardiovascular Disease

- Preceding tests plus pertinent previous cardiovascular laboratory tests as indicated (*e.g.*, resting 12-lead ECG, Holter ECG monitoring, coronary angiography, radionuclide or echocardiography studies, previous exercise tests)
- Carotid ultrasound and other peripheral vascular studies as indicated
- Chest radiograph, if heart failure is present or suspected
- Comprehensive blood chemistry panel and complete blood count as indicated by history and physical examination (see *Table 3.4*)

Patients with Pulmonary Disease

- Chest radiograph
- Pulmonary function tests (see *Table 3.5*)
- Carbon monoxide diffusing capacity
- Other specialized pulmonary studies (*e.g.*, oximetry or blood gas analysis)

ECG, electrocardiogram; HbA1C, glycolated hemoglobin; HDL, high-density lipoprotein; LDL, low-density lipoprotein.

Pooled Cohort Equations CV Risk Calculator as recommended by the American College of Cardiology (ACC)/American Heart Association (AHA) guidelines (15). (For ACC/AHA CVD Risk Calculator, go to http://tools.cardiosource.org /ASCVD-Risk-Estimator [6]). Data used to develop this risk calculator was derived from cohorts of non-Hispanic Whites and African Americans in the United States. Thus, an obvious limitation is recognized when using this tool in ethnic groups (*e.g.*, Asian Americans, Hispanic Americans, and American Indians) not represented by this data set.

Blood Pressure

Measurement of resting BP is an integral component of the preexercise evaluation. Subsequent decisions should be based on the average of two or more properly measured, seated BP readings recorded during each of two or more office visits (2,33). Specific techniques for measuring BP are critical to accuracy and detection of high BP and are presented in *Box 3.5*. Potential sources of error in BP assessment are presented in *Box 3.6*. In addition to high BP readings, unusual low readings should also be evaluated for clinical significance.

A classification scheme for hypertension in adults is detailed in *The Seventh Report of the Joint National Committee on Prevention, Detection, Evaluation, and Treatment of High Blood Pressure* (JNC 7) (38) (*Table 3.2*). The recently published *2014 Evidence-Based Guidelines for the Management of High Blood Pressure in Adults* (JNC 8) (19) specifically does not address the classification of

Box 3.5	Procedures for Assessment of Resting Blood Pressure

1. Patients should be seated quietly for at least 5 min in a chair with back support (rather than on an examination table) with their feet on the floor and their arms supported at heart level. Patients should refrain from smoking cigarettes or ingesting caffeine for at least 30 min preceding the measurement.
2. Measuring supine and standing values may be indicated under special circumstances.
3. Wrap cuff firmly around upper arm at heart level; align cuff with brachial artery.
4. The appropriate cuff size must be used to ensure accurate measurement. The bladder within the cuff should encircle at least 80% of the upper arm. Many adults require a large adult cuff.
5. Place stethoscope chest piece below the antecubital space over the brachial artery. Bell and diaphragm side of chest piece appear equally effective in assessing BP (22).
6. Quickly inflate cuff pressure to 20 mm Hg above the first Korotkoff sound.
7. Slowly release pressure at rate equal to 2–3 mm Hg $\cdot$ s^{-1}.
8. SBP is the point at which the first of two or more Korotkoff sounds is heard (phase 1), and DBP is the point before the disappearance of Korotkoff sounds (phase 5).
9. At least two measurements should be made (minimum of 1 min apart), and the average should be taken.
10. BP should be measured in both arms during the first examination. Higher pressure should be used when there is consistent interarm difference.
11. Provide to patients, verbally and in writing, their specific BP numbers and BP goals.

BP, blood pressure; DBP, diastolic blood pressure; SBP, systolic blood pressure.
Modified from (38). For additional, more detailed recommendations, see (33).

Box 3.6	Potential Sources of Error in Blood Pressure Assessment

- Inaccurate sphygmomanometer
- Improper cuff size
- Auditory acuity of technician
- Rate of inflation or deflation of cuff pressure
- Experience of technician
- Faulty equipment
- Improper stethoscope placement or pressure
- Not having the cuff at heart level
- Certain physiologic abnormalities (*e.g.*, damaged brachial artery, subclavian steal syndrome, arteriovenous fistula)
- Reaction time of technician[a]
- Background noise
- Allowing patient to hold treadmill handrails or flex elbow[a]

[a]Applies specifically during exercise testing.

prehypertension or hypertension in adults but rather recommends thresholds for pharmacologic treatment. Thus, the scheme proposed by the JNC 7 remains a widely accepted classification scheme (43). For recommendations on specific medications used in the management of hypertension in adults, see JNC 8 (19) and the American Society of Hypertension (ASH) and the International Society of Hypertension (ISH) Clinical Practice Guidelines (43).

The relationship between BP and risk for cardiovascular events is continuous, consistent, and independent of other risk factors. For individuals aged 40–70 yr, each increment of 20 mm Hg in systolic blood pressure (SBP) or 10 mm Hg in diastolic blood pressure (DBP) doubles the risk of CVD across the entire BP range of 115/75–185/115 mm Hg. Individuals with an SBP of 120–139 mm Hg and/or a DBP of 80–89 mm Hg have prehypertension and require health-promoting lifestyle modifications to prevent the development of hypertension (2,38).

Lifestyle modification including PA, weight reduction, a Dietary Approaches to Stop Hypertension (DASH) eating plan (*i.e.*, a diet rich in fruits, vegetables, low-fat dairy products with a reduced content of saturated and total fat), dietary sodium reduction (no more than 2 g sodium per day), and moderation of alcohol consumption remains the cornerstone of antihypertensive therapy. Pharmacologic therapy is added when lifestyle interventions have not proven effective in achieving the desired goal (2,10,19,38,43). However, most patients with hypertension who require drug therapy in addition to lifestyle modification require two or more antihypertensive medications to achieve the BP goal (43).

The main goal of BP treatment is to decrease the risk of CVD morbidity and mortality and renal morbidity. In general, the recommended BP goal for most patients is <140/90 mm Hg. There are specific segments of the population based on

TABLE 3.2

Classification and Management of Blood Pressure (BP) for Adults[a]

BP Classification	SBP (mm Hg)	DBP (mm Hg)	Lifestyle Modification	Initial Drug Therapy Without Compelling Indication	Initial Drug Therapy With Compelling Indications
Normal	<120	And <80	Encourage		
Prehypertension	120–139	Or 80–89	Yes	No antihypertensive drug indicated	Drug(s) for compelling indications[b]
Stage 1 hypertension	140–159	Or 90–99	Yes	Antihypertensive drug(s) indicated	Drug(s) for compelling indications[b] Other antihypertensive drugs, as needed
Stage 2 hypertension	≥160	Or ≥100	Yes	Antihypertensive drug(s) indicated Two-drug combination for most[c]	

[a]Treatment determined by highest BP category.
[b]Compelling indications include heart failure, known coronary artery disease, high coronary heart disease risk, diabetes mellitus, chronic kidney disease, and recurrent stroke prevention.
[c]Initial combined therapy should be used cautiously in those at risk for orthostatic hypotension.
DBP, diastolic blood pressure; SBP, systolic blood pressure.
Adapted from (19,38).

age and etiology (*e.g.*, DM, chronic kidney disease) in which the desired resting BP may be different than <140/90 mm Hg (38,43). Although there is a lack of consensus among professional organizations regarding the recommendations for lowering BP in older adults, most guidelines (*i.e.*, ACC Foundation/AHA Expert Consensus Document on Hypertension in the Elderly, ASH/ISH Clinical Practice Guidelines for the Management of Hypertension in the Community, European Society for Hypertension [ESH]/European Society of Cardiology [ESC]) consider the goal BP for patients 60–79 yr old to be <140/90 mm Hg which form the basis for the present American College of Sports Medicine recommendations (5,23,43). However, the recent JNC 8 guideline recommends initiating pharmacologic therapy for patients ≥60 yr (without DM or chronic kidney disease) at SBP ≥150 mm Hg or DBP ≥90 mm Hg and to treat to an SBP goal of <150 mm Hg and a DBP goal of <90 mm Hg. (19). Because of differences in the general health of very old patients, the BP goal may be higher than <140/90 mm Hg, and the decision to treat should be made on an individual basis (5,23,43).

Lipids and Lipoproteins

As emphasized in the Third Report of the Expert Panel on Detection, Evaluation, and Treatment of High Blood Cholesterol in Adults (Adult Treatment Panel III or ATP III) and subsequent updates by the National Heart, Lung, and Blood Institute (NHLBI), AHA/ACC, ESC and European Atherosclerosis Society (EAS), and the recent ACC/AHA Guidelines on the Treatment of Blood Cholesterol to Reduce Atherosclerotic Cardiovascular Risk in Adults, LDL-C is identified as the primary target for cholesterol-lowering therapy (16,35–37,39). This designation is based on a wide variety of evidence indicating elevated LDL-C is a powerful risk factor for CVD, and lowering of LDL-C results in a striking reduction in the incidence of CVD. *Table 3.3* summarizes the clinically accepted ATP III classifications of LDL-C, total cholesterol, and HDL-C and triglycerides; this classification of

TABLE 3.3	
Classification of LDL, Total, and HDL Cholesterol and Triglycerides (mg · dL^{-1})	
LDL Cholesterol	
<100	Optimal
100–129	Near optimal/above optimal
130–159	Borderline high
160–189	High
≥190	Very high
Total Cholesterol	
<200	Desirable
200–239	Borderline high
≥240	High
HDL Cholesterol	
<40	Low
≥60	High
Triglycerides	
<150	Normal
150–199	Borderline high
200–499	High
≥500	Very high

NOTE: To convert LDL, total, and HDL cholesterol from mg · dL^{-1} to mmol · L^{-1}, multiply by 0.0259.
To convert triglycerides from mg · dL^{-1} to mmol · L^{-1}, multiply by 0.0113.
HDL, high-density lipoprotein; LDL, low-density lipoprotein.
Adapted from (39).

lipoprotein and triglycerides is not specifically addressed in the 2013 ACC/AHA guidelines (37) and is similar to a classification scheme advocated by the National Lipid Association (18).

There is evidence of an association between elevated triglycerides and CVD risk, although adjustment for other risk factors, especially HDL-C, appears to attenuate this relationship (9,24). Nonfasting triglyceride levels have a stronger relationship with CVD risk than do fasting levels (21). Studies suggest some species of triglyceride-rich lipoproteins, notably small very low-density lipoproteins (VLDLs) and intermediate-density lipoproteins (IDLs), promote atherosclerosis and predispose to CVD. Because VLDL and IDL appear to have atherogenic potential similar to that of LDL-C, non–HDL-C (*i.e.*, VLDL plus IDL plus LDL-C; calculated as total cholesterol minus HDL-C) is recommended as a secondary target of therapy for individuals with elevated triglyceride levels (triglycerides ≥ 200 mg $\cdot$ dL^{-1}) (39). When the triglycerides are ≥ 500 mg $\cdot$ dL^{-1}, they become the primary target of therapy due to the increased risk of pancreatitis.

A low HDL-C is strongly and inversely associated with CVD risk. Clinical trials provide suggestive evidence that raising HDL-C reduces CVD risk. However, the mechanism explaining the role of low serum HDL-C in accelerating the CVD process remains unclear, and it remains uncertain whether raising HDL-C *per se*, independent of other changes in lipid and/or nonlipid risk factors, reduces the risk of CVD. In view of this, a specific HDL-C goal level to achieve with therapy has not been identified. Rather, current guidelines (18,35,37) emphasize that lifestyle and drug therapies used the management of atherogenic dyslipidemia may also provide the benefit of secondarily raising HDL-C levels.

The fundamental principle of guideline recommendations for the treatment of dyslipidemia is that the intensity of therapy should be adjusted to the individual's absolute risk for CVD (4,11,16–18,35–37,39). Therapeutic lifestyle changes are the cornerstone of therapy (10,37), with pharmacological therapy to lower LDL-C (primarily with hydroxymethylglutaryl-coenzyme A [HMG-CoA] reductase inhibitors [statins]) being used to achieve treatment goals when indicated. Similar to ATP III, guidelines for the management of dyslipidemias released by the ESC/EAS (35) and the National Lipid Association (18) recommend specific cut points and treatment goals for LDL-C based on CVD risk profile. The recent 2013 ACC/AHA Guideline on the Treatment of Blood Cholesterol to Reduce Atherosclerotic Cardiovascular Risk in Adults (37) represents a departure in approach (*i.e.*, not pursuing LDL-C targets) from other guideline statements by focusing solely on CVD risk reduction benefit demonstrated in randomized controlled clinical trials and by identifying individuals in primary or secondary prevention who would benefit most from initiation of moderate- or high-intensity statin therapy. For patients aged 40–75 yr without evident CVD or DM and with LDL-C levels of 70–189 mg $\cdot$ dL^{-1}, the 2013 ACC/AHA Guideline recommends use of the Pooled Cohort Equations CV Risk Calculator (15) to estimate 10-yr risk of a CVD event to inform therapy; high-intensity statin therapy is generally recommended for those with a 10-yr risk estimated to be $\geq 7.5\%$ (high risk), whereas moderate evidence exists to support statin use among individuals with an estimated 10-yr atherosclerotic cardiovascular disease (ASCVD) risk of 5%–<7.5% (intermediate risk). Moderate intensity or high intensity statin therapy, which typically reduce LDL-C levels by 30%–<50% and ≥50%, respectively should be used as initial lipid-lowering therapy based on risk level and treatment goals (37).

Blood Profile Analyses

Multiple analyses of blood profiles are commonly evaluated in clinical exercise programs. Such profiles may provide useful information about an individual's overall health status and ability to exercise and may help to explain certain ECG abnormalities. Because of varied methods of assaying blood samples, some caution is advised when comparing blood chemistries from different laboratories. *Table 3.4* gives normal ranges for selected blood chemistries, derived from a variety of sources. For many patients with CVD, medications for dyslipidemia and hypertension are common. Many of these medications act in the liver to lower blood cholesterol and in the kidneys to lower BP (see *Appendix A*). Although current recommendations do not suggest performing serial tests of liver function in patients receiving statin drugs, tests such as alanine transaminase (ALT) and aspartate transaminase (AST) may indicate the presence of liver abnormalities induced by the these agents. Periodic testing of renal function with tests such as creatinine, estimated glomerular filtration rate (GFR), blood urea nitrogen (BUN), BUN/creatinine ratio, and serum sodium and potassium levels is indicated in patients prescribed medications that may lead to alterations in renal function. Indication of volume depletion and potassium abnormalities can be seen in the sodium and potassium measurements.

Pulmonary Function

Pulmonary function testing with spirometry is recommended for all smokers >45 yr old and in any individual presenting with dyspnea (*i.e.*, shortness of breath), chronic cough, wheezing, or excessive mucus production (12). Spirometry is a simple and noninvasive test that can be performed easily. Indications for spirometry are listed in *Table 3.5*. When performing spirometry, standards for the performance of the test, as endorsed by the American Thoracic Society (ATS), should be followed (25).

Although many measurements can be made from a spirometric test, the most commonly used include the forced vital capacity (FVC), forced expiratory volume in one second ($FEV_{1.0}$), $FEV_{1.0}$/FVC ratio, and peak expiratory flow (PEF). Results from these measurements can help to identify the presence of restrictive or obstructive respiratory abnormalities, sometimes before symptoms or signs of disease are present. The $FEV_{1.0}$/FVC ratio is diminished with obstructive airway diseases (*e.g.*, asthma, chronic bronchitis, emphysema, chronic obstructive pulmonary disease [COPD]) but remains normal with restrictive disorders (*e.g.*, kyphoscoliosis, neuromuscular disease, pulmonary fibrosis, other interstitial lung diseases).

TABLE 3.4

Typical Ranges of Normal Values for Selected Blood Variables in Adults[a]

Variable	Men	Neutral	Women	SI Conversion Factor
Hemoglobin (g · dL⁻¹)	13.5–17.5		11.5–15.5	10 (g · L⁻¹)
Hematocrit (%)	40–52		36–48	0.01 (proportion of 1)
Red cell count (×10⁶ · μL⁻¹)	4.5–6.5 million		3.9–5.6 million	1 (×10¹² · L⁻¹)
White blood cell count (×10³ · μL⁻¹)		4–11 thousand		1 (×10⁹ · L⁻¹)
Platelet count (×10³ · μL⁻¹)		150–450 thousand		1 (×10⁹ · L⁻¹)
Fasting glucose[b] (mg · dL⁻¹)		60–99		0.0555 (mmol · L⁻¹)
HbA1C		≤6%		N/A
Blood urea nitrogen (BUN; mg · dL⁻¹)		4–24		0.357 (mmol · L⁻¹)
Creatinine (mg · dL⁻¹)		0.3–1.4		88.4 (μmol · L⁻¹)
BUN/creatinine ratio		7–27		
Uric acid (mg · dL⁻¹)		3.6–8.3		59.48 (μmol · L⁻¹)
Sodium (mEq · dL⁻¹)		135–150		1.0 (mmol · L⁻¹)
Potassium (mEq · dL⁻¹)		3.5–5.5		1.0 (mmol · L⁻¹)
Chloride (mEq · dL⁻¹)		98–110		1.0 (mmol · L⁻¹)
Osmolality (mOsm · kg⁻¹)		278–302		1.0 (mmol · kg⁻¹)
Calcium (mg · dL⁻¹)		8.5–10.5		0.25 (mmol · L⁻¹)
Calcium, ion (mg · dL⁻¹)		4.0–5.0		0.25 (mmol · L⁻¹)
Phosphorus (mg · dL⁻¹)		2.5–4.5		0.323 (mmol · L⁻¹)
Protein, total (g · dL⁻¹)		6.0–8.5		10 (g · L⁻¹)
Albumin (A) (g · dL⁻¹)		3.0–5.5		10 (g · L⁻¹)
Globulin (G) (g · dL⁻¹)		2.0–4.0		10 (g · L⁻¹)
A/G ratio		1.0–2.2		10
Iron, total (μg · dL⁻¹)		40–190	35–180	0.179 (μmol · L⁻¹)
Liver Function Tests				
Bilirubin (mg · dL⁻¹)		<1.5		17.1 (μmol · L⁻¹)
AST (U · L⁻¹)	8–46		7–34	1 (U · L⁻¹)
ALT (U · L⁻¹)	7–46		4–35	1 (U · L⁻¹)

[a]Certain variables must be interpreted in relation to the normal range of the issuing laboratory.
[b]Fasting blood glucose 100–125 mg · dL⁻¹ is considered impaired fasting glucose or prediabetes.
NOTE: For a complete list of Système International (SI) conversion factors, please see http://jama.ama-assn
.org/content/vol295/issue1/images/data/103/DC6/JAMA_auinst_si.dtl
ALT, alanine transaminase (formerly serum glutamic-pyruvic transaminase [SGPT]); AST, aspartate transaminase (formerly serum glutamic-oxaloacetic transaminase [SGOT]); HbA1C, glycolated hemoglobin; N/A, not applicable.

TABLE **3.5**

Indications for Spirometry

A. Indications for Spirometry

Diagnosis

To evaluate symptoms, signs, or abnormal laboratory tests
To measure the effect of disease on pulmonary function
To screen individuals at risk of having pulmonary disease
To assess preoperative risk
To assess prognosis
To assess health status before beginning strenuous physical activity programs

Monitoring

To assess therapeutic intervention
To describe the course of diseases that affect lung function
To monitor individuals exposed to injurious agents
To monitor for adverse reactions to drugs with known pulmonary toxicity

Disability/Impairment Evaluations

To assess patients as part of a rehabilitation program
To assess risks as part of an insurance evaluation
To assess individuals for legal reasons

Public Health

Epidemiologic surveys
Derivation of reference equations
Clinical research

B. The Global Initiative for Chronic Obstructive Lung Disease (GOLD) Spirometric Classification of COPD Severity Based on Postbronchodilator $FEV_{1.0}$

GOLD I	Mild	$FEV_{1.0}/FVC < 0.70$ $FEV_{1.0} \geq 80\%$ of predicted
GOLD II	Moderate	$FEV_{1.0}/FVC < 0.70$ $50\% \leq FEV_{1.0} < 80\%$ predicted
GOLD III	Severe	$FEV_{1.0}/FVC < 0.70$ $30\% \leq FEV_{1.0} < 50\%$ predicted
GOLD IV	Very severe	$FEV_{1.0}/FVC < 0.70$ $FEV_{1.0} < 30\%$ predicted respiratory failure

C. The American Thoracic Society and European Respiratory Society Classification of Severity of Any Spirometric Abnormality Based on $FEV_{1.0}$

Degree of Severity	$FEV_{1.0}$ % Predicted
Mild	Less than the LLN but ≥ 70
Moderate	60–69
Moderately severe	50–59
Severe	35–49
Very severe	<35

COPD, chronic obstructive pulmonary disease; $FEV_{1.0}$, forced expiratory volume in one second; FVC, forced vital capacity; respiratory failure defined as arterial partial pressure of oxygen (P_aO_2) <8.0 kPa (60 mm Hg) with or without arterial partial pressure of CO_2 (P_aCO_2) >6.7 kPa (50 mm Hg) while breathing air at sea level; LLN, lower limit of normal.

Modified from (32,34).

The Global Initiative for Chronic Obstructive Lung Disease classifies the presence and severity of COPD as seen in *Table 3.5* (14,34). The term *COPD* can be used when chronic bronchitis, emphysema, or both are present and spirometry documents an obstructive defect. A different approach for classifying the severity of obstructive and restrictive defects is that of the ATS and European Respiratory Society (ERS) Task Force on Standardisation of Lung Function Testing as presented in *Table 3.5* (32). This ATS/ERS Task Force prefers to use the largest available vital capacity (VC), whether it is obtained on inspiration (IVC), slow expiration (SVC), or forced expiration (FVC). An obstructive defect is defined by a reduced $FEV_{1.0}/FVC$ ratio below the fifth percentile of the predicted value. The use of the fifth percentile of the predicted value as the lower limit of normal does not lead to an overestimation of the presence of an obstructive defect in older individuals, which is more likely when a fixed value for $FEV_{1.0}/FVC$ ratio or a $FEV_{1.0}/FVC$ ratio of 0.7 is used as the dividing line between normal and abnormal (26). A restrictive defect is characterized by a reduction in the total lung capacity (TLC), as measured on a lung volume study, below the fifth percentile of the predicted value, and a normal $FEV_{1.0}/FVC$ ratio (26).

The spirometric classification of lung disease is useful in predicting health status, use of health resources, and mortality. Abnormal spirometry can also be indicative of an increased risk for lung cancer, heart attack, and stroke and can be used to identify patients in whom interventions such as smoking cessation and use of pharmacologic agents would be most beneficial. Spirometric testing is also valuable in identifying patients with chronic disease (*i.e.*, COPD and heart failure) who have diminished pulmonary function that may benefit from an inspiratory muscle training program (4,30).

The determination of the maximal voluntary ventilation (MVV) should also be obtained during routine spirometric testing (25,32). The MVV can be used to estimate breathing reserve during maximal exercise and should ideally be measured rather than estimated by multiplying the $FEV_{1.0}$ by a constant value as is often done in practice (32).

PARTICIPANT INSTRUCTIONS

Explicit instructions for participants before exercise testing increase test validity and data accuracy. Whenever possible, written instructions along with a description of the preexercise evaluation should be provided well in advance of the appointment so the client or patient can prepare adequately. When serial testing is performed, every effort should be made to ensure exercise testing procedures are consistent between/among assessments (3). The following points should be considered for inclusion in such preliminary instructions; however, specific instructions vary with test type and purpose:

- At a minimum, participants should refrain from ingesting food, alcohol, or caffeine or using tobacco products within 3 h of testing.
- Participants should be rested for the assessment, avoiding significant exertion or exercise on the day of the assessment.

- Clothing should permit freedom of movement and include walking or running shoes. Women should bring a loose-fitting, short-sleeved blouse that buttons down the front and should avoid restrictive undergarments.
- If the evaluation is on an outpatient basis, participants should be made aware that the exercise test may be fatiguing, and they may wish to have someone accompany them to the assessment to drive home afterward.
- If the exercise test is for diagnostic purposes, it may be helpful for patients to discontinue prescribed cardiovascular medications but only with physician approval. Currently, prescribed antianginal agents alter the hemodynamic response to exercise and significantly reduce the sensitivity of ECG changes for ischemia. Patients taking intermediate- or high-dose β-blocking agents may be asked to taper their medication over a 2- to 4-d period to minimize hyperadrenergic withdrawal responses (see *Appendix A*).
- If the exercise test is for functional or Ex R_x purposes, *patients should continue their medication regimen* on their usual schedule so that the exercise responses will be consistent with responses expected during exercise training.
- Participants should bring a list of their medications including dosage and frequency of administration to the assessment and should report the last actual dose taken. As an alternative, participants may wish to bring their medications with them for the exercise testing staff to record.
- Participants should be instructed to drink ample fluids over the 24-h period preceding the exercise test to ensure normal hydration before testing.

ONLINE RESOURCES

American College of Cardiology:
    http://www.cardiosource.org
    http://tools.cardiosource.org/ASCVD-Risk-Estimator/
American College of Sports Medicine Exercise is Medicine:
    http://www.exerciseismedicine.org
American Diabetes Association
    http://www.diabetes.org
American Heart Association:
    http://www.americanheart.org
European Society of Cardiology:
    http://www.escardio.org
National Heart, Lung, and Blood Institute Health Information for Professionals:
    http://www.nhlbi.nih.gov/health/indexpro.htm

REFERENCES

1. American Diabetes Association. 2. Classification and diagnosis of diabetes. *Diabetes Care.* 2015;38:S8–16.
2. Appel LJ, Brands MW, Daniels SR, et al. Dietary approaches to prevent and treat hypertension: a scientific statement from the American Heart Association. *Hypertension.* 2006;47(2):296–308.

3. Arena R, Myers J, Williams MA, et al. Assessment of functional capacity in clinical and research settings: a scientific statement from the American Heart Association Committee on Exercise, Rehabilitation, and Prevention of the Council on Clinical Cardiology and the Council on Cardiovascular Nursing. *Circulation*. 2007;116(3):329–43.

4. Arena R, Pinkstaff S, Wheeler E, Peberdy MA, Guazzi M, Myers J. Neuromuscular electrical stimulation and inspiratory muscle training as potential adjunctive rehabilitation options for patients with heart failure. *J Cardiopulm Rehabil Prev*. 2010;30(4):209–23.

5. Aronow WS, Fleg JL, Pepine CJ, et al. ACCF/AHA 2011 expert consensus document on hypertension in the elderly: a report of the American College of Cardiology Foundation Task Force on Clinical Expert Consensus documents developed in collaboration with the American Academy of Neurology, American Geriatrics Society, American Society for Preventive Cardiology, American Society of Hypertension, American Society of Nephrology, Association of Black Cardiologists, and European Society of Hypertension. *J Am Coll Cardiol*. 2011;57(20):2037–114.

6. *ASCVD risk estimator* [Internet].Washington (DC): American College of Cardiology/American Heart Association; [cited 2015 Aug 12]. Available from: http://tools.cardiosource.org/ASC-VD-Risk-Estimator

7. Bickley LS. *Bates' Pocket Guide to Physical Examination and History Taking*. 6th ed. Baltimore (MD): Lippincott Williams & Wilkins; 2008. 453 p.

8. Chobanian AV, Bakris GL, Black HR, et al. Seventh report of the Joint National Committee on Prevention, Detection, Evaluation, and Treatment of High Blood Pressure. *Hypertension*. 2003;42(6):1206–52.

9. Di Angelantonio E, Sarwar N, Perry P, et al. Major lipids, apolipoproteins, and risk of vascular disease. *JAMA*. 2009;302(18):1993–2000.

10. Eckel RH, Jakicic JM, Ard JD, et al. 2013 AHA/ACC guideline on lifestyle management to reduce cardiovascular risk: a report of the American College of Cardiology/American Heart Association Task Force on Practice Guidelines. *J Am Coll Cardiol*. 2014;63:2960–84.

11. Expert Panel on Detection, Evaluation, and Treatment of High Blood Cholesterol in Adults. Executive Summary of the Third Report of The National Cholesterol Education Program (NCEP) Expert Panel on Detection, Evaluation, and Treatment of High Blood Cholesterol in Adults (Adult Treatment Panel III). *JAMA*. 2001;285(19):2486–97.

12. Ferguson GT, Enright PL, Buist AS, Higgins MW. Office spirometry for lung health assessment in adults: a consensus statement from the National Lung Health Education Program. *Chest*. 2000;117(4):1146–61.

13. Gibbons RJ, Balady GJ, Bricker JT, et al. ACC/AHA 2002 guideline update for exercise testing: summary article. A report of the American College of Cardiology/American Heart Association Task Force on Practice Guidelines (Committee to Update the 1997 Exercise Testing Guidelines). *J Am Coll Cardiol*. 2002;40(8):1531–40.

14. Global Initiative for Chronic Obstructive Lung Disease Web site [Internet]. Global Initiative for Chronic Obstructive Lung Disease; [cited 2015 Aug 12]. Available from: http://www.goldcopd.org/

15. Goff DC Jr, Lloyd-Jones DM, Bennett G, et al. 2013 ACC/AHA guideline on the assessment of cardiovascular risk: a report of the American College of Cardiology/American Heart Association Task Force on Practice Guidelines. *J Am Coll Cardiol*. 2014;63:2935–59.

16. Grundy SM, Cleeman JI, Merz CN, et al. Implications of recent clinical trials for the National Cholesterol Education Program Adult Treatment Panel III Guidelines. *J Am Coll Cardiol*. 2004;44(3):720–32.

17. Hendel RC, Berman DS, Di Carli MF, et al. ACCF/ASNC/ACR/AHA/ASE/SCCT/SCMR/SNM 2009 appropriate use criteria for cardiac radionuclide imaging: a report of the American College of Cardiology Foundation Appropriate Use Criteria Task Force, the American Society of Nuclear Cardiology, the American College of Radiology, the American Heart Association, the American Society of Echocardiography, the Society of Cardiovascular Computed Tomography, the Society for Cardiovascular Magnetic Resonance, and the Society of Nuclear Medicine. *Circulation*. 2009;119(22):e561–87.

18. Jacobson TA, Ito MK, Maki KC, et al. National Lipid Association recommendations for patient-centered management of dyslipidemia: part 1 — executive summary. *J Clin Lipidol*. 2014; 8(5):473–88.

19. James PA, Oparil S, Carter BL, et al. 2014 evidence-based guideline for the management of high blood pressure in adults: report from the panel members appointed to the Eighth Joint National Committee (JNC 8). *JAMA*. 2014;311(5):507–20.

20. Jensen MD, Ryan DH, Apovian CM, et al. 2013 AHA/ACC/TOS Guidelines for the management of overweight and obesity in adults: a report of the American College of Cardiology/American Heart Association Task Force on Practice Guidelines and The Obesity Society. *J Am Coll Cardiol*. 2014;63(25):2985–3023.

21. Kannel WB, Vasan RS. Triglycerides as vascular risk factors: new epidemiologic insights. *Curr Opin Cardiol*. 2009;24(4):345–50.

22. Kantola I, Vesalainen R, Kangassalo K, Kariluoto A. Bell or diaphragm in the measurement of blood pressure? *J Hypertens*. 2005;23(3):499–503.

23. Mancia G, Fagard R, Narkiewicz K, et al. 2013 ESH/ESC guidelines for the management of arterial hypertension: the Task Force for the Management of Arterial Hypertension of the European Society of Hypertension (ESH) and of the European Society of Cardiology (ESC). *Eur Heart J*. 2013;34(28):2159–219.

24. Miller M, Stone NJ, Ballantyne C, et al. Triglycerides and cardiovascular disease: a scientific statement from the American Heart Association. *Circulation*. 2011;123(20):2292–333.

25. Miller MR, Hankinson J, Brusasco V, et al. Standardisation of spirometry. *Eur Respir J*. 2005;26(2):319–38.

26. Miller MR, Quanjer PH, Swanney MP, Ruppel G, Enright PL. Interpreting lung function data using 80% of predicted and fixed thresholds misclassifies more than 20% of patients. *Chest*. 2011;139(1):52–9.

27. Mozaffarian D, Benjamin EJ, Go AS, et al. Heart disease and stroke statistics — 2015 update: a report from the American Heart Association. *Circulation*. 2015;131(4):e29–322.

28. Myers J, Arena R, Franklin B, et al. Recommendations for clinical exercise laboratories: a scientific statement from the American Heart Association. *Circulation*. 2009;119(24):3144–61.

29. National Cholesterol Education Program (NCEP) Expert Panel on Detection, Evaluation, and Treatment of High Blood Cholesterol in Adults (Adult Treatment Panel III). Third Report of the National Cholesterol Education Program (NCEP) Expert Panel on Detection, Evaluation, and Treatment of High Blood Cholesterol in Adults (Adult Treatment Panel III) final report. *Circulation*. 2002;106(25):3143–421.

30. Nici L, Donner C, Wouters E, et al. American Thoracic Society/European Respiratory Society statement on pulmonary rehabilitation. *Am J Respir Crit Care Med*. 2006;173(12):1390–413.

31. Pate RR, Pratt M, Blair SN, et al. Physical activity and public health. A recommendation from the Centers for Disease Control and Prevention and the American College of Sports Medicine. *JAMA*. 1995;273(5):402–7.

32. Pellegrino R, Viegi G, Brusasco V, et al. Interpretative strategies for lung function tests. *Eur Respir J*. 2005;26(5):948–68.

33. Pickering TG, Hall JE, Appel LJ, et al. Recommendations for blood pressure measurement in humans and experimental animals: part 1: blood pressure measurement in humans: a statement for professionals from the Subcommittee of Professional and Public Education of the American Heart Association Council on High Blood Pressure Research. *Hypertension*. 2005;45(1):142–61.

34. Rabe KF, Hurd S, Anzueto A, et al. Global strategy for the diagnosis, management, and prevention of chronic obstructive pulmonary disease: GOLD executive summary. *Am J Respir Crit Care Med*. 2007;176(6):532–55.

35. Reiner Z, Catapano AL, De Backer G, et al. ESC/EAS guidelines for the management of dyslipidaemias: the Task Force for the management of dyslipidaemias of the European Society of Cardiology (ESC) and the European Atherosclerosis Society (EAS). *Eur Heart J*. 2011;32(14):1769–818.

36. Smith SC Jr, Allen J, Blair SN, et al. AHA/ACC guidelines for secondary prevention for patients with coronary and other atherosclerotic vascular disease: 2006 update: endorsed by the National Heart, Lung, and Blood Institute. *Circulation*. 2006;113(19):2363–72.

37. Stone NJ, Robinson JG, Lichtenstein AH, et al. 2013 ACC/AHA guideline on the treatment of blood cholesterol to reduce atherosclerotic cardiovascular risk in adults: a report of the American College of Cardiology/American Heart Association Task Force on Practice Guidelines. *Circulation*. 2014;129:S1–45.

38. The Seventh Report of the Joint National Committee on Prevention, Detection, Evaluation, and Treatment of High Blood Pressure [Internet]. Bethesda (MD): National High Blood Pressure Education Program; 2004 [cited 2015 Aug 12]. 104 p. Available from: http://www.nhlbi.nih.gov/guidelines/hypertension/jnc7full.pdf

39. *Third Report of the National Cholesterol Education Program (NCEP) Expert Panel on Detection, Evaluation, and Treatment of High Blood Cholesterol in Adults (Adult Treatment Panel III)* [Internet]. Bethesda (MD): National Cholesterol Education Program; 2004 [cited 2015 Aug 12]. 284 p. Available from: http://www.nhlbi.nih.gov/guidelines/cholesterol/index.htm

40. U.S. Department of Health and Human Services. *2008 Physical Activity Guidelines for Americans* [Internet]. Washington (DC): U.S. Department of Health and Human Services; 2008 [cited 2015 Aug 12]. Available from: http://health.gov/paguidelines/pdf/paguide.pdf

41. U.S. Preventive Services Task Force. Screening for coronary heart disease: recommendation statement. *Ann Intern Med.* 2004;140(7):569–72.

42. Verrill D, Graham H, Vitcenda M, Peno-Green L, Kramer V, Corbisiero T. Measuring behavioral outcomes in cardiopulmonary rehabilitation: an AACVPR statement. *J Cardiopulm Rehabil Prev.* 2009;29(3):193–203.

43. Weber MA, Schiffrin EL, White WB, et al. Clinical practice guidelines for the management of hypertension in the community: a statement by the American Society of Hypertension and the International Society of Hypertension. *J Clin Hypertens (Greenwich).* 2014;16(1):14–26.

Health-Related Physical Fitness Testing and Interpretation

INTRODUCTION

Evidence outlined in *Chapter 1* clearly supports the numerous health benefits that result from regular participation in physical activity (PA) and structured exercise programs. The health-related components of physical fitness have a strong relationship with overall health, are characterized by an ability to perform activities of daily living with vigor, and are associated with a lower prevalence of chronic disease and health conditions and their risk factors (95). Measures of health-related physical fitness are closely allied with disease prevention and health promotion and can be modified through regular participation in PA and structured exercise programs. A fundamental goal of primary and secondary prevention and rehabilitative programs should be the promotion of health; hence, exercise programs should focus on enhancement of the health-related components of physical fitness. Accordingly, the focus of this chapter is on the health-related components of physical fitness testing and interpretation (36,40).

Compared to previous editions of the *Guidelines*, the present version of *Chapter 4* does not include YMCA protocols or normative data, as their policy for permission has changed.

PURPOSES OF HEALTH-RELATED PHYSICAL FITNESS TESTING

Measurement of physical fitness is a common and appropriate practice in preventive and rehabilitative exercise programs. Minimally, a health-related physical fitness test must be both reliable and valid, and ideally, it should be relatively inexpensive. The information obtained from health-related physical fitness testing, in combination with the individual's medical and exercise history, is used for the following:

- Collecting baseline data and educating participants about their present health/fitness status relative to health-related standards and age- and sex-matched norms.
- Providing data that are helpful in development of individualized exercise prescriptions (Ex R_x) to address all health/fitness components.

- Collecting follow-up data that allow evaluation of progress following an Ex R_x and long-term monitoring as participants age.
- Motivating participants by establishing reasonable and attainable health/fitness goals (see *Chapter 12*).

BASIC PRINCIPLES AND GUIDELINES

Pretest Instructions

All pretest instructions should be provided and adhered to prior to arrival at the testing facility. The following steps should be taken to ensure client safety and comfort before administering a health-related physical fitness test:

- Perform the informed consent process and allow time for the individual undergoing assessment to have all questions adequately addressed (see *Figure 3.1*).
- Perform exercise preparticipation health screening (see *Chapter 2*).
- Complete a preexercise evaluation including a medical history and a cardiovascular disease (CVD) risk factor assessment (see *Chapter 3*). A minimal recommendation is that individuals complete a self-guided questionnaire such as the Physical Activity Readiness Questionnaire + (PAR-Q+) (see *Figure 2.1*). Other more detailed medical history forms may also be used.
- Follow the list of preliminary testing instructions for all clients located in *Chapter 3* under "Participant Instructions" section. These instructions may be modified to meet specific needs and circumstances.

Test Organization

The following should be accomplished before the client/patient arrives at the test site:

- Ensure consent and screening forms, data recording sheets, and any related testing documents are available in the client's file and available for the test's administration.
- Calibrate all equipment (*e.g.*, cycle ergometer, treadmill, sphygmomanometer) at least monthly, or more frequently based on use; certain equipment such as ventilatory expired gas analysis systems should be calibrated prior to each test according to manufacturers' specifications; and document equipment calibration. Skinfold calipers should be regularly checked for accuracy and sent to the manufacturer for calibration when needed.
- Ensure a room temperature between 68° F and 72° F (20° C and 22° C) and humidity of less than 60% with adequate airflow (60).

When multiple tests are to be administered, the organization of the testing session can be very important, depending on what physical fitness components are to be evaluated. Resting measurements such as heart rate (HR), blood pressure (BP), height, weight, and body composition should be obtained first. An optimal testing order for multiple health-related components of fitness (*i.e.*, cardiorespiratory fitness [CRF], muscular fitness, and flexibility) has not been established, but sufficient time should be allowed for HR and BP to return to baseline between tests conducted serially. Additionally, test procedures should be organized to follow in sequence without stressing the same muscle group repeatedly. To ensure reliability, the chosen order should be followed on subsequent testing sessions. Because certain medications (*e.g.*, β-blockers which lower HR) will affect some physical fitness test results, use of these medications should be noted (see *Appendix A*).

Test Environment

The environment is important for test validity and reliability. Test anxiety, emotions, room temperature, and ventilation should be controlled as much as possible. To minimize subject anxiety, the test procedures should be explained adequately and should not be rushed, and the test environment should be quiet and private. The room should be equipped with a comfortable seat and/or examination table to be used for resting BP and HR. The demeanor of personnel should be one of relaxed confidence to put the subject at ease. Finally, the exercise professional should be familiar with the emergency response plan (see *Appendix B*).

A COMPREHENSIVE HEALTH FITNESS EVALUATION

A comprehensive health/fitness assessment includes the following: (a) informed consent and exercise preparticipation health screening (see *Chapters 2* and *3*), (b) preexercise evaluation (see *Chapter 3*), (c) resting measurements, (d) circumference measurements and body composition analysis, (e) measurement of CRF, (f) measurement of muscular fitness, and (g) measurement of flexibility. Additional evaluations may be administered; however, the components of a health/fitness evaluation represent a comprehensive assessment that can usually be performed on the same day. The data accrued from the evaluation should be interpreted by a competent exercise professional and conveyed to the client. This information is central to educate the client about his or her current physical fitness status and to the development of the client's short- and long-term goals as well as forming the basis for the individualized Ex R$_x$ and subsequent evaluations to monitor progress.

For certain individuals, the risks of health-related physical fitness testing may outweigh the potential benefits. Although some assessments pose little risk (*e.g.*, body composition), others may have higher risks (*e.g.*, CRF and one repetition maximum [1-RM]) for some individuals. For these individuals, it is important to carefully assess risk versus benefit when deciding on whether a fitness test should be performed. Performing the preexercise evaluation with a careful review of prior medical history, as described in *Chapter 3*, helps identify potential contraindications and increases the safety of the health-related physical fitness assessment. See *Box 5.2* for a list of absolute and relative contraindications to exercise testing.

MEASUREMENT OF RESTING HEART RATE AND BLOOD PRESSURE

A comprehensive physical fitness assessment includes the measurement of resting HR and BP. HR can be determined using several techniques including pulse palpation, auscultation with a stethoscope, or the use of an HR monitor. The pulse palpation technique involves "feeling" the pulse by placing the second and third fingers (*e.g.*, index and middle fingers) most typically over the radial artery, located near the thumb side of the wrist. The pulse is counted for 30 or 60 s. The 30-s count is multiplied by 2 to determine the 1-min resting HR (beats per minute). For the auscultation method, the bell of the stethoscope should be placed to the left of the sternum just above the level of the nipple. The auscultation method is most accurate when the heart sounds are clearly audible, and the subject's torso is stable. Upon arrival to the testing facility, it is important to allow a client time to relax (at least 5 min) to allow resting HR and BP to stabilize. The measurement of resting BP is described elsewhere (see *Box 3.5*).

BODY COMPOSITION

It is well established that excess body fat, particularly when located centrally around the abdomen, is associated with many chronic conditions including hypertension, metabolic syndrome (Metsyn), Type 2 diabetes mellitus (T2DM), stroke, CVD, and dyslipidemia (102). Approximately two-thirds (68.5%) of American adults are classified as either overweight or obese (body mass index [BMI] $\geq$25 kg $\cdot$ m^{-2}), and more than a third (34.9%) are classified as obese (BMI $\geq$30 kg $\cdot$ m^{-2}) (85). Nearly one-third (31.8%) of American children and adolescents are overweight or obese (85) (see *Chapter 10*). The troubling data on overweight/obesity prevalence among the adult and pediatric populations and its health implications have precipitated an increased awareness in the value of identifying and treating individuals with excess body weight (24,29,65,115). Indeed in 2013, the American Medical Association labeled obesity as a disease (1).

It is important to recognize the health-related changes in body composition that accompany aging. Sarcopenia, the degenerative loss of muscle mass and strength as a result of aging and reduced PA, is associated with a reduced ability to perform activities of daily living and increases the risk of musculoskeletal injury (34,81). Thus, body composition measurement can be used to monitor changes in lean body mass, particularly among older adults.

Basic body composition can be expressed as the relative percentage of body mass that is fat and fat-free tissue using a two-compartment model. Body composition can be estimated with methods that vary in terms of complexity, cost, and accuracy (30,66). Different assessment techniques are briefly reviewed in this section, but details associated with obtaining measurements and calculating estimates of body fat for all of these techniques are beyond the scope of the *Guidelines*. Additional detailed information is available (38,42,45). Before collecting data for body composition assessment, the technician must be trained, experienced in the techniques, and already have demonstrated reliability in his or her measurements, independent of the technique being used.

Anthropometric Methods

Height, Weight, and Body Mass Index

Body weight should be measured using a calibrated balance beam or electronic scale with the client wearing minimal clothing and having empty pockets. Shoes should be removed prior to the use of a stadiometer for the measurement of height.

BMI or the Quetelet index is used to assess weight relative to height and is calculated by dividing body weight in kilograms by height in meters squared $(kg \cdot m^{-2})$. The Expert Panel on the Identification, Evaluation, and Treatment of Overweight and Obesity in Adults (31) defines a BMI of <18.5 $kg \cdot m^{-2}$ as underweight, 18.5–24.9 $kg \cdot m^{-2}$ as normal, 25.0–29.9 $kg \cdot m^{-2}$ as overweight, and ≥ 30.0 $kg \cdot m^{-2}$ as obese. Although BMI fails to distinguish between body fat, muscle mass, or bone, it is well accepted that with the exception of individuals with large amounts of muscle mass, those with a BMI >30 $kg \cdot m^{-2}$ have excess body fat. An increased risk of obesity-related diseases, health conditions, and mortality are associated with a BMI ≥ 30.0 $kg \cdot m^{-2}$ (*Table 4.1*) (31,93). This association is not perfect, as there is compelling evidence to indicate patients diagnosed with congestive heart failure (CHF) actually have improved survival when BMI is ≥ 30.0 $kg \cdot m^{-2}$, a phenomenon known as the "obesity paradox" (2,86).

TABLE 4.1

Classification of Disease Risk Based on Body Mass Index (BMI) and Waist Circumference

	BMI (kg · m⁻²)	Disease Risk[a] Relative to Normal Weight and Waist Circumference	
		Men, 102 cm Women, 88 cm	Men, 102 cm Women, 88 cm
Underweight	<18.5	—	—
Normal	18.5–24.9	—	—
Overweight	25.0–29.9	Increased	High
Obesity, class			
I	30.0–34.9	High	Very high
II	35.0–39.9	Very high	Very high
III	≥40.0	Extremely high	Extremely high

Dashes (—) indicate that no additional risk at these levels of BMI was assigned. Increased waist circumference can also be a marker for increased risk even in individuals of normal weight.
[a]Disease risk for Type 2 diabetes, hypertension, and cardiovascular disease.
Modified from (31).

Compared to individuals classified as obese, the link between BMI in the overweight range (25.0–29.9 kg $\cdot$ m^{-2}) and higher mortality risk is less clear. However, a BMI of 25.0–29.9 kg $\cdot$ m^{-2} is convincingly linked to an increased risk for other health issues such as T2DM, dyslipidemia, hypertension, and certain cancers (69). A BMI of <18.5 kg $\cdot$ m^{-2} also increases mortality risk (32). Although it has been suggested that BMI can predict percent body fat (35), because of the large standard error ($\pm$5% fat), other methods of body composition assessment should be used to estimate percent body fat during a physical fitness assessment (30).

Circumferences

The measurement of regional body circumference can be important to quantify body fat distribution, especially of the waist and hip. The pattern of body fat distribution is recognized as an important indicator of health and prognosis (26,96). Android obesity that is characterized by more fat on the trunk (*i.e.*, abdominal fat) increases the risk of hypertension, Metsyn, T2DM, dyslipidemia, CVD, and premature death compared with individuals who demonstrate gynoid or gynecoid obesity (*i.e.*, fat distributed in the hip and thigh) (92). Moreover, individuals with increased visceral fat (*i.e.*, fat within and surrounding thoracic and abdominal cavities) confer a higher risk for development of the Metsyn compared to distribution of fat within the subcutaneous compartment (33). Because of this, circumference (or girth) measurements may be used to provide a general representation of body fat distribution and subsequent risk. Equations are also available for both sexes and a range of age groups to predict body fat percentage from circumference measurements (standard error of estimate [SEE] = 2.5%–4.0%) (113,114). A cloth tape measure with a spring-loaded handle (*e.g.*, Gulick tape measure) standardizes the tension of the tape on the skin and improves consistency of measurement. Duplicate measurements are recommended at each site and should be obtained in a rotational instead of a consecutive order (*i.e.*, take one measurement at all sites being assessed and then repeat the sequence). An average of the two measures is used provided they do not differ by more than 5 mm. *Box 4.1* contains a description of the common measurement sites.

The waist-to-hip ratio (WHR) is the circumference of the waist divided by the circumference of the hips (see *Box 4.1* for waist and buttocks/hips measures) and has traditionally been used as a simple method for assessing body fat distribution and identifying individuals with higher amounts of abdominal fat (30,92). Health risk increases as WHR increases, and the standards for risk vary with age and sex. For example, health risk is *very high* for young men when WHR is >0.95 and for young women when WHR is >0.86. For individuals aged 60–69 yr, the WHR cutoff values are >1.03 for men and >0.90 for women for the same high-risk classification as young adults (45).

The waist circumference alone may be used as an indicator of obesity-related health risk because abdominal obesity is the primary issue (19,26); waist circumference may be superior to BMI for this purpose (28,51). Specifically, although BMI and waist circumference are correlated, waist circumference is a better measure of visceral adiposity which can be varied within a given BMI (28). Because visceral

Box 4.1	**Standardized Description of Circumference Sites and Procedures**
Abdomen:	With the subject standing, a horizontal measure is taken at the height of the iliac crest, usually at the level of the umbilicus.
Arm:	With the subject standing and arms hanging freely at the sides with hands facing the thigh, a horizontal measure is taken midway between the acromion and olecranon processes.
Buttocks/Hips:	With the subject standing and feet together, a horizontal measure is taken at the maximal circumference of the buttocks. This measure is used for the hip measure in the waist-to-hip ratio.
Calf:	With the subject standing (feet apart ~20 cm), a horizontal measure is taken at the level of the maximum circumference between the knee and the ankle, perpendicular to the long axis.
Forearm:	With the subject standing, arms hanging downward but slightly away from the trunk and palms facing anteriorly, a measure is taken perpendicular to the long axis at the maximal circumference.
Hips/Thigh:	With the subject standing, legs slightly apart (~10 cm), a horizontal measure is taken at the maximal circumference of the hip/proximal thigh, just below the gluteal fold.
Mid-Thigh:	With the subject standing and one foot on a bench so the knee is flexed at 90 degrees, a measure is taken midway between the inguinal crease and the proximal border of the patella, perpendicular to the long axis.
Waist:	With the subject standing, arms at the sides, feet together, and abdomen relaxed, a horizontal measure is taken at the narrowest part of the torso (above the umbilicus and below the xiphoid process). The National Obesity Task Force (NOTF) suggests obtaining a horizontal measure directly above the iliac crest as a method to enhance standardization (31). Unfortunately, current formulas are not predicated on the NOTF suggested site.

Procedures

- All measurements should be made with a flexible yet inelastic tape measure.
- The tape should be placed on the skin surface without compressing the subcutaneous adipose tissue.
- If a Gulick-type spring-loaded tape measure is used, the handle should be extended to the same marking with each trial.
- Take duplicate measures at each site and retest if duplicate measurements are not within 5 mm.
- Rotate through measurement sites or allow time for skin to regain normal texture.

Modified from (16).

adiposity is a greater risk for obesity-related diseases, waist circumference or WHR can be an important measure for health risk assessments (28). The Expert Panel on the Identification, Evaluation, and Treatment of Overweight and Obesity in Adults provides a classification of disease risk based on both BMI and waist circumference as shown in *Table 4.1* (31). Previous research demonstrated that the waist circumference thresholds shown in *Table 4.1* effectively identify individuals at increased health risk across the different BMI categories (50). Furthermore, risk criteria for adults based on more specific waist circumferences have been developed (*Table 4.2*) (13). It is important to note that these risk criteria are based on data derived from Caucasian men and women and may be different for other racial/ethnic groups. For example, African American men and women may have different cutpoints for specific BMI and waist circumferences (17,57). The Pennington Center Longitudinal Study found that BMI, body adiposity index, waist-to-height ratio, and WHR all correlated with mortality in Caucasians but not in African Americans. However, the risk of mortality associated with waist circumference was almost identical between races (57). Furthermore, the optimal BMI and waist circumference thresholds to identify cardiometabolic health risk differs between Caucasian and African American women and men (56).

Several methods for waist circumference measurement involving different anatomical sites are available. Practitioners should be aware of which anatomical location the waist circumference is measured in order to be consistent with certain disease risk stratification. For example, *Table 4.2* is based on data where the waist circumference was taken at the level of the iliac crest (13,51), whereas the Pennington Longitudinal Studies take waist circumference at the midpoint between the inferior border of the ribcage and the superior aspect of the iliac crest (17,56,57). Evidence indicates that all currently available waist circumference measurement techniques are equally reliable and effective in identifying individuals at increased health risk (103,117).

Skinfold Measurements

Although BMI and circumferences are anthropometric measures that may be used to assess health risk, they are not true measures of body composition.

TABLE 4.2		
Risk Criteria for Waist Circumference in Adults		
	Waist Circumference cm (in)	
Risk Category	**Women**	**Men**
Very low	<70 cm (<27.5 in)	<80 cm (31.5 in)
Low	70–89 (27.5–35.0)	80–99 (31.5–39.0)
High	90–110 (35.5–43.0)	100–120 (39.5–47.0)
Very high	>110 (>43.5)	>120 (>47.0)

Reprinted with permission from (13).

The skinfold technique is a method that estimates body fat percentage by determining the thickness of several folds of skin across the body. Body fat percentage determined from skinfold thickness measurements correlates well ($r = .70–.90$) with hydrodensitometry (42). The principle behind the skinfold technique is that the amount of subcutaneous fat is proportional to the total amount of body fat. It is assumed that approximately one-third of the total fat is located subcutaneously (72), but there is considerable variation in intramuscular, intermuscular, and internal organ fat deposits among individuals (22,72). The exact proportion of subcutaneous to total fat also varies with sex, age, and race (72,101). Therefore, regression equations used to convert sum of skinfolds to body density and to convert body density to percent body fat should consider these variables for reducing prediction error. *Box 4.2* presents a standardized description of skinfold sites and procedures. Additional detail of skinfold technique is described elsewhere (38,42,45). Skinfold assessment of body composition is dependent on the expertise of the technician, so proper training (*i.e.*, knowledge of anatomical landmarks) and ample practice of the technique is necessary to obtain accurate measurements. The accuracy of predicting percent body fat from skinfolds is approximately $\pm 3.5\%$, assuming appropriate techniques and equations have been used (45).

Factors that may contribute to measurement error within skinfold assessment include poor anatomical landmark identification, poor measurement technique, an inexperienced evaluator, an extremely obese or extremely lean subject, and an improperly calibrated caliper (43,44). Various regression equations have been developed to predict body density or percent body fat from skinfold measurements. *Box 4.3* lists generalized equations that allow calculation of body density for a wide range of individuals (43,48). Other equations have been published that are sex, age, race, fat, and sport specific (45). A useful alternative to using skinfolds to predict body fat is to just track change in measurements at individual skinfold sites or use the sum of skinfolds.

Densitometry

The estimate of total body fat percentage can be derived from a measurement of whole-body density using the ratio of body mass to body volume. Densitometry has been used as a reference or criterion standard for assessing body composition for many years, although dual-energy X-ray absorptiometry (DEXA) and multicompartment modeling have recently gained popularity as a criterion measure. The limiting factor in the measurement of body density is the accuracy of the body volume measurement because the measurement of body mass (weight) is considered to be highly accurate. Body volume can be measured by hydrodensitometry (underwater) weighing or by plethysmography.

Hydrodensitometry (underwater) weighing is based on Archimedes principle that states when a body is immersed in water, it is buoyed by a counterforce equal to the weight of the water displaced. This loss of weight in water allows for calculation of body volume. Bone and muscle tissues are denser than water, whereas

Box 4.2	Standardized Description of Skinfold Sites and Procedures

Skinfold Site

Abdominal	Vertical fold; 2 cm to the right side of the umbilicus
Triceps	Vertical fold; on the posterior midline of the upper arm, halfway between the acromion and olecranon processes, with the arm held freely to the side of the body
Biceps	Vertical fold; on the anterior aspect of the arm over the belly of the biceps muscle, 1 cm above the level used to mark the triceps site
Chest/Pectoral	Diagonal fold; one-half the distance between the anterior axillary line and the nipple (men), or one-third of the distance between the anterior axillary line and the nipple (women)
Medial calf	Vertical fold; at the maximum circumference of the calf on the midline of its medial border
Midaxillary	Vertical fold; on the midaxillary line at the level of the xiphoid process of the sternum. An alternate method is a horizontal fold taken at the level of the xiphoid/sternal border on the midaxillary line.
Subscapular	Diagonal fold (45-degree angle); 1–2 cm below the inferior angle of the scapula
Suprailiac	Diagonal fold; in line with the natural angle of the iliac crest taken in the anterior axillary line immediately superior to the iliac crest
Thigh	Vertical fold; on the anterior midline of the thigh, midway between the proximal border of the patella and the inguinal crease (hip)

Procedures

- All measurements should be made on the right side of the body with the subject standing upright.
- Caliper should be placed directly on the skin surface, 1 cm away from the thumb and finger, perpendicular to the skinfold, and halfway between the crest and the base of the fold.
- Pinch should be maintained while reading the caliper.
- Wait 1–2 s before reading caliper.
- Take duplicate measures at each site and retest if duplicate measurements are not within 1–2 mm.
- Rotate through measurement sites or allow time for skin to regain normal texture and thickness.

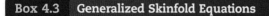

| Box 4.3 | Generalized Skinfold Equations |

MEN

■ **Seven-Site Formula** (chest, midaxillary, triceps, subscapular, abdomen, suprailiac, thigh)

Body density = $1.112 - 0.00043499$ (sum of seven skinfolds)
$+ 0.00000055$ (sum of seven skinfolds)^2
$- 0.00028826$ (age) *[SEE 0.008 or ~3.5% fat]*

■ **Three-Site Formula** (chest, abdomen, thigh)

Body density = $1.10938 - 0.0008267$ (sum of three skinfolds)
$+ 0.0000016$ (sum of three skinfolds)^2
$- 0.0002574$ (age) *[SEE 0.008 or ~3.4% fat]*

■ **Three-Site Formula** (chest, triceps, subscapular)

Body density = $1.1125025 - 0.0013125$ (sum of three skinfolds)
$+ 0.0000055$ (sum of three skinfolds)^2
$- 0.000244$ (age) *[SEE 0.008 or ~3.6% fat]*

WOMEN

■ **Seven-Site Formula** (chest, midaxillary, triceps, subscapular, abdomen, suprailiac, thigh)

Body density = $1.097 - 0.00046971$ (sum of seven skinfolds)
$+ 0.00000056$ (sum of seven skinfolds)^2
$- 0.00012828$ (age) *[SEE 0.008 or ~3.8% fat]*

■ **Three-Site Formula** (triceps, suprailiac, thigh)

Body density = $1.0994921 - 0.0009929$ (sum of three skinfolds)
$+ 0.0000023$ (sum of three skinfolds)^2
$- 0.0001329$ (age) *[SEE 0.009 or ~3.9% fat]*

■ **Three-Site Formula** (triceps, suprailiac, abdominal)

Body density = $1.089733 - 0.0009245$ (sum of three skinfolds)
$+ 0.0000025$ (sum of three skinfolds)^2
$- 0.0000979$ (age) *[SEE 0.009 or ~3.9% fat]*

SEE, standard error of estimate.
Adapted from (49,94).

fat tissue is less dense. Therefore, when two individuals have the same total body mass, the person with more fat-free mass (FFM) (*i.e.*, body mass − fat mass [FM]) weighs more in water and has a higher body density and lower percentage of body fat compared to the person with less FFM. Although hydrostatic weighing is a standard method for measuring body volume and, hence, body composition, it requires special equipment, the accurate measurement of residual volume, population-specific formulas, and significant cooperation by the subject (37). Body volume also can be measured by plethysmography (*i.e.*, air displacement in a closed chamber). Albeit expensive, this technology is well established and is thought to reduce the anxiety associated with submersion in water during hydrodensitometry in some individuals (27,37,71). For a more detailed explanation of these techniques, see (38,42,45).

Conversion of Body Density to Body Composition

Percent body fat can be estimated once body density has been determined. The most commonly used prediction equation to estimate percent body fat from body density was derived from the two-component model of body composition (108):

$$[(4.95 / Db) - 4.50] \times 100$$

The prediction of body fat from body density assumes the density of FM and FFM is consistent for the studied population. However, age, gender, race, and certain disease states may affect the density of FFM, with much of this variance related to the bone mineral density component of FFM. Because of this variance, population-specific, two-component model conversion formulas are also available for specific age, gender, ethnicity, training status, and disease condition (*Table 4.3*). Because of the significant effect of these factors on the validity of the conversion of body density to body fat, exercise professionals are encouraged to select the most specific formula possible for their clients (44).

Other Techniques

Additional body composition assessment techniques include DEXA and total body electrical conductivity (TOBEC), but these techniques have limited applicability in routine health/fitness testing because of cost and the need for highly trained personnel (42). Rather, bioelectrical impedance analysis (BIA) is occasionally used as an assessment technique in routine health/fitness testing. Generally, the accuracy of BIA is similar to skinfolds, as long as stringent protocol adherence (*e.g.*, assurance of normal hydration status) is followed, and the equations programmed into the analyzer are valid for the populations being tested (25,41). It should be noted, however, that the accuracy of the BIA method in individuals who are obese may be limited secondary to differences in body water distribution compared to those who are in the normal weight range (30).

Body Composition Norms

There are no universally accepted norms for body composition; however, *Tables 4.4* and *4.5*, which were developed using skinfold measurements, provide percentile values for percent body fat in men and women, respectively. A consensus opinion for an exact percent body fat value associated with optimal health risk has yet to be defined; however, a range of 10%–22% and 20%–32% for men and women, respectively, has long been viewed as satisfactory for health (71). More recent data support this range, although age and race, in addition to sex, impact what may be construed as a healthy percent body fat (35,58).

TABLE 4.3

Population-Specific Formulas for Conversion of Body Density to Percent Body Fat

	Population	Age	Gender	%BF[a]	FFBd[b] (g · cm^{-3})
ETHNICITY	African American	9–17	Women	(5.24 / Db) − 4.82	1.088
		19–45	Men	(4.86 / Db) − 4.39	1.106
		24–79	Women	(4.85 / Db) − 4.39	1.106
	American Indian	18–62	Men	(4.97 / Db) − 4.52	1.099
		18–60	Women	(4.81 / Db) − 4.34	1.108
	Asian Japanese Native	18–48	Men	(4.97 / Db) − 4.52	1.099
			Women	(4.76 / Db) − 4.28	1.111
		61–78	Men	(4.87 / Db) − 4.41	1.105
			Women	(4.95 / Db) − 4.50	1.100
	Singaporean (Chinese, Indian, Malay)		Men	(4.94 / Db) − 4.48	1.102
			Women	(4.84 / Db) − 4.37	1.107
	Caucasian	8–12	Men	(5.27 / Db) − 4.85	1.086
			Women	(5.27 / Db) − 4.85	1.086
		13–17	Men	(5.12 / Db) − 4.69	1.092
			Women	(5.19 / Db) − 4.76	1.090
		18–59	Men	(4.95 / Db) − 4.50	1.100
			Women	(4.96 / Db) − 4.51	1.101
		60–90	Men	(4.97 / Db) − 4.52	1.099
			Women	(5.02 / Db) − 4.57	1.098
	Hispanic		Men	NA	NA
		20–40	Women	(4.87 / Db) − 4.41	1.105
ATHLETES	Resistance trained	24 ± 4	Men	(5.21 / Db) − 4.78	1.089
		35 ± 6	Women	(4.97 / Db) − 4.52	1.099
	Endurance trained	21 ± 2	Men	(5.03 / Db) − 4.59	1.097
		21 ± 4	Women	(4.95 / Db) − 4.50	1.100
	All sports	18–22	Men	(5.12 / Db) − 4.68	1.093
		18–22	Women	(4.97 / Db) − 4.52	1.099
CLINICAL POPULATIONS[c]	Anorexia nervosa	15–44	Women	(4.96 / Db) − 4.51	1.101
	Cirrhosis				
	Childs A			(5.33 / Db) − 4.91	1.084
	Childs B			(5.48 / Db) − 5.08	1.078
	Childs C			(5.69 / Db) − 5.32	1.070
	Obesity	17–62	Women	(4.95 / Db) − 4.50	1.100
	Spinal cord injury (paraplegic/quadriplegic)	18–73	Men	(4.67 / Db) − 4.18	1.116
		18–73	Women	(4.70 / Db) − 4.22	1.114

[a]Multiply by 100 for percentage of body fat.

[b]FFBd, fat-free body density based on average values reported in selected research articles.

[c]There are insufficient multicomponent model data to estimate the average FFBd of the following clinical populations: coronary artery disease, heart/lung transplants, chronic obstructive pulmonary disease, cystic fibrosis, diabetes mellitus, thyroid disease, HIV/AIDS, cancer, kidney failure (dialysis), multiple sclerosis, and muscular dystrophy.

%BF, percentage of body fat; Db, body density; NA, no data available for this population subgroup.

Adapted with permission from (45).

			TABLE 4.4			

TABLE 4.4

Fitness Categories for Body Composition (% Body Fat) for Men by Age

%		20–29	30–39	40–49	50–59	60–69	70–79
		Age (year)					
99	Very lean[a]	4.2	7.3	9.5	11.0	11.9	13.6
95		6.4	10.3	12.9	14.8	16.2	15.5
90		7.9	12.4	15.0	17.0	18.1	17.5
85	Excellent	9.1	13.7	16.4	18.3	19.2	19.0
80		10.5	14.9	17.5	19.4	20.2	20.1
75		11.5	15.9	18.5	20.2	21.0	21.0
70	Good	12.6	16.8	19.3	21.0	21.7	21.6
65		13.8	17.7	20.1	21.7	22.4	22.3
60		14.8	18.4	20.8	22.3	23.0	22.9
55		15.8	19.2	21.4	23.0	23.6	23.7
50	Fair	16.6	20.0	22.1	23.6	24.2	24.1
45		17.5	20.7	22.8	24.2	24.9	24.7
40		18.6	21.6	23.5	24.9	25.6	25.3
35		19.7	22.4	24.2	25.6	26.4	25.8
30	Poor	20.7	23.2	24.9	26.3	27.0	26.5
25		22.0	24.1	25.7	27.1	27.9	27.1
20		23.3	25.1	26.6	28.1	28.8	28.4
15		24.9	26.4	27.8	29.2	29.8	29.4
10	Very poor	26.6	27.8	29.2	30.6	31.2	30.7
5		29.2	30.2	31.3	32.7	33.3	32.9
1		33.4	34.4	35.2	36.4	36.8	37.2
n =		1,844	10,099	15,073	9,255	2,851	522

Total *n* = 39,644.

[a]Very lean, no less than 3% body fat is recommended for men.

Adapted with permission from *Physical Fitness Assessments and Norms for Adults and Law Enforcement.* The Cooper Institute, Dallas, Texas. 2009. For more information: www.cooperinstitute.org

CARDIORESPIRATORY FITNESS

CRF is related to the ability to perform large muscle, dynamic, moderate-to-vigorous intensity exercise for prolonged periods of time. Performance of exercise at this level of physical exertion depends on the integrated physiologic and functional state of the respiratory, cardiovascular, and musculoskeletal systems. CRF is considered a health-related component of physical fitness because (a) low levels of CRF have been associated with a markedly increased risk of premature

TABLE 4.5

Fitness Categories for Body Composition (% Body Fat) for Women by Age

%		20–29	30–39	40–49	50–59	60–69	70–79
				Age (year)			
99	Very lean[a]	11.4	11.2	12.1	13.9	13.9	11.7
95		14.0	13.9	15.2	16.9	17.7	16.4
90	Excellent	15.1	15.5	16.8	19.1	20.2	18.3
85		16.1	16.5	18.3	20.8	22.0	21.2
80		16.8	17.5	19.5	22.3	23.3	22.5
75		17.6	18.3	20.6	23.6	24.6	23.7
70	Good	18.4	19.2	21.7	24.8	25.7	24.8
65		19.0	20.1	22.7	25.8	26.7	25.7
60		19.8	21.0	23.7	26.7	27.5	26.6
55		20.6	22.0	24.6	27.6	28.3	27.6
50	Fair	21.5	22.8	25.5	28.4	29.2	28.2
45		22.2	23.7	26.4	29.3	30.1	28.9
40		23.4	24.8	27.5	30.1	30.8	30.5
35		24.2	25.8	28.4	30.8	31.5	31.0
30	Poor	25.5	26.9	29.5	31.8	32.6	31.9
25		26.7	28.1	30.7	32.9	33.3	32.9
20		28.2	29.6	31.9	33.9	34.4	34.0
15		30.5	31.5	33.4	35.0	35.6	35.3
10	Very poor	33.5	33.6	35.1	36.1	36.6	36.4
5		36.6	36.2	37.1	37.6	38.2	38.1
1		38.6	39.0	39.1	39.8	40.3	40.2
n =		1,250	4,130	5,902	4,118	1,450	295

Total *n* = 17,145.

[a]Very lean, no less than 10%–13% body fat is recommended for women.

Adapted with permission from *Physical Fitness Assessments and Norms for Adults and Law Enforcement.* The Cooper Institute, Dallas, Texas. 2009. For more information: www.cooperinstitute.org

death from all causes and specifically from CVD; (b) increases in CRF are associated with a reduction in death from all causes; and (c) high levels of CRF are associated with higher levels of habitual PA, which in turn are associated with many health benefits (9,10,64,105,116). As such, the assessment of CRF is an important part of any primary or secondary prevention and rehabilitative programs, and the knowledge and skills to complete the assessment and interpret the subsequent results are an important responsibility of the exercise professional.

The Concept of Maximal Oxygen Uptake

Maximal volume of oxygen consumed per unit time ($\dot{V}O_{2max}$) is accepted as the criterion measure of CRF. This variable is typically expressed clinically in relative ($mL \cdot kg^{-1} \cdot min^{-1}$) as opposed to absolute ($mL \cdot min^{-1}$) terms, allowing for meaningful comparisons between/among individuals with differing body weight. $\dot{V}O_{2max}$ is the product of the maximal cardiac output ($\dot{Q}$; L blood $\cdot min^{-1}$) and arterial-venous oxygen difference ($mL\ O_2 \cdot L\ blood^{-1}$). Significant variation in $\dot{V}O_{2max}$ across populations and fitness levels results primarily from differences in $\dot{Q}$; therefore, $\dot{V}O_{2max}$ is closely related to the functional capacity of the heart. The designation of $\dot{V}O_{2max}$ implies an individual's true physiologic limit has been reached, and a plateau in $\dot{V}O_2$ may be observed between the final two work rates of a progressive exercise test. This plateau is not consistently observed during maximal exercise testing and rarely observed in individuals with CVD or pulmonary disease. Peak $\dot{V}O_2$ ($\dot{V}O_{2peak}$) is used when leveling off of $\dot{V}O_2$ does not occur, or maximum performance appears limited by local muscular factors rather than central circulatory dynamics (75). $\dot{V}O_{2peak}$ is commonly used to describe CRF in these and other populations with chronic diseases and health conditions (3).

Open circuit spirometry is used to measure $\dot{V}O_{2max}$ during a graded incremental or ramp exercise test to exhaustion, also called *indirect calorimetry*. In this procedure, the subject breathes through a low-resistance valve with his or her nose occluded (or through a nonlatex mask) while pulmonary ventilation and expired fractions of oxygen (O_2) and carbon dioxide (CO_2) are measured. In addition, the use of open circuit spirometry during maximal exercise testing may allow for the accurate assessment of an anaerobic/ventilatory threshold and direct measurement of $\dot{V}O_{2max}/\dot{V}O_{2peak}$. Many automated systems are currently available that provide ease of use and downloadable data of test results that save time and effort; however, system calibration is essential to obtain accurate results (82). The mode selected (*i.e.*, leg ergometer vs. treadmill) for the exercise test can impact the result (see *Chapter 5*). Administration of the test and interpretation of results should be reserved for trained professional personnel with a thorough understanding of exercise science. Because of costs associated with the equipment, space, and personnel needed to carry out these tests, direct measurement of $\dot{V}O_{2max}$ may not always be possible.

When direct measurement of $\dot{V}O_{2max}$ is not feasible, a variety of maximal and submaximal exercise tests can be used to estimate $\dot{V}O_{2max}$. These tests have been validated by examining (a) the correlation between directly measured $\dot{V}O_{2max}$ and the $\dot{V}O_{2max}$ estimated from physiologic responses to submaximal exercise (*e.g.*, HR at a specified power output) or (b) the correlation between directly measured $\dot{V}O_{2max}$ and field test performance (*e.g.*, time to run 1 or 1.5 mi [1.6 or 2.4 km]) or time to volitional fatigue using a standard graded exercise test protocol. It should be noted that there is the potential for a significant underestimation or overestimation of $\dot{V}O_{2max}$ by these types of indirect measurement techniques. Overestimation is more likely to occur when (a) the exercise protocol (see *Chapter 5*) chosen for testing is too aggressive for a given individual (*i.e.*, Bruce treadmill protocol in patients with CHF) or (b) when treadmill testing is employed and the individual heavily relies on handrail support (3). Every effort should be taken to choose the appropriate exercise protocol given an individual's characteristics and handrail use should be minimized during testing on a treadmill (82).

Maximal versus Submaximal Exercise Testing

The decision to use a maximal or submaximal exercise test depends largely on the reasons for the test, risk level of the client, and availability of appropriate equipment (see *Chapter 5*). Maximal tests require participants to exercise to the point of volitional fatigue, which may be inappropriate for some individuals and may require the need for emergency equipment (see *Appendix B*).

Exercise professionals often rely on submaximal exercise tests to assess CRF because maximal exercise testing is not always feasible in the health/fitness setting. The basic aim of submaximal exercise testing is to determine the HR response to one or more submaximal work rates and use the results to predict $\dot{V}O_{2max}$. Although the primary purpose of the test has traditionally been to predict $\dot{V}O_{2max}$ from the HR workload relationship, it is important to obtain additional indices of the client's response to exercise. The exercise professional should use the various submaximal measures of HR, BP, workload, rating of perceived exertion (RPE), and other subjective indices as valuable information regarding one's functional response to exercise. This information can be used to evaluate submaximal exercise responses over time in a controlled environment and make modifications the Ex R_x.

The most accurate estimate of $\dot{V}O_{2max}$ is achieved from the HR response to submaximal exercise tests if all of the following assumptions are achieved (38,44):

- A steady state HR is obtained for each exercise work rate.
- A linear relationship exists between HR and work rate.
- The difference between actual and predicted maximal HR is minimal.
- Mechanical efficiency (*i.e.*, $\dot{V}O_2$ at a given work rate) is the same for everyone.
- The subject is not on any medications that may alter the HR response to exercise (see *Appendix A*).
- The subject is not using high quantities of caffeine, ill, or in a high-temperature environment, all of which may alter the HR response.

Cardiorespiratory Test Sequence and Measures

After the initial screening process, selected baseline measurements should be obtained prior to the start of the exercise test. A minimum of HR, BP, and RPE should be measured during exercise tests. HR can be determined using the palpation or auscultation technique described earlier in this chapter. HR telemetry monitors with chest electrodes or radio telemetry have proven to be accurate and reliable, provided there is no outside electrical interference (67). When using palpation or auscultation during an exercise test, it is common to use 10-s or 15-s time intervals to measure HR once steady state is reached. Most protocols that use postexercise HR to assess CRF also use shorter time intervals due to the rapid and immediate decline in HR following the cessation of exercise.

BP should be measured at heart level with the subject's arm relaxed and not grasping a handrail (treadmill) or handlebar (cycle ergometer). Systolic (SBP) and diastolic (DBP) BP measurements can be used as indicators for stopping an exercise test (*Box 4.4*). To obtain accurate BP measures during exercise, follow the guidelines in *Chapter 3* (see *Box 3.5*) for resting BP; however, BP should be obtained in the exercise position. Several devices have been developed to automate BP measurements during exercise and demonstrate reasonable accuracy (82). These devices also typically allow for auditory confirmation of the automated BP measurement, which may improve confidence in the value obtained. If an automated BP system is used during exercise testing, calibration checks with manual BP measurements must be routinely performed to confirm accuracy of the automated readings (82).

RPE can be a valuable indicator for monitoring an individual's exercise tolerance. Although RPEs correlate with exercise HRs and work rates, large interindividual variability in RPE with healthy individuals as well as patient populations mandates caution in the universal application of RPE scales (118). The RPE scale was developed to allow the exerciser to subjectively rate his or her physical strain during exercise (12). Ratings can be influenced by psychological factors, mood states, environmental conditions (11), exercise modes, age (100), and thirst (98). Exercise professionals should therefore be careful to control as many variables as possible and refrain from comparing RPE responses across modalities and clients. Currently, two RPE scales are widely used: (a) the original Borg or category scale, which rates exercise intensity from 6 to 20 (*Table 4.6*), and (b) the category-ratio scale of 0–10 (see *Figure 5.2*). Both RPE scales are appropriate subjective tools (11).

TABLE **4.6**	
The Borg Rating of Perceived Exertion Scale	
6	No exertion at all
7	Extremely light
8	
9	Very light
10	
11	Light
12	
13	Somewhat hard
14	
15	Hard (heavy)
16	
17	Very hard
18	
19	Extremely hard
20	Maximal exertion

From (11). © Gunnar Borg. Reproduced with permission. The scale with correct instructions can be obtained from Borg Perception, Radisvagen 124, 16573 Hasselby, Sweden. See also the home page: http://www.borgperception.se/index.html.

During exercise testing, the RPE can be used as an indication of impending fatigue. Most apparently healthy subjects reach their subjective limit of fatigue at an RPE of 18–19 (very, very hard) on the category Borg scale, or 9–10 (very, very strong) on the category-ratio scale; therefore, RPE can be used to monitor progress toward maximal exertion during exercise testing (11).

Test Termination Criteria

Graded exercise testing (GXT), whether maximal or submaximal, is a safe procedure when subject prescreening and testing guidelines are adhered to and when administered by trained exercise professionals. Occasionally, for safety reasons, the test may have to be terminated prior to the subject reaching a measured or estimated $\dot{V}O_{2max}$, volitional fatigue, or a predetermined endpoint (*i.e.*, 50%–70% heart rate reserve [HRR] or 70%–85% age-predicted HR_{max}). Because of the individual variation in HR_{max}, the upper limit of 85% of an estimated HR_{max} may result in a maximal effort for some individuals and submaximal effort in others. General indications for stopping an exercise test are outlined in *Box 4.4*.

Modes of Testing

Commonly used modes for exercise testing include treadmills, cycle ergometers, steps, and field tests. The mode of exercise testing used is dependent on the setting, equipment available, and training of personnel. There are advantages and disadvantages of each exercise testing mode:

- *Field tests* consist of walking or running for a predetermined time or distance (*i.e.*, 1.5-mi [2.4 km] walk/run test; 1-mi and 6-min walk test). The advantages of

---

Box 4.4	General Indications for Stopping an Exercise Test[a]

- Onset of angina or angina-like symptoms
- Drop in SBP of ≥10 mm Hg with an increase in work rate or if SBP decreases below the value obtained in the same position prior to testing
- Excessive rise in BP: systolic pressure >250 mm Hg and/or diastolic pressure >115 mm Hg
- Shortness of breath, wheezing, leg cramps, or claudication
- Signs of poor perfusion: light-headedness, confusion, ataxia, pallor, cyanosis, nausea, or cold and clammy skin
- Failure of HR to increase with increased exercise intensity
- Noticeable change in heart rhythm by palpation or auscultation
- Subject requests to stop
- Physical or verbal manifestations of severe fatigue
- Failure of the testing equipment

[a]Assumes that testing is nondiagnostic and is being performed without electrocardiogram monitoring. For clinical testing, *Box 5.4* provides more definitive and specific termination criteria. BP, blood pressure; HR, heart rate; SBP, systolic blood pressure.

field tests are they are easy to administer to large numbers of individuals at one time, and little equipment (*e.g.*, a stopwatch) is needed. The disadvantages are some tests can be near-maximal or maximal for some individuals, particularly in individuals with low aerobic fitness, and potentially be unmonitored for test termination criteria (*Box 4.4*) or BP and HR responses. Therefore, these tests may be inappropriate for sedentary individuals or individuals at increased risk for cardiovascular and/or musculoskeletal complications. An individual's level of motivation and pacing ability also can have a profound impact on test results.

- *Motor-driven treadmills* can be used for submaximal and maximal testing and are often employed for diagnostic testing in the United States. They provide a familiar form of exercise to many and, if the correct protocol is chosen (*i.e.*, aggressive vs. conservative adjustments in workload), can accommodate the least physically fit to the fittest individuals across the continuum of walking to running speeds. Nevertheless, a practice session might be necessary in some cases to permit habituation and reduce anxiety. On the other hand, treadmills usually are expensive, not easily transportable, and potentially make some measurements (*e.g.*, BP, electrocardiogram [ECG]) more difficult, particularly while an individual is running. Treadmills must be calibrated periodically to ensure the accuracy of the test when $\dot{V}O_2$ is not directly measured (82). In addition, holding on to the support rail(s) should be discouraged to ensure accuracy of metabolic work output, particularly when $\dot{V}O_2$ is estimated as opposed to directly measured. Extensive handrail use often leads to significant overestimation of $\dot{V}O_2$.

- *Mechanically braked cycle ergometers* are also a viable test modality for submaximal and maximal testing and are frequently used for diagnostic testing, particularly in European laboratories (82). Advantages of this exercise mode include lower equipment expense, transportability, and greater ease in obtaining BP and ECG (if appropriate) measurements. Cycle ergometers also provide a non–weight-bearing test modality in which work rates are easily adjusted in small increments. The main disadvantage is cycling may be a less familiar mode of exercise to some individuals, often resulting in limiting localized muscle fatigue and an underestimation of $\dot{V}O_{2max}$. The cycle ergometer must be calibrated, and the subject must maintain the proper pedal rate because most tests require HR to be measured at specific work rates (82). Electronic cycle ergometers can deliver the same work rate across a range of pedal rates (*i.e.*, revolutions per minute, rpm), but calibration might require special equipment not available in some laboratories. If a cycle ergometer cannot be calibrated for any reason or if it does not provide a reasonable estimate of workload, it should not be used for fitness testing to predict CRF.

- *Step testing* is an inexpensive modality for predicting CRF by measuring the HR response to stepping at a fixed rate and/or a fixed step height or by measuring postexercise recovery HR. Step tests require little or no equipment, steps are easily transportable, stepping skill requires little practice, the test usually is of short duration, and stepping is advantageous for mass testing (110). Postexercise (recovery) HR decreases with improved CRF, and test results are easy to explain to participants (53). Special precautions may be needed for those who have balance problems or are extremely deconditioned. Some single-stage step tests require an energy cost of 7–9 metabolic equivalents (METs), which may exceed the maximal capacity of some participants (4). Therefore, the protocol chosen must be appropriate for the physical fitness level of the client. In addition, inadequate compliance to the step cadence and excessive fatigue in the lead limb may diminish the value of a step test. Most tests do not monitor HR and BP while stepping because of the difficulty of these measures during the test.

Field Tests

Two of the most widely used run/walk tests (subjects may run, walk, or use a combination of both to complete the test) for assessing CRF are the 1.5-mi (2.4 km) test for time and the Cooper 12-min test. The objective of the Cooper 12-min test is to cover the greatest distance in the allotted time period and for the 1.5-mi (2.4 km) test to cover the distance in the shortest period of time. $\dot{V}O_{2max}$ can be estimated from using the following equations:

1.5-mi run/walk test

$$\dot{V}O_{2max} \, (\text{mL} \cdot \text{kg}^{-1} \cdot \text{min}^{-1}) = 3.5 + 483 \, / \, 1.5 \text{ mi time (min)}$$

12-min walk/run test

$$\dot{V}O_{2max} \, (\text{mL} \cdot \text{kg}^{-1} \cdot \text{min}^{-1}) = (\text{distance in meters} - 504.9) \, / \, 44.73$$

The Rockport One-Mile Fitness Walking Test is another well-recognized field test for estimating CRF. In this test, an individual walks 1 mi (1.6 km) as fast as possible, preferably on a track or a level surface, and HR is obtained in the final minute. An alternative is to measure a 10-s HR immediately on completion of the 1-mi (1.6 km) walk, but this may overestimate the $\dot{V}O_{2max}$ compared to when HR is measured during the walk. $\dot{V}O_{2max}$ is estimated using the following regression equation (61):

$$\dot{V}O_{2max} \, (\text{mL} \cdot \text{kg}^{-1} \cdot \text{min}^{-1}) = 132.853 - (0.1692 \times \text{body mass in kg}) - (0.3877 \times \text{age in years}) + (6.315 \times \text{gender}) - (3.2649 \times \text{time in minutes}) - (0.1565 \times \text{HR})$$

$$(\text{SEE} = 5.0 \text{ mL} \cdot \text{kg}^{-1} \cdot \text{min}^{-1}; \text{gender} = 0 \text{ for female, 1 for male})$$

In addition to independently predicting morbidity and mortality (20,104), the 6-min walk test has been used to evaluate CRF in populations considered to have reduced CRF such as older adults and some clinical patient populations (*e.g.*, individuals with CHF or pulmonary disease). The American Thoracic Society has published guidelines on 6-min walk test procedures and interpretation (6). Even though the test is considered submaximal, it may result in near-maximal performance for those with low physical fitness levels or disease (52). Clients and patients completing less than 300 m (~984 ft) during the 6-min walk demonstrate a poorer short-term survival compared to those surpassing this threshold (14). Several multivariate equations are available to predict $\dot{V}O_{2 \, peak}$ from the 6-min walk; however, the following equation requires minimal clinical information (14):

$$\dot{V}O_{2peak} = \dot{V}O_2 \, \text{mL} \cdot \text{kg}^{-1} \cdot \text{min}^{-1} = (0.02 \times \text{distance [m]}) - (0.191 \times \text{age [yr]}) - (0.07 \times \text{weight [kg]}) + (0.09 \times \text{height [cm]}) + (0.26 \times \text{RPP [} \times 10^{-3}]) + 2.45$$

where m = distance in meters; yr = year; kg = kilogram; cm = centimeter; RPP = rate-pressure product (HR × SBP in mm Hg); SEE = 2.68 mL · kg^{-1} · min^{-1}

Submaximal Exercise Tests

Single-stage and multistage submaximal exercise tests are available to estimate $\dot{V}O_{2max}$ from simple HR measurements. Accurate measurement of HR is critical for valid testing. Although HR obtained by palpation is commonly used, the accuracy of this method depends on the experience and technique of the evaluator. It is recommended that an ECG, validated HR monitor, or a stethoscope be used to determine HR. The submaximal HR response is easily altered by a number of environmental (*e.g.*, heat, humidity; see *Chapter 8*), dietary (*e.g.*, caffeine, time since last meal), and behavioral (*e.g.*, anxiety, smoking, previous PA) factors. These variables must be controlled to have a valid estimate that can be used as a reference point in an individual's fitness program. In addition, the test mode (*e.g.*, cycle, treadmill, step) should be consistent with the primary exercise modality used by the participant to address specificity of training issues. Standardized procedures for submaximal testing are presented in *Box 4.5*. See *Chapter 5* for a list of incremental treadmill protocols that may be used to assess submaximal exercise responses.

Cycle Ergometer Tests

The Astrand-Ryhming cycle ergometer test is a single-stage test lasting 6 min (5). The pedal rate is set at 50 rpm. The goal is to obtain HR values between 125 and 170 beats · min^{-1}, with HR measured during the fifth and sixth minute of work. The average of the two HRs is then used to estimate $\dot{V}O_{2max}$ from a nomogram (*Figure 4.1*). The suggested work rate is based on sex and an individual's fitness status as follows:

men, unconditioned: 300 or 600 kg · m · min^{-1} (50 or 100 W)
men, conditioned: 600 or 900 kg · m · min^{-1} (100 or 150 W)
women, unconditioned: 300 or 450 kg · m · min^{-1} (50 or 75 W)
women, conditioned: 450 or 600 kg · m · min^{-1} (75 or 100 W)

Since HR$_{max}$ decreases with age, the value from the nomogram must be adjusted for age by multiplying the $\dot{V}O_{2max}$ value by the following correction factors (4):

AGE	CORRECTION FACTOR
15	1.10
25	1.00
35	0.87
40	0.83
45	0.78
50	0.75
55	0.71
60	0.68
65	0.65

| Box 4.5 | General Procedures for Submaximal Testing of Cardiorespiratory Fitness |

1. Obtain resting HR and BP immediately prior to exercise in the exercise posture.
2. The client should be familiarized with the ergometer or treadmill. If using a cycle ergometer, properly position the client on the ergometer (*i.e.*, upright posture, ~25-degree bend in the knee at maximal leg extension, and hands in proper position on handlebars) (89,90).
3. The exercise test should begin with a 2–3 min warm-up to acquaint the client with the cycle ergometer or treadmill and prepare him or her for the exercise intensity in the first stage of the test.
4. A specific protocol should consist of 2- or 3-min stages with appropriate increments in work rate.
5. HR should be monitored at least two times during each stage, near the end of the second and third minutes of each stage. If HR is >110 beats $\cdot$ min^{-1}, steady state HR (*i.e.*, two HRs within 5 beats $\cdot$ min^{-1}) should be reached before the workload is increased.
6. BP should be monitored in the last minute of each stage and repeated (verified) in the event of a hypotensive or hypertensive response.
7. RPE (using either the Borg category or category-ratio scale [see *Table 4.6* and *Figure 5.2*]) and additional rating scales should be monitored near the end of the last minute of each stage.
8. Client's appearance and symptoms should be monitored and recorded regularly.
9. The test should be terminated when the subject reaches 70% heart rate reserve (85% of age-predicted HR$_{max}$), fails to conform to the exercise test protocol, experiences adverse signs or symptoms, requests to stop, or experiences an emergency situation.
10. An appropriate cool-down/recovery period should be initiated consisting of either
    a. Continued exercise at a work rate equivalent to that of the first stage of the exercise test protocol or lower or
    b. A passive cool-down if the subject experiences signs of discomfort or an emergency situation occurs
11. All physiologic observations (*e.g.*, HR, BP, signs, and symptoms) should be continued for at least 5 min of recovery unless abnormal responses occur, which would warrant a longer posttest surveillance period. Continue low-level exercise until HR and BP stabilize but not necessarily until they reach preexercise levels.

BP, blood pressure; HR, heart rate; HR$_{max}$, maximal heart rate; RPE, rating of perceived exertion.

In contrast to the Astrand-Ryhming cycle ergometer single-stage test, Maritz et al. (73) devised a test where HR was measured at a series of submaximal work rates and extrapolated the HR response to the subject's age-predicted HR$_{max}$. This multistage method is a well-known assessment technique to estimate $\dot{V}O_{2max}$. The HR measured during the last minute of two steady state stages is plotted against work rate. The line generated from the plotted points is then extrapolated to the age-predicted HR$_{max}$,

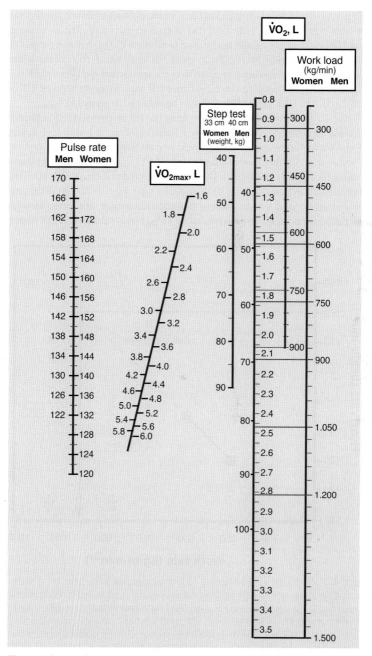

Figure 4.1 Modified Astrand-Ryhming nomogram. Used with permission from (5).

and a perpendicular line is dropped to the x-axis to estimate the work rate that would have been achieved if the individual had worked to maximum. HR measurements below 110 beats · min^{-1} should not be used to estimate $\dot{V}O_{2max}$ because there is more day-to-day and individual variability at lower HR levels which reduces the accuracy of prediction, and submaximal exercise tests are terminated if a client reaches 70% HRR (85% HR$_{max}$). Therefore, two consecutive HR measurements between 110 beats · min^{-1} and 70% HRR (85% HR$_{max}$) should be obtained to predict $\dot{V}O_{2max}$.

Figure 4.2 presents an example of graphing the HR response to two submaximal workloads to estimate $\dot{V}O_{2max}$. The two lines noted as ±1 standard deviation (SD) show what the estimated $\dot{V}O_{2max}$ would be if the subject's true HR$_{max}$ were 168 or 192 beats · min^{-1}, rather than 180 beats · min^{-1}. $\dot{V}O_{2max}$ is estimated from the work rate using the formula in *Table 6.3*. This equation is valid to estimate $\dot{V}O_2$ at submaximal steady state workloads (from 300 to 1,200 kg · m · min^{-1}) (50–200 W); therefore, caution must be used if extrapolating to workloads outside this range. However a larger part of the error involved in estimating $\dot{V}O_{2max}$ from submaximal HR responses

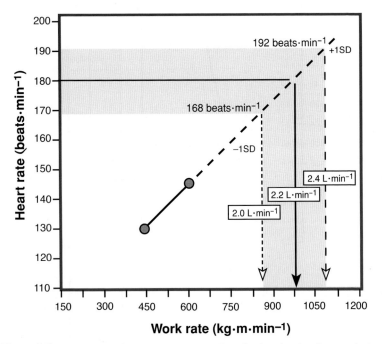

Figure 4.2 Heart rate (HR) responses to two submaximal work rates for a sedentary woman 40 yr of age weighing 64 kg. Maximal work load was estimated by extrapolating the HR response to the age-predicted HR$_{max}$ of 180 beats · min^{-1} (based on 220 − age). The work rate that would have been achieved at that HR was determined by dropping a line from that HR value to the x-axis. The other two lines estimate what the maximal work load would have been if the subject's true HR$_{max}$ was ±1 SD from the 180 beats · min^{-1} value. $\dot{V}O_{2max}$ estimated using the formula in *Chapter 6* and expressed in L · min^{-1} was 2.2 L · min^{-1}.

occurs as the result of estimating HR_{max} (see *Table 6.2*) (112). Accurate submaximal HR recording is also critical, as extrapolation magnifies even the smallest of errors. In addition, errors can be attributed to inaccurate pedaling cadence (workload), imprecise achievement of steady state HR, and the extrapolation of work rate to oxygen consumption at maximal intensities. Finally, the test administrator should recognize the error associated with age-predicted HR_{max} (see *Table 6.2*) and should monitor the subject throughout the test to ensure the test remains submaximal.

The modified YMCA protocol is a good example of a multistage submaximal cycle ergometer test that uses two to four 3-min stages of continuous exercise with a constant pedal rate of 50 rpm (38,88). Stage 1 requires participants to pedal against 0.5 kg of resistance (25 W; 150 kgm $\cdot$ min^{-1}). The workload for stage 2 is based on the steady state HR measured during the last minute of the initial stage:

- HR <80 bpm — change the resistance to 2.5 kg (125 W; 750 kgm $\cdot$ min^{-1})
- HR 80−89 bpm — change the resistance to 2.0 kg (100 W; 600 kgm $\cdot$ min^{-1})
- HR 90−100 bpm — change the resistance to 1.5 kg (75 W; 450 kgm $\cdot$ min^{-1})
- HR >100 bpm — change the resistance to 1.0 kg (50 W; 300 kgm $\cdot$ min^{-1})

Use stages 3 and 4 as needed to elicit two consecutive steady state HRs between 110 bpm and 70% HRR (85% HR_{max}). For stages 3 and 4, the resistance used in stage 2 is increased by 0.5 kg (25 W; 150 kgm $\cdot$ min^{-1}) per stage. Normative tables for the YMCA protocol are published elsewhere (120).

Treadmill Tests

The primary exercise modality for submaximal exercise testing traditionally has been the cycle ergometer, although treadmills are used in many settings. The same submaximal definition (70% HRR or 85% of age-predicted HR_{max}) is used, and the stages of the test should be 3 min or longer to ensure a steady state HR response at each stage. The HR values are extrapolated to age-predicted HR_{max}, and $\dot{V}O_{2max}$ is estimated using the formula in *Table 6.3* from the highest speed and/or grade that would have been achieved if the individual had worked to maximum. Most common treadmill protocols presented in *Figure 5.1* can be used, but the duration of each stage should be at least 3 min.

Step Tests

Step tests are also used to estimate $\dot{V}O_{2max}$. Astrand and Ryhming (5) used a single-step height of 33 cm (13 in) for women and 40 cm (15.7 in) for men at a rate of 22.5 steps $\cdot$ min^{-1} (when counting just the leading leg) for 5 min. These tests require $\dot{V}O_2$ of about 25.8 and 29.5 mL $\cdot$ kg^{-1} $\cdot$ min^{-1}, respectively. Because of this, step tests are not a good choice of modality for less fit or diseased clients. HR is measured in the last minute as described for the Astrand-Rhyming cycle ergometer test, and $\dot{V}O_{2max}$ is estimated from a nomogram (see *Figure 4.1*). Multistage step tests are also possible. Maritz et al. (73) used a single-step height of 12 in (30.5 cm) and four-step rates to systematically increase the work rate. A steady state HR is measured for each step rate, and a line formed from these HR values is extrapolated to age-predicted HR_{max}. The maximal work rate is determined as described for the YMCA cycle test. $\dot{V}O_{2max}$ can be estimated from the formula for stepping in *Table 6.3*. Such step tests should be modified to suit the population being tested. The Canadian Home Fitness Test has demonstrated that such testing can be performed on a large scale and at low cost (106).

Instead of estimating $\dot{V}O_{2max}$ from HR responses to submaximal work rates, a wide variety of step tests have been developed to categorize CRF based on an individual's recovery HR following a standardized step test. This eliminates the potential problem of taking HR during stepping. The 3-Minute YMCA Step Test is a good example of such a test. This test uses a 12-in (30.5 cm) bench, with a stepping rate of 24 steps $\cdot$ min^{-1} (estimated O_2 of 25.8 mL $\cdot$ kg^{-1} $\cdot$ min^{-1}). After stepping is completed, the subject immediately sits down, and HR is counted for 1 min. Counting must start within 5 s at the end of exercise. HR values are used to obtain a qualitative rating of fitness from published normative tables (120). The Queens College Step Test (also called the McArdle Step Test) requires participants to step at a rate of 24 steps $\cdot$ min^{-1} for men and 22 steps $\cdot$ min^{-1} for women for 3 min. The bench height is 16.25 in (41.25 cm). After stepping is completed, the subject remains standing. Wait 5 s, take a 15-s HR count, and multiply the HR by 4 to convert to beats $\cdot$ min^{-1}. $\dot{V}O_{2max}$ is calculated using the formulas below (76):

For men:

$$\dot{V}O_{2max} \text{ (mL} \cdot \text{kg}^{-1} \cdot \text{min}^{-1}) = 111.33 - (0.42 \times HR)$$

For women:

$$\dot{V}O_{2max} \text{ (mL} \cdot \text{kg}^{-1} \cdot \text{min}^{-1}) = 65.81 - (0.1847 \times HR)$$

where HR = heart rate (beats $\cdot$ min^{-1})

Interpretation of Results

Table 4.7 provides normative fitness categories and percentiles by age group for CRF from cardiopulmonary exercise testing on a treadmill with directly measured $\dot{V}O_{2max}$. This data was obtained from the Fitness Registry and the Importance of Exercise National Database (FRIEND) Registry for men and women who were considered free from known CVD. Research suggests that low CRF, usually defined as the lowest quartile or quintile on an exercise test, is associated with two- to fivefold increases in CVD or all-cause mortality, independent of other CVD risk factors (8,64,83,111).

Although submaximal exercise testing is not as precise as maximal exercise testing, it provides a general reflection of an individual's physical fitness at a lower cost, potentially reduced risk for adverse events, and requires less time and effort on the part of the subject. Some of the assumptions inherent in a submaximal test are more easily met (*e.g.*, steady state HR can be verified), whereas others (*e.g.*, estimated HR$_{max}$) introduce errors into the prediction of $\dot{V}O_{2max}$. Despite this, when an individual is given repeated submaximal exercise tests over the course of an Ex R$_x$, the HR response to a fixed work rate decreases. This indicates the individual's CRF has improved, independent of the accuracy of

TABLE 4.7

Cardiorespiratory Fitness Classifications ($\dot{V}O_{2max}$) by Age and Sex

$\dot{V}O_{2max}$ (mL $O_2 \cdot kg^{-1} \cdot min^{-1}$)

MEN						
		\multicolumn{5}{c}{Age Group (yr)}				
Percentile		20–29	30–39	40–49	50–59	60–69
95	Superior	66.3	59.8	55.6	50.7	43.0
90		61.8	56.5	52.1	45.6	40.3
85	Excellent	59.3	54.2	49.3	43.2	38.2
80		57.1	51.6	46.7	41.2	36.1
75		55.2	49.2	45.0	39.7	34.5
70	Good	53.7	48.0	43.9	38.2	32.9
65		52.1	46.6	42.1	36.3	31.6
60		50.2	45.2	40.3	35.1	30.5
55		49.0	43.8	38.9	33.8	29.1
50	Fair	48.0	42.4	37.8	32.6	28.2
45		46.5	41.3	36.7	31.6	27.2
40		44.9	39.6	35.7	30.7	26.6
35		43.5	38.5	34.6	29.5	25.7
30	Poor	41.9	37.4	33.3	28.4	24.6
25		40.1	35.9	31.9	27.1	23.7
20		38.1	34.1	30.5	26.1	22.4
15		35.4	32.7	29.0	24.4	21.2
10	Very poor	32.1	30.2	26.8	22.8	19.8
5		29.0	27.2	24.2	20.9	17.4
		(n = 513)	(n = 963)	(n = 1,327)	(n = 1,078)	(n = 593)
WOMEN						
		\multicolumn{5}{c}{Age Group (yr)}				
95	Superior	56.0	45.8	41.7	35.9	29.4
90		51.3	41.4	38.4	32.0	27.0
85	Excellent	48.3	39.3	36.0	30.2	25.6
80		46.5	37.5	34.0	28.6	24.6
75		44.7	36.1	32.4	27.6	23.8
70	Good	43.2	34.6	31.1	26.8	23.1
65		41.6	33.5	30.0	26.0	22.0
60		40.6	32.2	28.7	25.2	21.2
55		38.9	31.2	27.7	24.4	20.5
50	Fair	37.6	30.2	26.7	23.4	20.0
45		35.9	29.3	25.9	22.7	19.6
40		34.6	28.2	24.9	21.8	18.9

(continued)

TABLE 4.7

Cardiorespiratory Fitness Classifications ($\dot{V}O_{2max}$) by Age and Sex (Continued)

$\dot{V}O_{2max}$ (mL $O_2 \cdot kg^{-1} \cdot min^{-1}$)

		WOMEN				
		\multicolumn{5}{c}{Age Group (yr)}
Percentile		20–29	30–39	40–49	50–59	60–69
35		33.6	27.4	24.1	21.2	18.4
30	Poor	32.0	26.4	23.3	20.6	17.9
25		30.5	25.3	22.1	19.9	17.2
20		28.6	24.1	21.3	19.1	16.5
15		26.2	22.5	20.0	18.3	15.6
10	Very poor	23.9	20.9	18.8	17.3	14.6
5		21.7	19.0	17.0	16.0	13.4
		(n = 410)	(n = 608)	(n = 843)	(n = 805)	(n = 408)

Percentiles from cardiopulmonary exercise testing on a treadmill with measured $\dot{V}O_{2max}$ (mL $O_2 \cdot kg^{-1} \cdot min^{-1}$). Data obtained from the Fitness Registry and the Importance of Exercise National Database (FRIEND) Registry for men and women who were considered free from known CVD.

Adapted with permission from (55).

the $\dot{V}O_{2max}$ prediction. Despite differences in test accuracy and methodology, virtually all evaluations can establish a baseline and be used to track relative progress during exercise training.

Several regression equations for estimating CRF according to age and sex are also available. These equations produce a single expected aerobic capacity value for comparison to a measured response as opposed to percentiles. Of the available regression equations, research indicates prediction formulas derived from a Veterans Affairs cohort (predicted METs $= 18 - 0.15 \times$ age) and the St. James Women Take Heart project (predicted METs $= 14.7 - 0.13 \times$ age) may provide somewhat better prognostic information in men and women, respectively (59). These prediction equations may be useful when CRF testing is not possible.

MUSCULAR FITNESS

Muscular strength and endurance are health-related fitness components that may improve or maintain the following important health-related fitness characteristics (36,79,119):

- Bone mass, which is related to osteoporosis
- Muscle mass, which is related to sarcopenia
- Glucose tolerance, which is pertinent in both the prediabetic and diabetic state

- Musculotendinous integrity, which is related to a lower risk of injury including low back pain
- The ability to carry out the activities of daily living, which is related to perceived quality of life and self-efficacy among other indicators of mental health
- FFM and resting metabolic rate, which are related to weight management

The American College of Sports Medicine (ACSM) has melded the terms *muscular strength*, *endurance*, and *power* into a category termed *muscular fitness* and included it as an integral portion of total health-related fitness in the position stand on the quantity and quality of exercise for developing and maintaining fitness (37). Muscular strength refers to the muscle's ability to exert a maximal force on one occasion, muscular endurance is the muscle's ability to continue to perform successive exertions or repetitions against a submaximal load, and muscular power is the muscle's ability to exert force per unit of time (*i.e.*, rate) (95). Traditionally, tests allowing few (≤3) repetitions of a task prior to reaching muscular fatigue have been considered strength measures, whereas those in which numerous repetitions (>12) are performed prior to muscular fatigue were considered measures of muscular endurance. However, the performance of a maximal repetitions (*i.e.*, 4, 6, or 8 repetitions at a given resistance) across a wider range can also be used to predict muscle strength.

Rationale

Physical fitness tests of muscular strength and muscular endurance before commencing exercise training or as part of a health/fitness screening evaluation can provide valuable information on a client's baseline physical fitness level. For example, muscular fitness test results can be compared to established standards and can be helpful in identifying weaknesses in certain muscle groups or muscle imbalances that could be targeted in exercise training programs. The information obtained during baseline muscular fitness assessments can also serve as a basis for designing individualized exercise training programs. An equally useful application of physical fitness testing is to show a client's progressive improvements over time as a result of the training program and thus provide feedback that is often beneficial in promoting long-term exercise adherence.

Principles

Muscle function tests are very specific to the muscle group and joint(s) tested, the type of muscle action, velocity of muscle movement, type of equipment, and joint range of motion (ROM). Results of any one test are specific to the procedures used, and no single test exists for evaluating total body muscular endurance or strength. Individuals should participate in familiarization/practice sessions with test equipment and adhere to a specific protocol including a predetermined repetition duration and ROM in order to obtain a reliable score that can be used to track true physiologic adaptations over time. Moreover, a warm-up consisting of 5–10 min of light intensity aerobic exercise (*i.e.*, treadmill or cycle ergometer), dynamic stretching, and several light intensity repetitions of the specific testing exercise should precede muscular fitness testing. These warm-up activities increase muscle temperature and localized blood flow and promote appropriate cardiovascular responses for exercise. Standardized conditions for muscular fitness assessment include the following:

- Aerobic warm-up
- Equipment familiarization
- Strict posture
- Consistent repetition duration (movement speed)
- Full ROM
- Use of spotters (when necessary)

Change in muscular fitness over time can be based on the absolute value of the external load or resistance (*e.g.*, newtons, kilograms [kg], or pounds [lb]), but when comparisons are made between individuals, the values should be expressed as relative values (per kilogram of body weight [kg · kg^{-1}]). In both cases, caution must be used in the interpretation of the scores because the norms may not include a representative sample of the individual being measured, a standardized protocol may be absent, or the exact test being used (*e.g.*, free weight vs. machine weight) may differ. In addition, the biomechanics for a given resistance exercise may differ significantly when using equipment from different manufacturers, further impacting generalizability.

Muscular Strength

Although muscular strength refers to the external force (properly expressed in newtons, although kilograms and pounds are commonly used as well) that can be generated by a specific muscle or muscle group, it is commonly expressed in terms of resistance met or overcome. Strength can be assessed either statically (*i.e.*, no overt muscular movement at a given joint or group of joints) or dynamically (*i.e.*, movement of an external load or body part in which the muscle changes length). Static or isometric strength can be measured conveniently using a variety of devices including cable tensiometers and handgrip dynamometers. Measures of static strength are specific to the muscle group and joint angle involved in testing and thus may be limited in describing overall muscular strength. Despite this limitation, simple measurements such as handgrip strength have predicted mortality and functional status in older individuals (99,109). Peak force development in such tests is commonly referred to as the maximum voluntary contraction (MVC). Procedures for the grip strength test are described in *Box 4.6*, and grip strength norms are provided in *Table 4.8*.

Traditionally, the 1-RM, the greatest resistance that can be moved through the full ROM in a controlled manner with good posture, has been the standard for dynamic strength assessment. The exercise professional should be aware that 1-RM measurements may vary between different types of equipment (97). With appropriate testing familiarization, 1-RM is a reliable indicator of muscle strength

Box 4.6	Static Handgrip Strength Test Procedures

1. Adjust the grip bar so the second joint of the fingers fits snugly under the handle and takes the weight of the instrument. Set the dynamometer to zero.
2. The subject holds the handgrip dynamometer in line with the forearm at the level of the thigh, away from the body.
3. The subject squeezes the handgrip dynamometer as hard as possible without holding the breath (to avoid the Valsalva maneuver). Neither the hand nor the handgrip dynamometer should touch the body or any other object.
4. Repeat the test twice with each hand. The score is the highest of the two readings (to the nearest kilogram) for each hand added together.

Adapted from (18).

(68,91). A multiple repetition maximum (RM), such as 5- or 10-RM, can also be used as a measure of muscular strength. It is important when performing 5- to 10-RM that the exercise be performed to failure. When using a multiple RM (*i.e.*, 2- to 10-RM) to estimate the 1-RM, the prediction accuracy increases with the least number of repetitions (7,97). Tables and prediction equations are available to estimate 1-RM from multiple RM (7,74,97). It is possible to track strength gains over time without the need to estimate 1-RM. For example, if one were training with 6- to 8-RM, the performance of a 6-RM to muscular fatigue would provide an index of strength changes over time, independent of the true 1-RM.

TABLE 4.8

Fitness Categories for Grip Strength[a] by Sex and Age

Gender	M	F	M	F	M	F
Age (yr)	**15–19**		**20–29**		**30–39**	
Excellent	≥108	≥68	≥115	≥70	≥115	≥71
Very Good	98–107	60–67	104–114	63–69	104–114	63–70
Good	90–97	53–59	95–103	58–62	95–103	58–62
Fair	79–89	48–52	84–94	52–57	84–94	51–57
Poor	≤78	≤47	≤83	≤51	≤83	≤50
Age (yr)	**40–49**		**50–59**		**60–69**	
Excellent	≥108	≥69	≥101	≥61	≥100	≥54
Very Good	97–107	61–68	92–100	54–60	91–99	48–53
Good	88–96	54–60	84–91	49–53	84–90	45–47
Fair	80–87	49–53	76–83	45–48	73–83	41–44
Poor	≤79	≤48	≤75	≤44	≤72	≤40

[a]Norms use a combined score for the left and right hands.
Reprinted with permission from (18).

TABLE **4.9**

Fitness Categories for Upper Body Strength[a] for Men and Women by Age

Bench Press Weight Ratio = weight pushed in lb ÷ body weight in lb

		MEN					
		Age					
%		<20	20–29	30–39	40–49	50–59	60+
99	Superior	>1.76	>1.63	>1.35	>1.20	>1.05	>0.94
95		1.76	1.63	1.35	1.20	1.05	0.94
90		1.46	1.48	1.24	1.10	0.97	0.89
85	Excellent	1.38	1.37	1.17	1.04	0.93	0.84
80		1.34	1.32	1.12	1.00	0.90	0.82
75		1.29	1.26	1.08	0.96	0.87	0.79
70	Good	1.24	1.22	1.04	0.93	0.84	0.77
65		1.23	1.18	1.01	0.90	0.81	0.74
60		1.19	1.14	0.98	0.88	0.79	0.72
55		1.16	1.10	0.96	0.86	0.77	0.70
50	Fair	1.13	1.06	0.93	0.84	0.75	0.68
45		1.10	1.03	0.90	0.82	0.73	0.67
40		1.06	0.99	0.88	0.80	0.71	0.66
35		1.01	0.96	0.86	0.78	0.70	0.65
30	Poor	0.96	0.93	0.83	0.76	0.68	0.63
25		0.93	0.90	0.81	0.74	0.66	0.60
20		0.89	0.88	0.78	0.72	0.63	0.57
15		0.86	0.84	0.75	0.69	0.60	0.56
10	Very poor	0.81	0.80	0.71	0.65	0.57	0.53
5		0.76	0.72	0.65	0.59	0.53	0.49
1		<0.76	<0.72	<0.65	<0.59	<0.53	<0.49
n		60	425	1,909	2,090	1,279	343

Total n = 6,106

(continued)

A conservative approach to assessing maximal muscle strength should be considered in patients at high risk for or with known CVD, pulmonary, and metabolic diseases and health conditions. For these groups, assessment of 10- to 15-RM that approximates training recommendations may be prudent (119).

Valid measures of general upper body strength include the 1-RM values for bench press or shoulder press. Corresponding indices of lower body strength include 1-RM values for the leg press or leg extension. Norms based on resistance lifted divided by body mass for the bench press and leg press are provided

TABLE 4.9

Fitness Categories for Upper Body Strength[a] for Men and Women by Age (Continued)

Bench Press Weight Ratio = weight pushed in lb ÷ body weight in lb

		WOMEN					
				Age			
%		<20	20–29	30–39	40–49	50–59	60+
99	Superior	>0.88	>1.01	>0.82	>0.77	>0.68	>0.72
95		0.88	1.01	0.82	0.77	0.68	0.72
90		0.83	0.90	0.76	0.71	0.61	0.64
85	Excellent	0.81	0.83	0.72	0.66	0.57	0.59
80		0.77	0.80	0.70	0.62	0.55	0.54
75		0.76	0.77	0.65	0.60	0.53	0.53
70	Good	0.74	0.74	0.63	0.57	0.52	0.51
65		0.70	0.72	0.62	0.55	0.50	0.48
60		0.65	0.70	0.60	0.54	0.48	0.47
55		0.64	0.68	0.58	0.53	0.47	0.46
50	Fair	0.63	0.65	0.57	0.52	0.46	0.45
45		0.60	0.63	0.55	0.51	0.45	0.44
40		0.58	0.59	0.53	0.50	0.44	0.43
35		0.57	0.58	0.52	0.48	0.43	0.41
30	Poor	0.56	0.56	0.51	0.47	0.42	0.40
25		0.55	0.53	0.49	0.45	0.41	0.39
20		0.53	0.51	0.47	0.43	0.39	0.38
15		0.52	0.50	0.45	0.42	0.38	0.36
10	Very poor	0.50	0.48	0.42	0.38	0.37	0.33
5		0.41	0.44	0.39	0.35	0.31	0.26
1		<0.41	<0.44	<0.39	<0.35	<0.31	<0.26
n		20	191	379	333	189	42
Total n = 1,154							

[a]One repetition maximum (1-RM) bench press, with bench press weight ratio = weight pushed in pounds per body weight in pounds. 1-RM was measured using a Universal Dynamic Variable Resistance (DVR) machine.

Adapted with permission from *Physical Fitness Assessments and Norms for Adults and Law Enforcement*. The Cooper Institute, Dallas, Texas. 2009. For more information: www.cooperinstitute.org

in *Tables 4.9* and *4.10*, respectively. The normative data must be interpreted with caution because it was developed using universal dynamic variable resistance (DVR) multistation resistance machines which are no longer available for purchase. Free weights and other brands of resistance exercise machines which are more commonly used today may not provide the same weight–press

TABLE 4.10

Fitness Categories for Leg Strength by Age and Sex[a]

Leg Press Weight Ratio = weight pushed in lb ÷ body weight in lb

		MEN				
		Age (yr)				
Percentile		20–29	30–39	40–49	50–59	60+
90	Well above average	2.27	2.07	1.92	1.80	1.73
80	Above average	2.13	1.93	1.82	1.71	1.62
70		2.05	1.85	1.74	1.64	1.56
60	Average	1.97	1.77	1.68	1.58	1.49
50		1.91	1.71	1.62	1.52	1.43
40	Below average	1.83	1.65	1.57	1.46	1.38
30		1.74	1.59	1.51	1.39	1.30
20	Well below average	1.63	1.52	1.44	1.32	1.25
10		1.51	1.43	1.35	1.22	1.16
		WOMEN				
		Age (yr)				
Percentile		20–29	30–39	40–49	50–59	60+
90	Well above average	1.82	1.61	1.48	1.37	1.32
80	Above average	1.68	1.47	1.37	1.25	1.18
70		1.58	1.39	1.29	1.17	1.13
60	Average	1.50	1.33	1.23	1.10	1.04
50		1.44	1.27	1.18	1.05	0.99
40	Below average	1.37	1.21	1.13	0.99	0.93
30		1.27	1.15	1.08	0.95	0.88
20	Well below average	1.22	1.09	1.02	0.88	0.85
10		1.14	1.00	0.94	0.78	0.72

[a]One repetition maximum (1-RM) leg press with leg press weight ratio = weight pushed per body weight. 1-RM was measured using a Universal Dynamic Variable Resistance (DVR) machine. Study population for the data set was predominantly white and college educated.

Adapted from Institute for Aerobics Research, Dallas, 1994.

ratio and to date have not been validated (54). The basic steps in 1-RM (or any multiple RM) testing following familiarization/practice sessions are presented in *Box 4.7*.

Isokinetic testing involves the assessment of maximal muscle tension throughout an ROM set at a constant angular velocity (*e.g.*, 60 angles · s^{-1}). Equipment that allows control of the speed of joint rotation (degrees · s^{-1}) as well as the ability to test movement around various joints (*e.g.*, knee, hip, shoulder, elbow) is available from commercial sources. Such devices measure peak rotational force or torque,

Box 4.7	One Repetition Maximum (1-RM) and Multiple Repetition Maximum (RM) Test Procedures for Measurement of Muscular Strength

1. Testing should be completed only after the subject has participated in familiarization/practice sessions.
2. The subject should warm up by completing a number of submaximal repetitions of the specific exercise that will be used to determine the 1-RM.
3. Determine the 1-RM (or any multiple of 1-RM) within four trials with rest periods of 3–5 min between trials.
4. Select an initial weight that is within the subject's perceived capacity (~50%–70% of capacity).
5. Resistance is progressively increased by 5.0%–10.0% for upper body or 10.0%–20.0% for lower body exercise from the previous successful attempt until the subject cannot complete the selected repetition(s); all repetitions should be performed at the same speed of movement and ROM to instill consistency between trials.
6. The final weight lifted successfully is recorded as the absolute 1-RM or multiple RM.

ROM, range of motion.
Adapted from (7,70).

but an important drawback is that this equipment is substantially more expensive compared to other strength testing modalities (39).

Muscular Endurance

Muscular endurance is the ability of a muscle group to execute repeated muscle actions over a period of time sufficient to cause muscular fatigue or to maintain a specific percentage of the 1-RM for a prolonged period of time. If the total number of repetitions at a given amount of resistance is measured, the result is termed *absolute muscular endurance*. If the number of repetitions performed at a percentage of the 1-RM (*e.g.*, 70%) is used pre- and posttesting, the result is termed *relative muscular endurance*. A simple field test such as the maximum number of push-ups that can be performed without rest may be used to evaluate the endurance of upper body muscles (18). Procedures for conducting this push-up endurance test are presented in *Box 4.8*, and physical fitness categories are provided in *Table 4.11*. Previous editions of this publication included the curl-up (crunch) test as a simple field test for the measurement of muscular endurance. This edition of the *Guidelines* does not include the curl-up test in light of recent research suggesting that the test may not be sensitive enough to grade performance and may cause lower back injury (77,78,107). Most curl-up tests are only moderately related to abdominal endurance ($r = .46-.50$) and poorly related to abdominal strength ($r = -.21-.36$) (62,63).

Box 4.8	Push-up Test Procedures for Measurement of Muscular Endurance

1. The push-up test is administered with men starting in the standard "down" position (hands pointing forward and under the shoulder, back straight, head up, using the toes as the pivotal point) and women in the modified "knee push-up" position (legs together, lower leg in contact with mat with ankles plantar-flexed, back straight, hands shoulder width apart, head up, using the knees as the pivotal point).
2. The client/patient must raise the body by straightening the elbows and return to the "down" position, until the chin touches the mat. The stomach should not touch the mat.
3. For both men and women, the subject's back must be straight at all times, and the subject must push up to a straight arm position.
4. The maximal number of push-ups performed consecutively without rest is counted as the score.
5. The test is stopped when the client strains forcibly or unable to maintain the appropriate technique within two repetitions.

FLEXIBILITY

Flexibility is the ability to move a joint through its complete ROM. It is important in athletic performance (*e.g.*, ballet, gymnastics) and in the ability to carry out activities of daily living. Consequently, maintaining flexibility of all joints facilitates movement and may prevent injury; in contrast, when an activity moves the structures of a joint beyond its full ROM, tissue damage can occur.

Flexibility depends on a number of specific variables including distensibility of the joint capsule, adequate warm-up, and muscle viscosity. In addition, compliance

TABLE 4.11
Fitness Categories for the Push-up by Age and Sex

Category	Age (yr)									
	20–29		30–39		40–49		50–59		60–69	
Sex	M	W	M	W	M	W	M	W	M	W
Excellent	≥36	≥30	≥30	≥27	≥25	≥24	≥21	≥21	≥18	≥17
Very good	29–35	21–29	22–29	20–26	17–24	15–23	13–20	11–20	11–17	12–16
Good	22–28	15–20	17–21	13–19	13–16	11–14	10–12	7–10	8–10	5–11
Fair	17–21	10–14	12–16	8–12	10–12	5–10	7–9	2–6	5–7	2–4
Poor	≤16	≤9	≤11	≤7	≤9	≤4	≤6	≤1	≤4	≤1

M, men; W, women.
Reprinted with permission from (18).

(*i.e.*, tightness) of various other tissues such as ligaments and tendons affects the ROM. Just as muscular strength and endurance is specific to the muscles involved, flexibility is joint specific; therefore, no single flexibility test can be used to evaluate total body flexibility. Laboratory tests usually quantify flexibility in terms of ROM expressed in degrees. Common devices for this purpose include goniometers, electrogoniometers, the Leighton flexometer, inclinometers, and tape measures. Comprehensive instructions are available for the evaluation of flexibility of most anatomic joints (21,87). Visual estimates of ROM can be useful in fitness screening but are inaccurate relative to directly measured ROM. These estimates can include neck and trunk flexibility, hip flexibility, lower extremity flexibility, shoulder flexibility, and postural assessment.

A precise measurement of joint ROM can be assessed at most anatomic joints following strict procedures (21,87) and the proper use of a goniometer. Accurate measurements require in-depth knowledge of bone, muscle, and joint anatomy as well as experience in administering the evaluation. *Table 4.12* provides normative

TABLE **4.12**			
Range of Motion of Select Single-Joint Movements in Degrees			
	Degrees		**Degrees**
Shoulder Girdle Movement			
Flexion	90–120	Extension	20–60
Abduction	80–100		
Horizontal abduction	30–45	Horizontal adduction	90–135
Medial rotation	70–90	Lateral rotation	70–90
Elbow Movement			
Flexion	135–160		
Supination	75–90	Pronation	75–90
Trunk Movement			
Flexion	120–150	Extension	20–45
Lateral flexion	10–35	Rotation	20–40
Hip Movement			
Flexion	90–135	Extension	10–30
Abduction	30–50	Adduction	10–30
Medial rotation	30–45	Lateral rotation	45–60
Knee Movement			
Flexion	130–140	Extension	5–10
Ankle Movement			
Dorsiflexion	15–20	Plantar flexion	30–50
Inversion	10–30	Eversion	10–20

Adapted from (84).

Box 4.9	Canadian Trunk Forward Flexion (Sit-and-Reach) Test Procedures

Pretest: Clients/Patients should perform a short warm-up prior to this test and include some stretches (*e.g.*, modified hurdler's stretch). It is also recommended that the participant refrain from fast, jerky movements, which may increase the possibility of an injury. The participant's shoes should be removed.

1. The client sits without shoes and the soles of the feet flat against a sit-and-reach box with the zero mark at the 26 cm. Inner edges of the soles should be 6 in (15.2 cm) apart.
2. The client should slowly reach forward with both hands as far as possible, holding this position approximately 2 s. Be sure that the participant keeps the hands parallel and does not lead with one hand, or bounce. Fingertips can be overlapped and should be in contact with the measuring portion or yardstick of the sit-and-reach box.
3. The score is the most distant point reached with the fingertips. The best of two trials should be recorded. To assist with the best attempt, the client should exhale and drop the head between the arms when reaching. Testers should ensure that the knees of the participant stay extended; however, the participant's knees should not be pressed down by the test administrator. The client/patient should breathe normally during the test and should not hold his or her breath at any time. Norms for the Canadian test are presented in *Table 4.13*. Note that these norms use a sit-and-reach box in which the "zero" point is at the 26 cm mark. If a box is used in which the zero point is set at 23 cm (*e.g.*, Fitnessgram), subtract 3 cm from each value in this table.

Reprinted with permission from (18).

ROM values for select anatomic joints. Additional information can be found elsewhere (38,44).

The sit-and-reach test has been used commonly to assess low back and hamstring flexibility; however, its relationship to predict the incidence of low back pain is limited (48). The sit-and-reach test is suggested to be a better measure of hamstring flexibility than low back flexibility (47). The relative importance of hamstring flexibility to activities of daily living and sports performance, therefore, supports the inclusion of the sit-and-reach test for health-related fitness testing until a criterion measure evaluation of low back flexibility is available. Although limb and torso length disparity may impact sit-and-reach scoring, modified testing that establishes an individual zero point for each participant has not enhanced the predictive index for low back flexibility or low back pain (15,46,80).

Poor lower back and hip flexibility, in conjunction with poor abdominal strength and endurance or other causative factors, may contribute to development of muscular low back pain; however, this hypothesis remains to be substantiated (36). Methods for administering the sit-and-reach test are presented in *Box 4.9*. Normative data for the Canadian Trunk Forward Flexion test are presented in *Table 4.13*.

TABLE 4.13									
Fitness Categories for Canadian Trunk Forward Flexion Test Using a Sit-and-Reach Box (cm)^a by Age and Sex									
				Age (yr)					
Category	20–29		30–39		40–49		50–59		60–69	
Sex	**M**	**W**	**M**	**W**	**M**	**W**	**M**	**W**	**M**	**W**
Excellent	≥40	≥41	≥38	≥41	≥35	≥38	≥35	≥39	≥33	≥35
Very good	34–39	37–40	33–37	36–40	29–34	34–37	28–34	33–38	25–32	31–34
Good	30–33	33–36	28–32	32–35	24–28	30–33	24–27	30–32	20–24	27–30
Fair	25–29	28–32	23–27	27–31	18–23	25–29	16–23	25–29	15–19	23–26
Poor	≤24	≤27	≤22	≤26	≤17	≤24	≤15	≤24	≤14	≤22

^{a}These norms are based on a sit-and-reach box in which the "zero" point is set at 26 cm. When using a box in which the zero point is set at 23 cm, subtract 3 cm from each value in this table.
M, men; W, women.

Reprinted with permission from (18).

ONLINE RESOURCES

ACSM Certifications:
    http://acsm.org/certification
ACSM Exercise is Medicine Exercise Professionals:
    http://www.exerciseismedicine.org/support_page.php?p=91
American Heart Association:
    http://www.heart.org/HEARTORG/
Clinical Guidelines on the Identification, Evaluation, and Treatment of Overweight
    and Obesity in Adults: The Evidence Report (23): http://www.nhlbi.nih.gov/health
    -pro/guidelines/archive/clinical-guidelines-obesity-adults-evidence-report
The Cooper Institute Fitness Adult Education:
    http://www.cooperinstitute.org/education/
National Heart, Lung, and Blood Institute Health Information for Professionals:
    http://www.nhlbi.nih.gov/health/indexpro.htm
2008 Physical Activity Guidelines for Americans:
    http://www.health.gov/paguidelines/guidelines/
Fitness Testing Resources from Lippincott Williams & Wilkins:
    http://www.lww.com/search?ProductType=All+Products&search=fitness=testing

REFERENCES

1. American Medical Association. *AMA Adopts New Policies on Second Day of Voting at Annual Meeting* [Internet]. Chicago (IL): American Medical Association; 2013 [cited 2016 Jun 6]. Available from: http://www.ama-assn.org/ama/pub/news/news/2013/2013-06-18-new-ama-policies-annual-meeting.page

2. Arena R, Lavie C. The obesity paradox and outcome in heart failure: is excess bodyweight truly protective? *Future Cardiol.* 2010;6(1):1–6.

3. Arena R, Myers J, Williams MA, et al. Assessment of functional capacity in clinical and research settings: a scientific statement from the American Heart Association Committee on Exercise, Rehabilitation, and Prevention of the Council on Clinical Cardiology and the Council on Cardiovascular Nursing. *Circulation.* 2007;116(3):329–43.

4. Astrand PO. Aerobic work capacity in men and women with special reference to age. *Acta Physiol Scand.* 1960;49(Suppl 169):45–60.

5. Astrand PO, Ryhming I. A nomogram for calculation of aerobic capacity (physical fitness) from pulse rate during sub-maximal work. *J Appl Physiol.* 1954;7(2):218–21.

6. ATS Committee on Proficiency Standards for Clinical Pulmonary Function Laboratories. ATS statement: guidelines for the six-minute walk test. *Am J Respir Crit Care Med.* 2002;166(1):111–7.

7. Baechle TR, Earle RW, Wathen D. Resistance training. In: Baechle TR, Earle RW, editors. *Essentials of Strength Training and Conditioning.* 3rd ed. Champaign (IL): Human Kinetics; 2008. p. 381–412.

8. Balady GJ, Larson MG, Vasan RS, Leip EP, O'Donnell CJ, Levy D. Usefulness of exercise testing in the prediction of coronary disease risk among asymptomatic persons as a function of the Framingham risk score. *Circulation.* 2004;110(14):1920–5.

9. Blair SN, Kohl HW III, Barlow CE, Paffenbarger RS Jr, Gibbons LW, Macera CA. Changes in physical fitness and all-cause mortality. A prospective study of healthy and unhealthy men. *JAMA.* 1995;273(14):1093–8.

10. Blair SN, Kohl HW III, Paffenbarger RS Jr, Clark DG, Cooper KH, Gibbons LW. Physical fitness and all-cause mortality. A prospective study of healthy men and women. *JAMA.* 1989;262(17):2395–401.

11. Borg GA. *Borg's Perceived Exertion and Pain Scales.* Champaign (IL): Human Kinetics; 1998. 104 p.

12. Borg GA. Psychophysical bases of perceived exertion. *Med Sci Sports Exerc.* 1982;14(5):377–81.

13. Bray GA. Don't throw the baby out with the bath water. *Am J Clin Nutr.* 2004;79(3):347–9.

14. Cahalin LP, Mathier MA, Semigran MJ, Dec GW, DiSalvo TG. The six-minute walk test predicts peak oxygen uptake and survival in patients with advanced heart failure. *Chest.* 1996;110(2):325–32.

15. Cailliet R. *Low Back Pain Syndrome.* 4th ed. Philadelphia (PA): F.A. Davis; 1988. 341 p.

16. Callaway CW, Chumlea WC, Bouchard C, Himes JH, Lohman TG, Martin AD. Circumferences. In: Lohman TG, Roche AF, Martorell R, editors. *Anthropometric Standardization Reference Manual.* Champaign (IL): Human Kinetics; 1988. p. 39–80.

17. Camhi SM, Bray GA, Bouchard C, et al. The relationship of waist circumference and BMI to visceral, subcutaneous, and total body fat: sex and race differences. *Obesity (Silver Spring).* 2011;19(2):402–8.

18. Canadian Society for Exercise Physiology. *Physical Activity Training for Health (CSEP-PATH) Resource Manual.* Ottawa, Ontario (Canada): Canadian Society for Exercise Physiology; 2013. 210 p.

19. Canoy D. Distribution of body fat and risk of coronary heart disease in men and women. *Curr Opin Cardiol.* 2008;23(6):591–8.

20. Casanova C, Cote C, Marin JM, et al. Distance and oxygen desaturation during the 6-min walk test as predictors of long-term mortality in patients with COPD. *Chest.* 2008;134(4):746–52.

21. Clarkson HM. *Musculoskeletal Assessment: Joint Range of Motion and Manual Muscle Strength.* 2nd ed. Baltimore (MD): Lippincott Williams & Wilkins; 2000. 432 p.

22. Clarys JP, Martin AD, Drinkwater DT, Marfell-Jones MJ. The skinfold: myth and reality. *J Sports Sci.* 1987;5(1):3–33.

23. *Clinical Guidelines on the Identification, Evaluation, and Treatment of Overweight and Obesity in Adults: The Evidence Report* [Internet]. Bethesda (MD): National Institutes of Health; National Heart, Lung, and Blood Institute; 2008 [cited 2016 Jun 6]. Available from: http://www.nhlbi.nih.gov /guidelines/obesity/ob_gdlns.htm

24. Daniels SR, Jacobson MS, McCrindle BW, Eckel RH, Sanner BM. American Heart Association Childhood Obesity Research Summit Report. *Circulation.* 2009;119(15):e489–517.

25. Dehghan M, Merchant A. Is bioelectrical impedance accurate for use in large epidemiological studies? *Nutr J.* 2008;7:26.

26. de Koning L, Merchant AT, Pogue J, Anand SS. Waist circumference and waist-to-hip ratio as predictors of cardiovascular events: meta-regression analysis of prospective studies. *Eur Heart J.* 2007;28(7):850–6.

27. Dempster P, Aitkens S. A new air displacement method for the determination of human body composition. *Med Sci Sports Exerc*. 1995;27(12):1692–7.

28. Després JP. Body fat distribution and risk of cardiovascular disease: an update. *Circulation*. 2012;126(10):1301–13.

29. Donnelly JE, Blair SN, Jakicic JM, et al. American College of Sports Medicine position stand. Appropriate physical activity intervention strategies for weight loss and prevention of weight regain for adults. *Med Sci Sports Exerc*. 2009;41(2):459–71.

30. Duren DL, Sherwood RJ, Czerwinski SA, et al. Body composition methods: comparisons and interpretation. *J Diabetes Sci Technol*. 2008;2(6):1139–46.

31. Expert Panel on the Identification, Evaluation, and Treatment of Overweight and Obesity in Adults. Executive summary of the clinical guidelines on the identification, evaluation, and treatment of overweight and obesity in adults. *Arch Intern Med*. 1998;158(17):1855–67.

32. Flegal KM, Graubard BI, Williamson DF, Gail MH. Excess deaths associated with underweight, overweight, and obesity. *JAMA*. 2005;293(15):1861–7.

33. Fox CS, Massaro JM, Hoffmann U, et al. Abdominal visceral and subcutaneous adipose tissue compartments: association with metabolic risk factors in the Framingham Heart Study. *Circulation*. 2007;116(1):39–48.

34. Freiberger E, Sieber C, Pfeifer K. Physical activity, exercise, and sarcopenia — future challenges. *Wien Med Wochenschr*. 2011;161(17–18):416–25.

35. Gallagher D, Heymsfield SB, Heo M, Jebb SA, Murgatroyd PR, Sakamoto Y. Healthy percentage body fat ranges: an approach for developing guidelines based on body mass index. *Am J Clin Nutr*. 2000;72(3):694–701.

36. Garber CE, Blissmer B, Deschenes MR, et al. American College of Sports Medicine position stand. The quantity and quality of exercise for developing and maintaining cardiorespiratory, musculoskeletal, and neuromotor fitness in apparently healthy adults: guidance for prescribing exercise. *Med Sci Sports Exerc*. 2011;43(7):1334–559.

37. Going BS. *Densitometry*. In: Roche AF, editor. *Human Body Composition*. Champaign (IL): Human Kinetics; 1996. p. 3–23.

38. Haff GG, Dumke C. *Laboratory Manual for Exercise Physiology*. Champaign (IL): Human Kinetics; 2012. 449 p.

39. Hall SJ. *Basic Biomechanics*. 6th ed. New York (NY): McGraw-Hill; 2012. 560 p.

40. Haskell WL, Lee IM, Pate RR, et al. Physical activity and public health: updated recommendation for adults from the American College of Sports Medicine and the American Heart Association. *Circulation*. 2007;116(9):1081–93.

41. Hendel HW, Gotfredsen A, Højgaard L, Andersen T, Hilsted J. Change in fat-free mass assessed by bioelectrical impedance, total body potassium and dual energy X-ray absorptiometry during prolonged weight loss. *Scand J Clin Lab Invest*. 1996;56(8):671–9.

42. Heymsfield S. *Human Body Composition*. 2nd ed. Champaign (IL): Human Kinetics; 2005. 523 p.

43. Heyward VH. Practical body composition assessment for children, adults, and older adults. *Int J Sport Nutr*. 1998;8(3):285–307.

44. Heyward VH, Gibson A. *Advanced Fitness Assessment and Exercise Prescription*. 7th ed. Champaign (IL): Human Kinetics; 2014. 552 p.

45. Heyward VH, Wagner D. *Applied Body Composition Assessment*. 2nd ed. Champaign (IL): Human Kinetics; 2004. 280 p.

46. Hoeger WW, Hopkins D. A comparison of the sit and reach and the modified sit and reach in the measurement of flexibility in women. *Res Q Exerc Sport*. 1992;63(2):191–5.

47. Jackson AW, Baker A. The relationship of the sit and reach test to criterion measures of hamstring and back flexibility in young females. *Res Q Exerc Sport*. 1986;57(3):183–6.

48. Jackson AW, Morrow JR Jr, Bril PA, Kohl HW III, Gordon NF, Blair SN. Relations of sit-up and sit-and-reach tests to low back pain in adults. *J Orthop Sports Phys Ther*. 1998;27(1):22–6.

49. Jackson AW, Pollock M. Practical assessment of body composition. *Phys Sportsmed*. 1985;13(5):76,80,82–90.

50. Janssen I, Katzmarzyk PT, Ross R. Body mass index, waist circumference, and health risk: evidence in support of current National Institutes of Health guidelines. *Arch Intern Med*. 2002;162(18):2074–9.

51. Janssen I, Katzmarzyk PT, Ross R. Waist circumference and not body mass index explains obesity-related health risk. *Am J Clin Nutr*. 2004;79(3):379–84.

52. Jehn M, Halle M, Schuster T, et al. The 6-min walk test in heart failure: is it a max or sub-maximum exercise test? *Eur J Appl Physiol*. 2009;107(3):317–23.

53. Jette M, Campbell J, Mongeon J, Routhier R. The Canadian Home Fitness Test as a predictor for aerobic capacity. *Can Med Assoc J*. 1976;114(8):680–2.

54. Kaminsky LA, American College of Sports Medicine. *ACSM's Health-Related Physical Fitness Assessment Manual*. 4th ed. Baltimore (MD): Lippincott Williams & Wilkins; 2014. 192 p.

55. Kaminsky LA, Arena R, Myers J. Reference standards for cardiorespiratory fitness measured with cardiopulmonary exercise testing: data from the Fitness Registry and the Importance of Exercise National Database. *Mayo Clin Proc*. 2015;90(11):1515–23.

56. Katzmarzyk PT, Bray GA, Greenway FL, et al. Racial differences in abdominal depot-specific adiposity in white and African American adults. *Am J Clin Nutr*. 2010;91(1):7–15.

57. Katzmarzyk PT, Mire E, Bray GA, Greenway FL, Heymsfield SB, Bouchard C. Anthropometric markers of obesity and mortality in white and African American adults: the Pennington center longitudinal study. *Obesity (Silver Spring)*. 2013;21(5):1070–5.

58. Kelly TL, Wilson KE, Heymsfield SB. Dual energy X-Ray absorptiometry body composition reference values from NHANES. *PLoS One*. 2009;4(9):e7038.

59. Kim ES, Ishwaran H, Blackstone E, Lauer MS. External prognostic validations and comparisons of age- and gender-adjusted exercise capacity predictions. *J Am Coll Cardiol*. 2007;50(19):1867–75.

60. Kingma B, Frijns A, van Marken LW. The thermoneutral zone: implications for metabolic studies. *Front Biosci (Elite Ed)*. 2012;4:1975–85.

61. Kline GM, Porcari JP, Hintermeister R, et al. Estimation of $\dot{V}O_{2max}$ from a one-mile track walk, gender, age, and body weight. *Med Sci Sports Exerc*. 1987;19(3):253–9.

62. Knudson D. The validity of recent curl-up tests in young adults. *J Strength Cond Res*. 2001; 15(1):81–5.

63. Knudson D, Johnston D. Validity and reliability of a bench trunk-curl test of abdominal endurance. *J Strength Cond Res*. 1995;9(3):165–9.

64. Kodama S, Saito K, Tanaka S, et al. Cardiorespiratory fitness as a quantitative predictor of all-cause mortality and cardiovascular events in healthy men and women: a meta-analysis. *JAMA*. 2009;301(19):2024–35.

65. Kumanyika SK, Obarzanek E, Stettler N, et al. Population-based prevention of obesity: the need for comprehensive promotion of healthful eating, physical activity, and energy balance: a scientific statement from American Heart Association Council on Epidemiology and Prevention, Interdisciplinary Committee for Prevention (formerly the Expert Panel on Population and Prevention Science). *Circulation*. 2008;118(4):428–64.

66. Lee SY, Gallagher D. Assessment methods in human body composition. *Curr Opin Clin Nutr Metab Care*. 2008;11(5):566–72.

67. Leger L, Thivierge M. Heart rate monitors: validity, stability, and functionality. *Phys Sportsmed*. 1988;16(5):143,146,148,149,151.

68. Levinger I, Goodman C, Hare DL, Jerums G, Toia D, Selig S. The reliability of the 1RM strength test for untrained middle-aged individuals. *J Sci Med Sport*. 2009;12(2):310–6.

69. Lewis CE, McTigue KM, Burke LE, et al. Mortality, health outcomes, and body mass index in the overweight range: a science advisory from the American Heart Association. *Circulation*. 2009;119(25):3263–71.

70. Logan P, Fornasiero D, Abernathy P. Protocols for the assessment of isoinertial strength. In: Gore CJ, editor. *Physiological Tests for Elite Athletes*. Champaign (IL): Human Kinetics; 2000. p. 200–21.

71. Lohman TG. Body composition methodology in sports medicine. *Phys Sportsmed*. 1982;10(12):46–7.

72. Lohman TG. Skinfolds and body density and their relation to body fatness: a review. *Hum Biol*. 1981;53(2):181–225.

73. Maritz JS, Morrison JF, Peter J, Strydom NB, Wyndham CH. A practical method of estimating an individual's maximal oxygen intake. *Ergonomics*. 1961;4:97–122.

74. Mayhew JL, Ball TE, Arnold MD, Bowen JC. Relative muscular endurance performance as a predictor of bench press strength in college men and women. *J Strength Cond Res*. 1992;6:200–6.

75. McArdle WD, Katch FI, Katch VL. *Exercise Physiology : Nutrition, Energy, and Human Performance*. Philadelphia (PA): Wolters Kluwer Health/Lippincott Williams & Wilkins; 2015.

76. McArdle WD, Katch FI, Pechar GS, Jacobson L, Ruck S. Reliability and interrelationships between maximal oxygen intake, physical work capacity and step-test scores in college women. *Med Sci Sports*. 1972;4(4):182–6.

77. McGill S. Core training: evidence translating to better performance and injury prevention. *Strength Cond J*. 2010;32:33–46.

78. McGill SM. *Ultimate Back Fitness and Performance*. Waterloo, Ontario (Canada): Backfitpro Inc.; 2013. 325 p.

79. Melov S, Tarnopolsky MA, Beckman K, Felkey K, Hubbard A. Resistance exercise reverses aging in human skeletal muscle. *PLoS One*. 2007;2(5):e465.

80. Minkler S, Patterson P. The validity of the modified sit-and-reach test in college-age students. *Res Q Exerc Sport*. 1994;65(2):189–92.

81. Montero-Fernández N, Serra Rexach J. Role of exercise on sarcopenia in the elderly. *Eur J Phys Rehabil Med*. 2013;49(1):131–43.

82. Myers J, Arena R, Franklin B, et al. Recommendations for clinical exercise laboratories: a scientific statement from the American Heart Association. *Circulation*. 2009;119(24):3144–61.

83. Myers J, Prakash M, Froelicher V, Do D, Partington S, Atwood JE. Exercise capacity and mortality among men referred for exercise testing. *N Engl J Med*. 2002;346(11):793–801.

84. Norkin CC, Levangie PK. *Joint Structure & Function: A Comprehensive Analysis*. 2nd ed. Philadelphia (PA): Davis; 1992. 512 p.

85. Ogden CL, Carroll MD, Kit BK, Flegal KM. Prevalence of childhood and adult obesity in the United States, 2011-2012. *JAMA*. 2014;311(8):806–14.

86. Oreopoulos A, Padwal R, Kalantar-Zadeh K, Fonarow GC, Norris CM, McAlister FA. Body mass index and mortality in heart failure: a meta-analysis. *Am Heart J*. 2008;156(1):13–22.

87. Palmer ML, Epler M. *Fundamentals of Musculoskeletal Assessment Techniques*. 2nd ed. Baltimore (MD): Lippincott Williams & Wilkins; 1998. 415 p.

88. Pescatello, L, Arena R, Riebe D, Thompson P, American College of Sports Medicine. *ACSM's Guidelines for Exercise Testing and Prescription*. 9th ed. Baltimore (MD): Lippincott Williams & Wilkins; 2014. 480 p.

89. Peveler WW. Effects of saddle height on economy in cycling. *J Strength Cond Res*. 2008;22(4):1355–9.

90. Peveler WW, Pounders JD, Bishop PA. Effects of saddle height on anaerobic power production in cycling. *J Strength Cond Res*. 2007;21(4):1023–7.

91. Phillips WT, Batterham AM, Valenzuela JE, Burkett LN. Reliability of maximal strength testing in older adults. *Arch Phys Med Rehabil*. 2004;85(2):329–34.

92. Pi-Sunyer FX. The epidemiology of central fat distribution in relation to disease. *Nutr Rev*. 2004;62(7 Pt 2):S120–6.

93. Poirier P, Giles TD, Bray GA, et al. Obesity and cardiovascular disease: pathophysiology, evaluation, and effect of weight loss: an update of the 1997 American Heart Association Scientific Statement on Obesity and Heart Disease from the Obesity Committee of the Council on Nutrition, Physical Activity, and Metabolism. *Circulation*. 2006;113(6):898–918.

94. Pollack ML, Schmidt DH, Jackson AS. Measurement of cardiorespiratory fitness and body composition in the clinical setting. *Compr Ther*. 1980;6(9):12–27.

95. President's Council on Physical Fitness and Sports. *Definitions — Health, Fitness, and Physical Activity* [Internet]. Washington (DC): President's Council on Physical Fitness and Sports; 2000 [cited 2012 Jan 7]. Available from: http://purl.access.gpo.gov/GPO/LPS21074

96. Reis JP, Macera CA, Araneta MR, Lindsay SP, Marshall SJ, Wingard DL. Comparison of overall obesity and body fat distribution in predicting risk of mortality. *Obesity (Silver Spring)*. 2009;17(6):1232–9.

97. Reynolds JM, Gordon TJ, Robergs RA. Prediction of one repetition maximum strength from multiple repetition maximum testing and anthropometry. *J Strength Cond Res*. 2006;20(3):584–92.

98. Riebe D, Maresh CM, Armstrong LE, et al. Effects of oral and intravenous rehydration on ratings of perceived exertion and thirst. *Med Sci Sports Exerc*. 1997;29(1):117–24.

99. Rijk JM, Roos PR, Deckx L, van den Akker M, Buntinx F. Prognostic value of handgrip strength in people aged 60 years and older: a systematic review and meta-analysis. *Geriatr Gerontol Int.* 2015.

100. Robertson, RJ, Noble, BJ. Perception of physical exertion: methods, mediators, and applications. *Exerc Sport Sci Rev.* 1997;25:407–52.

101. Roche AF. Anthropometry and ultrasound. In: Roche AF, Heymsfield S, Lohman T, editors. *Human Body Composition.* Champaign (IL): Human Kinetics; 1996. p. 167–89.

102. Roger VL, Go AS, Lloyd-Jones DM, et al. Heart Disease and Stroke Statistics — 2012 update: a report from the American Heart Association. *Circulation.* 2012;125(1):e2–e220.

103. Ross R, Berentzen T, Bradshaw AJ, et al. Does the relationship between waist circumference, morbidity and mortality depend on measurement protocol for waist circumference? *Obes Rev.* 2008;9(4):312–25.

104. Salzman SH. The 6-min walk test: clinical and research role, technique, coding, and reimbursement. *Chest.* 2009;135(5):1345–52.

105. Sesso HD, Paffenbarger RS Jr, Lee IM. Physical activity and coronary heart disease in men: the Harvard Alumni Health Study. *Circulation.* 2000;102(9):975–80.

106. Shephard RJ, Thomas S, Weller I. The Canadian Home Fitness Test. 1991 update. *Sports Med.* 1991;11(6):358–66.

107. Shields M, Tremblay MS, Laviolette M, Craig CL, Janssen I, Connor Gorber S. Fitness of Canadian adults: results from the 2007-2009 Canadian Health Measures Survey. *Health Rep.* 2010;21(1):21–35.

108. Siri WE. Body composition from fluid spaces and density: analysis of methods. *Nutrition.* 1961;9(5):480, 91; discussion 480, 492.

109. Stenholm S, Mehta NK, Elo IT, Heliövaara M, Koskinen S, Aromaa A. Obesity and muscle strength as long-term determinants of all-cause mortality — a 33-year follow-up of the Mini-Finland Health Examination Survey. *Int J Obes.* 2014;38(8):1126–32.

110. Swain DP, American College of Sports Medicine. *ACSM's Resource Manual for Guidelines for Exercise Testing and Prescription.* 7th ed. Baltimore (MD): Lippincott Williams & Wilkins; 2014. 896 p.

111. Swift DL, Lavie CJ, Johannsen NM, et al. Physical activity, cardiorespiratory fitness, and exercise training in primary and secondary coronary prevention. *Circ J.* 2013;77(2):281–92.

112. Tanaka H, Monahan KD, Seals DR. Age-predicted maximal heart rate revisited. *J Am Coll Cardiol.* 2001;37(1):153–6.

113. Tran ZV, Weltman A. Generalized equation for predicting body density of women from girth measurements. *Med Sci Sports Exerc.* 1989;21(1):101–4.

114. Tran ZV, Weltman A. Predicting body composition of men from girth measurements. *Hum Biol.* 1988;60(1):167–75.

115. U.S. Preventive Services Task Force, Barton M. Screening for obesity in children and adolescents: US Preventive Services Task Force recommendation statement. *Pediatrics.* 2010;125(2):361–7.

116. Wang CY, Haskell WL, Farrell SW, et al. Cardiorespiratory fitness levels among US adults 20–49 years of age: findings from the 1999–2004 National Health and Nutrition Examination Survey. *Am J Epidemiol.* 2010;171(4):426–35.

117. Wang J, Thornton JC, Bari S, et al. Comparisons of waist circumferences measured at 4 sites. *Am J Clin Nutr.* 2003;77(2):379–84.

118. Whaley MH, Brubaker PH, Kaminsky LA, Miller CR. Validity of rating of perceived exertion during graded exercise testing in apparently healthy adults and cardiac patients. *J Cardiopulm Rehabil.* 1997;17(4):261–7.

119. Williams MA, Haskell WL, Ades PA, et al. Resistance exercise in individuals with and without cardiovascular disease: 2007 update: a scientific statement from the American Heart Association Council on Clinical Cardiology and Council on Nutrition, Physical Activity, and Metabolism. *Circulation.* 2007;116(5):572–84.

120. YMCA of the USA, Golding LA. *YMCA Fitness Testing and Assessment Manual.* 4th ed. Champaign (IL): Human Kinetics; 2000. 247 p.

Clinical Exercise Testing and Interpretation

CHAPTER 5

INTRODUCTION

Clinical exercise testing has been part of the differential diagnosis of patients with suspected ischemic heart disease (IHD) for more than 50 yr. Although there are several indications for clinical exercise testing, most tests are likely performed as part of the diagnosis and evaluation of IHD. There are several evidence-based statements from professional organizations related to the conduct and application of clinical exercise testing. This chapter briefly summarizes these statements with a focus on noninvasive, symptom-limited, maximal exercise tests in adults with heart disease. Individuals who regularly perform or supervise clinical exercise tests should be familiar with the professional statements referenced in this chapter, especially those related to the conditions that are regularly presented in their clinic.

During a clinical exercise test, patients are monitored while performing incremental (most common) or constant work rate exercise using standardized protocols and procedures and typically using a treadmill or a stationary cycle ergometer (3,17,44). The purpose is to observe physiological responses to increasing or sustained metabolic demand. The clinical exercise test typically continues until the patient reaches a sign (*e.g.*, ST-segment depression) or symptom-limited (*e.g.*, angina, fatigue) maximal level of exertion. A clinical exercise test is often referred to as a graded exercise test (GXT), exercise stress test, or an exercise tolerance test (ETT). When an exercise test includes the analysis of expired gases during exercise, it is termed a *cardiopulmonary exercise test* (most often abbreviated CPX or CPET) or exercise metabolic test.

INDICATIONS FOR A CLINICAL EXERCISE TEST

Indications for clinical exercise testing encompass three general categories: (a) diagnosis (*e.g.*, presence of disease or abnormal physiologic response), (b) prognosis (*e.g.*, risk for an adverse event), and (c) evaluation of the physiologic response to exercise (*e.g.*, blood pressure [BP] and peak exercise capacity). The most common diagnostic indication is the assessment of symptoms suggestive of IHD. The American College of Cardiology (ACC) and the American Heart Association (AHA) recommend a logistic approach to determining the type of test to be used in the evaluation of someone presenting with stable chest pain (21). In this approach, a symptom-limited maximal exercise test with electrocardiographic monitoring only (*i.e.*, without adjunctive cardiac imaging) should initially be considered when the diagnosis of IHD is not certain, the patient has an interpretable resting electrocardiogram (ECG) (see "Electrocardiogram" section), and the patient is able to exercise (21,39).

Current evidence does not support the routine use of clinical exercise testing (with or without imaging) to screen for IHD or the risk of IHD-related events in asymptomatic individuals who have a very low or low pretest probability of IHD (21,43) nor individuals with a high pretest probability of IHD based on age, symptoms, and gender (21). Pretest likelihood of IHD is described in *Table 5.1*. The evidence also does not support the use of exercise testing with ECG alone to diagnose IHD in individuals on digitalis therapy with ST-segment depression on their resting ECG and for those who meet the ECG criteria for left ventricular hypertrophy with ST-segment depression on their resting ECG (21). Additionally, the exercise test with ECG alone is not useful for the diagnosis of IHD in patients with Wolff-Parkinson-White, ventricular pacing, >1 mm of ST-segment depression on their resting ECG, or left bundle branch block (21). Although these ECG abnormalities limit the utility of the exercise test with ECG alone in the diagnosis of IHD, there may be other indications in which a test with ECG alone is appropriate, such as the measurement of exercise capacity.

The clinical utility of exercise testing is described in several evidence-based guideline statements aimed at specific cardiac diagnoses (*Box 5.1*). In addition

TABLE 5.1					
Pretest Likelihood of Ischemic Heart Disease[a]					
Age	Sex	Typical/ Definite Angina Pectoris	Atypical/ Probable Angina Pectoris	Nonanginal Chest Pain	Asymptomatic
30 to 39 yr	Men	Intermediate	Intermediate	Low	Very low
	Women	Intermediate	Very low	Very low	Very low
40 to 49 yr	Men	High	Intermediate	Intermediate	Low
	Women	Intermediate	Low	Very low	Very low
50 to 59 yr	Men	High	Intermediate	Intermediate	Low
	Women	Intermediate	Intermediate	Low	Very low
60 to 69 yr	Men	High	Intermediate	Intermediate	Low
	Women	High	Intermediate	Intermediate	Low

[a]No data exist for patients who are <30 or >69 yr, but it can be assumed that prevalence of ischemic heart disease increases with age. In a few cases, patients with ages at the extremes of the decades listed may have probabilities slightly outside the high or low range. High indicates >90%; intermediate, 10%–90%; low, <10%; and very low, <5%.

Reprinted with permission from (21).

Box 5.1	**Select Evidence-Based Recommendations Regarding the Utility of Clinical Exercise Testing among Patients with Heart Disease**

Circumstance: Patients with ST-Segment Elevation Myocardial Infarction (STEMI) (2)

Recommendation: "Noninvasive testing for ischemia should be performed before discharge to assess the presence and extent of inducible ischemia in patients with STEMI who have not had coronary angiography and do not have high-risk clinical features for which coronary angiography would be warranted." (*class I — should be performed*)

Comment: "Exercise testing early after STEMI may also be performed to (a) assess functional capacity and the ability to perform tasks at home and at work, (b) evaluate the efficacy of medical therapy, and (c) assess the risk of a subsequent cardiac event. Symptom-limited exercise testing is a key feature of the intake evaluation for enrollment in a program of cardiac rehabilitation ≥2 wk after discharge."

Comment: "Low-level exercise testing after MI appears to be safe if patients have undergone in-hospital cardiac rehabilitation, including low-level exercise; have had no symptoms of angina or HF; and have a stable baseline ECG 48–72 h before the test. Two different protocols have been used for early post-MI exercise testing: the traditional submaximal exercise test (done at 3–5 d in patients without complications) or a symptom-limited exercise test (done at 5 d or later) without stopping at a prespecified target heart rate or metabolic equivalent level."

Comment: "[P]atients without complications who have not undergone coronary angiography and who might be potential candidates for revascularization should undergo provocative testing before hospital discharge. In patients with noninfarct coronary artery disease who have undergone successful PCI of the infarct artery and have an uncomplicated course, it is reasonable to proceed with discharge and plans for close clinical follow-up with stress imaging within 3 to 6 weeks."

Circumstance: Risk Stratification before Discharge in the Absence of Invasive Intervention in Patients with Non–ST-Segment Elevation (NSTE) Acute Coronary Syndrome (ACS) (6)

Recommendation: "Noninvasive stress testing is recommended in low and intermediate-risk patients who have been free of ischemia at rest or with low-level activity for a minimum of 12 to 24 hours." (*class I — should be performed*)

Recommendation: "[Low-level or symptom-limited] treadmill exercise testing is useful in patients able to exercise in whom the ECG is free of resting ST changes that may interfere with interpretation." (*class I — should be performed*)

Comment: "Low- and intermediate-risk patients with NSTE-ACS may undergo symptom-limited stress testing, provided they have been asymptomatic and clinically stable at 12 to 24 hours for those with [unstable angina] and 2 to 5 days for patients at similar risk with NSTEMI."

(continued)

| Box 5.1 | Select Evidence-Based Recommendations Regarding the Utility of Clinical Exercise Testing among Patients with Heart Disease (*Continued*) |

Circumstance: Ischemic Heart Disease (IHD) (15)

Indication: Initial diagnosis of suspected IHD

Recommendation: "Standard exercise ECG testing is recommended for patients with an intermediate pretest probability of IHD who have an interpretable ECG and at least moderate physical functioning or no disabling comorbidity." (*class I — should be performed*)

Recommendation: "Standard exercise ECG testing is not recommended for patients who have an uninterpretable ECG or are incapable of at least moderate physical functioning or have disabling comorbidity." (*class III — no benefit*)

Indication: Risk assessment in patients with stable IHD

Recommendation: "Standard exercise ECG testing is recommended for risk assessment in patients with [stable IHD] who are able to exercise to an adequate workload and have an interpretable ECG." (*class I — should be performed*)

Indication: Diagnostic assessment in symptomatic patients with known stable IHD

Recommendation: "Standard exercise ECG testing is recommended in patients with known [stable IHD] who have new or worsening symptoms not consistent with [unstable angina] and who have (a) at least moderate physical functioning and no disabling comorbidity and (b) an interpretable ECG." (*class I — should be performed*)

Indication: Prognosis and exercise prescription in patients with stable IHD

Recommendation: "For all patients, risk assessment with a physical activity history and/or an exercise test is recommended to guide prognosis and prescription." (*class I — should be performed*)

Indication: Follow-up assessment in asymptomatic patients with known stable IHD

Recommendation: "Standard exercise ECG testing performed at 1 yr or longer intervals might be considered for follow-up assessment in patients with [stable IHD] who have had prior evidence of silent ischemia or are at high risk for a recurrent cardiac event and are able to exercise to an adequate workload and have an interpretable ECG." (*class IIb — may be considered*)

Recommendation: "In patients who have no new or worsening symptoms or no prior evidence of silent ischemia and are not at high risk for a recurrent cardiac event, the usefulness of annual surveillance exercise ECG testing is not well established." (*class IIb — may be considered*)

Circumstance: Preoperative Cardiovascular Evaluation (16)

Recommendation: "For patients with elevated risk and unknown functional capacity, it may be reasonable to perform exercise testing to assess for functional capacity if it will change management." (*class IIb — may be considered*)

Recommendation: "Routine screening with noninvasive stress testing is not useful for patients at low risk for noncardiac surgery." (*class III — no benefit*)

Recommendation: "Cardiopulmonary exercise testing may be considered for patients undergoing elevated risk procedures in whom functional capacity is unknown." (*class IIb — may be considered*)

(continued)

Box 5.1 (continued)

Recommendation: "Routine screening with noninvasive stress testing is not useful for patients undergoing low-risk noncardiac surgery." (class III — no benefit)

Circumstance: Adults with Chronic Heart Failure (HF)

Recommendation: "Maximal exercise testing with or without measurement of respiratory gas exchange and/or blood oxygen saturation is reasonable in patients presenting with HF to help determine whether HF is the cause of exercise limitation when the contribution of HF is uncertain." (class IIa — reasonable to perform) (26)

Recommendation: "Maximal exercise testing with measurement of respiratory gas exchange is reasonable to identify high-risk patients presenting with HF who are candidates for cardiac transplantation or other advanced treatments." (class IIa — reasonable to perform) (26)

Recommendation: "Exercise testing should be considered [in patients with HF]: (i) To detect reversible myocardial ischemia; (ii) As part of the evaluation of patients for heart transplantation and mechanical circulatory support; (iii) To aid in the prescription of exercise training; (iv) To obtain prognostic information." (class IIa — should be considered) (36)

Circumstance: Percutaneous Coronary Intervention (PCI) (31)

Recommendation: "In patients entering a formal cardiac rehabilitation program after PCI, treadmill exercise testing is reasonable." (class IIa — reasonable to perform)

Recommendation: "Routine periodic stress testing of asymptomatic patients after PCI without specific clinical indications should not be performed." (class III — no benefit)

Circumstance: Valvular Heart Disease (VHD) (49)

Recommendation: "Exercise testing is reasonable in selected patients with asymptomatic severe VHD to 1) confirm the absence of symptoms, or 2) assess the hemodynamic response to exercise, or 3) determine prognosis." (class IIa — reasonable to perform)

Recommendation: "Exercise testing is reasonable to assess physiological changes with exercise and to confirm the absence of symptoms in asymptomatic patients with a calcified aortic valve and an aortic velocity 4.0 m per second or greater or mean pressure gradient 40 mm Hg or higher (stage C)." (class IIa — reasonable to perform)

Recommendation: "Exercise testing should not be performed in symptomatic patients with AS when the aortic velocity is 4.0 m per second or greater or mean pressure gradient is 40 mm Hg or higher (stage D)." (class III — may be harmful)

Comment: "Exercise testing may be helpful in clarifying symptom status in patients with severe AS."

Comment: "Exercise stress testing can be used to assess symptomatic status and functional capacity in patients with AR."

Recommendation: "Exercise testing with Doppler or invasive hemodynamic assessment is recommended to evaluate the response of the mean mitral gradient and pulmonary artery pressure in patients with mitral stenosis when there is a discrepancy between resting Doppler echocardiographic findings and clinical symptoms or signs." (class I — should be performed)

(continued)

Box 5.1	Select Evidence-Based Recommendations Regarding the Utility of Clinical Exercise Testing among Patients with Heart Disease (*Continued*)

Recommendation: "Exercise hemodynamics with either Doppler echocardiography or cardiac catheterization is reasonable in symptomatic patients with chronic primary MR where there is a discrepancy between symptoms and the severity of MR at rest (stages B and C)." (*class IIa — reasonable to perform*)

Recommendation: "Exercise testing may be considered for the assessment of exercise capacity in patients with severe TR with no or minimal symptoms (stage C)." (*class IIb — may be considered*)

Recommendation: "Exercise testing is reasonable in asymptomatic patients with severe AS (stage C) . . . or severe valve regurgitation (stage C) before pregnancy." (*class IIa — reasonable to perform*)

Comment: "Evaluation for concurrent [coronary artery disease] in patients with AS is problematic, and standard ECG exercise testing is not adequate."

AR, aortic regurgitation; AS, aortic stenosis; ECG, electrocardiogram; MI, myocardial infarction; MR, mitral regurgitation; NSTEMI, non–ST-segment elevation myocardial infarction; TR, tricuspid regurgitation.

to indications listed in *Box 5.1*, an exercise test can be useful in the evaluation of patients who present to emergency departments with chest pain. This practice (a) appears to be safe in patients who are at low-to-intermediate risk for IHD and have been appropriately screened by a physician, (b) may improve the accuracy of diagnosing acute coronary syndrome, and (c) may reduce the cost of care by reducing the need for additional tests and length of stay (5). Generally, exercise testing may be appropriate for patients whose symptoms have resolved, have a normal ECG, and had no change in enzymes reflecting cardiac muscle damage. Exercise testing in this setting (often called a *chest pain unit*) should be performed only as part of well-defined clinical care pathway (5).

Additional indications that might warrant the use of a clinical exercise test include the assessment of various pulmonary diseases (*e.g.*, chronic obstructive pulmonary disease) (3,13), exercise intolerance and unexplained dyspnea (3,10,13), exercise-induced bronchoconstriction (3,13,52), exercise-induced arrhythmias (21), pacemaker or heart rate (HR) response to exercise (21), preoperative risk evaluation (3,13,16), claudication in peripheral arterial disease (58), disability evaluation (3,10,13), and physical activity (PA) counseling (3,13,21).

In addition to the diagnostic utility, data from a clinical exercise test can be useful to predict prognosis. There is an inverse relationship between cardiorespiratory fitness (CRF) measured from an exercise test and the risk of mortality among apparently healthy individuals (8); patients at risk for IHD (47); and those with diagnosed heart disease (3,10,28), heart failure (3,10), and lung disease (7,14,24,40).

In addition to CRF, other measures from an exercise test have been associated with prognosis, such as the chronotropic response during or after an exercise test (12,30,42,50).

Clinical exercise testing is useful in guiding recommendations for return to work after a cardiac event (see *Chapter 9*) as well as developing an exercise prescription (Ex R$_x$) in those with known heart disease (21). In addition, the maximal exercise test is the gold standard to objectively measure exercise capacity. Although exercise time and/or peak workload achieved during an exercise test can be used to estimate peak metabolic equivalents (METs), the best measurement of exercise capacity is via respiratory gas analysis using open circuit indirect calorimetry for the determination of maximal volume of oxygen consumed per unit of time ($\dot{V}O_{2max}$) (8,21).

CONDUCTING THE CLINICAL EXERCISE TEST

When administering clinical exercise tests, it is important to consider contraindications, the exercise test protocol and mode, test endpoint indicators, safety, medications, and staff and facility emergency preparedness (17,44). The AHA (17) has outlined both absolute and relative contraindications to clinical exercise testing (*Box 5.2*). These contraindications are intended to avoid unstable ischemic, rhythm, or hemodynamic conditions or other situations in which the risk associated with undergoing the exercise test is likely to exceed the information to be gained from it.

Prior to the exercise test, patients should be provided informed consent to ensure that they understand the purpose, expectations, and risks associated with the test (see *Chapter 3*) (44). The extent and quality of data obtained from a symptom-limited maximal exercise test depends on the patient's ability and willingness to provide a maximal exertion; therefore, it is important to educate the patient about what he or she may experience during the test (*e.g.*, fatigue, dyspnea, chest pain) (44). Prior to performing an exercise test, the medical history (including current and recent symptoms), current medications (see *Appendix A*), and indications for the test should be noted (44). Lastly, the resting ECG should be examined for abnormalities that may preclude testing, such as new-onset atrial fibrillation or new repolarization changes (44). Also, if the purpose of the exercise test is the assessment of exercise-induced myocardial ischemia, the resting ECG must allow for interpretation of exercise-induced repolarization changes (21,44); otherwise, consideration should be given to adjunctive imaging procedures such as nuclear or echocardiographic imaging (21). These additional imaging procedures are not necessary if the exercise test is being conducted for reasons other than the assessment of myocardial ischemia.

Testing Staff

Over the past several decades, there has been a transition in many exercise testing laboratories from tests being administered by physicians to nonphysician allied

Box 5.2	Contraindications to Symptom-Limited Maximal Exercise Testing

Absolute Contraindications

- Acute myocardial infarction within 2 d
- Ongoing unstable angina
- Uncontrolled cardiac arrhythmia with hemodynamic compromise
- Active endocarditis
- Symptomatic severe aortic stenosis
- Decompensated heart failure
- Acute pulmonary embolism, pulmonary infarction, or deep venous thrombosis
- Acute myocarditis or pericarditis
- Acute aortic dissection
- Physical disability that precludes safe and adequate testing

Relative Contraindications

- Known obstructive left main coronary artery stenosis
- Moderate to severe aortic stenosis with uncertain relationship to symptoms
- Tachyarrhythmias with uncontrolled ventricular rates
- Acquired advanced or complete heart block
- Recent stroke or transient ischemia attack
- Mental impairment with limited ability to cooperate
- Resting hypertension with systolic >200 mm Hg or diastolic >110 mm Hg
- Uncorrected medical conditions, such as significant anemia, important electrolyte imbalance, and hyperthyroidism

Reprinted with permission from (17).

health professionals, such as clinical exercise physiologists, nurses, physical therapists, and physician assistants. This shift from physician to nonphysician staff has occurred to contain staffing costs and improve utilization of physician time (46). These allied health care professionals are not intended to replace the knowledge and skills of a physician (46). The overall supervision of clinical exercise testing laboratories as well as the interpretation of test results remains the legal responsibility of the supervising physician (44,46,57).

According to the ACC and AHA, the nonphysician allied health care professional who administers clinical exercise tests should have cognitive skills similar to, although not as extensive as, the physician who provides the final interpretation (57). These skills are presented in *Box 5.3*. In addition, this individual should perform at least 50 exercise tests with preceptor supervision (57). However, 200 supervised exercise tests before independence has also been recommended (46). Recommendations for maintenance of competency vary from between 25 (57) and 50 (46) exercise tests per year. Appropriately trained nonphysician staff can safely administer maximal clinical exercise tests when a qualified physician is "in the immediate vicinity . . . and available for emergencies" (46) and who later reviews and provides final interpretation of the test results (44). There are no differences

Box 5.3	**Cognitive Skills Required to Competently Supervise Clinical Exercise Tests**

- Knowledge of appropriate indications for exercise testing
- Knowledge of alternative physiologic cardiovascular tests
- Knowledge of appropriate contraindications, risks, and risk assessment of testing
- Knowledge to promptly recognize and treat complications of exercise testing
- Competence in cardiopulmonary resuscitation and successful completion of an American Heart Association–sponsored course in advanced cardiovascular life support and renewal on a regular basis
- Knowledge of various exercise protocols and indications for each
- Knowledge of basic cardiovascular and exercise physiology including hemodynamic response to exercise
- Knowledge of cardiac arrhythmias and the ability to recognize and treat serious arrhythmias (see *Appendix C*)
- Knowledge of cardiovascular drugs and how they can affect exercise performance, hemodynamics, and the electrocardiogram (see *Appendix A*)
- Knowledge of the effects of age and disease on hemodynamic and the electrocardiographic response to exercise
- Knowledge of principles and details of exercise testing including proper lead placement and skin preparation
- Knowledge of endpoints of exercise testing and indications to terminate exercise testing

Adapted from (57).

in morbidity and mortality rates related to maximal exercise testing when the testing is performed by an appropriately trained allied health professional compared to a physician (46). Although the AHA does define high-risk patient groups in which they recommend that a physician provide "personal supervision" (*i.e.*, the physician is directly present in the exercise testing room) (46), empirical evidence suggests that "direct supervision" (*i.e.*, the physician is available within the vicinity of the exercise testing room) (46) and "general supervision" (*i.e.*, the physician is available by phone) (46) are the models employed in the majority of noninvasive clinical exercise testing laboratories in the United States, regardless of the disease severity of patients being tested.

In addition to the test administrator (physician or nonphysician), at least one support technician should assist with testing (44). This person should have knowledge and skills in obtaining informed consent and medical history, skin preparation and ECG electrode placement, equipment operation, the measurement of BP at rest and during exercise, and effective patient interaction skills (44).

Testing Mode and Protocol

The mode selected for the exercise test can impact the results and should be selected based on the test purpose and patient preference (17). In the United States, treadmill is the most frequently used mode, whereas a cycle ergometer is more common in Europe. With the potential exception of highly trained cyclists, peak exercise capacity (*e.g.*, peak oxygen consumption [$\dot{V}O_{2peak}$]) can be 5%–20% lower during a maximal exercise test performed on a cycle ergometer compared to a treadmill due to regional muscle fatigue (3,8,17,44). This range of 5%–20% suggests interstudy and interindividual variability. Based on anecdotal evidence, a 10% difference is typically used by clinicians when comparing peak exercise responses between cycle ergometry and treadmill exercise. Optimally, the same exercise mode would be used at each time point when tracking a patient's response over time. Other exercise testing modes may be considered as needed, such as arm ergometry, dual-action ergometry, or seated stepping ergometry. These can be useful options for patients with balance issues, amputation, extreme obesity, and other mobility deficiencies.

The use of a standardized exercise protocol, such as those shown in *Figure 5.1*, represents a convenient and repeatable way to conduct the exercise test, for both the patient and the clinician supervising the test. There are few guidelines for the selection of the exercise protocol. Most clinicians select a protocol with an initial level of exertion that is submaximal with increments of work that are of similar magnitude. The Bruce treadmill protocol is the most widely used exercise protocol in the United States (48). This will likely continue due to physician familiarity and the breadth of research based on the Bruce protocol (19,34,45).

When performing a sign- and symptom-limited maximal exercise test, it is often recommended that the selected exercise testing protocol results in a total exercise duration of 6–12 min (17,21,44). To assist in the protocol selection, the patient's medical and PA history and symptomology should be considered. The aerobic requirements associated with the first stage of the Bruce protocol (~5 METs) and the large increases between stages (~3 METs) make it less than optimal for persons who may have a low functional capacity. As such, the Bruce protocol can result in extensive handrail support and over an estimation of the patient's peak exercise capacity based on the exercise duration or peak workload achieved (23,34). In response to these limitations, modifications of the Bruce protocol and other treadmill and cycle ergometry protocols have been developed, including patient-specific ramping protocols (18,23,27,45,54). *Figure 5.1* shows some common protocols and the estimated metabolic requirement for each.

Monitoring and Test Termination

Variables that are typically monitored during clinical exercise testing include HR; ECG; cardiac rhythm; BP; perceived exertion; and clinical signs and patient-reported symptoms suggestive of myocardial ischemia, inadequate blood perfusion, inadequate gas diffusion, and limitations in pulmonary ventilation (17,21,44). Measurement of expired gases through open circuit spirometry during a CPET and oxygen saturation of blood through pulse oximetry and/or arterial blood gases are also obtained when indicated (3,8,10,44).

METS	CYCLE ERGOMETER	RAMP		MODIFIED BRUCE 3 min Stages		BRUCE 3 min Stages		NAUGHTON 2 min Stages		MODIFIED NAUGHTON (CHF) 2 min Stages	
				MPH	%GR	MPH	%GR				
21	FOR 70 KG BODY WEIGHT										
20				6.0	22	6.0	22				
19	1 WATT = 6.1 Kpm/min										
18				5.5	20	5.5	20				
17											
16											
15	Kpm/min			5.0	18	5.0	18				
14	1500	PER 30 SEC								MPH	%GR
13		MPH	%GR	4.2	16	4.2	16			3.0	25
		3.0	25.0								
		3.0	24.0								
12	1350	3.0	23.0							3.0	22.5
		3.0	22.0								
11	1200	3.0	21.0							3.0	20
		3.0	20.0								
10	1050	3.0	19.0	3.4	14	3.4	14			3.0	17.5
		3.0	18.0								
		3.0	17.0								
9	900	3.0	16.0					MPH	%GR	3.0	15
		3.0	15.0								
8		3.0	14.0					2	17.5	3.0	12.5
	750	3.0	13.0								
7		3.0	12.0	2.5	12	2.5	12	2	14.0	3.0	10
		3.0	11.0								
	600	3.0	10.0								
6		3.0	9.0							3.0	7.5
		3.0	8.0					2	10.5		
5	450	3.0	7.0	1.7	10	1.7	10			2.0	10.5
		3.0	6.0					2	7.0		
		3.0	5.0								
4	300	3.0	4.0					2	3.5	2.0	7.0
		3.0	3.0								
3		3.0	2.0	1.7	5			2	0	2.0	3.5
	150	3.0	1.0								
2		3.0	0	1.7	0			1	0	1.5	0
		2.5	0								
		2.0	0								
1		1.5	0							1.0	0
		1.0	0								
		0.5	0								

Figure 5.1 Common treadmill and stationary cycle ergometry protocols used in symptom-limited maximal exercise testing with exercise workload and metabolic demand. MET, metabolic equivalents of task; MPH, miles per hour; %GR, percent grade; KPM, kilopond meter; min, minute; kg, kilogram; CHF, congestive heart failure. METs reflect the estimated value for each stage. Modified with permission from (17).

Table 5.2 outlines best practices for monitoring during a symptom-limited maximal exercise test. A high-quality ECG tracing can be obtained during an exercise test. However, this requires more attention to preparation of the patient and lead placement than is typically required for a resting ECG. A thorough discussion of ECG preparation is provided by Fletcher et al. (17). HR and BP should be assessed and an

TABLE 5.2

Best Practices for Monitoring during a Symptom-Limited Maximal Exercise Test

Variable	Before Exercise Test	During Exercise Test	After Exercise Test
Electrocardiogram	Monitor continuously; record in supine position and position of exercise (e.g., standing).	Monitor continuously; record during the last 5–10 s of each stage or every 2 min (ramp protocol).	Monitor continuously; record immediately postexercise, after 60 s of recovery and then every 2 min.
Heart rate[a]	Monitor continuously; record in supine position and position of exercise (e.g., standing).	Monitor continuously; record during the last 5–10 s of each minute.	Monitor continuously; record during the last 5–10 s of each minute.
Blood pressure[a,b]	Monitor continuously; record in supine position and position of exercise (e.g., standing).	Measure and record during the last 30–60 s of each stage or every 2 min (ramp protocol).	Measure and record immediately postexercise, after 60 s of recovery and then every 2 min.
Signs and symptoms	Monitor continuously; record as observed.	Monitor continuously; record as observed.	Monitor continuously; record as observed or as symptoms resolve.
Rating of perceived exertion	Explain scale.	Record during the last 5–10 s each stage or every 2 min (ramp protocol).	Obtain peak exercise shortly after exercise is terminated.

[a]In addition, heart rate and blood pressure should be assessed and recorded whenever adverse symptoms or abnormal electrocardiogram changes occur.
[b]An unchanged or decreasing systolic blood pressure with increasing workloads should be retaken (i.e., verified immediately).

Adapted and used with permission from Brubaker PH, Kaminsky LA, Whaley MH. *Coronary Artery Disease: Essentials of Prevention and Rehabilitation Programs.* Champaign (IL): Human Kinetics; 2002. 364 p.

ECG recorded regularly during the test (e.g., each stage or every 2–3 min) at peak exercise and regularly through at least 6 min of recovery (17,21,44). It can also be helpful to assess the patient's perceived exertion regularly during the exercise test and at peak exercise. Throughout the test, the ECG should be continuously monitored for repolarization changes suggestive of myocardial ischemia and dysrhythmias (17,21,44).

During the test and through postexercise recovery, the clinician should also monitor the patient for untoward symptoms, such as light-headedness, angina, dyspnea, claudication (if suspected by history), and fatigue (see *Table 2.1*) (17,21,44). In the case of chest pain that is suspected to be angina pectoris, the timing, character, magnitude, and resolution should be described (44). The appearance of symptoms should be correlated with HR, BP, and ECG abnormalities (when present). Standardized scales to assess perceived exertion (see *Table 4.6* and *Figure 5.2*), angina, dyspnea, and claudication (*Figure 5.3*) are available. Although scales to assess these symptoms have been recommended by the AHA (44), some clinical exercise testing laboratories use a 10-point visual analog pain scale (see *Figure 11.1*).

The analysis of expired gas during a CPET overcomes the potential inaccuracies associated with estimating exercise capacity from peak workload (*e.g.*, treadmill speed and grade). The direct measurement of $\dot{V}O_2$ is the most accurate measure of exercise capacity and is a useful index of overall cardiopulmonary health (3,10).

Borg CR10 Scale®

0	Nothing at all	
0.3		
0.5	Extremely weak	Just noticeable
0.7		
1	Very weak	
1.5		
2	Weak	Light
2.5		
3	Moderate	
4		
5	Strong	Heavy
6		
7	Very strong	
8		
9		
10	Extremely strong	"Maximal"
11		
{		
•	Absolute maximum	Highest possible

Figure 5.2 The Borg category–ratio scale. Printed with permission from Borg G, Borg E. *The Borg CR Scales Folder.* Hässelby (Sweden): Borg Perception; 2010.

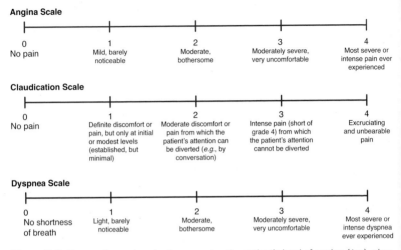

Figure 5.3 Frequently used scales for assessing the patient's level of angina (*top*), claudication (*middle*), and dyspnea (*bottom*).

The CPET provides additional data that is not available without expired gas analysis, such as the respiratory exchange ratio (RER), ventilatory-derived anaerobic threshold (VAT), and the rate of change of minute ventilation (volume of expired air per unit time [$\dot{V}E$] to change in volume of carbon dioxide exhaled [$\dot{V}CO_2$] during exercise (*i.e.*, $\dot{V}E/\dot{V}CO_2$ slope; an indicator of ventilatory efficiency). The CPET is useful in the differentiation of the cause of exertional dyspnea and the risk stratification of many patient groups, particularly those with heart failure (3,8,10). There are several extensive resources available on CPET (3,10,37).

Oxygen desaturation may be a cause of exertional dyspnea in some patients. Although measurement of the partial pressure of arterial oxygen (P_aO_2) and partial pressure of carbon dioxide in arterial blood (P_aCO_2) via the measurement of arterial blood gases is the gold standard, pulse oximetry provides a noninvasive, indirect measure of arterial oxygen saturation (SpO_2). In patients with pulmonary disease, direct measurements of percent saturation of arterial oxygen (SaO_2) correlate reasonably well with SpO_2 ($\pm 2\%$–3%) provided SpO_2 remains $>85\%$ (3,10). An absolute decrease in $SpO_2 \geq 5\%$ during exercise is considered an abnormal response suggestive of exercise-induced hypoxemia, and follow-up testing with arterial blood gases may be indicated (3,10). An $SpO_2 \leq 80\%$ with signs or symptoms of hypoxemia is an indication to stop a test (3). The measurement of SpO_2 with pulse oximetry through a fingertip probe can be affected by low perfusion or low pulse wave, dyshemoglobinemias (*i.e.*, hemoglobin abnormalities), low oxygen saturation, very dark skin tone, nail polish, acrylic nails (55), and movement during exercise. Alternate probe locations such as the earlobe or forehead can be helpful.

Box 5.4	Indications for Terminating a Symptom-Limited Maximal Exercise Test

Absolute Indications

- ST elevation (>1.0 mm) in leads without preexisting Q waves because of prior MI (other than aVR, aVL, or V_1)
- Drop in systolic blood pressure of >10 mm Hg, despite an increase in workload, when accompanied by other evidence of ischemia
- Moderate-to-severe angina
- Central nervous system symptoms (*e.g.*, ataxia, dizziness, or near syncope)
- Signs of poor perfusion (cyanosis or pallor)
- Sustained ventricular tachycardia or other arrhythmia, including second- or third-degree atrioventricular block, that interferes with normal maintenance of cardiac output during exercise
- Technical difficulties monitoring the ECG or systolic blood pressure
- The subject's request to stop

Relative Indications

- Marked ST displacement (horizontal or downsloping of >2 mm, measured 60 to 80 ms after the J point in a patient with suspected ischemia)
- Drop in systolic blood pressure >10 mm Hg (persistently below baseline) despite an increase in workload, *in the absence* of other evidence of ischemia
- Increasing chest pain
- Fatigue, shortness of breath, wheezing, leg cramps, or claudication
- Arrhythmias other than sustained ventricular tachycardia, including multifocal ectopy, ventricular triplets, supraventricular tachycardia, and bradyarrhythmias that have the potential to become more complex or to interfere with hemodynamic stability
- Exaggerated hypertensive response (systolic blood pressure >250 mm Hg or diastolic blood pressure >115 mm Hg)
- Development of bundle-branch block that cannot be distinguished from ventricular tachycardia
- SpO_2 ≤80% (3)

ECG, electrocardiogram; MI, myocardial infarction; SpO_2, percent saturation of arterial oxygen.
Adapted with permission from (21).

Termination criteria for clinical exercise testing have been established by the AHA and ACC (17) (*Box 5.4*). When the goal is a symptom-limited maximal exercise test, a predetermined intensity, such as an 85% of the age-predicted maximal heart rate (HR_{max}) should not be used as a reason to end the test (17,21). Failure to continue a test until the patient attains maximal exertion or a clinical limitation will result in an underestimation of the patient's peak exercise capacity. Some clinicians view the achievement of 85% of the age-predicted HR_{max} as adequate level of stress for revealing exertional ischemia; however, the sensitivity of exercise test results is increased when the HR achieved is greater than 85% of predicted (17).

Postexercise

The sensitivity of the exercise test for the diagnosis of IHD can be maximized when the patient is placed in a seated or supine position immediately following exercise (17,44). Therefore, if the primary indication of the test is suspected IHD and nonsignificant repolarization changes are observed at peak exercise, then immediate supine recovery without active recovery should be considered. However, exercise cessation can cause an excessive drop in venous return resulting in profound hypotension during recovery and ischemia secondary to decreased perfusion pressure into the myocardium. Therefore, continuation of low-intensity active recovery during the postexercise period is often practiced in order to support venous return and hemodynamic stability. Each laboratory should develop standardized procedures for the postexercise recovery period (active vs. inactive and monitoring duration) with the laboratory's medical director that considers the indication for the exercise test and the patient's status during the test.

Safety

Although untoward events do occur, clinical exercise testing is generally safe when performed by appropriately trained clinicians. The classic data of Rochmis and Blackburn (56) reported a rate of serious complications (morbidity or mortality) of 34 events per 10,000 tests. Excluding studies of patients tested with a history of life-threatening ventricular arrhythmias, among 17 studies, serious complications during clinical exercise tests ranged from 0 to 35 events per 10,000 tests, with rates typically higher among patients known to have higher mortality rates, such as patients with heart failure (46). However, prior studies might overestimate the risk of today's patients given advances in medicine, such as the implantable cardioverter defibrillator (46).

In tests that are performed to assess the likelihood of IHD, some physicians might request that select patients withhold medications that are known to limit the hemodynamic response to exercise (*e.g.*, β-adrenergic blocking agents) because they may limit test sensitivity (17,21). However, for most test indications, patients are encouraged to continue to take their medications on the day of testing (21). If the indication for the exercise test is to evaluate the effectiveness (*e.g.*, change in exercise capacity) of medical therapy, then patients should be instructed to continue their normal medical regimen (21).

INTERPRETING THE CLINICAL EXERCISE TEST

Multiple factors should be considered during the interpretation of exercise test data including patient symptoms, ECG responses, exercise capacity, hemodynamic responses, and the combination of multiple responses, as reflected by exercise test scores such as the Duke Treadmill Score (discussed later).

Heart Rate Response

The normal HR response to incremental exercise is to increase with increasing workloads at a rate of ≈ 10 beats $\cdot$ min^{-1} per 1 MET (17). HR$_{max}$ decreases with age and is attenuated in patients on β-adrenergic blocking agents. Several equations have been published to predict HR$_{max}$ in individuals who are not taking a β-adrenergic blocking agent (see *Table 6.2*) (17). All estimates have large interindividual variability with standard deviations of 10 beats or more (11).

Among patients referred for testing secondary to IHD and in the absence of β-adrenergic blocking agents, failure to achieve an age-predicted HR$_{max}$ $\geq 85\%$ in the presence of maximal effort is an indicator of chronotropic incompetence and is independently associated with increased risk of morbidity and mortality (17). An abnormal chronotropic response provides prognostic information that is independent of myocardial perfusion. The combination of a myocardial perfusion abnormality and an abnormal chronotropic response suggests a worse prognosis than either abnormality alone (29).

The rate of decline in HR following exercise provides independent information related to prognosis (17). A failure of the HR to decrease by at least 12 beats during the first minute or 22 beats by the end of the second minute of active postexercise recovery is strongly associated with an increased risk of mortality in patients diagnosed with or at increased risk for IHD (17,29). The failure of HR to recover adequately may be related to the inability of the parasympathetic nervous system to reassert vagal control of HR, which is known to predispose individuals to ventricular dysrhythmias (29).

Blood Pressure Response

The normal systolic blood pressure (SBP) response to exercise is to increase with increasing workloads at a rate of ~ 10 mm Hg per 1 MET (17). On average, this response is greater among men; increases with age; and is attenuated in patients on vasodilators, calcium channel blockers, angiotensin-converting enzyme inhibitors, and α- and β-adrenergic blockers. Specific SBP responses are defined in the following:

- Hypertensive response: An SBP >250 mm Hg is a relative indication to stop a test (see *Box 5.4*) (17). An SBP ≥ 210 mm Hg in men and ≥ 190 mm Hg in women during exercise is considered an exaggerated response (17). A peak SBP >250 mm Hg or an increase in SBP >140 mm Hg during exercise above the pretest resting value is predictive of future resting hypertension (53).
- Hypotensive response: A decrease of SBP below the pretest resting value or by >10 mm Hg after a preliminary increase, particularly in the presence of other indices of ischemia, is abnormal and often associated with myocardial ischemia, left ventricular dysfunction, and an increased risk of subsequent cardiac events (17).

- Blunted response: In patients with a limited ability to augment cardiac output ($\dot{Q}$), the response of SBP during exercise will be slower compared to normal.
- Postexercise response: SBP typically returns to preexercise levels or lower by 6 min of recovery (17). Studies have demonstrated that a delay in the recovery of SBP is highly related both to ischemic abnormalities and to a poor prognosis (4,35).

There is normally no change or a slight decrease in diastolic blood pressure (DBP) during an exercise test. A peak DBP >90 mm Hg or an increase in DBP >10 mm Hg during exercise above the pretest resting value is considered an abnormal response (17) and may occur with exertional ischemia (53). A DBP >115 mm Hg is an exaggerated response and a relative indication to stop a test (see *Box 5.4*) (17).

Rate-Pressure Product

Rate-pressure product (also known as *double product*) is calculated by multiplying the values for HR and SBP that occur at the same time during rest or exercise. Rate-pressure product is a surrogate for myocardial oxygen uptake (17). There is a linear relationship between myocardial oxygen uptake and both coronary blood flow and exercise intensity (17). Coronary blood flow increases due to increased myocardial oxygen demand as a result of increases in HR and myocardial contractility. If coronary blood flow supply is impaired, which can occur in obstructive IHD, then signs or symptoms of myocardial ischemia may be present. The point during exercise when this occurs is the ischemic threshold. Rate-pressure product is a repeatable estimate of the ischemic threshold and more reliable than external workload (17). The normal range for peak rate-pressure product is 25,000–40,000 mm Hg $\cdot$ beats $\cdot$ min^{-1} (17). Rate-pressure product at peak exercise and at the ischemic threshold (when applicable) should be reported.

Electrocardiogram

The normal response of the ECG during exercise includes the following (17):

- P-wave: increased magnitude among inferior leads
- PR segment: shortens and slopes downward among inferior leads
- QRS: Duration decreases, septal Q-waves increase among lateral leads, R waves decrease, and S waves increase among inferior leads.
- J point (J junction): depresses below isoelectric line with upsloping ST segments that reach the isoelectric line within 80 ms
- T-wave: decreases amplitude in early exercise, returns to preexercise amplitude at higher exercise intensities, and may exceed preexercise amplitude in recovery
- QT interval: Absolute QT interval decreases. The QT interval corrected for HR increases with early exercise and then decreases at higher HRs.

Box 5.5	**Considerations That May Necessitate Adjunctive Imaging When the Indication Is the Assessment of Ischemic Heart Disease (21)**

- Resting ST-segment depression >1.0 mm
- Ventricular paced rhythm
- Left ventricular hypertrophy with repolarization abnormalities
- Left bundle-branch block
- Leads V1 through V3 will not be interpretable with right bundle-branch block.
- Wolff-Parkinson-White
- Digitalis therapy

ST-segment changes (*i.e.*, depression and elevation) are widely accepted criteria for myocardial ischemia and injury. The interpretation of ST segments may be affected by the resting ECG configuration and the presence of digitalis therapy (17,21). Considerations that may indicate that an exercise test with ECG only would be inadequate for the diagnosis of IHD are shown in *Box 5.5*.

Abnormal responses of the ST segment during exercise include the following (17):

- To be clinically meaningful, ST-segment depression or elevation should be present in at least three consecutive cardiac cycles within the same lead. The level of the ST segment should be compared relative to the end of the PR segment. Automated computer-averaged complexes should be visually confirmed.
- Horizontal or downsloping ST-segment depression ≥1 mm (0.1 mV) at 80 ms after the J point is a strong indicator of myocardial ischemia.
- Clinically significant ST-segment depression that occurs during postexercise recovery is an indicator of myocardial ischemia.
- ST-segment depression at a low workload or low rate-pressure product is associated with worse prognosis and increased likelihood for multivessel disease.
- When ST-segment depression is present in the upright resting ECG, only additional ST-segment depression during exercise is considered for ischemia.
- When ST-segment elevation is present in the upright resting ECG, only ST-segment depression below the isoelectric line during exercise is considered for ischemia.
- Upsloping ST-segment depression ≥2 mm (0.2 mV) at 80 ms after the J point may represent myocardial ischemia, especially in the presence of angina. However, this response has a low positive predictive value; it is often categorized as equivocal.
- Among patients after myocardial infarction (MI), exercise-induced ST-segment elevation (>1 mm or >0.1 mV for 60 ms) in leads with Q waves is an abnormal response and may represent reversible ischemia or wall motion abnormalities.
- Among patients without prior MI, exercise-induced ST-segment elevation most often represents transient combined endocardial and subepicardial ischemia but may also be due to acute coronary spasm.

■ Repolarization changes (ST-segment depression or T-wave inversion) that normalize with exercise may represent exercise-induced myocardial ischemia but is considered a normal response in young subjects with early repolarization on the resting ECG.

In general, dysrhythmias that increase in frequency or complexity with progressive exercise intensity and are associated with ischemia or with hemodynamic instability are more likely to cause a poor outcome than isolated dysrhythmias (17). The clinical significance of ventricular ectopy during exercise has varied. Although ventricular ectopy is more common with some pathologies, such as cardiomyopathy, in general, frequent and complex ventricular ectopy during exercise and especially in recovery are associated with increased risk for cardiac arrest (17). Sustained ventricular tachycardia is an absolute criterion to terminate a test. There are several relative termination criteria related to atrial and ventricular dysrhythmias and blocks that should be considered based on the presence of signs or symptoms of myocardial ischemia or inadequate perfusion (17) (see *Box 5.4*).

Symptoms

Symptoms that are consistent with myocardial ischemia (*e.g.*, angina, dyspnea) or hemodynamic instability (*e.g.*, light-headedness) should be noted and correlated with ECG, HR, and BP abnormalities (when present). It is important to recognize that dyspnea can be an anginal equivalent. Exercise-induced angina is associated with an increased risk for IHD (17). This risk is greater when ST-segment depression is also present (17). Compared to angina or leg fatigue, an exercise test that is limited by dyspnea has been associated with a worse prognosis (17).

Exercise Capacity

Evaluating exercise capacity is an important aspect of exercise testing. A high exercise capacity is indicative of a high peak $\dot{Q}$ and therefore suggests the absence of serious limitations of left ventricular function. Within the past two decades, several studies have been published demonstrating the importance of exercise capacity relative to the prognosis of patients with heart failure or cardiovascular disease (3,8,10,37). Either absolute or age- and gender-normalized exercise capacity is highly related to survival (8,37). A significant issue relative to exercise capacity is the imprecision of estimating exercise capacity from exercise time or peak workload (8). The standard error in estimating exercise capacity from various published prediction equations is at least ±1 MET (18,19,23,27,45,53). This measurement error is less meaningful in young, healthy individuals with a peak exercise capacity of 13–15 METs (7%–8% error) but more significant in individuals with reduced exercise capacities typical of those observed in patients with cardiac or pulmonary disease (4–8 METs; 13%–25% error). Estimating exercise capacity on a treadmill is confounded when patients use the handrail for support which will result in an overestimation of their exercise capacity (34). Although equations exist to predict exercise capacity from an exercise test using handrail support, the standard error of the estimate remains large (34). Safety of treadmill walking is always an important consideration, and allowing a patient to use the handrail should be determined on a case-by-case basis.

In addition to describing a patient's exercise capacity as estimated peak METs or measured $\dot{V}O_{2peak}$, exercise capacity is frequently expressed relative to age- and sex-based norms (3,10,37) (*Figure 5.4*). This is especially true for $\dot{V}O_{2peak}$. Several equations exist to estimate $\dot{V}O_{2max}$ based on select demographics (*e.g.*, gender, age, height, weight) (3). Reference tables are also available to provide a percentile ranking for an individual's measured exercise capacity by gender and age categories (see *Table 4.7*). The vast majority of these references are based on apparently healthy individuals. In order to provide a comparative reference specific to patients with established heart disease, Ades et al. (1) developed nomograms stratified by age, gender, and heart disease diagnosis based on patients with heart disease entering cardiac rehabilitation. *Figure 5.5* provides a nomogram to determine predicted $\dot{V}O_{2peak}$ in patients referred for cardiac rehabilitation and have either a medical (*i.e.*, angina, MI) or surgical (*i.e.*, coronary artery bypass graft [CABG], percutaneous coronary intervention [PCI], valve) indication for participation (1).

Cardiopulmonary Exercise Testing

A major advantage of measuring gas exchange during exercise is a more accurate measurement of exercise capacity. Several thorough reviews on CPET are available (3,10,14). In addition to a more accurate measurement of exercise capacity, CPET data may be particularly useful in defining prognosis and defining the timing of cardiac transplantation and other advanced therapies in patients with heart failure. CPET is also helpful in the differential diagnosis of patients with suspected cardiovascular and respiratory diseases (3,10,14). In addition to $\dot{V}O_{2peak}$, the slope of the change in $\dot{V}E$ to change in carbon dioxide ($\dot{V}CO_2$) production (*i.e.*, $\dot{V}E$–$\dot{V}CO_2$ slope) during an exercise test is related to prognosis, especially in patients with heart failure (3,10,14). Other variables that can be determined through the measurement of respiratory gas exchange include the VAT, oxygen pulse, slope of the change in work rate to change in $\dot{V}O_2$, oxygen uptake efficiency slope (OUES), partial pressure of end-tidal CO_2, breathing reserve, and the RER (3,10,14). CPET is particularly useful in identifying whether the cause of dyspnea has a cardiac or pulmonary etiology (3,10).

Maximal versus Peak Cardiorespiratory Stress

When an exercise test is performed as part of the evaluation of IHD, patients should be encouraged to exercise to their maximal level of exertion or until a clinical indication to stop the test is observed. However, the determination of what constitutes "maximal" effort, although important for interpreting test results, can

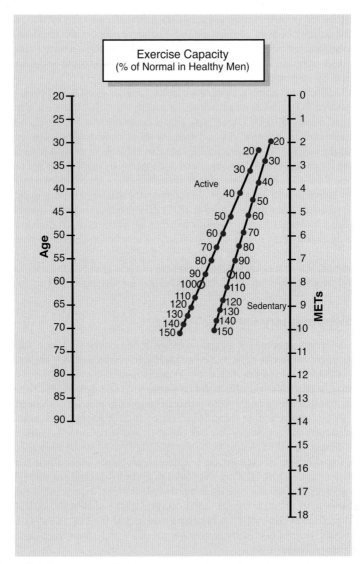

Figure 5.4 Nomograms to identify percentage of normal exercise capacity compared to apparently healthy men and women. METs, metabolic equivalents. Reprinted with permission from (22) and (41). (*continued*)

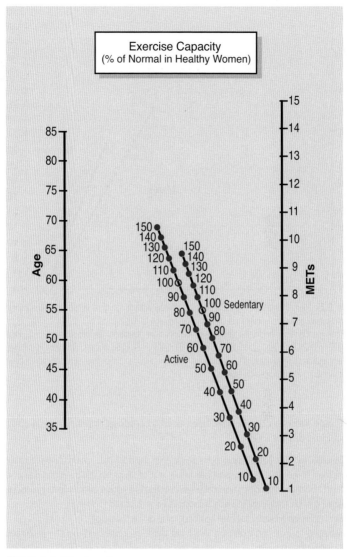

Figure 5.4 (*Continued*)

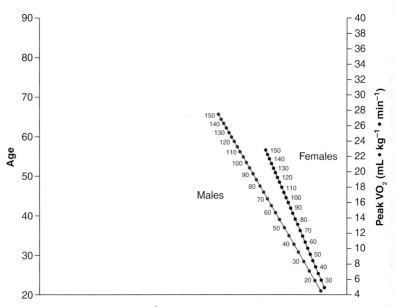

Figure 5.5 Percentage-predicted $\dot{V}O_{2peak}$ in those with a medical or surgical diagnosis. No-mogram for all patients, separated by sex, related age to measured $\dot{V}O_{2peak}$ (mL · kg^{-1} · min^{-1}), giving the percentage of predicted value. Regression equation for predicted $\dot{V}O_{2peak}$ for men is $33.97 - 0.242 \times$ age, and for women, $21.693 - 0.116 \times$ age. Drawing a straight line between age and measured $\dot{V}O_{2peak}$ allows the determination of the percentage of predicted $\dot{V}O_{2peak}$. Used with permission from (1).

be difficult. Various criteria have been used to confirm that a maximal effort has been elicited during a GXT:

- A plateau in $\dot{V}O_2$ (or failure to increase $\dot{V}O_2$ by 150 mL · min^{-1}) with increased workload (59,60). This criterion has fallen out of favor because a plateau is not consistently observed during maximal exercise testing with a continuous protocol (51).
- Failure of HR to increase with increases in workload (59)
- A postexercise venous lactate concentration >8.0 mmol · L^{-1} (41)
- A rating of perceived exertion (RPE) at peak exercise >17 on the 6–20 scale or >7 on the 0–10 scale
- A peak RER ≥1.10. Peak RER is perhaps the most accurate and objective non-invasive indicator of subject effort during a GXT (10).

There is no consensus on the number of criteria that should be met in order to call a test maximal (38). In addition, interindividual and interprotocol variability may limit the validity of these criteria (38). In the absence of data supporting that an individual reached their physiologic maximum, data at peak exercise are commonly described as "peak" (*e.g.*, HR$_{peak}$, $\dot{V}O_{2peak}$) instead of "maximal" (*e.g.*, HR$_{max}$, $\dot{V}O_{2max}$) (3,8,17).

DIAGNOSTIC VALUE OF EXERCISE TESTING FOR THE DETECTION OF ISCHEMIC HEART DISEASE

The diagnostic value of the clinical exercise test for the detection of IHD is influenced by the principles of conditional probability (*i.e.*, the probability of identifying a patient with IHD given the probability of IHD in the underlying population). The factors that determine the diagnostic value of exercise testing (and other diagnostic tests) are the sensitivity and specificity of the test procedure and prevalence of IHD in the population tested (21).

Sensitivity, Specificity, and Predictive Value

Sensitivity refers to the ability to positively identify patients who truly have IHD (21). Exercise ECG sensitivity for the detection of IHD has traditionally been based on angiographic evidence of a coronary artery stenosis ≥70% in at least one vessel. In a true positive (TP) test, the test is positive for myocardial ischemia (*e.g.*, ≥1.0 mm of horizontal or downsloping ST-segment depression), and the patient truly has IHD. Conversely, in a false negative (FN) test, the test is negative for myocardial ischemia, but the patient truly has IHD (21).

Common factors that contribute to FN exercise tests are summarized in *Box 5.6*. The sensitivity of an exercise test is decreased by inadequate myocardial stress, medications that attenuate the cardiac demand to exercise or reduce myocardial ischemia (*e.g.*, β-adrenergic blockers, nitrates, calcium channel blocking agents), and insufficient ECG lead monitoring. In many clinics, a test is not classified as "negative," unless the patient has attained an adequate level of myocardial stress based on achieving ≥85% of predicted HR_{max} (17,21) and/or a peak rate-pressure product ≥25,000 mm Hg · beats · min^{-1}. Preexisting ECG changes such as left ventricular hypertrophy, left bundle-branch block (LBBB), or the preexcitation syndrome (Wolff-Parkinson-White syndrome or W-P-W) limit the ability to interpret exercise-induced ST-segment changes (21).

Specificity refers to the ability to correctly identify patients who do not have IHD. In a true negative (TN) test, the test is negative for myocardial ischemia

Box 5.6	Causes of False Negative Symptom-Limited Maximal Exercise Test Results for the Diagnosis of Ischemic Heart Disease

- Failure to reach an ischemic threshold
- Monitoring an insufficient number of leads to detect ECG changes
- Failure to recognize non-ECG signs and symptoms that may be associated with underlying CVD (*e.g.*, exertional hypotension)
- Angiographically significant CVD compensated by collateral circulation
- Musculoskeletal limitations to exercise preceding cardiac abnormalities
- Technical or observer error

CVD, cardiovascular disease; ECG, electrocardiogram.

Box 5.7	Causes of False Positive Symptom-Limited Maximal Exercise Test Results for the Diagnosis of Ischemic Heart Disease

- ST-segment depression > 1.0 mm at rest
- Left ventricular hypertrophy
- Accelerated conduction defects (*e.g.*, Wolff-Parkinson-White syndrome)
- Digitalis therapy
- Nonischemic cardiomyopathy
- Hypokalemia
- Vasoregulatory abnormalities
- Mitral valve prolapse
- Pericardial disorders
- Technical or observer error
- Coronary spasm
- Anemia

and the patient is free of IHD (21). Conversely, in a false positive (FP) test result, the test is positive for myocardial ischemia, but the patient does not have IHD. Conditions that may cause an abnormal exercise ECG response in the absence of significant IHD are shown in *Box 5.7* (21).

Reported values for the specificity and sensitivity of exercise testing with ECG only vary because of differences in disease prevalence of the cohort studied, test protocols, ECG criteria for a positive test, and the angiographic definition of IHD. In studies that accounted for these variables, the pooled results show a sensitivity of 68% and specificity of 77% (21). Sensitivity, however, is somewhat lower, and specificity is higher when workup bias (*i.e.*, only assessing individuals with a higher likelihood for IHD) is removed (20).

The predictive value of clinical exercise testing is a measure of how accurately a test result (positive or negative) correctly identifies the presence or absence of IHD in patients (21) and is calculated from sensitivity and specificity (*Box 5.8*).

Box 5.8	Sensitivity, Specificity, and Predictive Value of Symptom-Limited Maximal Exercise Testing for the Diagnosis of Ischemic Heart Disease (IHD)

Sensitivity = [TP / (TP + FN)] × 100
- The percentage of patients with IHD who have a positive test

Specificity = [TN / (FP + TN)] × 100
- The percentage of patients without IHD who have a negative test

Positive predictive value = [TP / (TP + FP)] × 100
- The percentage of positive tests that correctly identify patients with IHD

Negative predictive value = [TN / (TN + FN)] × 100
- The percentage of negative tests that correct identify patients without IHD

FN, false negative; FP, false positive; TN, true negative; TP, true positive.

The positive predictive value is the percentage of individuals with an abnormal test who truly have IHD (21). The negative predictive value is the percentage of individuals with a negative test who are free of IHD (21).

Clinical Exercise Test Data and Prognosis

First introduced in 1991 when the Duke Treadmill Score was published (33), the implementation of various exercise test scores that combine information derived during the exercise test into a single prognostic estimate has gained popularity. The most widely accepted and used of these prognostic scores is the Duke Treadmill Score or the related Duke Treadmill Nomogram (17,21). Both are appropriate for patients with or without a history of IHD being considered for coronary angiography without a history of a MI or revascularization procedure. The Duke Score/Nomogram (*Figure 5.6*) considers exercise capacity, the

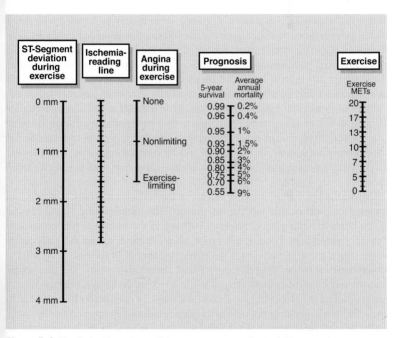

Figure 5.6 The Duke Nomogram. This nomogram uses five variables to estimate prognosis for a given individual. First, the observed amount of ST-segment depression is marked on the ST-segment deviation line. Second, the observed degree of angina is marked on the line for angina, and these two points are connected. Third, the point where this line intersects the ischemia reading line is noted. Fourth, the observed exercise tolerance is marked on the line for exercise capacity. Finally, the mark on the ischemia reading line is connected to the mark on the exercise capacity line, and the estimated 5-yr survival or average annual mortality rate is read from the point at which this line intersects the prognosis scale. Reprinted with permission from (33).

magnitude of ST-segment depression, and the presence and severity of angina pectoris. The calculated score is related to annual and 5-yr survival rates and allows the categorization of patients into low-, moderate-, and high-risk subgroups. This categorization may help the physician choose between more conservative or more aggressive therapies. Physicians may also use prognosis estimates based on other hemodynamic findings, such as chronotropic incompetence or an abnormal HR recovery, to guide their clinical decisions (17,21). Each of these abnormalities of exercise testing contributes independent prognostic information. Although there is a general belief that physicians informally integrate much of this information without the specific calculation of an exercise test score, estimates of the presence of IHD provided by scores are superior to physician estimates and analysis of ST-segment changes alone (32).

CLINICAL EXERCISE TESTS WITH IMAGING

When the resting ECG is abnormal, exercise testing may be coupled with other techniques designed to either augment the information provided by the ECG or to replace the ECG when resting abnormalities (see *Box 5.5*) make evaluation of changes during exercise impossible. Various radioisotopes can be used to evaluate the presence of a myocardial perfusion abnormality, which is the initiating event in exertional ischemia and the beginning of the "ischemic cascade," or abnormalities of ventricular function that often occur with MI or myocardial ischemia (17,21). When exercise testing is coupled with myocardial perfusion imaging (*e.g.*, nuclear stress test) or echocardiography, all other aspects of the exercise test should remain the same, including HR and BP monitoring during and after exercise, symptom evaluation, rhythm monitoring, and symptom-limited maximal exertion.

Myocardial perfusion imaging can be performed with a variety of agents and imaging approaches, although the two most common isotopes are ^{201}thallium and ^{199m}technetium sestamibi (Cardiolite). Delivery of the isotope is proportional to coronary blood flow. These agents cross cell membranes of metabolically active tissue either actively (thallium) or passively (sestamibi). In the case of an MI, the isotope does not cross the cell membrane of the necrotic tissue, and thus a permanent reduction of isotope activity is observed on the image, referred to as a nonreversible, or fixed, perfusion defect. In the case of exertional myocardial ischemia, the tissue uptake in the ischemic region is reduced during exercise by virtue of the relative reduction of blood flow (and thus isotope) to the ischemic tissue. This abnormality is reversed when myocardial perfusion is evaluated at rest. This is called a reversible, or transient, perfusion defect and is diagnostic of exertional myocardial ischemia.

Echocardiography can also be used as an adjunct during an exercise test and is often called *stress echocardiography*. Echocardiographic examination allows evaluation of wall motion, wall thickness, and valve function. Although it is theoretically possible to perform an echocardiography during the course of upright cycle ergometer exercise, it is technically challenging. Typical practice is to have the patient lie down on their left side immediately following completion of the exercise test (treadmill or upright cycle ergometer) or for exercise to involve recumbent cycle ergometry. This allows optimization of the echocardiographic window to the heart. Regional wall motion is assessed for various segments of the left ventricle. Deterioration in regional wall motion with exercise (compared to rest) is a sign of myocardial ischemia. Left ventricular ejection fraction (LVEF) is also measured before and after exercise.

Imaging techniques, such as radionuclide myocardial perfusion imaging and echocardiography, allow the physician to identify the location and magnitude of myocardial ischemia. In patients incapable of exercising, it is also possible to perform either myocardial perfusion imaging or stress echocardiography with pharmacologic stress. These techniques are beyond the scope of this chapter.

FIELD WALKING TESTS

This chapter focuses on the traditional sign/symptom-limited, maximal exercise test with ECG monitoring that is performed in a clinical laboratory, often with a treadmill or cycle ergometer. However, non–laboratory-based clinical exercise tests are also frequently used in patients with chronic disease. These are generally classified as field or hallway walking tests and are typically considered submaximal. Similar to maximal exercise tests, field walking tests are used to evaluate exercise capacity, estimate prognosis, and evaluate response to treatment (8,9,25). The most common among the field walking tests is the 6-min walk test (6MWT), but evidence has been building for other field walking tests, such as the incremental and endurance shuttle walk tests (25). The 6MWT was originally developed to assess patients with pulmonary disease (25); however, it has been applied in various patient groups and is a popular tool to assess patients with heart failure.

The advantages of field walking tests are the simplicity and minimal cost, often requiring just a hallway. In addition, because the patient walks at a self-selected pace, a field walking test might be more representative of a patient's ability to perform activities of daily living (8,25). Additional discussion of field walking tests is provided in *Chapter 4*.

ONLINE RESOURCES

American Thoracic Society: statements, guidelines, and reports
  https://www.thoracic.org/statements/
American College of Cardiology: guidelines
  http://www.acc.org/guidelines
American Heart Association: guidelines and statements
  http://my.americanheart.org/professional/StatementsGuidelines
  /Statements-Guidelines_UCM_316885_SubHomePage.jsp

REFERENCES

1. Ades PA, Savage PD, Brawner CA, et al. Aerobic capacity in patients entering cardiac rehabilitation. *Circulation*. 2006;113(23):2706–12.
2. American College of Emergency Physicians, Society for Cardiovascular Angiography and Interventions. 2013 ACCF/AHA guideline for the management of ST-elevation myocardial infarction: a report of the American College of Cardiology Foundation/American Heart Association Task Force on Practice Guidelines. *J Am Coll Cardiol*. 2013;61(4):e78–140.
3. American Thoracic Society, American College of Chest Physicians. ATS/ACCP statement on cardiopulmonary exercise testing. *Am J Respir Crit Care Med*. 2003;167(2):211–77.
4. Amon KW, Richards KL, Crawford MH. Usefulness of the postexercise response of systolic blood pressure in the diagnosis of coronary artery disease. *Circulation*. 1984;70(6):951–6.
5. Amsterdam EA, Kirk JD, Bluemke DA, et al. Testing of low-risk patients presenting to the emergency department with chest pain: a scientific statement from the American Heart Association. *Circulation*. 2010;122(17):1756–76.
6. Amsterdam EA, Wenger NK, Brindis RG, et al. 2014 AHA/ACC guideline for the management of patients with non-ST-elevation acute coronary syndromes: executive summary: a report of the American College of Cardiology/American Heart Association Task Force on Practice Guidelines. *Circulation*. 2014;130(25):2354–94.
7. Arena R, Lavie CJ, Milani RV, Myers J, Guazzi M. Cardiopulmonary exercise testing in patients with pulmonary arterial hypertension: an evidence-based review. *J Heart Lung Transplant*. 2010;29(2):159–73.
8. Arena R, Myers J, Williams MA, et al. Assessment of functional capacity in clinical and research settings: a scientific statement from the American Heart Association Committee on Exercise, Rehabilitation, and Prevention of the Council on Clinical Cardiology and the Council on Cardiovascular Nursing. *Circulation*. 2007;116(3):329–43.
9. ATS Committee on Proficiency Standards for Clinical Pulmonary Function Laboratories. ATS statement: guidelines for the six-minute walk test. *Am J Respir Crit Care Med*. 2002;166(1):111–7.
10. Balady GJ, Arena R, Sietsema K, et al. Clinician's guide to cardiopulmonary exercise testing in adults. A scientific statement from the American Heart Association. *Circulation*. 2010;122(2):191–225.
11. Brawner CA, Ehrman JK, Schairer JR, Cao JJ, Keteyian SJ. Predicting maximum heart rate among patients with coronary heart disease receiving beta-adrenergic blockade therapy. *Am Heart J*. 2004;148(5):910–4.
12. Cole CR, Blackstone EH, Pashkow FJ, Snader CE, Lauer MS. Heart-rate recovery immediately after exercise as a predictor of mortality. *N Engl J Med*. 1999;341(18):1351–7.
13. ERS Task Force, Palange P, Ward SA, et al. Recommendations on the use of exercise testing in clinical practice. *Eur Respir J*. 2007;29(1):185–209.
14. Ferrazza AM, Martolini D, Valli G, Palange P. Cardiopulmonary exercise testing in the functional and prognostic evaluation of patients with pulmonary diseases. *Respiration*. 2009;77(1):3–17.
15. Fihn SD, Gardin JM, Abrams J, et al. 2012 ACCF/AHA/ACP/AATS/PCNA/SCAI/STS Guideline for the diagnosis and management of patients with stable ischemic heart disease: a report of the American College of Cardiology Foundation/American Heart Association Task Force on Practice Guidelines, and the American College of Physicians, American Association for Thoracic Surgery, Preventive Cardiovascular Nurses Association, Society for Cardiovascular Angiography and Interventions, and Society of Thoracic Surgeons. *J Am Coll Cardiol*. 2012;60(24):e44–164.
16. Fleisher LA, Fleischmann KE, Auerbach AD, et al. 2014 ACC/AHA guideline on perioperative cardiovascular evaluation and management of patients undergoing noncardiac surgery: executive summary: a report of the American College of Cardiology/American Heart Association Task Force on Practice Guidelines. *Circulation*. 2014;130(24):2215–45.
17. Fletcher GF, Ades PA, Kligfield P, et al. Exercise standards for testing and training: a scientific statement from the American Heart Association. *Circulation*. 2013;128(8):873–934.
18. Foster C, Crowe AJ, Daines E, et al. Predicting functional capacity during treadmill testing independent of exercise protocol. *Med Sci Sports Exerc*. 1996;28(6):752–6.
19. Foster C, Jackson AS, Pollock ML, et al. Generalized equations for predicting functional capacity from treadmill performance. *Am Heart J*. 1984;107(6):1229–34.

20. Froelicher VF, Lehmann KG, Thomas R, et al. The electrocardiographic exercise test in a population with reduced workup bias: diagnostic performance, computerized interpretation, and multivariable prediction. Veterans Affairs Cooperative Study in Health Services #016 (QUEXTA) Study Group. Quantitative exercise testing and angiography. *Ann Intern Med*. 1998;128(12 Pt 1):965–74.

21. Gibbons RJ, Balady GJ, Bricker JT, et al. ACC/AHA 2002 guideline update for exercise testing: summary article. A report of the American College of Cardiology/American Heart Association Task Force on Practice Guidelines (Committee to Update the 1997 Exercise Testing Guidelines). *J Am Coll Cardiol*. 2002;40(8):1531–40.

22. Gulati M, Black HR, Shaw LJ, et al. The prognostic value of a nomogram for exercise capacity in women. *N Engl J Med*. 2005;353(5):468–75.

23. Haskell WL, Savin W, Oldridge N, DeBusk R. Factors influencing estimated oxygen uptake during exercise testing soon after myocardial infarction. *Am J Cardiol*. 1982;50(2):299–304.

24. Hiraga T, Maekura R, Okuda Y, et al. Prognostic predictors for survival in patients with COPD using cardiopulmonary exercise testing. *Clin Physiol Funct Imaging*. 2003;23(6):324–31.

25. Holland AE, Spruit MA, Troosters T, et al. An official European Respiratory Society/American Thoracic Society technical standard: field walking tests in chronic respiratory disease. *Eur Respir J*. 2014;44(6):1428–46.

26. Hunt SA, Abraham WT, Chin MH, et al. ACC/AHA 2005 guideline update for the diagnosis and management of chronic heart failure in the adult: a report of the American College of Cardiology/American Heart Association Task Force on Practice Guidelines (Writing Committee to Update the 2001 Guidelines for the Evaluation and Management of Heart Failure): developed in collaboration with the American College of Chest Physicians and the International Society for Heart and Lung Transplantation: endorsed by the Heart Rhythm Society. *Circulation*. 2005;112(12):e154–235.

27. Kaminsky LA, Whaley MH. Evaluation of a new standardized ramp protocol: the BSU/Bruce Ramp protocol. *J Cardiopulm Rehabil*. 1998;18(6):438–44.

28. Keteyian SJ, Brawner CA, Savage PD et al. Peak aerobic capacity predicts prognosis in patients with coronary heart disease. *Am Heart J*. 2008;156(2):292–300.

29. Lauer MS. Exercise electrocardiogram testing and prognosis. Novel markers and predictive instruments. *Cardiol Clin*. 2001;19(3):401–14.

30. Lauer MS, Francis GS, Okin PM, et al. Impaired chronotropic response to exercise stress testing as a predictor of mortality. *JAMA*. 1999;281(6):524–9.

31. Levine GN, Bates ER, Blankenship JC, et al. 2011 ACCF/AHA/SCAI guideline for percutaneous coronary intervention. A report of the American College of Cardiology Foundation/American Heart Association Task Force on Practice Guidelines and the Society for Cardiovascular Angiography and Interventions. *J Am Coll Cardiol*. 2011;58(24):e44–122.

32. Lipinski M, Froelicher V, Atwood E, et al. Comparison of treadmill scores with physician estimates of diagnosis and prognosis in patients with coronary artery disease. *Am Heart J*. 2002;143(4):650–8.

33. Mark DB, Shaw L, Harrell FE Jr, et al. Prognostic value of a treadmill exercise score in outpatients with suspected coronary artery disease. *N Engl J Med*. 1991;325(12):849–53.

34. McConnell TR, Foster C, Conlin NC, Thompson NN. Prediction of functional capacity during treadmill testing: effect of handrail support. *J Cardiopulm Rehabil*. 1991;11(4):255–60.

35. McHam SA, Marwick TH, Pashkow FJ, Lauer MS. Delayed systolic blood pressure recovery after graded exercise: an independent correlate of angiographic coronary disease. *J Am Coll Cardiol*. 1999;34(3):754–9.

36. McMurray JJ, Adamopoulos S, Anker SD, et al. ESC guidelines for the diagnosis and treatment of acute and chronic heart failure 2012: the Task Force for the Diagnosis and Treatment of Acute and Chronic Heart Failure 2012 of the European Society of Cardiology. Developed in collaboration with the Heart Failure Association (HFA) of the ESC. *Eur Heart J*. 2012;33(14):1787–847.

37. Mezzani A, Agostoni P, Cohen-Solal A, et al. Standards for the use of cardiopulmonary exercise testing for the functional evaluation of cardiac patients: a report from the Exercise Physiology Section of the European Association for Cardiovascular Prevention and Rehabilitation. *Eur J Cardiovasc Prev Rehabil*. 2009;16(3):249–67.

38. Midgley AW, McNaughton LR, Polman R, Marchant D. Criteria for determination of maximal oxygen uptake: a brief critique and recommendations for future research. *Sports Med*. 2007;37(12):1019–28.

39. Mieres JH, Gulati M, Bairey Merz N, et al. Role of noninvasive testing in the clinical evaluation of women with suspected ischemic heart disease: a consensus statement from the American Heart Association. *Circulation*. 2014;130(4):350–79.

40. Miki K, Maekura R, Hiraga T, et al. Impairments and prognostic factors for survival in patients with idiopathic pulmonary fibrosis. *Respir Med*. 2003;97(5):482–90.

41. Morris CK, Myers J, Froelicher VF, Kawaguchi T, Ueshima K, Hideg A. Nomogram based on metabolic equivalents and age for assessing aerobic exercise capacity in men. *J Am Coll Cardiol*. 1993;22(1):175–82.

42. Morshedi-Meibodi A, Larson MG, Levy D, O'Donnell CJ, Vasan RS. Heart rate recovery after treadmill exercise testing and risk of cardiovascular disease events (The Framingham Heart Study). *Am J Cardiol*. 2002;90(8):848–52.

43. Moyer VA, U.S. Preventive Services Task Force. Screening for coronary heart disease with electrocardiography: U.S. Preventive Services Task Force recommendation statement. *Ann Intern Med*. 2012;157(7):512–8.

44. Myers J, Arena R, Franklin B, et al. Recommendations for clinical exercise laboratories: a scientific statement from the American Heart Association. *Circulation*. 2009;119(24):3144–61.

45. Myers J, Bellin D. Ramp exercise protocols for clinical and cardiopulmonary exercise testing. *Sports Med*. 2000;30(1):23–9.

46. Myers J, Forman DE, Balady GJ, et al. Supervision of exercise testing by nonphysicians: a scientific statement from the American Heart Association. *Circulation*. 2014;130(12):1014–27.

47. Myers J, Prakash M, Froelicher V, Do D, Partington S, Atwood JE. Exercise capacity and mortality among men referred for exercise testing. *N Engl J Med*. 2002;346(11):793–801.

48. Myers J, Voodi L, Umann T, Froelicher VF. A survey of exercise testing: methods, utilization, interpretation, and safety in the VAHCS. *J Cardiopulm Rehabil*. 2000;20(4):251–8.

49. Nishimura RA, Otto CM, Bonow RO, et al. 2014 AHA/ACC guideline for the management of patients with valvular heart disease: executive summary: a report of the American College of Cardiology/American Heart Association Task Force on Practice Guidelines. *J Am Coll Cardiol*. 2014;63(22):2438–88.

50. Nissinen SI, Mäkikallio TH, Seppänen T, et al. Heart rate recovery after exercise as a predictor of mortality among survivors of acute myocardial infarction. *Am J Cardiol*. 2003;91(6):711–4.

51. Noakes TD. Maximal oxygen uptake: "classical" versus "contemporary" viewpoints: a rebuttal. *Med Sci Sports Exerc*. 1998;30(9):1381–98.

52. Parsons JP, Hallstrand TS, Mastronarde JG, et al. An official American Thoracic Society clinical practice guideline: exercise-induced bronchoconstriction. *Am J Respir Crit Care Med*. 2013;187(9):1016–27.

53. Pescatello LS, Franklin BA, Fagard R, et al. American College of Sports Medicine position stand. Exercise and hypertension. *Med Sci Sports Exerc*. 2004;36(3):533–53.

54. Peterson MJ, Pieper CF, Morey MC. Accuracy of VO2(max) prediction equations in older adults. *Med Sci Sports Exerc*. 2003;35(1):145–9.

55. Pretto JJ, Roebuck T, Beckert L, Hamilton G. Clinical use of pulse oximetry: official guidelines from the Thoracic Society of Australia and New Zealand. *Respirology*. 2014;19(1):38–46.

56. Rochmis P, Blackburn H. Exercise tests. A survey of procedures, safety, and litigation experience in approximately 170,000 tests. *JAMA*. 1971;217(8):1061–6.

57. Rodgers GP, Ayanian JZ, Balady G, et al. American College of Cardiology/American Heart Association Clinical Competence statement on stress testing. A report of the American College of Cardiology/American Heart Association/American College of Physicians-American Society of Internal Medicine Task Force on Clinical Competence. *Circulation*. 2000 Oct 3;102(14):1726–38.

58. Rooke TW, Hirsch AT, Misra S, et al. Management of patients with peripheral artery disease (compilation of 2005 and 2011 ACCF/AHA Guideline Recommendations): a report of the American College of Cardiology Foundation/American Heart Association Task Force on Practice Guidelines. *J Am Coll Cardiol*. 2013;61(14):1555–70.

59. Taylor HL, Buskirk E, Henschel A. Maximal oxygen intake as an objective measure of cardio-respiratory performance. *J Appl Physiol*. 1955;8(1):73–80.

60. Wasserman K, Whipp BJ, Koyl SN, Beaver WL. Anaerobic threshold and respiratory gas exchange during exercise. *J Appl Physiol*. 1973;35(2):236–43.

CHAPTER 6

General Principles of Exercise Prescription

AN INTRODUCTION TO THE PRINCIPLES OF EXERCISE PRESCRIPTION

The scientific evidence demonstrating the beneficial effects of exercise is indisputable, and the benefits of exercise far outweigh the risks in most adults (19,37,75,80) (see *Chapters 1* and *2*). An exercise training program ideally is designed to meet *individual* health and physical fitness goals within the context of individual health status, function, and the respective physical and social environment. The principles of exercise prescription (Ex R_x) presented in this chapter are intended to guide exercise professionals in the development of an *individually* tailored Ex R_x for the apparently healthy adult whose goal is to improve physical fitness and health. Recreational and competitive athletes will benefit from more advanced training techniques than are presented in this chapter. This chapter employs the *F*requency (how often), *I*ntensity (how hard), *T*ime (duration or how long), *T*ype (mode or what kind), total *V*olume (amount), and *P*rogression (advancement) or the FITT-VP principle of Ex R_x and provides recommendations on exercise pattern to be consistent with the American College of Sports Medicine (ACSM) recommendations made in its companion evidence-based position stand (37).

The FITT-VP principles of Ex R_x presented in this chapter are based on the application of the existing scientific evidence on the physiologic, psychological, and health benefits of exercise (37) (see *Chapter 1*). Nonetheless, some individuals may not respond as expected because there is appreciable individual variability in the magnitude of response to a particular exercise regimen (37,91,94). Furthermore, the FITT-VP principle of Ex R_x may not apply in certain cases because of individual characteristics (*e.g.*, health status, physical ability, age) or athletic and performance goals. Accommodations to the Ex R_x should be made for individuals with clinical conditions and healthy individuals with special considerations, as indicated in other related chapters of the *Guidelines* (see *Chapters 7, 9, 10*, and *11*).

For most adults, an exercise program including aerobic, resistance, flexibility, and neuromotor exercise training is indispensable to improve and maintain physical fitness and health (37). The FITT-VP Ex R_x guidelines present recommended targets for exercise derived from the available scientific evidence showing most

143

individuals will realize benefit when following the stated quantity and quality of exercise. However, some individuals will want or need to include only some of the health-related components of physical fitness in their training regimen or exercise less than suggested by the guidelines presented in this chapter. Even if an individual cannot meet the recommended targets in this chapter, performing some exercise is beneficial, especially in inactive or deconditioned individuals, and, for that reason, should be encouraged except where there are safety concerns.

The guidelines presented in this chapter are consistent with other evidence-based exercise recommendations, including relevant ACSM position stands (4,5,28,37,50,72) and other professional scientific statements (19,80,106,109).

GENERAL CONSIDERATIONS FOR EXERCISE PRESCRIPTION

A program of regular exercise for most adults should include a variety of exercises *beyond* activities performed as part of daily living (37). The optimal Ex R_x should address cardiorespiratory (aerobic) fitness (CRF), muscular strength and endurance, flexibility, body composition, and neuromotor fitness. Separately, a reduction in the time spent in sedentary activities (*e.g.*, television watching, computer use, sitting in a car or at a desk) is important for the health of both physically active and inactive individuals. As detailed elsewhere, long periods of sedentary activity are associated with elevated risks of cardiovascular disease (CVD) mortality, worsened cardiometabolic disease biomarkers, and depression (19,29,37,76). The adverse health effect of prolonged sedentary activity not only is more pronounced in inactive adults but also applies to those adults who are currently meeting the physical activity (PA) recommendations (12,19,29,37,76). When periods of physical inactivity are broken up by short bouts of standing or PA (*e.g.*, a very short walk around the office or home), the adverse effects of physical inactivity are reduced (9,19,29,37,76). Therefore, the Ex R_x should include a plan to decrease periods of physical inactivity in addition to an increase in PA (19,29,37,76).

Musculoskeletal injuries (MSIs) are of concern to adults and may be reduced by including a warm-up and cool-down, stretching exercises, and gradual progression of volume and intensity (37) (see *Chapter 1*). The risk of CVD complications, a concern in middle-aged and older adults, can be minimized by (a) following the preparticipation health screening and evaluation procedures outlined in *Chapters 2* and *3*, respectively; (b) beginning a new program of exercise at light-to-moderate intensity; and (c) employing a gradual progression of the quantity and quality of exercise (37). Also important to the Ex R_x are behavioral interventions that may reduce barriers and enhance the adoption and adherence to exercise participation (see *Chapter 12*).

Bone health is of great importance to younger and older adults (see *Chapters 7* and *11*), especially among women. The ACSM recommends loading exercises (*i.e.*, weight bearing and resistance exercise) to maintain bone health (3–5,37,72), and these types of exercises should be part of an exercise program, particularly in individuals at risk for low bone density (*i.e.*, osteopenia) and osteoporosis.

Box 6.1	Components of the Exercise Training Session

Warm-up: at least 5–10 min of light-to-moderate intensity cardiorespiratory and muscular endurance activities
Conditioning: at least 20–60 min of aerobic, resistance, neuromotor, and/or sports activities (exercise bouts of 10 min are acceptable if the individual accumulates at least 20–60 min $\cdot$ d^{-1} of daily aerobic exercise)
Cool-down: at least 5–10 min of light-to-moderate intensity cardiorespiratory and muscular endurance activities
Stretching: at least 10 min of stretching exercises performed after the warm-up or cool-down phase

Adapted from (37,107).

An individual's goals, physical ability, physical fitness, health status, schedule, physical and social environment, and available equipment and facilities should be considered when designing the FITT-VP principle of Ex R$_x$. *Box 6.1* provides general recommendations for the components to be included in an exercise training session for apparently healthy adults. This chapter presents the scientific evidence-based recommendations for aerobic, resistance, flexibility, and neuromotor exercise training based on a combination of the FITT-VP principles of Ex R$_x$. The following sections present specific recommendations for the Ex R$_x$ to improve health and fitness.

COMPONENTS OF THE EXERCISE TRAINING SESSION

A single exercise session should include the following phases:

- Warm-up
- Conditioning and/or sports-related exercise
- Cool-down
- Stretching

The warm-up phase consists of a minimum of 5–10 min of light-to-moderate intensity aerobic and muscular endurance activity (see *Table 6.1* for definitions of exercise intensity). The warm-up is a transitional phase that allows the body to adjust to the changing physiologic, biomechanical, and bioenergetic demands of the conditioning or sports phase of the exercise session. Warming up also improves range of motion (ROM) and may reduce the risk of injury (37). A dynamic, cardiorespiratory endurance exercise warm-up is superior to static flexibility exercises for the purpose of enhancing the *performance* of cardiorespiratory endurance, aerobic exercise, sports, or resistance exercise, especially activities that are of long duration or with many repetitions (37).

The conditioning phase includes aerobic, resistance, flexibility, and neuromotor exercise, and/or sports activities. Specifics about these modes of

TABLE 6.1

Methods of Estimating Intensity of Cardiorespiratory and Resistance Exercise

Intensity	Cardiorespiratory Endurance Exercise											Resistance Exercise
	Relative Intensity			Perceived Exertion (Rating on 6-20 RPE Scale)	Intensity (%VO₂ₘₐₓ) Relative to Maximal Exercise Capacity in MET			Absolute Intensity	Absolute Intensity (MET) by Age			Relative Intensity
	%HRR or %V̇O₂R	%HR$_{max}$	%V̇O₂max		20 METs %V̇O₂max	10 METs %V̇O₂max	5 METs %V̇O₂max	METs	Young (20–39 yr)	Middle Age (40–64 yr)	Older (≥65 yr)	% One Repetition Maximum
Very light	<30	<57	<37	Very light (RPE <9)	<34	<37	<44	<2.0	<2.4	<2.0	<1.6	<30
Light	30–39	57–63	37–45	Very light to fairly light (RPE 9–11)	34–42	37–45	44–51	2.0–2.9	2.4–4.7	2.0–3.9	1.6–3.1	30–49
Moderate	40–59	64–76	46–63	Fairly light to somewhat hard (RPE 12–13)	43–61	46–63	52–67	3.0–5.9	4.8–7.1	4.0–5.9	3.2–4.7	50–69
Vigorous	60–89	77–95	64–90	Somewhat hard to very hard (RPE 14–17)	62–90	64–90	68–91	6.0–8.7	7.2–10.1	6.0–8.4	4.8–6.7	70–84
Near maximal to maximal	≥90	≥96	≥91	≥ Very hard (RPE ≥18)	≥91	≥91	≥92	≥8.8	≥10.2	≥8.5	≥6.8	≥85

HR$_{max}$, maximal heart rate; HRR, heart rate reserve; MET, metabolic equivalent; RPE, rating of perceived exertion; V̇O₂ₘₐₓ, maximum oxygen consumption; V̇O₂R, oxygen uptake reserve. Adapted from (37).

exercise are discussed in subsequent sections of this chapter. The conditioning phase is followed by a cool-down period involving aerobic and muscular endurance activity of light-to-moderate intensity lasting at least 5–10 min. The purpose of the cool-down period is to allow for a gradual recovery of heart rate (HR) and blood pressure (BP) and removal of metabolic end products from the muscles used during the more intense exercise conditioning phase.

The stretching phase is distinct from the warm-up and cool-down phases and may be performed following the warm-up or cool-down, as warmer muscles improve ROM (37).

AEROBIC (CARDIORESPIRATORY ENDURANCE) EXERCISE

Frequency of Exercise

The frequency of PA (*i.e.*, the number of days per week dedicated to an exercise program) is an important contributor to health/fitness benefits that result from exercise. Aerobic exercise is recommended on 3–5 d $\cdot$ wk^{-1} for most adults, with the frequency varying with the intensity of exercise (37,50,72,80,107). Improvements in CRF are attenuated with exercise frequencies $<$3 d $\cdot$ wk^{-1} and plateau in improvement with exercise done $>$5 d $\cdot$ wk^{-1} (37). Vigorous intensity exercise performed $>$5 d $\cdot$ wk^{-1} might increase the incidence of MSI, so this amount of vigorous intensity PA is not recommended for adults who are not well conditioned (37,75). Nevertheless, if a variety of exercise modes placing different impact stresses on the body (*e.g.*, running, cycling), or using different muscle groups (*e.g.*, swimming, running), are included in the exercise program, daily vigorous intensity PA may be recommended for some individuals. Alternatively, a weekly combination of 3–5 d $\cdot$ wk^{-1} of moderate and vigorous intensity exercise can be performed, which may be more suitable for most individuals (37,72,107).

Exercise done only once or twice per week at moderate-to-vigorous intensity can bring health/fitness benefits, especially with large volumes of exercise (37). Despite the possible benefits, exercising one to two times per week is not recommended for most adults because the risk of MSI, and adverse cardiovascular events are higher in individuals who are not physically active on a regular basis and those who engage in unaccustomed vigorous exercise (37).

AEROBIC EXERCISE FREQUENCY RECOMMENDATION

Moderate intensity aerobic exercise done at least 5 d $\cdot$ wk^{-1}, or vigorous intensity aerobic exercise done at least 3 d $\cdot$ wk^{-1}, or a weekly combination of 3–5 d $\cdot$ wk^{-1} of moderate and vigorous intensity exercise is recommended for most adults to achieve and maintain health/fitness benefits.

Intensity of Exercise

There is a positive dose response of health/fitness benefits that results from increasing exercise intensity (37). The overload principle of training states exercise below a minimum intensity, or *threshold*, will not challenge the body sufficiently to result in changes in physiologic parameters, including increased maximal volume of oxygen consumed per unit of time ($\dot{V}O_{2max}$) (37). However, the minimum threshold of intensity for benefit seems to vary depending on an individual's current CRF level and other factors such as age, health status, physiologic differences, genetics, habitual PA, and social and psychological factors (37,94,98,99). Therefore, precisely defining an exact threshold to improve CRF may be difficult (37,98). For example, individuals with an exercise capacity of 11–14 metabolic equivalents (METs) seemingly require an exercise intensity of at least 45% oxygen uptake reserve ($\dot{V}O_2R$) to increase $\dot{V}O_{2max}$, but no threshold is apparent in individuals with a baseline fitness of <11 METs (37,98). Highly trained athletes may need to exercise at "near maximal" (i.e., 95%–100% $\dot{V}O_{2max}$) training intensities to improve $\dot{V}O_{2max}$, whereas 70%–80% $\dot{V}O_{2max}$ may provide a sufficient stimulus in moderately trained athletes (37,98).

Interval training involves varying the exercise intensity at fixed intervals during a single exercise session, which can increase the total volume and/or average exercise intensity performed during that session. Improvements in CRF and cardiometabolic biomarkers with short-term (≤3 mo) interval training are similar or superior to steady state moderate-to-vigorous intensity exercise in healthy adults and individuals with metabolic, cardiovascular, or pulmonary disease (37,43,53,63,88,104,112).

During interval training, several aspects of the Ex R_x can be varied depending on the goals of the training session and physical fitness level of the client or patient. These variables include the exercise mode; the number, duration, and intensity of the work and recovery intervals; the number of repetitions of the intervals; and the duration of the between-interval rest period (20). Studies of high intensity interval training (HIIT) and sprint interval training (SIT) demonstrate improvements in CRF, cardiometabolic biomarkers, and other fitness and health-related physiological variables when including repeated alternating short (<45–240 s) bouts of vigorous-to-near maximal intensity exercise followed by equal or longer bouts (60–360 s) of light-to-moderate intensity aerobic exercise (6,20–22,27,31,33,45,48,53,58,70,71,112). Training responses to HIIT have been reported across a wide range of modalities and work: active recovery interval ratios (20,21,43,117).

■ **AEROBIC EXERCISE INTENSITY RECOMMENDATION**

Moderate (*e.g.*, 40%–59% heart rate reserve [HRR] or $\dot{V}O_2R$) to vigorous (*e.g.*, 60%–89% HRR or $\dot{V}O_2R$) intensity aerobic exercise is recommended for most adults, and light (*e.g.*, 30%–39% HRR or $\dot{V}O_2R$) to moderate intensity aerobic exercise can be beneficial in individuals who are deconditioned. Interval training may be an effective way to increase the total volume and/or average exercise intensity performed during an exercise session and may be beneficial for adults.

Methods of Estimating Intensity of Exercise

Several effective methods for prescribing exercise intensity result in improvements in CRF that can be recommended for individualized Ex R$_x$ (37). *Table 6.1* shows the approximate classification of exercise intensity commonly used in practice. One method of determining exercise intensity is not necessarily equivalent to the intensity derived using another method because no studies have compared all of the methods of measurement of exercise intensity simultaneously. Moreover, the relationship among measures of actual energy expenditure (EE) and the absolute (*i.e.*, $\dot{V}O_2$ and METs) and relative methods to prescribe exercise intensity (*i.e.*, %HRR, maximal heart rate [%HR$_{max}$], and %$\dot{V}O_{2max}$) can vary considerably depending on exercise test protocol, exercise mode, exercise intensity, medications, and characteristics of the client or patient (*i.e.*, resting HR, physical fitness level, age, and body composition) as well as other factors (37,54).

The HRR, $\dot{V}O_2$R, and threshold (ventilatory threshold [VT] and respiratory compensation point [RCP]) methods are recommended for Ex R$_x$ because exercise intensity can be underestimated or overestimated when using an HR-dependent method (*i.e.*, %HR$_{max}$) or $\dot{V}O_2$ (*i.e.*, %$\dot{V}O_{2max}$) (37,70,96). Furthermore, the accuracy of any of these methods may be influenced by the method of measurement or estimation used (37). Therefore, direct measurement of the physiologic responses to exercise through an incremental (graded) cardiopulmonary exercise test is the preferred method for Ex R$_x$ whenever possible.

The formula "220 − age" is commonly used to predict HR$_{max}$ (35). This formula is simple to use but can underestimate or overestimate measured HR$_{max}$ (38,47,101,118). Specialized regression equations for estimating HR$_{max}$ may be superior to the equation of 220 − age in some individuals (38,51,101,118). Although these equations are promising, they cannot yet be recommended for universal application, although they may be applied to populations similar to those in which they were derived (37). *Table 6.2* shows some of the more commonly used equations to estimate HR$_{max}$. For greater accuracy in determining exercise intensity for

---

TABLE 6.2		
Commonly Used Equations for Estimating Maximal Heart Rate		
Author	**Equation**	**Population**
Fox et al. (35)	HR$_{max}$ = 220 − age	Small group of men and women
Astrand (8)	HR$_{max}$ = 216.6 − (0.84 × age)	Men and women age 4–34 yr
Tanaka et al. (101)	HR$_{max}$ = 208 − (0.7 × age)	Healthy men and women
Gellish et al. (38)	HR$_{max}$ = 207 − (0.7 × age)	Men and women participants in an adult fitness program with broad range of age and fitness levels
Gulati et al. (47)	HR$_{max}$ = 206 − (0.88 × age)	Asymptomatic middle-aged women referred for stress testing

HR$_{max}$, maximal heart rate.

the Ex R_x, using the directly measured HR_{max} is preferred to estimated methods, but when not feasible, estimation of HR_{max} is acceptable.

Measured or estimated measures of absolute exercise intensity include caloric expenditure (kcal $\cdot$ min^{-1}), absolute oxygen uptake (mL $\cdot$ min^{-1} or L $\cdot$ min^{-1}), and METs. These absolute measures can result in misclassification of exercise intensity (*e.g.*, moderate and vigorous intensity) because they do not take into consideration individual factors such as body weight, sex, and fitness level (1,2,55). Measurement error, and consequently misclassification, is greater when using estimated rather than directly measured absolute EE and under free living compared to laboratory conditions (1,2,55). For example, an older individual working at 6 METs may be exercising at a vigorous-to-maximal intensity, whereas a younger individual working at the same absolute intensity may be exercising at a moderate intensity (55). Therefore, for individual Ex R_x, a *relative* measure of intensity (*i.e.*, the energy cost of the activity relative to the individual's peak or maximal capacity such as %$\dot{V}O_2$ [*i.e.*, $\dot{V}O_2$ mL $\cdot$ kg^{-1} $\cdot$ min^{-1}], HRR, and $\dot{V}O_2$R, or using a threshold method, [*i.e.*, VT or RCP]) is more appropriate, especially for older, deconditioned individuals and people with chronic diseases (55,70,72).

A summary of methods for calculating exercise intensity using HR, $\dot{V}O_2$, and METs is presented in *Box 6.2*. Intensity of exercise training is usually determined as a range, so the calculation using the formula presented in *Box 6.2* needs to be repeated twice (*i.e.*, once for the lower limit of the desired intensity range and once for the upper limit of the desired intensity range). The prescribed exercise intensity

Box 6.2	**Summary of Methods for Prescribing Exercise Intensity Using Heart Rate (HR), Oxygen Uptake (O₂), and Metabolic Equivalents (METs)**

- HRR method: Target HR (THR) = [($HR_{max/peak}$[a] $-$ HR_{rest}) $\times$ % intensity desired] + HR_{rest}
- $\dot{V}O_2$R method: Target $\dot{V}O_2$R[c] = [($\dot{V}O_{2max/peak}$[b] $-$ $\dot{V}O_{2rest}$) $\times$ % intensity desired] + $\dot{V}O_{rest}$
- HR method: Target HR = $HR_{max/peak}$[a] $\times$ % intensity desired
- $\dot{V}O_2$ method: Target $\dot{V}O_2$[c] = $\dot{V}O_{2max/peak}$[b] $-$ % intensity desired
- MET method: Target MET[c] = [($\dot{V}O_{2max/peak}$[b]) / 3.5 mL $\cdot$ kg^{-1} $\cdot$ min^{-1}] $\times$ % intensity desired

[a]$HR_{max/peak}$ is the highest value obtained during maximal/peak exercise or it can be estimated by 220 $-$ age or some other prediction equation (see *Table 6.2*).
[b]$\dot{V}O_{2max/peak}$ is the highest value obtained during maximal/peak exercise or it can be estimated from a submaximal exercise test. See "The Concept of Maximal Oxygen Uptake" section in *Chapter 4* for the distinction between $\dot{V}O_{2max}$ and $\dot{V}O_{2peak}$.
[c]Activities at the target $\dot{V}O_2$ and MET can be determined using a compendium of physical activity (1,2) or metabolic calculations (46) (see *Table 6.3*).
$HR_{max/peak}$, maximal or peak heart rate; HRR, heart rate reserve; HR_{rest}, resting heart rate; $\dot{V}O_{2max/peak}$, maximal or peak volume of oxygen consumed per unit of time; $\dot{V}O_2$R, oxygen uptake reserve; $\dot{V}O_{2rest}$, resting volume of oxygen consumed per unit of time.

range for an individual should be determined by taking various factors into consideration, including age, habitual PA level, physical fitness level, and health status. Examples illustrating the use of several methods for prescribing exercise intensity are found in *Figure 6.1*. The reader is directed to additional resources (34,70) including other ACSM publications (37,97) for further explanation and examples using these additional methods of prescribing exercise intensity.

When using $\dot{V}O_2$ or METs to prescribe exercise, activities within the desired intensity range can be identified by using a compendium of PAs (1,2) or metabolic calculations (46) (see *Table 6.3* and *Figure 6.1*). There are metabolic equations for estimation of EE during walking, running, cycling, and stepping. Although there are preliminary equations for other modes of exercise such as the elliptical trainer, there are insufficient data to recommend these for universal use at this time. A direct method of Ex R_x by plotting the relationship between HR and $\dot{V}O_2$ may be used when HR and $\dot{V}O_2$ are measured during an exercise test (*Figure 6.2* on page 156). This method may be particularly useful when prescribing exercise in individuals taking medications such as β-blockers or who have a chronic disease or health condition such as diabetes mellitus or atherosclerotic CVD that alters the HR response to exercise (see *Appendix A* and *Chapters 9* and *10*). However, in some individuals with CVD or chronotropic incompetence, a deviation in the linear relationship between HR and $\dot{V}O_2$ may occur, so the use of a threshold method may be superior (70).

Measures of perceived effort and affective valence (*i.e.*, the pleasantness of exercise) can be used to modulate or refine the prescribed exercise intensity. These measures include the Borg Rating of Perceived Exertion (RPE) Scales (15–17,74), OMNI Scales (85,86,110), Talk Test (77), and Feeling Scale (49). The Talk Test is a valid and reliable measure of exercise intensity that is a reasonable surrogate of the lactate threshold, VT, and RCP across a broad range of individuals and can now be recommended as an effective primary method for prescribing and monitoring exercise intensity (10,18,44,56,65,73,78,81,87,115). The other methods (*i.e.*, RPE, OMNI, Feeling Scale) are recommended as adjunct methods for prescribing and monitoring exercise due to the need for further research to validate these methods (37).

Exercise Time (Duration)

Exercise time/duration is prescribed as a measure of the amount of time PA is performed (*i.e.*, time per session, per day, and per week). Most adults are recommended to accumulate 30–60 min $\cdot$ d^{-1} ($\geq$150 min $\cdot$ wk^{-1}) of moderate intensity exercise, 20–60 min $\cdot$ d^{-1} ($\geq$75 min $\cdot$ wk^{-1}) of vigorous intensity exercise, or a combination of moderate and vigorous intensity exercise per day to attain the volumes of exercise recommended in the following discussion (37,107). However, less than 20 min of exercise per day can be beneficial, especially in previously sedentary individuals (37,107). For weight management, longer durations of exercise ($\geq$60–90 min $\cdot$ d^{-1}) may be needed, especially in individuals who spend large amounts of time in sedentary behaviors (28). See *Chapter 10* and the ACSM position stand on overweight and obesity (28) for additional information regarding the Ex R_x recommendations for promoting and maintaining weight loss.

TABLE 6.3

Metabolic Calculations for the Estimation of Energy Expenditure ($\dot{V}O_{2max}$ [mL · kg^{-1} · min^{-1}]) during Common Physical Activities

Sum of Resting + Horizontal + Vertical/ Resistance Components

Activity	Resting Component	Horizontal Component	Vertical Component/ Resistance Component	Limitations
Walking	3.5	0.1 × speed[a]	1.8 × speed[a] × grade[b]	Most accurate for speeds of 1.9–3.7 mi · h^{-1} (50–100 m · min^{-1})
Running	3.5	0.2 × speed[a]	0.9 × speed[a] × grade[b]	Most accurate for speeds >5 mi · h^{-1} (134 m · min^{-1})
Stepping	3.5	0.2 × steps · min^{-1}	1.33 × (1.8 × step height[c] × steps · min^{-1})	Most accurate for stepping rates of 12–30 steps · min^{-1}
Leg cycling	3.5	3.5	(1.8 × work rate[d]/body mass[e]	Most accurate for work rates of 300–1,200 kg · m · min^{-1} (50–200 W)
Arm cycling	3.5	—	(3 × work rate[d])/ body mass[e]	Most accurate for work rates between 150–750 kg · m · min^{-1} (25–125 W)

[a]Speed in m · min^{-1}.
[b]Grade is grade percentage expressed in decimal format (*e.g.*, 10% = 0.10).
[c]Step height in m.
Multiply by the following conversion factors:
  lb to kg: 0.454; in to cm: 2.54; ft to m: 0.3048; mi to km: 1.609; mi · h^{-1} to m · min^{-1}: 26.8; kg · m · min^{-1} to W: 0.164; W to kg · m · min^{-1}: 6.12; O$_{2max}$ L · min^{-1} to kcal · min^{-1}: 4.9; O$_2$ MET to mL · kg^{-1} · min^{-1}: 3.5.
[d]Work rate in kilogram meters per minute (kg · m · min^{-1}) is calculated as resistance (kg) × distance per revolution of flywheel × pedal frequency per minute. Note: Distance per revolution is 6 m for Monark leg ergometer, 3 m for the Tunturi and BodyGuard ergometers, and 2.4 m for Monark arm ergometer.
[e]Body mass in kg.
$\dot{V}O_{2max}$, maximal volume of oxygen consumed per unit of time.

Adapted from (7).

Heart Rate Reserve (HRR) Method

Available test data:

HR_{rest}: 70 beats $\cdot$ min^{-1}

HR_{max}: 180 beats $\cdot$ min^{-1}

Desired exercise intensity range: 50%–60%

Formula: Target Heart Rate (THR) = [(HR_{max} − HR_{rest}) × % intensity] + HR_{rest}

1) Calculation of HRR:

HRR = (HR_{max} − HR_{rest})

HRR = (180 beats $\cdot$ min^{-1} − 70 beats $\cdot$ min^{-1}) = 110 beats $\cdot$ min^{-1}

2) Determination of exercise intensity as %HRR:

Convert desired %HRR into a decimal by dividing by 100

%HRR = desired intensity × HRR

%HRR = 0.5 × 110 beats $\cdot$ min^{-1} = 55 beats $\cdot$ min^{-1}

%HRR = 0.6 × 110 beats $\cdot$ min^{-1} = 66 beats $\cdot$ min^{-1}

3) Determine THR range:

THR = (%HRR) + HR_{rest}

To determine lower limit of THR range:

THR = 55 beats $\cdot$ min^{-1} + 70 beats $\cdot$ min^{-1} = 125 beats $\cdot$ min^{-1}

To determine upper limit of THR range:

THR = 66 beats $\cdot$ min^{-1} + 70 beats $\cdot$ min^{-1} = 136 beats $\cdot$ min^{-1}

THR range: 125 beats $\cdot$ min^{-1} to 136 beats $\cdot$ min^{-1}

$\dot{V}O_2$ Reserve ($\dot{V}O_2R$) Method

Available test data:

$\dot{V}O_{2max}$: 30 mL $\cdot$ kg^{-1} $\cdot$ min^{-1}

$\dot{V}O_{2rest}$: 3.5 mL $\cdot$ kg^{-1} $\cdot$ min^{-1}

Desired exercise intensity range: 50%–60%

Formula: Target $\dot{V}O_2$ = [($\dot{V}O_{2max}$ − $\dot{V}O_{2rest}$) × % intensity] + $\dot{V}O_{2rest}$

1) Calculation of $\dot{V}O_2R$:

$\dot{V}O_2R$ = $\dot{V}O_{2max}$ − $\dot{V}O_{2rest}$

$\dot{V}O_2R$ = 30 mL $\cdot$ kg^{-1} $\cdot$ min^{-1} − 3.5 mL $\cdot$ kg^{-1} $\cdot$ min^{-1}

$\dot{V}O_2R$ = 26.5 mL $\cdot$ kg^{-1} $\cdot$ min^{-1}

2) Determination of exercise intensity as %$\dot{V}O_2R$:

Convert desired intensity (%$\dot{V}O_2R$) into a decimal by dividing by 100

%$\dot{V}O_2R$ = desired intensity × %$\dot{V}O_2R$

Calculate %$\dot{V}O_2R$:

%$\dot{V}O_2R$ = 0.5 × 26.5 mL $\cdot$ kg^{-1} $\cdot$ min^{-1} = 13.3 mL $\cdot$ kg^{-1} $\cdot$ min^{-1}

%$\dot{V}O_2R$ = 0.6 × 26.5 mL $\cdot$ kg^{-1} $\cdot$ min^{-1} = 15.9 mL $\cdot$ kg^{-1} $\cdot$ min^{-1}

3) Determine target $\dot{V}O_2R$ range:

(%$\dot{V}O_2R$) + $\dot{V}O_{2rest}$

To determine the lower target $\dot{V}O_2$ range:

Target $\dot{V}O_2$ = 13.3 mL $\cdot$ kg^{-1} $\cdot$ min^{-1} + 3.5 mL $\cdot$ kg^{-1} $\cdot$ min^{-1} = 16.8 mL $\cdot$ kg^{-1} $\cdot$ min^{-1}

To determine upper target $\dot{V}O_2$ range:

Target $\dot{V}O_2$ = 15.9 mL $\cdot$ kg^{-1} $\cdot$ min^{-1} + 3.5 mL $\cdot$ kg^1 $\cdot$ min^{-1} = 19.4 mL $\cdot$ kg^{-1} $\cdot$ min^{-1}

Target $\dot{V}O_2$ range: 16.8 mL $\cdot$ kg^{-1} $\cdot$ min^{-1} to 19.4 mL $\cdot$ kg^{-1} $\cdot$ min^{-1}

Figure 6.1 Examples of the application of various methods for prescribing exercise intensity. EE, energy expenditure; HR_{max}, maximal heart rate; HR_{rest}, resting heart rate; MET, metabolic equivalent; $\dot{V}O_2$, volume of oxygen consumed per unit of time; $\dot{V}O_{2max}$, maximal volume of oxygen consumed per unit of time; $\dot{V}O_{2rest}$, resting volume of oxygen consumed per unit of time. Adapted from (102). (*continued*)

    4) Determine MET target range (optional):
       1 MET = 3.5 mL $\cdot$ kg^{-1} $\cdot$ min^{-1}
       Calculate lower MET target:
          16.8 mL $\cdot$ kg^{-1} $\cdot$ min^{-1}/3.5 mL $\cdot$ kg^{-1} $\cdot$ min^{-1} = 4.8 METs
       Calculate upper MET target:
          19.4 mL $\cdot$ kg^{-1} $\cdot$ min^{-1}/3.5 mL $\cdot$ kg^{-1} $\cdot$ min^{-1} = 5.5 METs
    5) Identify physical activities requiring EE within the target range from compendium of physical activities (1,2) or by using metabolic calculations shown in *Table 6.3* or reference (46). Also see the following examples of use of metabolic equations.

%HR$_{max}$ (Measured or Estimated) Method:
   Available data:
     A man 45 yr of age
   Desired exercise intensity: 70%–80%
   Formula: THR = HR$_{max}$ × desired %
   Calculate estimated HR$_{max}$ (if measured HR$_{max}$ not available):
     HR$_{max}$ = 220 − age
     HR$_{max}$ = 220 − 45 = 175 beats $\cdot$ min^{-1}
     1) Determine THR range:
       THR = Desired % × HR$_{max}$
       Convert desired % HR$_{max}$ into a decimal by dividing by 100
       Determine lower limit of THR range:
          THR = 175 beats $\cdot$ min^{-1} × 0.70 = 123 beats $\cdot$ min^{-1}
       Determine upper limit of THR range:
          THR = 175 beats $\cdot$ min^{-1} × 0.80 = 140 beats $\cdot$ min^{-1}
       THR range: 123 beats $\cdot$ min^{-1} to 140 beats $\cdot$ min^{-1}

%$\dot{V}O_2$ (Measured or Estimated) Method
   Available data:
     A woman 45 yr of age
     Estimated $\dot{V}O_{2max}$: 30 mL $\cdot$ kg^{-1} $\cdot$ min^{-1}
   Desired $\dot{V}O_2$ range: 50%–60%
   Formula: $\dot{V}O_{2max}$ × desired %
   Determine target $\dot{V}O_2$ range:
     Target $\dot{V}O_2$ = Desired % × $\dot{V}O_{2max}$
       Convert desired intensity (%$\dot{V}O_2$) into a decimal by dividing by 100
       Determine lower limit of target $\dot{V}O_2$ range:
          Target $\dot{V}O_2$ = 0.50 × 30 mL $\cdot$ kg^{-1} $\cdot$ min^{-1} = 15 mL $\cdot$ kg^{-1} $\cdot$ min^{-1}
   Determine upper limit of target $\dot{V}O_{2max}$ range:
     Target $\dot{V}O_2$ = 0.60 × 30 mL $\cdot$ kg^{-1} $\cdot$ min^{-1} = 18 mL $\cdot$ kg^{-1} $\cdot$ min^{-1}
     Target $\dot{V}O_2$ range: 15 mL $\cdot$ kg^{-1} $\cdot$ min^{-1} to 18 mL $\cdot$ kg^{-1} $\cdot$ min^{-1}
     1) Determine MET target range (optional):
       1 MET = 3.5 mL $\cdot$ kg^{-1} $\cdot$ min^{-1}
       Calculate lower MET target:
          15.0 mL $\cdot$ kg^{-1} $\cdot$ min^{-1}/3.5 mL $\cdot$ kg^{-1} $\cdot$ min^{-1} = 4.3 METs
       Calculate upper MET target:
          18.0 mL $\cdot$ kg^{-1} $\cdot$ min^{-1}/3.5 mL $\cdot$ kg^{-1} $\cdot$ min^{-1} = 5.1 METs

Figure 6.1 (*Continued*)

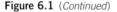

2) Identify physical activities requiring EE within the target range from compendium of physical activities (1,2) or by using metabolic calculations shown in *Table 6.3* and reference (46). See the following examples of use of metabolic equations.

Using metabolic calculations (46) *or (Table 6.3) to determine running speed on a treadmill*
Available data:

A man 32 yr of age
Weight: 130 lb (59 kg)
Height: 70 in (177.8 cm)
$\dot{V}O_{2max}$: 54 mL $\cdot$ kg^{-1} $\cdot$ min^{-1}
Desired treadmill grade: 2.5%
Desired exercise intensity: 80%
Formula: $\dot{V}O_2 = 3.5 + (0.2 \times$ speed$) + (0.9 \times$ speed $\times$ % grade$)$

1. Determine target $\dot{V}O_2$:
   Target $\dot{V}O_2$ = desired % $\times \dot{V}O_{2max}$
   Target $\dot{V}O_2 = 0.80 \times 54$ mL $\cdot$ kg^{-1} $\cdot$ min^{-1} = 43.2 mL $\cdot$ kg^{-1} $\cdot$ min^{-1}
2. Determine treadmill speed:
   $\dot{V}O_2 = 3.5 + (0.2 \times$ speed$) + (0.9 \times$ speed $\times$ % grade$)$
   43.2 mL $\cdot$ kg^{-1} $\cdot$ min^{-1} = 3.5 + (0.2 $\times$ speed) + (0.9 $\times$ speed $\times$ 0.025)
   39.7 = (0.2 $\times$ speed) + (0.9 $\times$ speed $\times$ 0.025)
   39.7 = (0.2 $\times$ speed) + (0.0225 $\times$ speed)
   39.7 = 0.2225 $\times$ speed
   178.4 m $\cdot$ min^{-1} = speed
   Speed on treadmill: 10.7 km $\cdot$ h^{-1} (6.7 mi $\cdot$ h^{1})

Using metabolic calculations (46) *(Table 6.3) to determine % grade during walking on a treadmill*
Available data:

A man 54 yr of age who is moderately physically active
Weight: 190 lb (86.4 kg)
Height: 70 in (177.8 cm)
Desired walking speed: 2.5 mi $\cdot$ h^{-1} (4 km $\cdot$ h^{-1}; 67 m $\cdot$ min^{-1})
Desired MET: 5 METs
Formula: $\dot{V}O_2 = 3.5 + (0.1 \times$ speed$) + (1.8 \times$ speed $\times$ % grade$)$

1. Determine target $\dot{V}O_2$:
   Target $\dot{V}O_2$ = MET $\times$ 3.5 mL $\cdot$ kg^{-1} $\cdot$ min^{-1}
   Target $\dot{V}O_2 = 5 \times 3.5$ mL $\cdot$ kg^{-1} $\cdot$ min^{-1} = 17.5 mL $\cdot$ kg^{-1} $\cdot$ min^{-1}
2. Determine treadmill grade:
   $\dot{V}O_2 = 3.5 + (0.1 \times$ speed$) + (1.8 \times$ speed $\times$ % grade$)$
   17.5 mL $\cdot$ kg^{-1} $\cdot$ min^{-1} = 3.5 + (0.1 $\times$ 67 m $\cdot$ s^{-1}) +
   (1.8 $\times$ 67 m $\cdot$ s^{-1} $\times$ % grade)
   14 = (0.1 $\times$ 67 m $\cdot$ s^{-1}) + (1.8 $\times$ 67 m $\cdot$ s^{-1} $\times$ % grade)
   14 = 6.7 + (120.6 $\times$ % grade)
   7.3 = 120.6 $\times$ % grade
   0.06 = % grade
   % grade = 6%

Figure 6.1 (*Continued*)

Using metabolic calculations (46) *(Table 6.3) to determine target work rate (kg· m · min⁻¹)*
on a Monarch leg cycle ergometer
  Available data:
    A woman 42 yr of age
    Weight: 190 lb (86.4 kg)
    Height: 70 in (177.8 cm)
  Desired $\dot{V}O_2$: 18 kg · m · min⁻¹
  Formula: $\dot{V}O_2 = 7.0 + (1.8 \times$ work rate)/body mass
      1. Calculate work rate on cycle ergometer:
          $\dot{V}O_2 = 7.0 + (1.8 \times$ work rate)/body mass
            18 mL · kg⁻¹ · min⁻¹ = 7.0 + (1.8 × work rate)/86.4 kg
            11 = (1.8 × work rate)/86.4
            950.4 = 1.8 × work rate
            528 = work rate
          Work rate = 528 kg · m · min⁻¹ = 86.6 W

Figure 6.1 (*Continued*)

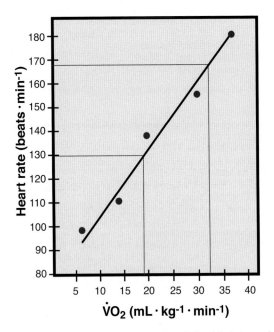

Figure 6.2 Prescribing exercise heart rate using the relationship between heart rate and
$\dot{V}O_2$. A line of best fit has been drawn through the data points on this plot of HR and $\dot{V}O_2$
during a hypothetical exercise test in which $\dot{V}O_{2max}$ was observed to be 38 mL · kg⁻¹ ·
min⁻¹ and HR$_{max}$ was 184 beats · min⁻¹. A THR range was determined by finding the HR
that corresponds to 50% and 85% $\dot{V}O_{2max}$. For this individual, 50% $\dot{V}O_{2max}$ was ~19 mL ·
kg⁻¹ · min⁻¹, and 85% $\dot{V}O_{2max}$ was ~32 mL · kg⁻¹ · min⁻¹. The corresponding THR range
is 130–168 beats · min⁻¹ (7).

The recommended time/duration of PA may be performed continuously (*i.e.*, one session) or intermittently and can be accumulated over the course of a day in one or more sessions that total at least 10 min per session. Exercise bouts of <10 min may yield favorable adaptations in very deconditioned individuals or when done as part of a high intensity aerobic interval program, but further study is needed to confirm the effectiveness of these shorter durations of exercise (37,41,94).

■ **AEROBIC EXERCISE TIME (DURATION) RECOMMENDATION**

Most adults should accumulate 30–60 min $\cdot$ d^{-1} ($\geq$150 min $\cdot$ wk^{-1}) of moderate intensity exercise, 20–60 min $\cdot$ d^{-1} ($\geq$75 min $\cdot$ wk^{-1}) of vigorous intensity exercise or a combination of moderate and vigorous intensity exercise daily to attain the recommended targeted volumes of exercise. This recommended amount of exercise may be accumulated in one continuous exercise session or in bouts of $\geq$10 min over the course of a day. Durations of exercise less than recommended can be beneficial in some individuals.

Type (Mode)

Rhythmic, aerobic type exercises involving large muscle groups are recommended for improving CRF (37). The modes of PA that result in improvement and maintenance of CRF are found in *Table 6.4*. The principle of specificity of training should be kept in mind when selecting the exercise modalities to be included in the Ex R$_x$. The specificity principle states that the physiologic adaptations to exercise are specific to the type of exercise performed (37).

Table 6.4 shows aerobic or cardiorespiratory endurance exercises categorized by the intensity and skill demands. Type A exercises, recommended for all adults, require little skill to perform, and the intensity can easily be modified to accommodate a wide range of physical fitness levels. Type B exercises are typically performed at a vigorous intensity and are recommended for individuals who are at least of average physical fitness and who have been doing some exercise on a regular basis. Type C exercises require skill to perform and therefore are best for individuals who have reasonably developed motor skills and physical fitness to perform the exercises safely. Type D exercises are recreational sports that can improve physical fitness but which are generally recommended as ancillary PAs performed in addition to recommended conditioning PAs. Type D PAs are recommended only for individuals who possess adequate motor skills and physical fitness to perform the sport; however, many of these sports may be modified to accommodate individuals of lower skill and physical fitness levels.

■ AEROBIC EXERCISE TYPE RECOMMENDATION

FITT

Rhythmic, aerobic exercise of at least moderate intensity that involves large muscle groups and requires little skill to perform is recommended for all adults to improve health and CRF. Other exercise and sports requiring skill to perform or higher levels of fitness are recommended only for individuals possessing adequate skill and fitness to perform the activity.

Exercise Volume (Quantity)

Exercise volume is the product of *F*requency, *I*ntensity, and *T*ime (duration) or FIT of exercise. Evidence supports the important role of exercise volume in realizing health/fitness outcomes, particularly with respect to body composition and weight management. Thus, exercise volume may be used to estimate the gross EE of an individual's Ex R_x. MET-min $\cdot$ wk^{-1} and kcal $\cdot$ wk^{-1} can be used to estimate exercise volume in a standardized manner. *Box 6.3* shows the definition and calculations for METs, MET-min, and kcal $\cdot$ min^{-1} for a wide array of PAs. These variables can also be estimated using previously published tables (1,2). MET-min and kcal $\cdot$ min^{-1}

TABLE 6.4

Modes of Aerobic (Cardiorespiratory Endurance) Exercises to Improve Physical Fitness

Exercise Group	Exercise Description	Recommended for	Examples
A	Endurance activities requiring minimal skill or physical fitness to perform	All adults	Walking, leisurely cycling, aqua-aerobics, slow dancing
B	Vigorous intensity endurance activities requiring minimal skill	Adults (as per the preparticipation screening guidelines in *Chapter 2*) who are habitually physically active and/or at least average physical fitness	Jogging, running, rowing, aerobics, spinning, elliptical exercise, stepping exercise, fast dancing
C	Endurance activities requiring skill to perform	Adults with acquired skill and/or at least average physical fitness levels	Swimming, cross-country skiing, skating
D	Recreational sports	Adults with a regular exercise program and at least average physical fitness	Racquet sports, basketball, soccer, downhill skiing, hiking

Adapted from (7).

Box 6.3   Calculation of METs, MET-min^{-1}, and kcal · min^{-1}

Metabolic Equivalents (METs): An index of energy expenditure (EE). "A MET is the ratio of the rate of energy expended during an activity to the rate of energy expended at rest. . . . [One] MET is the rate of EE while sitting at rest . . . by convention . . . [1 MET is equal to] an oxygen uptake of 3.5 [mL · kg^{-1} · min^{-1}]" (80).

MET-min: An index of EE that quantifies the total amount of physical activity performed in a standardized manner across individuals and types of activities (80). Calculated as the product of the number of METs associated with one or more physical activities and the number of minutes the activities were performed (*i.e.*, METs × min), usually standardized per week or per day as a measure of exercise volume.

Kilocalorie (kcal): The energy needed to increase the temperature of 1 kg of water by 1° C. To convert METs to kcal · min^{-1}, it is necessary to know an individual's body weight, kcal · min^{-1} = [(METs × 3.5 mL · kg^{-1} · min^{-1} × body wt in kg) ÷ 1,000)] × 5. Usually standardized as kilocalorie per week or per day as a measure of exercise volume.

Example:
Jogging (at ~7 METs) for 30 min on 3 d · wk^{-1} for a 70-kg male:
7 METs × 30 min × 3 times per week = 630 MET-min · wk^{-1}
[(7 METs × 3.5 mL · kg^{-1} · min^{-1} × 70 kg) ÷ 1,000)] × 5 = 8.575 kcal · min^{-1}
8.575 kcal · min^{-1} × 30 min × 3 times per week = 771.75 kcal · wk^{-1}

Adapted from (37).

---

can then be used to calculate MET-min · wk^{-1} and kcal · wk^{-1} that are accumulated as part of an exercise program to evaluate whether the exercise volume is within the ranges described later in this chapter that will likely result in health/fitness benefits.

The results of epidemiologic studies and randomized clinical trials have demonstrated a dose-response association between the volume of exercise and health/fitness outcomes (*i.e.*, with greater amounts of PA, the health/fitness benefits also increase) (24,37,94,107). Whether or not there is a minimum or maximum amount of exercise that is needed to attain health/fitness benefits is not clear. However, a total EE of ≥500–1,000 MET-min · wk^{-1} is consistently associated with lower rates of CVD and premature mortality. Thus, ≥500–1,000 MET-min · wk^{-1} is a reasonable target volume for an exercise program for most adults (37,107). This volume is approximately equal to (a) 1,000 kcal · wk^{-1} of moderate intensity PA (or about 150 min · wk^{-1}), (b) an exercise intensity of 3–5.9 METs (for individuals weighing ~68–91 kg [~150–200 lb]), and (c) 10 MET-h · wk^{-1} (37,107). Lower volumes of exercise (*i.e.*, 4 kcal · kg^{-1} · wk^{-1} or 330 kcal · wk^{-1}) can result in health/fitness benefits in some individuals, especially in those who are deconditioned (24,37,107). Even lower volumes of exercise may have benefit, but evidence is lacking to make definitive recommendations (37).

Pedometers are effective tools for promoting PA and can be used to approximate exercise volume in steps per day (105). The goal of 10,000 steps $\cdot$ d^{-1} is often cited, but achieving a pedometer step count of at least 5,400–7,900 steps $\cdot$ d^{-1} can meet recommended exercise targets, with the higher end of the range showing more consistent benefit (37,105). For this reason and the imprecision of step counting devices, a target of at least 7,000 steps is recommended for most people. To achieve step counts of 7,000 steps $\cdot$ d^{-1}, one can estimate total exercise volume by considering the following: (a) walking 100 steps $\cdot$ min^{-1} provides a very rough approximation of moderate intensity exercise; (b) walking 1 mi $\cdot$ d^{-1} yields about 2,000 steps $\cdot$ d^{-1}; and (c) walking at a moderate intensity for 30 min $\cdot$ d^{-1} yields about 3,000–4,000 steps $\cdot$ d^{-1} (11,37,57,105). Higher step counts may be necessary for weight management. A population-based study estimated men may require 11,000–12,000 steps $\cdot$ d^{-1} and women 8,000–12,000 steps $\cdot$ d^{-1}, respectively, to maintain a normal weight (37,105). Because of the substantial errors of prediction when using pedometer step counts, using steps per minute combined with currently recommended time/durations of exercise (*e.g.*, 100 steps $\cdot$ min^{-1} for 30 min $\cdot$ session^{-1} and 150 min $\cdot$ wk^{-1}) is judicious (37).

■ AEROBIC EXERCISE VOLUME RECOMMENDATION

A target volume of ≥500–1,000 MET-min $\cdot$ wk^{-1} is recommended for most adults. This volume is approximately equal to 1,000 kcal $\cdot$ wk^{-1} of moderate intensity PA, ~150 min $\cdot$ wk^{-1} of moderate intensity exercise, or pedometer counts of ≥5,400–7,900 steps $\cdot$ d^{-1}. Because of the substantial errors in prediction when using pedometer step counts, use steps per day combined with currently recommended time/durations of exercise. Lower exercise volumes can have health/fitness benefits for deconditioned individuals; however, greater volumes may be needed for weight management.

Rate of Progression

The recommended rate of progression in an exercise program depends on the individual's health status, physical fitness, training responses, and exercise program goals. Progression may consist of increasing any of the components of the FITT principle of Ex R$_x$ as tolerated by the individual. During the initial phase of the exercise program, applying the principle of "start low and go slow" is prudent to reduce risks of adverse cardiovascular events and MSI as well as to enhance adoption and adherence to exercise (see *Chapters 1* and *2*) (37). Initiating exercise at a light-to-moderate intensity in currently inactive individuals and then increasing exercise time/duration (*i.e.*, minutes per session) as tolerated is recommended. An increase in exercise time/duration per session of 5–10 min every 1–2 wk over the first 4–6 wk of an exercise training program is reasonable for the average adult (37). After the individual has been exercising regularly for ≥1 mo, the FIT of exercise is gradually adjusted upward over the next 4–8 mo — or longer for older adults and very deconditioned individuals — to meet the recommended quantity and quality of exercise presented in the *Guidelines*. Any progression in the FITT-VP principle of Ex R$_x$ should be made gradually, avoiding large increases in any of the FITT-VP components to minimize risks of muscular soreness, injury, undue fatigue, and the long-term risk of overtraining. Following any adjustments in the Ex R$_x$, the individual should be monitored for any adverse effects of the increased volume, such as excessive shortness of breath, fatigue, and muscle soreness, and downward adjustments should be made if the exercise is not well tolerated (37).

■ **THE FITT-VP PRINCIPLE OF EX R$_x$ SUMMARY**

The FITT-VP principle of Ex R$_x$ features an individually tailored exercise program that includes specification of the Frequency (F), Intensity (I), Time or duration (T), Type or mode (T), Volume (V), and Progression (P) of exercise to be performed. The exact composition of FITT-VP will vary depending on the characteristics and goals of the individual. The FITT-VP principle of Ex R$_x$ will need to be revised according to the individual response, need, limitation, and adaptations to exercise as well as evolution of the goals and objectives of the exercise program. *Table 6.5* summarizes the FITT-VP principle of Ex R$_x$ recommendations for aerobic exercise.

MUSCULAR FITNESS

The ACSM uses the phrase "muscular fitness" to refer collectively to muscular strength, endurance, and power. Each component of muscular fitness improves consequent to an appropriately designed resistance training regimen and correctly performed resistance exercises. As the trained muscles strengthen and enlarge (*i.e.*, hypertrophy), the resistance training stimulus must be progressively increased (*i.e.*, progressive resistance exercise) if additional gains are to be accrued. To optimize the efficacy of resistance training, the FITT-VP principle of Ex R$_x$ should be tailored to the individual's goals (4,37).

Muscular strength and endurance are often the foundation of a general training regimen focusing on health/fitness outcomes for young and middle-aged adults; however, muscular power should be equally emphasized. Older adults (≥65 yr old) may particularly benefit from power training because this element of muscle fitness declines most rapidly with aging, and insufficient power has been associated with a greater risk of accidental falls (14,23). Importantly, aged individuals can safely perform the fast-velocity muscular contractions, or repetitions, that optimally develop muscular power (83).

TABLE 6.5

Aerobic (Cardiovascular Endurance) Exercise Evidence-Based Recommendations

FITT-VP	Evidence-Based Recommendation
*F*requency	■ ≥5 d · wk^{-1} of moderate exercise, or ≥3 d · wk^{-1} of vigorous exercise, or a combination of moderate and vigorous exercise on ≥3–5 d · wk^{-1} is recommended.
*I*ntensity	■ Moderate and/or vigorous intensity is recommended for most adults. ■ Light-to-moderate intensity exercise may be beneficial in deconditioned individuals.
*T*ime	■ 30–60 min · d^{-1} of purposeful moderate exercise, or 20–60 min · d^{-1} of vigorous exercise, or a combination of moderate and vigorous exercise per day is recommended for most adults. ■ <20 min of exercise per day can be beneficial, especially in previously sedentary individuals.
*T*ype	■ Regular, purposeful exercise that involves major muscle groups and is continuous and rhythmic in nature is recommended.
*V*olume	■ A target volume of ≥500–1,000 MET-min · wk^{-1} is recommended. ■ Increasing pedometer step counts by ≥2,000 steps · d^{-1} to reach a daily step count ≥7,000 steps · d^{-1} steps is beneficial. ■ Exercising below these volumes may still be beneficial for individuals unable or unwilling to reach this amount of exercise.
*P*attern	■ Exercise may be performed in one continuous session, in one interval session, or in multiple sessions of ≥10 min to accumulate the desired duration and volume of exercise per day. ■ Exercise bouts of <10 min may yield favorable adaptations in very deconditioned individuals.
*P*rogression	■ A gradual progression of exercise volume by adjusting exercise duration, frequency, and/or intensity is reasonable until the desired exercise goal (maintenance) is attained. ■ This approach of "start low and go slow" may enhance adherence and reduce risks of musculoskeletal injury and adverse cardiac events.

Adapted from (37).

■ **GOALS FOR A HEALTH-RELATED RESISTANCE TRAINING PROGRAM**

For adults of all ages, the goals of a health-related resistance training program should be to (a) make activities of daily living (ADL) (*e.g.*, stair climbing, carrying bags of groceries) less stressful physiologically and (b) effectively manage, attenuate, and even prevent chronic diseases and health conditions such as osteoporosis, Type 2 diabetes mellitus, and obesity. For these reasons, although resistance training is important across the age span, its importance becomes even greater with age (5,37,72).

The guidelines described in this chapter for resistance training are dedicated to improving health and are most appropriate for an overall or general physical fitness program that includes but does not necessarily emphasize muscle development (4,37).

Frequency of Resistance Exercise

For general muscular fitness, particularly among those who are untrained or recreationally trained (*i.e.*, not engaged in a formal training program), an individual should resistance train each major muscle group (*i.e.*, the muscle groups of the chest, shoulders, upper and lower back, abdomen, hips, and legs) 2–3 d · wk^{-1} with at least 48 h separating the exercise training sessions for the same muscle group (4,37). Depending on the individual's daily schedule, all muscle groups to be trained may be done so in the same session (*i.e.*, whole body), or each session may "split" the body into selected muscle groups so that only a few of those groups are trained in any one session (4,37). For example, muscles of the lower body may be trained on Mondays and Thursdays, and upper body muscles may be trained on Tuesdays and Fridays. This split weight training routine entails 4 d · wk^{-1} to train each muscle group two times per week. The split and whole body methods are effective as long as each muscle group is trained 2–3 d · wk^{-1}. Having these different resistance training options provides the individual with more flexibility in scheduling, which may help to improve the likelihood of adherence to a resistance training regimen.

■ **RESISTANCE TRAINING FREQUENCY RECOMMENDATION**

Resistance training of each major muscle group 2–3 d · wk^{-1} with at least 48 h separating the exercise training sessions for the same muscle group is recommended for all adults.

Types of Resistance Exercises

Many types of resistance training equipment can effectively be used to improve muscular fitness including free weights, machines with stacked weights or pneumatic resistance, and resistance bands. Resistance training regimens should focus on multijoint or compound exercises that affect more than one muscle group (*e.g.*, chest press, shoulder press, pull-down, rows, push-ups, leg press, squats, deadlifts), single-joint exercises targeting major muscle groups (*e.g.*, biceps curls, triceps extensions, quadriceps extensions, leg curls, calf raises), and exercises that affect core muscles (*e.g.*, planks and bridges) (4,37).

To avoid creating muscle imbalances that may lead to injury, opposing muscle groups (*i.e.*, agonists and antagonists), such as the chest and upper back or the quadriceps and hamstring muscles, should be included in the resistance training routine (4,37). Examples of these types of resistance exercises are chest presses and dumbbell rows to target the muscles of the chest and upper back and leg extensions and leg curls to exercise the quadriceps and hamstring muscles or biceps curls and triceps extensions to work the muscles of the upper arms.

■ **TYPES OF RESISTANCE EXERCISES**

Many types of resistance training equipment can effectively be used to improve muscular fitness. Both multijoint and single-joint exercises targeting agonist and antagonist muscle groups are recommended for all adults as part of a comprehensive resistance training program.

Volume of Resistance Exercise (Sets and Repetitions)

Each muscle group should be trained for a total of two to four sets. The sets may be derived from the same exercise or from a combination of exercises affecting the same muscle group (4,37). For example, the pectoral muscles of the chest region may be trained either with four sets of bench presses or with two sets of bench presses and two sets of push-ups (79). A reasonable rest interval between sets is 2–3 min. Using different exercises to train the same muscle group adds variety and may prevent long-term mental "staleness"; however, evidence that these factors improve adherence to a training program is lacking (37).

Completing four sets per muscle group is more effective than two sets; however, even a single set per muscle group will significantly improve muscular strength, particularly among novices (4,37,79). The first set of a resistance exercise is responsible for the majority of the benefits derived from a series of sets (60,61). By completing one set of two different exercises that affect the same muscle group, the muscle has executed two sets. For example, bench presses and push-ups affect the pectoralis muscles of the chest so that by completing one set of each, the muscle group has performed a total of two sets. Moreover, compound exercises such as the bench press and push-ups also train the triceps muscle group. From a practical standpoint of program adherence, each individual should carefully assess his or her daily schedule, time demands, and level of commitment to determine how many sets per muscle should be performed during resistance training sessions. The adoption of a resistance training program that realistically will be maintained over the long term is of paramount importance.

The resistance training intensity and number of repetitions performed with each set are inversely related. That is, the greater the intensity or resistance, the fewer the number of repetitions that will need to be completed. To improve muscular strength, mass, and — to some extent — endurance, a resistance exercise that allows an individual to complete 8–12 repetitions per set should be selected.

This repetition number translates to a resistance that is ~60%–80% of the individual's one repetition maximum (1-RM) or the greatest amount of weight lifted for a single repetition. For example, if an individual's 1-RM in the shoulder press is 100 lb (45.5 kg), then, when performing that exercise during the training sessions, he or she should choose a resistance between 60 and 80 lb (27–36 kg). If an individual performs multiple sets per exercise, the number of repetitions completed before fatigue occurs will be at or close to 12 repetitions with the first set and will decline to about 8 repetitions during the last set for that exercise. Each set should be performed with proper technique and to the point of muscle fatigue but not failure because exerting muscles to the point of failure increases the likelihood of injury or debilitating residual muscle soreness, particularly among novices (4,37,79). Maximal strength gains follow a dose-response curve. Among the untrained, significant strength gains are realized with as few as one set per muscle group per session, whereas additional strength gains peak at a volume of four sets per muscle group at 60% of 1-RM, three times a week (84). Individuals interested in maximal strength gains should gradually progress from one to four sets as tolerated. Those who are recreationally or moderately trained achieve the greatest strength improvements with a training intensity of 80% of 1-RM, with four sets for each major muscle group at a training frequency of twice per week (84).

To improve muscular endurance rather than strength and mass, a higher number of repetitions, perhaps 15–25, should be performed per set along with shorter rest intervals and fewer sets (*i.e.*, one or two sets per muscle group) (4,37). This regimen necessitates a lower intensity of resistance, typically of no more than 50% 1-RM. Similarly, older and very deconditioned individuals who are more susceptible to musculotendinous injury should begin a resistance training program conducting more repetitions (*i.e.*, 10–15) at a very light-to-light intensity of 40%–50% of 1-RM or an RPE of 5–6 on a 10-point scale (4,37,72) assuming the individual has the capacity to use this intensity while maintaining proper lifting technique. Subsequent to a period of adaptation to resistance training and improved musculotendinous conditioning, older individuals may choose to follow guidelines for younger adults (*i.e.*, higher intensity with 8–12 repetitions per set) (37) (see *Chapter 7*).

■ **VOLUME OF RESISTANCE EXERCISE (SETS AND REPETITIONS) RECOMMENDATION**

Ideally, adults should train each muscle group for a total of 2–4 sets with 8–12 repetitions per set with a rest interval of 2–3 min between sets to improve muscular fitness. However, even a single set per muscle group will significantly improve muscular strength, particularly among novices. Older adults or deconditioned individuals should begin a training regimen with ≥1 set of 10–15 repetitions of very light-to-light intensity (*i.e.*, 40%–50% 1-RM) resistance exercise for muscular fitness improvements.

Resistance Exercise Technique

To ensure optimal health/fitness gains and minimize the chance of injury, each resistance exercise should be performed with proper technique regardless of training status or age. The exercises should be executed using correct form and technique, including performing the repetitions deliberately and in a controlled manner, moving through the full ROM of the joint, and employing proper breathing techniques (*i.e.*, exhalation during the concentric phase and inhalation during the eccentric phase and avoid the Valsalva maneuver) (4,37). However, resistance training composed exclusively of eccentric or lengthening contractions conducted at very high intensities (*e.g.*, >100% 1-RM) is not recommended because of the significant chance of injury, severe muscle soreness, and serious complications such as rhabdomyolysis (*i.e.*, muscle damage resulting in excretion of myoglobin into the urine that may harm kidney function) that can ensue (4,37). Similarly, for those with orthopedic injuries or pain, a symptom-limited ROM should be used when executing sets of resistance exercises. Individuals who are naïve to resistance training should receive instruction on proper technique from a qualified health/fitness professional (*e.g.*, ACSM Certified Exercise Physiologist[SM], ACSM Certified Personal Trainer®) on each exercise used during resistance training sessions (4,37).

■ RESISTANCE EXERCISE TECHNIQUE RECOMMENDATIONS

All individuals should perform resistance training using correct technique. Proper resistance exercise techniques employ controlled movements through the full ROM and involve concentric and eccentric muscle actions.

Progression/Maintenance

As adaptations to a resistance exercise training program occur, the participant should continue to subject the muscles to overload or greater stimuli to continue to increase muscular strength and mass. This "progressive overload" principle may be performed in several ways. The most common approach is to increase the amount of resistance lifted during training. For example, if an individual is using 100 lb (45.5 kg) of resistance for a given exercise, and his or her muscles have adapted to the point to which 12 repetitions are performed with minimal effort, then the resistance should be increased so that no more than 12 repetitions are completed without significant muscle fatigue and difficulty in completing the last repetition of that set while maintaining proper form/technique. Other ways to progressively overload muscles include performing more sets per muscle group and increasing the number of days per week the muscle groups are trained (4,37).

On the other hand, if the individual has attained the desired levels of muscular strength and mass and he or she seeks to simply maintain that level of muscular fitness, it is not necessary to progressively increase the training stimulus. That is, increasing the overload by adding resistance, sets, or training sessions per week is not required during a resistance training program focused on maintaining muscle fitness. Muscular strength may be maintained by training muscle groups as little as 1 d · wk^{-1} as long as the training intensity or the resistance lifted is held constant (4,37).

The FITT-VP principle of Ex R$_x$ for resistance training is summarized in *Table 6.6*. Because these guidelines are most appropriate for a general fitness program, a more rigorous training program must be employed if one's goal is to maximally increase muscular strength and mass, particularly among competitive athletes in sports such as football and basketball. Exercise professionals who are interested in the ability to maximally develop muscular strength and mass are referred to the ACSM position stand on progression models in resistance training for healthy adults for additional information (4,37).

■ **PROGRESSION/MAINTENANCE OF RESISTANCE TRAINING RECOMMENDATION**

As muscles adapt to a resistance exercise training program, the participant should continue to subject them to overload to continue to increase muscular strength and mass by gradually increasing resistance, number of sets, or frequency of training.

FLEXIBILITY EXERCISE (STRETCHING)

Joint ROM or flexibility can be improved across all age groups by engaging in flexibility exercises (37,72). The ROM around a joint is improved immediately after performing flexibility exercise and shows chronic improvement after about 3–4 wk of regular stretching at a frequency of at least 2–3 times · wk^{-1} (37). Postural stability and balance can also be improved by engaging in flexibility exercises, especially when combined with resistance exercise (37).

The goal of a flexibility program is to develop ROM in the major muscle/tendon groups in accordance with individualized goals. Certain performance standards discussed later in this chapter enhance the effectiveness of flexibility exercises. It is most effective to perform flexibility exercise when the muscle temperature is increased through warm-up exercises (37).

Static stretching exercises may result in a short-term decrease in muscle strength, power, and sports performance when performed immediately prior to the muscle strength and power activity, especially with longer duration (>45 s) stretching (93). This negative effect is particularly apparent when strength and power are important to performance (37,68). Less clear, however, is the mechanism responsible for the noted decreases (25). Before definitive recommendations

TABLE 6.6	
Resistance Exercise Evidence-Based Recommendations	
FITT-VP	**Evidence-Based Recommendation**
Frequency	■ Each major muscle group should be trained on 2–3 d · wk^{-1}.
Intensity	■ 60%–70% 1-RM (moderate-to-vigorous intensity) for novice to intermediate exercisers to improve strength ■ Experienced strength trainers can gradually increase to ≥80% 1-RM (vigorous-to-very vigorous intensity) to improve strength. ■ 40%–50% 1-RM (very light-to-light intensity) for older individuals beginning exercise to improve strength ■ 40%–50% 1-RM (very light-to-light intensity) may be beneficial for improving strength in sedentary individuals beginning a resistance training program. ■ <50% 1-RM (light-to-moderate intensity) to improve muscular endurance ■ 20%–50% 1-RM in older adults to improve power
Time	■ No specific duration of training has been identified for effectiveness.
Type	■ Resistance exercises involving each major muscle group are recommended. ■ Multijoint exercises affecting more than one muscle group and targeting agonist and antagonist muscle groups are recommended for all adults. ■ Single-joint exercises targeting major muscle groups may also be included in a resistance training program, typically after performing multijoint exercise(s) for that particular muscle group. ■ A variety of exercise equipment and/or body weight can be used to perform these exercises.
Repetitions	■ 8–12 repetitions are recommended to improve strength and power in most adults. ■ 10–15 repetitions are effective in improving strength in middle-aged and older individuals starting exercise. ■ 15–25 repetitions are recommended to improve muscular endurance.
Sets	■ 2–4 sets are recommended for most adults to improve strength and power. ■ A single set of resistance exercise can be effective especially among older and novice exercisers. ■ ≤2 sets are effective in improving muscular endurance.
Pattern	■ Rest intervals of 2–3 min between each set of repetitions are effective. ■ A rest of ≥48 h between sessions for any single muscle group is recommended.
Progression	■ A gradual progression of greater resistance, and/or more repetitions per set, and/or increasing frequency is recommended.

1-RM, one repetition maximum.

Adapted from (37).

can be made, more research is needed on the immediate effects of flexibility exercises on the performance of fitness-related activities. Nevertheless, it is reasonable, based on the available evidence, to recommend individuals engaging in a general fitness program perform flexibility exercise following cardiorespiratory or resistance exercise — or alternatively — as a stand-alone program (37).

■ FLEXIBILITY EXERCISE RECOMMENDATION

ROM is improved acutely and chronically following flexibility exercises. Flexibility exercises are most effective when the muscles are warm. Static stretching exercises may acutely reduce power and strength, so it is recommended that flexibility exercises be performed after exercise and sports where strength and power are important for performance.

Types of Flexibility Exercises

Flexibility exercise should target the major muscle tendon units of the shoulder girdle, chest, neck, trunk, lower back, hips, posterior and anterior legs, and ankles (37). *Box 6.4* shows the several types of flexibility exercises that can improve ROM. Properly performed ballistic stretching is equally as effective as static stretching in increasing joint ROM and may be considered for adults who engage in activities

---

Box 6.4   Flexibility Exercise Definitions

Ballistic methods or "bouncing" stretches use the momentum of the moving body segment to produce the stretch (116).

Dynamic or slow movement stretching involves a gradual transition from one body position to another and a progressive increase in reach and range of motion as the movement is repeated several times (69).

Static stretching involves slowly stretching a muscle/tendon group and holding the position for a period of time (*i.e.*, 10–30 s). Static stretches can be active or passive (114).

Active static stretching involves holding the stretched position using the strength of the agonist muscle as is common in many forms of yoga (37).

Passive static stretching involves assuming a position while holding a limb or other part of the body with or without the assistance of a partner or device (such as elastic bands or a ballet barre) (37).

Proprioceptive neuromuscular facilitation (PNF) methods take several forms but typically involve an isometric contraction of the selected muscle/tendon group followed by a static stretching of the same group (*i.e.*, contract-relax) (82,92).

Adapted from (37).

that involve ballistic movements such as basketball (26,37,66,116). Both proprioceptive neuromuscular facilitation (PNF) techniques that require a partner to perform and static stretching are superior to dynamic or slow movement stretching in increasing ROM around a joint (37). PNF techniques typically involve an isometric contraction followed by a static stretch in the same muscle/tendon group (*i.e.*, contract-relax).

■ **FLEXIBILITY TYPE RECOMMENDATION**

A series of flexibility exercises targeting the major muscle tendon units should be performed. A variety of static, dynamic, and PNF flexibility exercises can improve ROM around a joint.

Volume of Flexibility Exercise (Time, Repetitions, and Frequency)

Holding a stretch for 10–30 s to the point of tightness or slight discomfort enhances joint ROM, and although not entirely conclusive (36), there seems to be little additional benefit resulting from holding the stretch for a longer duration (37). However, in older adults, stretching for 30–60 s may result in greater flexibility gains than shorter duration stretches (37) (see *Chapter 7*). For PNF stretches, it is recommended that the individuals of all ages hold a light-to-moderate contraction (*i.e.*, 20%–75% of maximum voluntary contraction) for 3–6 s, followed by an assisted stretch for 10–30 s (37). Flexibility exercises should be repeated two to four times to accumulate a total of 60 s of stretching for each flexibility exercise by adjusting time/duration and repetitions according to individual needs (37). The goal of 60 s of stretch time can be attained by, for example, two 30-s stretches or four 15-s stretches (37). Performing flexibility exercises $\geq$2–3 d $\cdot$ wk^{-1} will improve ROM, but stretching exercises are most effective when performed daily (37). A stretching routine following these guidelines can be completed by most individuals in $\leq$10 min (37). A summary of the FITT-VP principle of Ex R$_x$ for flexibility exercise is found in *Table 6.7*.

■ **FLEXIBILITY VOLUME RECOMMENDATION**

A total of 60 s of flexibility exercise per joint is recommended. Holding a single flexibility exercise for 10–30 s to the point of tightness or slight discomfort is effective. Older adults can benefit from holding the stretch for 30–60 s. A 20%–75% maximum voluntary contraction held for 3–6 s followed by a 10- to 30-s assisted stretch is recommended for PNF techniques. Performing flexibility exercises $\geq$2–3 d $\cdot$ wk^{-1} is recommended with daily flexibility exercise being most effective.

TABLE 6.7	
Flexibility Exercise Evidence-Based Recommendations	
FITT-VP	**Evidence-Based Recommendation**
*F*requency	■ ≥2–3 d · wk^{-1} with daily being most effective
*I*ntensity	■ Stretch to the point of feeling tightness or slight discomfort.
*T*ime	■ Holding a static stretch for 10–30 s is recommended for most adults. ■ In older individuals, holding a stretch for 30–60 s may confer greater benefit. ■ For proprioceptive neuromuscular facilitation (PNF) stretching, a 3–6 s light-to-moderate contraction (*e.g.,* 20%–75% of maximum voluntary contraction) followed by a 10- to 30-s assisted stretch is desirable.
*T*ype	■ A series of flexibility exercises for each of the major muscle-tendon units is recommended. ■ Static flexibility (*i.e.,* active or passive), dynamic flexibility, ballistic flexibility, and PNF are each effective.
*V*olume	■ A reasonable target is to perform 60 s of total stretching time for each flexibility exercise.
*P*attern	■ Repetition of each flexibility exercise 2–4 times is recommended. ■ Flexibility exercise is most effective when the muscle is warmed through light-to-moderate aerobic activity or passively through external methods such as moist heat packs or hot baths.
*P*rogression	■ Methods for optimal progression are unknown.

Adapted from (37).

NEUROMOTOR EXERCISE

Neuromotor exercise training involves motor skills such as balance, coordination, gait, and agility and proprioceptive training and is sometimes called *functional fitness training*. Other multifaceted PAs sometimes considered to be neuromotor exercise involve varying combinations of neuromotor, resistance, and flexibility exercise and include tai ji (tai chi), qigong, and yoga. For older individuals, the benefits of neuromotor exercise training include improvements in balance, agility, and muscle strength and reduces the risk of falls and the fear of falling (5,37,72) (see *Chapter 7*). There are few studies on the benefits of neuromotor training in younger adults, although limited data suggest that balance and agility training may result in reduced injury in athletes (37). Because of a lack of research on middle-aged and younger adults, definitive recommendations for the benefit of neuromotor exercise training cannot be made.

The optimal effectiveness of the various types of neuromotor exercise, doses (*i.e.,* FIT), and training regimens are not known for adults of any age (37,72). Studies that have resulted in neuromotor improvements have mostly employed training frequencies of ≥2–3 d · wk^{-1} with exercise sessions of

TABLE 6.8	
Neuromotor Exercise Evidence-Based Recommendations	
FITT-VP	**Evidence-Based Recommendation**
*F*requency	■ ≥2–3 d · wk^{-1} is recommended.
*I*ntensity	■ An effective intensity of neuromotor exercise has not been determined.
*T*ime	■ ≥20–30 min · d^{-1} may be needed.
*T*ype	■ Exercises involving motor skills (*e.g.,* balance, agility, coordination, gait), proprioceptive exercise training, and multifaceted activities (*e.g.,* tai chi, yoga) are recommended for older individuals to improve and maintain physical function and reduce falls in those at risk for falling. ■ The effectiveness of neuromotor exercise training in younger and middle-aged individuals has not been established, but there is probable benefit.
*V*olume	■ The optimal volume (*e.g.,* number of repetitions, intensity) is not known.
*P*attern	■ The optimal pattern of performing neuromotor exercise is not known.
*P*rogression	■ Methods for optimal progression are not known.

Adapted from (37).

≥20–30 min duration for a total of ≥60 min of neuromotor exercise per week (37,72). There is no available evidence concerning the number of repetitions of exercises needed, the intensity of the exercise, or optimal methods for progression. A summary of the FITT-VP principle of Ex R$_x$ for neuromotor exercise is found in *Table 6.8*.

■ **NEUROMOTOR EXERCISE RECOMMENDATIONS**

Neuromotor exercises involving balance, agility, coordination, and gait are recommended on ≥2–3 d · wk^{-1} for older individuals and are likely beneficial for younger adults as well. The optimal duration or number of repetitions of these exercises is not known, but neuromotor exercise routines of ≥20–30 min in duration for a total of ≥60 min of neuromotor exercise per week are effective.

SEDENTARY BEHAVIOR AND BRIEF ACTIVITY BREAKS

Sedentary behaviors can have adverse health effects, even among those who regularly exercise (12,29,59,62,76). Moreover, there is increasing evidence that concurrently reducing sedentary time results in health benefits that are additive to exercise (29,39,52,64,67,76,113). Sedentary behavior negatively impacts cardiometabolic markers, body composition, and physical function, and these effects might be attenuated by interspersing brief PA breaks (*e.g.*, 1–5 min of standing and walking) (13,30,39,40,64,90,95,100). Although currently there are many gaps in the scientific knowledge about sedentary behavior and activity breaks (42,103), there is sufficient evidence as outlined earlier to propose limiting sedentary time and adding brief PA breaks during sedentary pastimes (37). Therefore, adding short PA breaks throughout the day may be considered as a part of the Ex R_x (89). Although the frequency, intensity, time (duration), and type of brief PA breaks have not been clearly identified (67), standing or engaging in light-to-moderate walking or other PA once or more per hour to breakup sedentary stretches may be encouraged.

EXERCISE PROGRAM SUPERVISION

The exercise professional may determine the level of supervision that is optimal for an individual by evaluating information derived from the preparticipation health screening (see *Chapter 2*) and the preexercise evaluation (see *Chapter 3*). Supervision by an experienced exercise professional can enhance adherence to exercise and may improve safety for individuals with chronic diseases and health conditions (37,72,111). Individualized exercise instruction may be especially helpful for sedentary adults and persons with a chronic disease who are initiating a new exercise program (37,72).

ONLINE RESOURCES

2008 Physical Activity Guidelines for Americans (107):
   http://www.health.gov/PAguidelines/
ACSM Exercise Is Medicine:
   http://www.exerciseismedicine.org
ACSM position stand on progression models in resistance training (4):
   http://www.acsm.org
ACSM position stand on the quantity and quality of exercise (37):
   http://www.acsm.org
American Heart Association:
   http://www.heart.org
Compendium of Physical Activities:
   https://sites.google.com/site/compendiumofphysicalactivities/
National Institutes on Aging Exercise and Physical Activity Guide (108):
   http://www.nia.nih.gov/HealthInformation/Publications/
National Strength and Conditioning Association:
   http://www.nsca-lift.org
Shape Up America:
   http://www.shapeup.org

REFERENCES

1. Ainsworth BE, Haskell WL, Leon AS, et al. Compendium of physical activities: classification of energy costs of human physical activities. *Med Sci Sports Exerc*. 1993;25(1):71–80.

2. Ainsworth BE, Haskell WL, Whitt MC, et al. Compendium of physical activities: an update of activity codes and MET intensities. *Med Sci Sports Exerc*. 2000;32(9 Suppl):S498–504.

3. American College of Sports Medicine. American College of Sports Medicine position stand. Osteoporosis and exercise. *Med Sci Sports Exerc*. 1995;27(4):i–vii.

4. American College of Sports Medicine. American College of Sports Medicine position stand. Progression models in resistance training for healthy adults. *Med Sci Sports Exerc*. 2009;41(3):687–708.

5. American College of Sports Medicine, Chodzko-Zajko WJ, Proctor DN, et al. American College of Sports Medicine position stand. Exercise and physical activity for older adults. *Med Sci Sports Exerc*. 2009;41(7):1510–30.

6. Angadi SS, Mookadam F, Lee CD, Tucker WJ, Haykowsky MJ, Gaesser GA. High-intensity interval training vs. moderate-intensity continuous exercise training in heart failure with preserved ejection fraction: a pilot study. *J Appl Physiol*. 2015;119(6):753–8.

7. Armstrong LE, Brubaker PH, Whaley MH, Otto RM, American College of Sports Medicine. *ACSM's Guidelines for Exercise Testing and Prescription*. 7th ed. Baltimore (MD): Lippincott Williams & Wilkins; 2005. 366 p.

8. Astrand PO. *Experimental Studies of Physical Working Capacity in Relation to Sex and Age*. Copenhagen (Denmark): Musksgaard; 1952. 171 p.

9. Bailey DP, Locke CD. Breaking up prolonged sitting with light-intensity walking improves postprandial glycemia, but breaking up sitting with standing does not. *J Sci Med Sport*. 2015; 18(3):294–8.

10. Ballweg J, Foster C, Porcari J, Haible S, Aminaka N, Mikat RP. Reliability of the talk test as a surrogate of ventilatory and respiratory compensation thresholds. *J Sports Sci Med*. 2013;12(3):610–1.

11. Bassett DR Jr, Wyatt HR, Thompson H, Peters JC, Hill JO. Pedometer-measured physical activity and health behaviors in U.S. adults. *Med Sci Sports Exerc*. 2010;42(10):1819–25.

12. Biswas A, Oh PI, Faulkner GE, et al. Sedentary time and its association with risk for disease incidence, mortality, and hospitalization in adults: a systematic review and meta-analysis. *Ann Intern Med*. 2015;162(2):123–32.

13. Blankenship JM, Granados K, Braun B. Effects of subtracting sitting versus adding exercise on glycemic control and variability in sedentary office workers. *Appl Physiol Nutr Metab*. 2014;39(11):1286–93.

14. Bonnefoy M, Jauffret M, Jusot JF. Muscle power of lower extremities in relation to functional ability and nutritional status in very elderly people. *J Nutr Health Aging*. 2007;11(3):223–8.

15. Borg GA. Perceived exertion. *Exerc Sport Sci Rev*. 1974;2:131–53.

16. Borg GA, Hassmen P, Lagerstrom M. Perceived exertion related to heart rate and blood lactate during arm and leg exercise. *Eur J Appl Physiol Occup Physiol*. 1987;56(6):679–85.

17. Borg GA, Ljunggren G, Ceci R. The increase of perceived exertion, aches and pain in the legs, heart rate and blood lactate during exercise on a bicycle ergometer. *Eur J Appl Physiol Occup Physiol*. 1985;54(4):343–9.

18. Brawner CA, Vanzant MA, Ehrman JK, et al. Guiding exercise using the talk test among patients with coronary artery disease. *J Cardiopulm Rehabil*. 2006;26(2):72–5; quiz 76–7.

19. Brown WJ, Bauman AE, Bull FC, Burton NW. *Development of Evidence-Based Physical Activity Recommendations for Adults (18-64 Years)* [Internet]. Canberra (Australia): Australian Government Department of Health; 2012 [cited 2015 Sept 23]. 170 p. Available from: http://www.health.gov.au/internet/main/publishing.nsf/Content/health-pubhlth-strateg-phys-act-guidelines/$File/DEB-PAR-Adults-18-64years.pdf

20. Buchheit M, Laursen PB. High-intensity interval training, solutions to the programming puzzle. Part I: cardiopulmonary emphasis. *Sports Med*. 2013;43(5):313–38.

21. Buchheit M, Laursen PB. High-intensity interval training, solutions to the programming puzzle. Part II: anaerobic energy, neuromuscular load and practical applications. *Sports Med*. 2013;43(10):927–54.

22. Burgomaster KA, Howarth KR, Phillips SM, et al. Similar metabolic adaptations during exercise after low volume sprint interval and traditional endurance training in humans. *J Physiol.* 2008;586(1):151–60.

23. Chan BK, Marshall LM, Winters KM, Faulkner KA, Schwartz AV, Orwoll ES. Incident fall risk and physical activity and physical performance among older men: the Osteoporotic Fractures in Men Study. *Am J Epidemiol.* 2007;165(6):696–703.

24. Church TS, Earnest CP, Skinner JS, Blair SN. Effects of different doses of physical activity on cardiorespiratory fitness among sedentary, overweight or obese postmenopausal women with elevated blood pressure: a randomized controlled trial. *JAMA.* 2007;297(19):2081–91.

25. Clark L, O'Leary CB, Hong J, Lockard M. The acute effects of stretching on presynaptic inhibition and peak power. *J Sports Med Phys Fitness.* 2014;54(5):605–10.

26. Covert CA, Alexander MP, Petronis JJ, Davis DS. Comparison of ballistic and static stretching on hamstring muscle length using an equal stretching dose. *J Strength Cond Res.* 2010;24(11):3008–14.

27. Currie KD, Dubberley JB, McKelvie RS, MacDonald MJ. Low-volume, high-intensity interval training in patients with CAD. *Med Sci Sports Exerc.* 2013;45(8):1436–42.

28. Donnelly JE, Blair SN, Jakicic JM, et al. American College of Sports Medicine position stand. Appropriate physical activity intervention strategies for weight loss and prevention of weight regain for adults. *Med Sci Sports Exerc.* 2009;41(2):459–71.

29. Dunstan DW, Howard B, Healy GN, Owen N. Too much sitting — a health hazard. *Diabetes Res Clin Pract.* 2012;97(3):368–76.

30. Duvivier BM, Schaper NC, Bremers MA, et al. Minimal intensity physical activity (standing and walking) of longer duration improves insulin action and plasma lipids more than shorter periods of moderate to vigorous exercise (cycling) in sedentary subjects when energy expenditure is comparable. *PLoS One.* 2013;8(2):e55542.

31. Edge J, Bishop D, Goodman C, Dawson B. Effects of high- and moderate-intensity training on metabolism and repeated sprints. *Med Sci Sports Exerc.* 2005;37(11):1975–82.

32. Ehrman JK, American College of Sports Medicine. *ACSM's Resource Manual for Guidelines for Exercise Testing and Prescription.* 6th ed. Baltimore (MD): Lippincott Williams & Wilkins; 2009. 868 p.

33. Elliott AD, Rajopadhyaya K, Bentley DJ, Beltrame JF, Aromataris EC. Interval training versus continuous exercise in patients with coronary artery disease: a meta-analysis. *Heart Lung Circ.* 2015;24(2):149–57.

34. Fletcher GF, Ades PA, Kligfield P, et al. Exercise standards for testing and training: a scientific statement from the American Heart Association. *Circulation.* 2013;128(8):873–934.

35. Fox SM III, Naughton JP, Haskell WL. Physical activity and the prevention of coronary heart disease. *Ann Clin Res.* 1971;3(6):404–32.

36. Freitas SR, Vilarinho D, Rocha Vaz J, Bruno PM, Costa PB, Mil-homens P. Responses to static stretching are dependent on stretch intensity and duration. *Clin Physiol Funct Imaging.* 2015;35(6):478–84.

37. Garber CE, Blissmer B, Deschenes MR, et al. American College of Sports Medicine position stand. The quantity and quality of exercise for developing and maintaining cardiorespiratory, musculoskeletal, and neuromotor fitness in apparently healthy adults: guidance for prescribing exercise. *Med Sci Sports Exerc.* 2011;43(7):1334–59.

38. Gellish RL, Goslin BR, Olson RE, McDonald A, Russi GD, Moudgil VK. Longitudinal modeling of the relationship between age and maximal heart rate. *Med Sci Sports Exerc.* 2007;39(5):822–9.

39. Gennuso KP, Gangnon RE, Thraen-Borowski KM, Colbert LH. Dose-response relationships between sedentary behaviour and the metabolic syndrome and its components. *Diabetologia.* 2015;58(3):485–92.

40. Gianoudis J, Bailey CA, Daly RM. Associations between sedentary behaviour and body composition, muscle function and sarcopenia in community-dwelling older adults. *Osteoporos Int.* 2015;26(2):571–9.

41. Gibala MJ, Gillen JB, Percival ME. Physiological and health-related adaptations to low-volume interval training: influences of nutrition and sex. *Sports Med.* 2014;44(2 Suppl):S127–37.

42. Gibbs BB, Hergenroeder AL, Katzmarzyk PT, Lee IM, Jakicic JM. Definition, measurement, and health risks associated with sedentary behavior. *Med Sci Sports Exerc.* 2015;47(6):1295–300.

43. Gillen JB, Gibala MJ. Is high-intensity interval training a time-efficient exercise strategy to improve health and fitness? *Appl Physiol Nutr Metab*. 2014;39(3):409–12.

44. Gillespie BD, McCormick JJ, Mermier CM, Gibson AL. Talk test as a practical method to estimate exercise intensity in highly trained competitive male cyclists. *J Strength Cond Res*. 2015; 29(4):894–8.

45. Gist NH, Fedewa MV, Dishman RK, Cureton KJ. Sprint interval training effects on aerobic capacity: a systematic review and meta-analysis. *Sports Med*. 2014;44(2):269–279.

46. Glass S, Dwyer GB, American College of Sports Medicine. *ACSM's Metabolic Calculations Handbook*. Baltimore (MD): Lippincott Williams & Wilkins; 2007. 128 p.

47. Gulati M, Shaw LJ, Thisted RA, Black HR, Merz CN, Arnsdorf MF. Heart rate response to exercise stress testing in asymptomatic women. The St. James Women Take Heart Project. *Circulation*. 2010;122(2):130–7.

48. Gunnarsson TP, Bangsbo J. The 10-20-30 training concept improves performance and health profile in moderately trained runners. *J Apply Physiol (1985)*. 2012;113(1):16–24.

49. Hardy CJ, Rejeski WJ. Not what, but how one feels: the measurement of affect during exercise. *J Sport Exer Psych*. 1989;11:304–17.

50. Haskell WL, Lee IM, Pate RR, et al. Physical activity and public health: updated recommendation for adults from the American College of Sports Medicine and the American Heart Association. *Med Sci Sports Exerc*. 2007;39(8):1423–34.

51. Hawkins S, Wiswell R. Rate and mechanism of maximal oxygen consumption decline with aging: implications for exercise training. *Sports Med*. 2003;33(12):877–88.

52. Healy GN, Dunstan DW, Salmon J, et al. Breaks in sedentary time: beneficial associations with metabolic risk. *Diabetes Care*. 2008;31(4):661–6.

53. Helgerud J, Høydal K, Wang E, et al. Aerobic high-intensity intervals improve $\dot{V}O_{2max}$ more than moderate training. *Med Sci Sports Exerc*. 2007;39(4):665–71.

54. Hill M, Talbot C, Price M. Predicted maximal heart rate for upper body exercise testing. *Clin Physiol Funct Imaging*. 2016;36(2):155–8.

55. Howley ET. Type of activity: resistance, aerobic and leisure versus occupational physical activity. *Med Sci Sports Exerc*. 2001;33(6 Suppl):S364, 9; discussion S419–20.

56. Jeanes EM, Foster C, Porcari JP, Gibson M, Doberstein S. Translation of exercise testing to exercise prescription using the talk test. *J Strength Cond Res*. 2011;25(3):590–6.

57. Kang M, Marshall SJ, Barreira TV, Lee JO. Effect of pedometer-based physical activity interventions: a meta-analysis. *Res Q Exerc Sport*. 2009;80(3):648–55.

58. Kiviniemi AM, Tulppo MP, Eskelinen JJ, et al. Cardiac autonomic function and high-intensity interval training in middle-age men. *Med Sci Sports Exerc*. 2014;46(10):1960–7.

59. Kohl HW III, Craig CL, Lambert EV, et al. The pandemic of physical inactivity: global action for public health. *Lancet*. 2012;380(9838):294–305.

60. Krieger JW. Single versus multiple sets of resistance exercise: a meta-regression. *J Strength Cond Res*. 2009;23(6):1890–901.

61. Krieger JW. Single vs. multiple sets of resistance exercise for muscle hypertrophy: a meta-analysis. *J Strength Cond Res*. 2010;24(4):1150–9.

62. Lee IM, Shiroma EJ, Lobelo F, et al. Effect of physical inactivity on major non-communicable diseases worldwide: an analysis of burden of disease and life expectancy. *Lancet*. 2012;380(9838): 219–29.

63. Little JP, Francois ME. High-intensity interval training for improving postprandial hyperglycemia. *Res Q Exerc Sport*. 2014;85(4):451–6.

64. Lyden K, Keadle SK, Staudenmayer J, Braun B, Freedson PS. Discrete features of sedentary behavior impact cardiometabolic risk factors. *Med Sci Sports Exerc*. 2015;47(5):1079–86.

65. Lyon E, Menke M, Foster C, Porcari JP, Gibson M, Bubbers T. Translation of incremental talk test responses to steady-state exercise training intensity. *J Cardiopulm Rehabil Prev*. 2014;34(4): 271–5.

66. Mahieu NN, McNair P, De Muynck M, et al. Effect of static and ballistic stretching on the muscle-tendon tissue properties. *Med Sci Sports Exerc*. 2007;39(3):494–501.

67. Manini TM, Carr LJ, King AC, Marshall S, Robinson TN, Rejeski WJ. Interventions to reduce sedentary behavior. *Med Sci Sports Exerc*. 2015;47(6):1306–10.

68. McHugh MP, Cosgrave CH. To stretch or not to stretch: the role of stretching in injury prevention and performance. *Scand J Med Sci Sports*. 2010;20(2):169–81.

69. McMillian DJ, Moore JH, Hatler BS, Taylor DC. Dynamic vs. static-stretching warm up: the effect on power and agility performance. *J Strength Cond Res*. 2006;20(3):492–9.

70. Mezzani A, Hamm LF, Jones AM, et al. Aerobic exercise intensity assessment and prescription in cardiac rehabilitation: a joint position statement of the European Association for Cardiovascular Prevention and Rehabilitation, the American Association of Cardiovascular and Pulmonary Rehabilitation and the Canadian Association of Cardiac Rehabilitation. *Eur J Prev Cardiol*. 2013;20(3):442–67.

71. Nakahara H, Ueda SY, Miyamoto T. Low-frequency severe-intensity interval training improves cardiorespiratory functions. *Med Sci Sports Exerc*. 2015;47(4):789–98.

72. Nelson ME, Rejeski WJ, Blair SN, et al. Physical activity and public health in older adults: recommendation from the American College of Sports Medicine and the American Heart Association. *Med Sci Sports Exerc*. 2007;39(8):1435–45.

73. Nielsen SG, Buus L, Hage T, Olsen H, Walsøe M, Vinther A. The graded cycling test combined with the talk test is reliable for patients with ischemic heart disease. *J Cardiopulm Rehabil Prev*. 2014;34(4):276–80.

74. Noble BJ, Borg GA, Jacobs I, Ceci R, Kaiser P. A category-ratio perceived exertion scale: relationship to blood and muscle lactates and heart rate. *Med Sci Sports Exerc*. 1983;15(6):523–8.

75. O'Donovan G, Blazevich AJ, Boreham C, et al. The ABC of Physical Activity for Health: a consensus statement from the British Association of Sport and Exercise Sciences. *J Sports Sci*. 2010;28(6):573–91.

76. Owen N, Healy GN, Matthews CE, Dunstan DW. Too much sitting: the population health science of sedentary behavior. *Exerc Sport Sci Rev*. 2010;38(3):105–13.

77. Persinger R, Foster C, Gibson M, Fater DC, Porcari JP. Consistency of the talk test for exercise prescription. *Med Sci Sports Exerc*. 2004;36(9):1632–6.

78. Petersen AK, Maribo T, Hjortdal VE, Laustsen S. Intertester reliability of the talk test in a cardiac rehabilitation population. *J Cardiopulm Rehabil Prev*. 2014;34(1):49–53.

79. Peterson MD, Rhea MR, Alvar BA. Applications of the dose-response for muscular strength development: a review of meta-analytic efficacy and reliability for designing training prescription. *J Strength Cond Res*. 2005;19(4):950–8.

80. Physical Activity Guidelines Advisory Committee. *Physical Activity Guidelines Advisory Committee Report, 2008* [Internet]. Washington (DC): U.S. Department of Health and Human Services; 2008 [updated Sep 24]. 683 p. Available from: http://health.gov/paguidelines/pdf/paguide.pdf

81. Reed JL, Pipe AL. The talk test: a useful tool for prescribing and monitoring exercise intensity. *Curr Opin Cardiol*. 2014;29(5):475–80.

82. Rees SS, Murphy AJ, Watsford ML, McLachlan KA, Coutts AJ. Effects of proprioceptive neuromuscular facilitation stretching on stiffness and force-producing characteristics of the ankle in active women. *J Strength Cond Res*. 2007;21(2):572–7.

83. Reid KF, Fielding RA. Skeletal muscle power: a critical determinant of physical functioning in older adults. *Exerc Sport Sci Rev*. 2012;40(1):4–12.

84. Rhea MR, Alvar BA, Burkett LN, Ball SD. A meta-analysis to determine the dose response for strength development. *Med Sci Sports Exerc*. 2003;35(3):456–64.

85. Robertson RJ, Goss FL, Dube J, et al. Validation of the adult OMNI scale of perceived exertion for cycle ergometer exercise. *Med Sci Sports Exerc*. 2004;36(1):102–8.

86. Robertson RJ, Goss FL, Rutkowski J, et al. Concurrent validation of the OMNI perceived exertion scale for resistance exercise. *Med Sci Sports Exerc*. 2003;35(2):333–41.

87. Rodríguez-Marroyo JA, Villa JG, García-López J, Foster C. Relationship between the talk test and ventilatory thresholds in well-trained cyclists. *J Strength Cond Res*. 2013;27(7):1942–9.

88. Roxburgh BH, Nolan PB, Weatherwax RM, Dalleck LC. Is moderate intensity exercise training combined with high intensity interval training more effective at improving cardiorespiratory fitness than moderate intensity exercise training alone? *J Sports Sci Med*. 2014;13(3):702–7.

89. Rutten GM, Savelberg HH, Biddle SJ, Kremers SP. Interrupting long periods of sitting: good STUFF. *Int J Behav Nutr Phys Act*. 2013;10:1.

90. Sardinha LB, Santos DA, Silva AM, Baptista F, Owen N. Breaking-up sedentary time is associated with physical function in older adults. *J Gerontol A Biol Sci Med Sci.* 2015;70(1):119–24.

91. Scharhag-Rosenberger F, Walitzek S, Kindermann W, Meyer T. Differences in adaptations to 1 year of aerobic endurance training: individual patterns of nonresponse. *Scand J Med Sci Sports.* 2012;22(1):113–8.

92. Sharman MJ, Cresswell AG, Riek S. Proprioceptive neuromuscular facilitation stretching: mechanisms and clinical implications. *Sports Med.* 2006;36(11):929–39.

93. Simic L, Sarabon N, Markovic G. Does pre-exercise static stretching inhibit maximal muscular performance? A meta-analytical review. *Scand J Med Sci Sports.* 2013;23(2):131–48.

94. Sisson SB, Katzmarzyk PT, Earnest CP, Bouchard C, Blair SN, Church TS. Volume of exercise and fitness nonresponse in sedentary, postmenopausal women. *Med Sci Sports Exerc.* 2009;41(3):539–45.

95. Stephens BR, Granados K, Zderic TW, Hamilton MT, Braun B. Effects of 1 day of inactivity on insulin action in healthy men and women: interaction with energy intake. *Metabolism.* 2011;60(7):941–9.

96. Swain DP. Energy cost calculations for exercise prescription: an update. *Sports Med.* 2000; 30(1):17–22.

97. Swain DP, American College of Sports Medicine. *ACSM's Resource Manual for Guidelines for Exercise Testing and Prescription.* 7th ed. Baltimore (MD): Lippincott Williams & Wilkins; 2014. 896 p.

98. Swain DP, Franklin BA. VO(2) reserve and the minimal intensity for improving cardiorespiratory fitness. *Med Sci Sports Exerc.* 2002;34(1):152–7.

99. Swain DP, Leuholtz BC. Heart rate reserve is equivalent to %VO2 reserve, not to %VO2max. *Med Sci Sports Exerc.* 1997;29(3):410–4.

100. Swartz AM, Squires L, Strath SJ. Energy expenditure of interruptions to sedentary behavior. *Int J Behav Nutr Phys Act.* 2011;8:69.

101. Tanaka H, Monahan KD, Seals DR. Age-predicted maximal heart rate revisited. *J Am Coll Cardiol.* 2001;37(1):153–6.

102. Thompson WR, Gordon NF, Pescatello LS, American College of Sports Medicine. *ACSM's Guidelines for Exercise Testing and Prescription.* 8th ed. Baltimore (MD): Lippincott Williams & Wilkins; 2010. 400 p.

103. Thyfault JP, Du M, Kraus WE, Levine JA, Booth FW. Physiology of sedentary behavior and its relationship to health outcomes. *Med Sci Sports Exerc.* 2015;47(6):1301–5.

104. Tschentscher M, Eichinger J, Egger A, Droese S, Schönfelder M, Niebauer J. High-intensity interval training is not superior to other forms of endurance training during cardiac rehabilitation. *Eur J Prev Cardiol.* 2016;23(1):14–20.

105. Tudor-Locke C, Hatano Y, Pangrazi RP, Kang M. Revisiting "how many steps are enough?" *Med Sci Sports Exerc.* 2008;40(7 Suppl):S537–43.

106. U.S. Department of Agriculture. *Report of the Dietary Guidelines Advisory Committee on the Dietary Guidelines for Americans, 2010* [Internet]. Washington (DC): U.S. Government Printing Office; 2010 [updated Jul 13]. Available from: http://www.cnpp.usda.gov/DGAs2010 -DGACReport.htm

107. U.S. Department of Health and Human Services. *2008 Physical Activity Guidelines for Americans* [Internet]. Washington (DC): U.S. Department of Health and Human Services; 2008 [updated Oct]. Available from: http://health.gov/paguidelines/pdf/paguide.pdf

108. U.S. Department of Health and Human Services. *Exercise & Physical Activity: Your Everyday Guide from the National Institute on Aging* [Internet]. Bethesda (MD): National Institute on Aging, National Institutes of Health; 2010 [updated Oct 20]. Available from: http://www .nia.nih.gov/HealthInformation/Publications/ExerciseGuide/

109. U.S. Department of Health and Human Services, United States Department of Agriculture, United States Dietary Guidelines Advisory Committee. *Dietary Guidelines for Americans, 2005.* 6th ed. Washington (DC): Government Printing Office; 2005. 71 p.

110. Utter AC, Robertson RJ, Green JM, Suminski RR, McAnulty SR, Nieman DC. Validation of the Adult OMNI Scale of perceived exertion for walking/running exercise. *Med Sci Sports Exerc.* 2004;36(10):1776–80.

111. Warburton DE, Bredin SS, Charlesworth SA, Foulds HJ, McKenzie DC, Shephard RJ. Evidence-based risk recommendations for best practices in the training of qualified exercise professionals working with clinical populations. *Appl Physiol Nutr Metab*. 2011;36(1 Suppl): S232–65.

112. Weston KS, Wisløff U, Coombes JS. High-intensity interval training in patients with lifestyle-induced cardiometabolic disease: a systematic review and meta-analysis. *Br J Sports Med*. 2014;48(46):1227–34.

113. Wilmot EG, Edwardson CL, Achana FA, et al. Sedentary time in adults and the association with diabetes, cardiovascular disease and death: systematic review and meta-analysis. *Diabetologia*. 2012;55(11):2895–905.

114. Winters MV, Blake CG, Trost JS, et al. Passive versus active stretching of hip flexor muscles in subjects with limited hip extension: a randomized clinical trial. *Phys Ther*. 2004;84(9):800–7.

115. Woltmann ML, Foster C, Porcari JP, et al. Evidence that the talk test can be used to regulate exercise intensity. *J Strength Cond Res*. 2015;29(5):1248–54.

116. Woolstenhulme MT, Griffiths CM, Woolstenhulme EM, Parcell AC. Ballistic stretching increases flexibility and acute vertical jump height when combined with basketball activity. *J Strength Cond Res*. 2006;20(4):799–803.

117. Zadow EK, Gordon N, Abbiss CR, Peiffer JJ. Pacing, the missing piece of the puzzle to high-intensity interval training. *Int J Sports Med*. 2015;36(3):215–9.

118. Zhu N, Suarez-Lopez JR, Sidney S, et al. Longitudinal examination of age-predicted symptom-limited exercise maximum HR. *Med Sci Sports Exerc*. 2010;42(8):1519–27.

Exercise Prescription for Healthy Populations with Special Considerations

This chapter contains the exercise prescription (Ex R_x) guidelines and recommendations for healthy populations with special considerations. The Ex R_x guidelines and recommendations are presented using the Frequency, Intensity, Time, and Type (FITT) principle of Ex R_x based on available literature. Specifically, this chapter focuses on children and adolescents, individuals with low back pain (LBP), pregnant women, and older adults.

CHILDREN AND ADOLESCENTS

Children and adolescents (defined as individuals aged 6–17 yr) are more physically active than their adult counterparts. However, only the youngest children (aged 6–7 yr) consistently meet the national physical activity (PA) recommendations (119), and most young individuals 10 yr and older do not meet prevailing PA guidelines. The *2008 Physical Activity Guidelines for Americans* call for children and adolescents to engage in at least 60 min · d^{-1} of moderate-to-vigorous intensity PA and to include vigorous intensity PA, resistance exercise, and bone loading activity on at least 3 d · wk^{-1} (119). In the United States, 42% of children aged 6–11 yr and 8% of adolescents aged 12–19 yr (116) meet the recommended guidelines.

In addition to the PA guidelines, expert panels from the National Heart, Lung, and Blood Institute and the American Academy of Pediatrics also recommend that children limit total entertainment screen time to <2 h · d^{-1} (6,38). Excess screen time has been linked to increased adiposity; decreased fitness; and elevated blood pressure, blood lipids, and glycohemoglobin levels in youth aged 5–17 yr (115). Yet, nationally, only slightly more than half of children aged 6–11 yr met this recommendation according to recent data from the National Health and Nutrition Examination Survey (NHANES) (40). Perhaps most importantly, the PA and sedentary behavior patterns of children track into adulthood, so it is vital that youth initiate and maintain a physically active lifestyle from an early age (19,113).

Children and adolescents are physiologically adaptive to aerobic exercise training (102), resistance training (17), and bone loading exercise (112). In fact, evidence suggests that prepubescent children who participate in resistance training can achieve relative strength gains similar to those seen in adolescents (70). Furthermore, exercise training produces improvements in cardiometabolic risk factors, weight control, bone strength, and psychosocial well-being and may help prevent sports-related injuries; thus, the benefits of exercise are much greater than the risks (*e.g.*, overuse injuries, concussion) (39,93). Recent evidence also supports the concept that PA and physical fitness are positively associated with cognition and academic achievement (35).

Most young individuals are healthy and able to start moderate intensity exercise training without medical screening. Vigorous exercise can be initiated after safely participating in moderate exercise. However, because prepubescent children have immature skeletons, younger children should not participate in excessive amounts of vigorous intensity exercise. Physiologic responses to acute, graded exercise are qualitatively similar to those seen in adults. However, there are important quantitative differences, many of which are related to the effects of body mass, muscle mass, and height. In addition, it is notable children have a much lower anaerobic capacity than adults limiting their ability to perform sustained vigorous intensity exercise (18).

Exercise Testing

Generally, the adult guidelines for standard exercise testing apply to children and adolescents (see *Chapter 6*). However, physiologic responses during exercise differ from those of adults (*Table 7.1*) so that the following issues should be considered (87,127):

- Exercise testing for clinical purposes is generally not indicated for children or adolescents unless there is a health concern.
- The exercise testing protocol should be based on the reason the test is being performed and the functional capability of the child or adolescent.
- Children and adolescents should be familiarized with the test protocol before testing to minimize stress and maximize the potential for a successful test.
- Treadmill and cycle ergometers should be available for testing. Treadmills tend to elicit a higher peak oxygen uptake ($\dot{V}O_{2peak}$) and maximal heart rate (HR_{max}). Cycle ergometers provide less risk for injury but need to be correctly sized for the child or adolescent.
- Children and adolescents may require extra motivation and support during the test compared to adults.

In addition, health/fitness testing may be performed outside of the clinical setting. In school-based settings, the FITNESSGRAM test battery may be used to assess the components of health-related fitness (95). The components of the FITNESSGRAM test battery include body composition (*i.e.*, body mass index [BMI], skinfold measurements, or bioelectrical impedance analysis),

TABLE 7.1	
Physiologic Responses to Acute Exercise in Children Compared to Adults (61,110)	
Variable	**Response**
Absolute oxygen uptake	Lower
Relative oxygen uptake	Higher
Heart rate	Higher
Cardiac output	Lower
Stroke volume	Lower
Systolic blood pressure	Lower
Diastolic blood pressure	Lower
Respiratory rate	Higher
Tidal volume	Lower
Minute ventilation	Lower
Respiratory exchange ratio	Lower

cardiorespiratory fitness (CRF) (*i.e.*, 1-mi walk/run and progressive aerobic cardiovascular endurance run [PACER]), muscular fitness (*i.e.*, curl-up test, trunk lift test, pull-ups, and push-up test), and flexibility (*i.e.*, back-saver sit-and-reach test and shoulder stretch) (95). Age- and gender-specific, criterion-referenced standards are available which allow results to be compared across demographic characteristics (95).

Due to the strong correlation between health and fitness, tests that evaluate aerobic and muscular fitness remain important screening tools. However, tracking behavior, especially through objective methods such as pedometers or accelerometers, provides a more appropriate gauge for evaluating PA levels. Although not designed to capture PA intensities, pedometers provide an unobtrusive and low-cost option for estimating daily locomotor activity, and recent research using national databases from Canada and the United States have translated the 60-min · d^{-1} guideline into a step-per-day recommendation of 9,000–12,000 steps. (2,27,117).

Exercise Prescription

The Ex R$_x$ guidelines outlined in this chapter for children and adolescents establish the minimal amount of PA needed to achieve the health/fitness benefits associated with regular PA (119). Children and adolescents should be encouraged to participate in various PAs that are enjoyable and age-appropriate. PA in young children should include unstructured active play, which typically consists of sporadic bursts of moderate and vigorous intensity PA alternating with brief periods of rest. It is important to recognize that these small bouts of PA, however brief, count toward FITT recommendations.

■ FITT RECOMMENDATIONS FOR CHILDREN AND ADOLESCENTS (119)

FITT	Aerobic	Resistance	Bone Strengthening
Frequency	Daily	$\geq$3 d · wk^{-1}	$\geq$3 d · wk^{-1}
Intensity	Most should be moderate (noticeable increase in HR and breathing) to vigorous intensity (substantial increases in HR and breathing). Include vigorous intensity at least 3 d · wk^{-1}.	Use of body weight as resistance or 8–15 submaximal repetitions of an exercise to the point of moderate fatigue with good mechanical form	N/A
Time	As part of $\geq$60 min · d^{-1} of exercise	As part of $\geq$60 min · d^{-1} of exercise	As part of $\geq$60 min · d^{-1} of exercise
Type	Enjoyable and developmentally appropriate activities, including running, brisk walking, swimming, dancing, bicycling, and sports such as soccer, basketball, or tennis	Muscle strengthening physical activities can be unstructured (e.g., playing on playground equipment, climbing trees, tug-of-war) or structured (e.g., lifting weights, working with resistance bands).	Bone strengthening activities include running, jump rope, basketball, tennis, resistance training, and hopscotch.

HR, heart rate

Special Considerations

■ Children and adolescents may safely participate in strength training activities provided they receive proper instruction and supervision. Generally, adult guidelines for resistance training may be applied (see *Chapter 6*).

■ Because of immature thermoregulatory systems, youth should avoid sustained, heavy exercise in exceptionally hot humid environments, be properly hydrated, and appropriately modify activities. See *Chapter 8* and the American College of Sports Medicine (ACSM) position stand (10) on exercising in the heat and fluid replacement for additional information.

■ Children and adolescents who are overweight or physically inactive may not be able to achieve 60 min · d^{-1} of moderate-to-vigorous intensity PA. These individuals should start out with moderate intensity PA as tolerated and gradually increase the frequency and time of PA to achieve the 60-min · d^{-1} goal. Vigorous intensity PA can then be gradually added at least 3 d · wk^{-1}.

- Children and adolescents with diseases or disabilities such as asthma, diabetes mellitus, obesity, cystic fibrosis, and cerebral palsy should have their Ex R_x tailored to their condition, symptoms, and physical fitness level (see *Chapters 10* and *11*).
- Efforts should be made to decrease sedentary activities (*i.e.*, television watching, Web surfing, and playing video games) and increase activities that promote life-long activity and fitness (*i.e.*, walking and cycling).

ONLINE RESOURCES

U.S. Department of Health and Human Services. *2008 Physical Activity Guidelines for Americans* [Internet]. Washington (DC): U.S. Department of Health and Human Services; 2008 (119):
http://www.health.gov/paguidelines/guidelines

U.S. Department of Health and Human Services. *Physical Activity Guidelines Advisory Committee report, 2008.* Washington (DC): U.S. Department of Health and Human Services; 2008 (93):
http://www.health.gov/paguidelines/guidelines/#committee

LOW BACK PAIN

LBP is defined as pain, muscle tension, or stiffness localized below the rib margin and above the inferior gluteal folds, with or without leg pain (14,121). LBP is a major public health problem, with the lifetime prevalence reported as high as 84% (5). Anywhere between 4% and 33% of the adult population experience LBP at any given point in time (42), and recurrent episodes of LBP can occur in over 70% of cases (45). Approximately 20% of cases become chronic, and about 10% of the cases progress to a disability (5).

Individuals with LBP can be classified into one of three broad categories: (a) LBP potentially associated with another specific spinal cause (*e.g.*, cancer, fracture, infection, ankylosing spondylitis or cauda equina syndrome); (b) LBP potentially associated with radiculopathy or spinal stenosis; and (c) and nonspecific LBP, which encompass over 85% of all cases (25). For prognosis and outcome purposes, LBP can be described as acute (<6 wk), subacute (6–12 wk), and chronic (>12 wk) (5,34).

Approximately 90% of acute low back episodes resolve within 6 wk regardless of treatment (118). To reduce the probability of disability, individuals with LBP should stay active by continue ordinary activity within pain limits, avoid bed rest, and return to work as soon as possible (128). If disabling pain continues beyond 6 wk, a multidisciplinary approach that includes addressing psychosocial factors is recommended (34). Many individuals with LBP have fear, anxiety, or misinformation regarding their LBP, exacerbating a persistent pain state (96). A combination of therapeutic and aerobic exercise, in conjunction with pain education, improves individual attitudes, outcomes, perceptions, and pain thresholds (72,81). Psychosocial factors that increase the risk of developing or perpetuating long-term disability and work loss associated with LBP can be found in *Box 7.1.*

Box 7.1	**Psychosocial Factors for Long-Term Disability and Work Loss Associated with Low Back Pain** (103)

- A negative attitude that back pain is harmful or potentially severely disabling
- Fear avoidance behavior and reduced activity levels
- An expectation that passive, rather than active, treatment will be beneficial
- A tendency to depression, low morale, and social withdrawal
- Social or financial problems

Current literature does not support a definitive cause for initial bouts of LBP (34). However, previous LBP is one of the strongest predictors for future back pain episodes (14). Recurrent episodes of LBP tend toward increased severity and duration, higher levels of disability, including work disability, and higher medical and indemnity costs (22,123). Current guidelines place a heavy emphasis on preventive measures and early interventions to minimize the risk of an acute LBP episode from becoming chronic and/or disabling (52). Current best evidence guidelines for treating LBP indicate PA as a key component in managing the condition (3,25,114).

Some considerations must be given to individuals with LBP who are fearful of pain or reinjury and thus avoid PA as well as to those individuals who persist in PA despite worsening symptoms (58,98). Individuals with LBP who are fearful of pain or reinjury often misinterpret any aggravation of symptoms as a worsening of their spinal condition and hold the mistaken belief that pain means tissue damage (105). In contrast, those with LBP who persist in PA may not allow injured tissues the time that is needed to heal. Both behaviors are associated with chronic pain (58).

When LBP is a symptom of another serious pathology (*e.g.*, cancer), exercise testing and prescription should be guided by considerations related to the primary condition. For all other causes, and in the absence of a comorbid condition (*e.g.*, cardiovascular disease [CVD] with its associated risk factors), recommendations for exercise testing and prescription are similar as for healthy individuals (see *Chapter 6*). Given that the vast majority of LBP cases are nonspecific, the focus of the Ex R_x recommendations presented here will address individuals with LBP that is not associated with trauma or any specific underlying conditions (*e.g.*, cancer or infection).

Exercise Testing

Individuals with acute or subacute LBP appear to vary in their individual levels of PA independent of their pain-related disability. However, chronic LBP with high levels of disability may lead to low levels of PA (71). Individual beliefs about the back pain will often influence one's willingness to exercise (66). As such, exercise testing and subsequent activities may be symptom limited in the first weeks following symptom onset (1,98).

Cardiorespiratory Fitness

Avoidance behavior due to pain may result in decreased PA, which may lead to the unavoidable consequence of reduced CRF (59). Current evidence, however, has failed to find a clear relationship between CRF and pain (122).

Few studies have subjected individuals with LBP to exercise tests to exhaustion (37). Submaximal exercise tests are considered reliable and valid for individuals with LBP (98), however, actual or anticipated pain may limit submaximal testing as often as maximal testing (37,64,98,108,109). Therefore, the choice of maximal versus submaximal testing in individuals with LBP should be guided by the same considerations as for the general population (see *Chapter 4*).

Muscular Strength and Endurance

Individuals with LBP frequently have deficits in trunk muscle strength and endurance (43,63,74) and neuromuscular imbalance (44,99); however, the role these play in the development and progression of LBP remains unclear (63,86). Decreases in muscular strength and endurance may be independent of the period and intensity of LBP (32,129).

General testing of muscular strength and endurance in individuals with LBP should be guided by the same considerations as for the general population (see *Chapter 4*). In addition, tests of the strength and endurance of the trunk musculature (*e.g.*, isokinetic dynamometers with back attachments, selectorized machines, and back hyperextension benches) are commonly assessed in individuals with LBP (53). However, the reliability of these tests is questionable because of considerable learning effect in particular between the first and second sessions (53,120). Performance of muscular strength and endurance assessments is often limited by actual or anticipated fear of reinjury in individuals with LBP (69).

Flexibility

There is no clear relationship between gross spinal flexibility and LBP or associated disability (3). A range of studies have shown associations between measures of spine flexibility, hip flexibility, and LBP (78), yet the nature of these associations is likely complex and requires further study. There appears to be some justification, although based on relatively weak evidence, for flexibility testing in the lower limbs, and in particular the hips of individuals with LBP (34,62). In general, flexibility testing in individuals with LBP should be guided by the same considerations as for the general population (see *Chapter 4*). It is essential, however, to identify whether the assessment is limited by stretch tolerance of the target structures or exacerbation of LBP symptoms.

Exercise Prescription

Current guidelines for the management of LBP consistently recommend staying physically active and avoiding bed rest (5,21,34,52,128). Although it may be best to avoid exercise in the first few days immediately following an acute and severe episode of LBP so as not to exacerbate symptoms (1,25,62), individuals with subacute and chronic LBP, as well as recurrent LBP, are encouraged to be physically active (1). Within 2 wk of an acute LBP episode, activities can be carefully introduced. Regular walking is a good way to encourage individuals with LBP to participate in activity that does not worsen symptoms (52). Aerobic exercise, particularly walking, biking, and swimming, has the best evidence of efficacy among exercise regimens, whether for acute, subacute, or chronic LBP patients (62,118).

Although there is agreement that exercise helps in the treatment of chronic back pain, there is no commonly prescribed exercise intervention that has demonstrated superiority (52). When recommendations are provided, they should follow very closely with the recommendations for the general population (see *Chapter 6*), combining resistance, aerobic, and flexibility exercise (1). In chronic LBP, exercise programs that incorporate individual tailoring, supervision, stretching, and strengthening are associated with the best outcomes (25,60). Furthermore, the evidence supporting the multidimensional nature of nonspecific chronic LBP shows most favorable outcomes with an individualized approach that addresses psychological distress, fear avoidance beliefs, self-efficacy in controlling pain, and coping strategies (86).

Special Considerations

- Trunk coordination, strengthening, and endurance exercises can be used to reduce LBP and disability in individuals with subacute and chronic LBP with movement coordination impairments (34). However, there is insufficient evidence for any benefit of emphasizing single-dimension therapies such as abdominal strengthening (62,86).
- Individual response to back pain symptoms can be improved by providing assurance, encouraging activity, and emphasizing that more than 90% of LBP complaints resolve without any specific therapies (62).
- There is a lack of agreement on the definition, components, and assessment techniques related to core stability. Furthermore, the majority of tests used to assess core stability have not demonstrated validity (73,75).
- Abdominal bracing (cocontraction of trunk muscles) (77) should be used with extreme caution because the increases in spinal compression that occur with abdominal bracing may cause further harm to the individual (4).
- Certain exercises or positions may aggravate symptoms of LBP. Walking, especially downhill, may aggravate symptoms in individuals with spinal stenosis (97).
- Certain individuals with LBP may experience a "peripheralization" of symptoms, that is, a spread of pain into the lower limbs with certain sustained or repeated movements of the lumbar spine (76). Limits should be placed on any activity or exercise that causes spread of symptoms (114).
- Repeated movements and exercises such as prone push-ups that promote centralization (*i.e.*, a reduction of pain in the lower limb from distal to proximal) are encouraged to reduce symptoms in patients with acute LBP with related lower extremity pain (34).

- Flexibility exercises are generally encouraged as part of an overall exercise program. Hip and lower limb flexibility should be promoted, although no stretching intervention studies have shown efficacy in treating or preventing LBP (36). It is generally not recommended to use trunk flexibility as a treatment goal in LBP (111).
- Consider progressive, low intensity aerobic exercise for individuals with chronic LBP with generalized pain (pain in more than one body area) and moderate-to-high intensity aerobic exercise for individuals with chronic LBP without generalized pain (34).

OLDER ADULTS

The term *older adult* defines individuals aged ≥65 yr and individuals aged 50–64 yr with clinically significant conditions or physical limitations that affect movement, physical fitness, or PA and represents a diverse spectrum of ages and physiologic capabilities (107). Because physiologic aging does not occur uniformly across the population, individuals of similar chronological age may differ dramatically in their response to exercise. In addition, it is difficult to distinguish the effects of aging on physiologic function from the effects of deconditioning or disease (*Table 7.2* provides a list of age-related changes in key physiologic variables). Therefore, health and functional status are often better indicators of the ability to engage in PA than chronological age.

TABLE 7.2	
Effects of Aging on Selected Physiologic and Health-Related Variables (107)	
Variable	**Change**
Resting heart rate	Unchanged
Maximum heart rate	Lower
Maximum cardiac output	Lower
Resting and exercise blood pressure	Higher
Absolute and relative maximum oxygen uptake reserve ($\dot{V}O_2R_{max}$ L · min^{-1} and mL · kg^{-1} · min^{-1})	Lower
Residual volume	Higher
Vital capacity	Lower
Reaction time	Slower
Muscular strength	Lower
Flexibility	Lower
Bone mass	Lower
Fat-free body mass	Lower
% Body fat	Higher
Glucose tolerance	Lower
Recovery time	Longer

Overwhelming evidence exists that supports the benefits of PA in (a) slowing physiologic changes of aging that impair exercise capacity, (b) optimizing age-related changes in body composition, (c) promoting psychological and cognitive well-being, (d) managing chronic diseases, (e) reducing the risks of physical disability, and (f) increasing longevity (9,106). Despite these benefits, older adults are the least physically active of all age groups. Today, only 11% of individuals aged ≥65 yr report engaging in aerobic and muscle strengthening activities that meet federal guidelines, and less than 5% of individuals aged 85 yr and older meet these same guidelines (41).

Exercise Testing

Most older adults do not require an exercise test prior to initiating a moderate intensity PA program (see *Chapter 2*). However, if exercise testing is recommended, it should be noted that the associated electrocardiogram (ECG) has higher sensitivity (*i.e.*, ~84%) and lower specificity (*i.e.*, ~70%) than in younger age groups (*i.e.*, <50% sensitivity and >80% specificity), producing a higher rate of false positive outcomes. This situation may be related to the greater frequency of left ventricular hypertrophy (LVH) and the increased presence of conduction disturbances among older rather than younger adults (49).

Although there are no specific exercise test termination criteria for older adults beyond those presented for all adults in *Chapter 4*, the increased prevalence of cardiovascular, metabolic, and orthopedic problems among older adults increases the overall likelihood of an early test termination. Therefore, exercise testing in older adults may require subtle differences in both protocol and methodology and should only be performed when indicated by a physician or other health care provider. Special considerations when testing older adults include the following (107):

- Initial workload should be light (*i.e.*, <3 metabolic equivalents [METs]) and workload increments should be small (*i.e.*, 0.5–1.0 MET) for those with low work capacities. The modified Naughton treadmill protocol is a good example of such a protocol (see *Figure 5.1*).
- A cycle ergometer may be preferable to a treadmill for those with poor balance, poor neuromotor coordination, impaired vision, impaired gait patterns, weight-bearing limitations, and/or orthopedic problems. However, local muscle fatigue may be a factor for premature test termination when using a cycle ergometer.
- Adding a treadmill handrail support may be required because of reduced balance, decreased muscular strength, poor neuromotor coordination, and fear. However, handrail support for gait abnormalities will reduce the accuracy of estimating peak MET capacity based on the exercise duration or peak workload achieved.
- Treadmill workload may need to be adapted according to walking ability by increasing grade rather than speed.
- Many older adults exceed the age-predicted HR_{max} during a maximal exercise test, which should be taken into account when considering test termination.
- The influence of prescribed medications on the ECG and hemodynamic responses to exercise may differ from usual expectations (see *Appendix A*).

The oldest segment of the population ($\geq$75 yr) and individuals with mobility limitations most likely have one or more chronic medical conditions. Additionally, the likelihood of physical limitations increases with age. The exercise testing approach described earlier may not be applicable for the oldest segment of the population and for individuals with mobility limitations. Currently, there is a paucity of evidence demonstrating increased mortality or cardiovascular event risk during exercise or exercise testing in this segment of the population, therefore eliminating the need for exercise testing unless medically indicated (*e.g.*, symptomatic CVD, uncontrolled diabetes). Otherwise, individuals free from CVD symptoms should be able to initiate a light intensity ($<$3 METs) exercise program without undue risk (50).

Physical Performance Testing

Physical performance testing has largely replaced exercise stress testing for the assessment of functional status of older adults (55). Some test batteries have been developed and validated as correlates of underlying fitness domains, whereas others have been developed and validated as predictors of subsequent disability, institutionalization, and death. Physical performance testing is appealing in that most performance tests require little space, equipment, and cost; can be administered by lay or health/fitness personnel with minimal training; and are considered extremely safe in healthy and clinical populations (23,101). The most widely used physical performance tests have identified cutpoints indicative of functional limitations associated with poorer health status that can be targeted for an exercise intervention. Some of the most commonly used physical performance tests are described in *Table 7.3*. Before performing these assessments, (a) carefully consider the specific population for which each test was developed, (b) be aware of known floor or ceiling effects, and (c) understand the context (*i.e.*, the sample, age, health status, and intervention) in which change scores or predictive capabilities are attributed.

The *Senior Fitness Test* was developed using a large, healthy community-dwelling sample and has published normative data for men and women aged 60–94 yr for items representing upper and lower body strength, upper and lower body flexibility, CRF, agility, and dynamic balance (101). Senior Fitness investigators have now published thresholds for each test item that define for adults ages 65–85 yr the level of capacity needed at their current age, within each domain of functional fitness, to remain independent to age 90 yr (100). The Short Physical Performance Battery (SPPB) (56), a test of lower extremity functioning, is best known for its predictive capabilities for disability, institutionalization, and death, but it also has known ceiling effects that limit its use as an outcome for exercise interventions in generally healthy older adults. A change of 0.5 point in the SPPB is considered a small meaningful change, whereas a change of 1.0 point is considered a substantial change (54). Usual gait speed, widely considered the simplest test of walking ability, has comparable predictive validity to the SPPB (90), but its sensitivity to change with exercise interventions has not been consistent. A change in usual gait speed of 0.05 m $\cdot$ s^{-1} is considered a small meaningful change, and a change of 0.10 m $\cdot$ s^{-1} is considered a substantial change (54).

TABLE 7.3

Commonly Used Physical Performance Tests

Measure and Description	Administration Time	Cutpoint Indicative of Lower Function
Senior Fitness Test (101) Seven items: 30 s chair stand, 30 s arm curls, 8 ft up and go, 6-min walk, 2-min step test, sit and reach, and back scratch with normative scales for each test	30 min total Individual items range from 2 to 10 min each	≤25th percentile of age-based norms
Short Physical Performance Battery (56) A test of lower extremity functioning that combines scores from usual gait speed and timed tests of balance and chair stands; scores range from 0 to 12 with higher score indicating better functioning.	10 min	10 points
Usual Gait Speed Usually assessed as the better of two trials of time to walk a short distance (3–10 m) at a usual pace	<2 min	$1 \text{ m} \cdot \text{s}^{-1}$
6-Min Walk Test Widely used as an indicator of cardiorespiratory endurance; assessed as the most distance an individual can walk in 6 min. A change of 50 m is considered a substantial change (54).	<10 min	≤25th percentile of age-based norms
Continuous Scale Physical Performance Test (29) Two versions — long and short — are available. Each consists of serial performance of daily living tasks, such as carrying a weighted pot of water, donning and removing a jacket, getting down and up from the floor, climbing stairs, carrying groceries, and others, performed within an environmental context that represent underlying physical domains. Scores range from 0 to 100 with higher scores representing better functioning.	60 min	57 points

Exercise Prescription

The general principles of Ex R$_x$ apply to adults of all ages (see *Chapter 6*). The relative adaptations to exercise and the percentage of improvement in the components of physical fitness among older adults are comparable with those reported in younger adults and are important for maintaining health and functional ability and attenuating many of the physiologic changes that are associated with aging (see *Table 7.2*). Low aerobic capacity, muscle weakness, and deconditioning are more common in older adults than in any other age group and contribute to loss of independence (9), and therefore, an appropriate Ex R$_x$ should include aerobic, muscle strengthening/endurance, and flexibility exercises. Individuals who are frequent fallers or have mobility limitations may also benefit from specific neuromotor exercises to improve balance, agility, and proprioceptive training (*e.g.*, tai chi), in addition to the other components of health-related physical fitness. However, age should not be a barrier to PA because positive improvements are attainable at any age.

For Ex R$_x$, an important distinction between older adults and their younger counterparts should be made relative to intensity. For apparently healthy adults, moderate and vigorous intensity PAs are defined relative to METs, with moderate intensity activities defined as 3–5.9 METs and vigorous intensity activities as ≥6 METs. In contrast for older adults, activities should be defined relative to an individual's physical fitness within the context of a perceived 10-point physical exertion scale which ranges from 0 (an effort equivalent to sitting) to 10 (an all-out effort), with moderate intensity defined as 5 or 6 and vigorous intensity as ≥7. A moderate intensity PA should produce a noticeable increase in HR and breathing, whereas a vigorous intensity PA should produce a large increase in HR or breathing (85).

Neuromotor (Balance) Exercises for Frequent Fallers or Individuals with Mobility Limitations

There are no specific recommendations regarding specific frequency, intensity, or type of exercises that incorporate neuromotor training into an Ex R$_x$. However, neuromotor exercise training, which combines balance, agility, and proprioceptive training, is effective in reducing and preventing falls if performed 2–3 d · wk^{-1} (9,46). General recommendations include using the following: (a) progressively difficult postures that gradually reduce the base of support (*e.g.*, two-legged stand, semitandem stand, tandem stand, one-legged stand); (b) dynamic movements that perturb the center of gravity (*e.g.*, tandem walk, circle turns); (c) stressing postural muscle groups (*e.g.*, heel, toe stands); (d) reducing sensory input (*e.g.*, standing with eyes closed); and (e) tai chi. Multimodal exercise programs that include two or more components of strength, balance, endurance, or flexibility exercises have been shown to reduce fall rates and the number of people falling (124). Exercise done in supervised groups, such as tai chi, or individually prescribed home programs have all been shown to be effective at reducing fall risk. (51); however, there may be times when supervision of these activities is warranted (9).

■ **FITT RECOMMENDATIONS FOR OLDER ADULTS** (9,46,85)

	Aerobic	Resistance	Flexibility
Frequency	≥5 d · wk^{-1} for moderate intensity; ≥3 d · wk^{-1} for vigorous intensity; 3–5 d · wk^{-1} for a combination of moderate and vigorous intensity	≥2 d · wk^{-1}	≥2 d · wk^{-1}
Intensity	On a scale of 0–10 for level of physical exertion, 5–6 for moderate intensity and 7–8 for vigorous intensity	Light intensity (*i.e.,* 40%–50% 1-RM) for beginners; progress to moderate-to-vigorous intensity (60%–80% 1-RM); alternatively, moderate (5–6) to vigorous (7–8) intensity on a 0–10 scale	Stretch to the point of feeling tightness or slight discomfort.
Time	30–60 min · d^{-1} of moderate intensity exercise; 20–30 min · d^{-1} of vigorous intensity exercise; or an equivalent combination of moderate and vigorous intensity exercise; may be accumulated in bouts of at least 10 min each	8–10 exercises involving the major muscle groups; 1–3 sets of 8–12 repetitions each	Hold stretch for 30–60 s.
Type	Any modality that does not impose excessive orthopedic stress such as walking. Aquatic exercise and stationary cycle exercise may be advantageous for those with limited tolerance for weight-bearing activity.	Progressive weight-training programs or weight-bearing calisthenics, stair climbing, and other strengthening activities that use the major muscle groups	Any physical activities that maintain or increase flexibility using slow movements that terminate in static stretches for each muscle group rather than rapid ballistic movements.

1-RM, one repetition maximum

Special Considerations for Exercise Programming

There are numerous considerations that should be taken into account to maximize the effective development of an exercise program, including the following:

- Intensity and duration of PA should be light at the beginning, in particular for older adults who are highly deconditioned, functionally limited, or have chronic conditions that affect their ability to perform physical tasks.
- Progression of PA should be individualized and tailored to tolerance and preference; a conservative approach may be necessary for the older adults who are highly deconditioned or physically limited.
- Muscular strength decreases rapidly with age, especially for those aged >50 yr. Although resistance training is important across the lifespan, it becomes more important with increasing age (9,46,85).
- For strength training involving use of selectorized machines or free weights, initial training sessions should be supervised and monitored by personnel who are sensitive to the special needs of older adults.
- Older adults may particularly benefit from power training because this element of muscle fitness declines most rapidly with aging, and insufficient power has been associated with a greater risk of accidental falls (20,24). Increasing muscle power in healthy older adults should include both single- and multiple-joint exercises (one to three sets) using light-to-moderate loading (30%–60% of 1-RM) for 6–10 repetitions with high velocity.
- Individuals with sarcopenia, a marker of frailty, need to increase muscular strength before they are physiologically capable of engaging in aerobic training.
- If chronic conditions preclude activity at the recommended minimum amount, older adults should perform PA as tolerated to avoid being sedentary.
- Older adults should gradually exceed the recommended minimum amounts of PA and attempt continued progression if they desire to improve and/or maintain their physical fitness.
- Older adults should consider exceeding the recommended minimum amounts of PA to improve management of chronic diseases and health conditions for which a higher level of PA is known to confer a therapeutic benefit.
- Moderate intensity PA should be encouraged for individuals with cognitive decline given the known benefits of PA on cognition. Individuals with significant cognitive impairment can engage in PA but may require individualized assistance.
- Structured PA sessions should end with an appropriate cool-down, particularly among individuals with CVD. The cool-down should include a gradual reduction of effort and intensity and, optimally, flexibility exercises.
- Incorporation of behavioral strategies such as social support, self-efficacy, the ability to make healthy choices, and perceived safety all may enhance participation in a regular exercise program (see *Chapter 12*).
- The exercise professional should also provide regular feedback, positive reinforcement, and other behavioral/programmatic strategies to enhance adherence.

ONLINE RESOURCES

Continuous Scale Physical Functional Performance Battery (28):
    http://www.rehabmeasures.org/Lists/RehabMeasures/DispForm.aspx?ID=1125
Short Physical Performance Battery (12):
    http://www.grc.nia.nih.gov/branches/ledb/sppb/index.htm

PREGNANCY

Healthy pregnant women without exercise contraindications (*Box 7.2*) are encouraged to exercise throughout pregnancy (7,33,93). Not only are the health benefits of exercise during pregnancy well recognized (*Box 7.3*), but also the short- and long-term risks associated with sedentary behavior are of increasing concern (33). In their respective guidelines, the American College of Obstetricians and Gynecologists (7,11) and the US Department of Health and Human Services (119)

Box 7.2	Contraindications for Exercising during Pregnancy

Relative

- Severe anemia
- Unevaluated maternal cardiac dysrhythmia
- Chronic bronchitis
- Poorly controlled Type 1 diabetes mellitus
- Extreme morbid obesity
- Extreme underweight
- History of extremely sedentary lifestyle
- Intrauterine growth restriction in current pregnancy
- Poorly controlled hypertension
- Orthopedic limitations
- Poorly controlled seizure disorder
- Poorly controlled hyperthyroidism
- Heavy smoker

Absolute

- Hemodynamically significant heart disease
- Restrictive lung disease
- Incompetent cervix/cerclage
- Multiple gestation at risk for premature labor
- Persistent second or third trimester bleeding
- Placenta previa after 26 wk of gestation
- Premature labor during the current pregnancy
- Ruptured membranes
- Preeclampsia/pregnancy-induced hypertension

Reprinted with permission from (7).

Box 7.3	**Benefits of Exercise during Pregnancy** (8,13,30,31,57,80,84,89)

- Prevention of excessive gestational weight gain
- Prevention of gestational diabetes mellitus
- Decreased risk of preeclampsia
- Decreased incidence/symptoms of low back pain
- Decreased risk of urinary incontinence
- Prevention/improvement of depressive symptoms
- Maintenance of fitness
- Prevention of postpartum weight retention

outline the importance of exercise during pregnancy and provide evidence-based guidance on Ex R_x for the minimization of risk and promotion of health benefits. With appropriate modifications and progression, pregnancy is an opportunity for sedentary women to adopt PA behavior (93).

Exercise Testing

Maximal exercise testing should not be performed on women who are pregnant unless medically necessary (7,11,33,65). If a maximal exercise test is warranted, the test should be performed with physician supervision after the woman has been medically evaluated for contraindications to exercise (see *Box 7.2*).

The acute physiologic responses to exercise are generally increased during pregnancy compared to nonpregnancy (127) (*Table 7.4*). Because of the physiological changes that accompany pregnancy, assumptions of submaximal protocols in predicting maximal aerobic capacity may be compromised (79) and are therefore

TABLE **7.4**	
Physiologic Responses to Acute Exercise during Pregnancy Compared to Nonpregnancy (127)	
Oxygen uptake (during weight-dependent exercise)	Increase
Heart rate	Increase
Stroke volume	Increase
Cardiac output	Increase
Tidal volume	Increase
Minute ventilation	Increase
Ventilatory equivalent for oxygen ($\dot{V}E/\dot{V}O_2$)	Increase
Ventilatory equivalent for carbon dioxide ($\dot{V}E/\dot{V}CO_2$)	Increase
Systolic blood pressure	No change/decrease
Diastolic blood pressure	No change/decrease

most appropriately used in determining the effectiveness of training rather than accurately estimating maximal aerobic power.

Exercise Prescription

In the absence of obstetric or medical complications, the exercise recommendations during pregnancy are consistent with recommendations for healthy adults: accumulation of at least 150 min $\cdot$ wk^{-1} of moderate intensity aerobic exercise or 75 min $\cdot$ wk^{-1} of vigorous intensity aerobic exercise spread across most days of the week (119). Ex R$_x$ for pregnant women should be modified according to the woman's prior exercise history as well as symptoms, discomforts, and abilities across the time course of pregnancy. The Canadian Society for Exercise Physiologists Physical Activity Readiness Medical Examination for Pregnancy (*PARmed-X for Pregnancy*) or the electronic Physical Activity Readiness Medical Examination (*ePARmed-X+*) should be used for the health screening of pregnant women before their participation in exercise programs (*Figure 7.1*) (88). All pregnant women should be educated on the warning signs for when to stop exercise (*Box 7.4*).

Research on the effects of resistance exercise during pregnancy is limited but shows that compared to sedentary controls, resistance training either has no effect (*e.g.*, no difference in gestational age, preterm labor, or cesarian delivery; delivery of normal birth weight infants at term) or produces better outcomes (*e.g.*, lower incidence of LBP; shorter labor duration; shorter recovery time/faster return to activity in postpartum) (15,16,47,68,91,126).

Exercise Training Considerations

- Although there is no ideal number of days, exercise frequency during pregnancy should be regular, occurring throughout the week, and adjusted based on total exercise volume (*i.e.*, number of days may vary based on intensity and duration of exercise). For previously inactive women, lower

Box 7.4	Warning Signs to Stop Exercise during Pregnancy

- Vaginal bleeding or (amniotic) fluid leakage
- Shortness of breath prior to exertion
- Dizziness, feeling faint, or headache
- Chest pain
- Muscle weakness
- Calf pain or swelling
- Decreased fetal movement
- Preterm labor

Reprinted with permission from (7).

Physical Activity Readiness
Medical Examination for
Pregnancy (2002)

PARmed-X for PREGNANCY PHYSICAL ACTIVITY READINESS MEDICAL EXAMINATION

PARmed-X for PREGNANCY is a guideline for health screening prior to participation in a prenatal fitness class or other exercise.

Healthy women with uncomplicated pregnancies can integrate physical activity into their daily living and can participate without significant risks either to themselves or to their unborn child. Postulated benefits of such programs include improved aerobic and muscular fitness, promotion of appropriate weight gain, and facilitation of labour. Regular exercise may also help to prevent gestational glucose intolerance and pregnancy-induced hypertension.

The safety of prenatal exercise programs depends on an adequate level of maternal-fetal physiological reserve. PARmed-X for PREGNANCY is a convenient checklist and prescription for use by health care providers to evaluate pregnant patients who want to enter a prenatal fitness program and for ongoing medical surveillance of exercising pregnant patients.

Instructions for use of the 4-page PARmed-X for PREGNANCY are the following:

1. The patient should fill out the section on PATIENT INFORMATION and the PRE-EXERCISE HEALTH CHECKLIST (PART 1, 2, 3, and 4 on p. 1) and give the form to the health care provider monitoring her pregnancy.

2. The health care provider should check the information provided by the patient for accuracy and fill out SECTION C on CONTRAINDICATIONS (p. 2) based on current medical information.

3. If no exercise contraindications exist, the HEALTH EVALUATION FORM (p. 3) should be completed, signed by the health care provider, and given by the patient to her prenatal fitness professional.

In addition to prudent medical care, participation in appropriate types, intensities and amounts of exercise is recommended to increase the likelihood of a beneficial pregnancy outcome. PARmed-X for PREGNANCY provides recommendations for individualized exercise prescription (p. 3) and program safety (p. 4).

NOTE: Sections A and B should be completed by the patient before the appointment with the health care provider.

A PATIENT INFORMATION

NAME _____

ADDRESS _____

TELEPHONE_____ BIRTHDATE_____ HEALTH INSURANCE No. _____

NAME OF   PRENATAL FITNESS
PRENATAL FITNESS PROFESSIONAL_____ PROFESSIONAL?S PHONE NUMBER_____

B PRE-EXERCISE HEALTH CHECKLIST

PART 1: GENERAL HEALTH STATUS

In the past, have you experienced (check YES or NO):

		YES	NO
1.	Miscarriage in an earlier pregnacy?	❏	❏
2.	Other pregnancy complications?	❏	❏
3.	I have completed a PAR-Q within the last 30 days.	❏	❏

If you answered YES to question 1 or 2, please explain:

Number of previous pregnancies? _____

PART 2: STATUS OF CURRENT PREGNANCY

Due Date: _____

During this pregnancy, have you experienced:

		YES	NO
1.	Marked fatigue?	❏	❏
2.	Bleeding from the vagina ("spotting")?	❏	❏
3.	Unexplained faintness or dizziness?	❏	❏
4.	Unexplained abdominal pain?	❏	❏
5.	Sudden swelling of ankles, hands or face?	❏	❏
6.	Persistent headaches or problems with headaches?	❏	❏
7.	Swelling, pain or redness in the calf of one leg?	❏	❏
8.	Absence of fetal movement after 6th month?	❏	❏
9.	Failure to gain weight after 5th month?	❏	❏

If you answered YES to any of the above questions, please explain:

PART 3: ACTIVITY HABITS DURING THE PAST MONTH

1. List only regular fitness/recreational activities:

_____

INTENSITY	FREQUENCY (times/week)			TIME (minutes/day)		
	1-2	2-4	4+	<20	20-40	40+
Heavy	___	___	___	___	___	___
Medium	___	___	___	___	___	___
Light	___	___	___	___	___	___

2. Does your regular occupation (job/home) activity involve:

		YES	NO
	Heavy Lifting?	❏	❏
	Frequent walking/stair climbing?	❏	❏
	Occasional walking (>once/hr)?	❏	❏
	Prolonged standing?	❏	❏
	Mainly sitting?	❏	❏
	Normal daily activity?	❏	❏
3.	Do you currently smoke tobacco?*	❏	❏
4.	Do you consume alcohol?*	❏	❏

PART 4: PHYSICAL ACTIVITY INTENTIONS

What physical activity do you intend to do?

_____

Is this a change from what you currently do? ❏ YES ❏ NO

*NOTE: PREGNANT WOMEN ARE STRONGLY ADVISED NOT TO SMOKE OR CONSUME ALCOHOL DURING PREGNANCY AND DURING LACTATION.

CSEP SCPE © Canadian Society for Exercise Physiology
Société canadienne de physiologie de l'exercice

Supported by: Health Santé
Canada Canada

Figure 7.1 Physical Activity Readiness Medical Examination for Pregnancy (PARmed-X for Pregnancy). Reprinted with permission from (88). (*continued*)

PARmed-X for PREGNANCY **PHYSICAL ACTIVITY READINESS MEDICAL EXAMINATION**

C CONTRAINDICATIONS TO EXERCISE: to be completed by your health care provider

Absolute Contraindications			Relative Contraindications		
Does the patient have:			Does the patient have:		
	YES	NO		YES	NO
1. Ruptured membranes, premature labour?	❏	❏	1. History of spontaneous abortion or premature labour in previous pregnancies?	❏	❏
2. Persistent second or third trimester bleeding/placenta previa?	❏	❏	2. Mild/moderate cardiovascular or respiratory disease (e.g., chronic hypertension, asthma)?	❏	❏
3. Pregnancy-induced hypertension or pre-eclampsia?	❏	❏	3. Anemia or iron deficiency? (Hb < 100 g/L)?	❏	❏
4. Incompetent cervix?	❏	❏	4. Malnutrition or eating disorder (anorexia, bulimia)?	❏	❏
5. Evidence of intrauterine growth restriction?	❏	❏	5. Twin pregnancy after 28th week?		
6. High-order pregnancy (e.g., triplets)?	❏	❏	6. Other significant medical condition?	❏	❏
7. Uncontrolled Type I diabetes, hypertension or thyroid disease, other serious cardiovascular, respiratory or systemic disorder?	❏	❏	Please specify: _____		
			NOTE: Risk may exceed benefits of regular physical activity. The decision to be physically active or not should be made with qualified medical advice.		
PHYSICAL ACTIVITY RECOMMENDATION:	❏ Recommended/Approved		❏ Contraindicated		

Figure 7.1 (*Continued*)

intensity and/or duration is recommended rather than reduced or irregular frequency.

- HR ranges corresponding to moderate intensity exercise have been developed (*Box 7.5*); however, due to HR variability, rating of perceived exertion (RPE) may also be used to monitor exercise intensity during pregnancy (94).
- Exercise may be accumulated in shorter bouts (*e.g.*, 15 min) or performed continuously. A 10- to 15-min warm-up and a 10- to 15-min cool-down of light intensity PA are suggested before and after each exercise session, respectively (33).
- Previously inactive women should progress from 15 min $\cdot$ d^{-1} ($\sim$3 d $\cdot$ wk^{-1}) at the appropriate RPE or target HR (33) to approximately 30 min $\cdot$ d^{-1} on most days of the week (11). Exercise goals and progression may vary at different time points during pregnancy, and exercise routines should remain flexible. Substitution of activity may be necessary given that physiological adaptations change over the time course of pregnancy (26).
- Women who habitually participate in resistance training should continue during pregnancy and should discuss how to adjust their routine with their health care provider (90).
- Kegel exercises and those that strengthen the pelvic floor are recommended to decrease the risk of incontinence during and after pregnancy (82).

Special Considerations

- PA in the supine position should be avoided (7) or modified after week 16 of pregnancy. Due to the weight of the growing fetus, exertion or prolonged periods in the supine position may reduce venous return and subsequent cardiac output.
- Women who are pregnant should avoid exercising in a hot humid environment, be well hydrated at all times, and dress appropriately to avoid heat stress. See

Box 7.5	Heart Rate Ranges that Correspond to Moderate Intensity Exercise for Low-Risk Normal Weight Women Who Are Pregnant and to Light Intensity Exercise for Low-Risk Women Who Are Pregnant and Overweight or Obese (33,83)

Prepregnancy BMI <25 kg · m^{-2}

Age (yr)	Fitness Level[a]	Heart Rate Range (beats · min^{-1})[a]
<20	—	140–155
20–29	Unfit	129–144
	Active	135–150
	Fit	145–160
30–39	Unfit	128–144
	Active	130–145
	Fit	140–156

BMI ≥25 kg · m^{-2}

Age (yr)	Heart Rate Range (beats · min^{-1})[b]
20–29	102–124
30–39	101–120

[a]Fitness level defined as: Unfit, bottom 25th percentile of $\dot{V}O_{2peak}$; Active, middle 50th percentile of $\dot{V}O_{2peak}$; Fit, top 25th percentile of $\dot{V}O_{2peak}$.
[b]Target heart rate ranges were derived from peak exercise tests in medically prescreened low-risk women who were pregnant (83).
BMI, body mass index.

Chapter 8 as well as the ACSM position stand (10) on exercising in the heat and fluid replacement for additional information.

■ During pregnancy, the metabolic demand increases by ~300 kcal · d^{-1}. Women should increase caloric intake to meet the caloric costs of pregnancy and exercise. Intake above or below recommended levels with concomitant changes in weight gain during pregnancy may be associated with adverse maternal and fetal outcomes (125). In order to avoid excessive weight gain during pregnancy, consult appropriate weight gain guidelines based on prepregnancy BMI, available from the Institute of Medicine and the National Research Council (125).

■ PA may help regulate weight gain during pregnancy (92). However, women who exercise above recommended levels should be monitored to ensure adequate caloric intake and weight gain (7,93).

■ Women who are pregnant and severely obese or have gestational diabetes mellitus or hypertension should consult their physician before beginning an exercise program, and their exercise program should be adjusted to their medical condition, symptoms, and physical fitness level. Exercise may be beneficial as an adjunct therapy for weight control (8) and in primary prevention of preeclampsia (8,48) and gestational diabetes (7,84), especially for women who are obese (67).

■ FITT RECOMMENDATIONS FOR WOMEN WHO ARE PREGNANT (11,93,104)

<table>
<tr><td>FITT</td><td>**Aerobic**</td><td>**Resistance**</td><td>**Flexibility**</td></tr>
<tr><td>Frequency</td><td>$\geq$3–5 d · wk^{-1}</td><td>2–3 nonconsecutive d · wk^{-1}</td><td>$\geq$2–3 d · wk^{-1} with daily being most effective</td></tr>
<tr><td>Intensity</td><td>Moderate intensity (3–5.9 METs; RPE of 12–13 on the 6–20 scale); vigorous intensity exercise ($\geq$6 METs; RPE 14–17 on the 6–20 scale) for women who were highly active prior to pregnancy or for women who progress to higher fitness levels during pregnancy</td><td>Intensity that permits multiple submaximal repetitions (*i.e.*, 8–10 or 12–15 repetitions) to be performed to a point of moderate fatigue</td><td>Stretch to the point of feeling tightness or slight discomfort.</td></tr>
<tr><td>Time</td><td>~30 min · d^{-1} of accumulated moderate intensity exercise to total at least 150 min · wk^{-1} or 75 min · wk^{-1} of vigorous intensity aerobic exercise</td><td>One set for beginners; two to three sets for intermediate and advanced; target major muscle groups (104)</td><td>Hold static stretch for 10–30 s.</td></tr>
<tr><td>Type</td><td>A variety of weight- and non–weight-bearing activities are well tolerated during pregnancy (*e.g.*, hiking, group exercise, swimming).</td><td>A variety of machines, free weights, and body weight exercises are well tolerated during pregnancy (*e.g.*, upright chest press, dumbbells, lunges).</td><td>A series of static (*i.e.*, active or passive) and dynamic flexibility exercises for each muscle-tendon unit.</td></tr>
</table>

METs, metabolic equivalents; RPE, rating of perceived exertion

- Women who are pregnant should avoid contact sports and sports/activities that may cause loss of balance or trauma to the mother or fetus. Examples of sports/activities to avoid include soccer, basketball, ice hockey, roller blading, horseback riding, skiing/snowboarding, scuba diving, and (vigorous intensity) racquet sports.
- In any activity, avoid using the Valsalva maneuver, prolonged isometric contraction, and motionless standing.

- PA can be resumed after pregnancy but should be done so gradually because of normal deconditioning in the initial postpartum period. Generally, gradual exercise may begin ~4–6 wk after a normal vaginal delivery or about 8–10 wk (with medical clearance) after a cesarean section delivery (82). Women with higher CRF levels and more rigorous exercise routines prior to and during pregnancy may be able to resume exercise sooner (91). Light-to-moderate intensity exercise in the postpartum period is important for return to prepregnancy BMI (67) and does not interfere with breastfeeding (82).

ONLINE RESOURCES

The American Congress of Obstetricians and Gynecologists:
  http://www.acog.org
The Canadian Society for Exercise Physiology (PARmed-X for Pregnancy) (88):
  http://www.csep.ca/english/view.asp?x=698

REFERENCES

1. Abenhaim L, Rossignol M, Valat JP, et al. The role of activity in the therapeutic management of back pain. Report of the International Paris Task Force on Back Pain. *Spine.* 2000;25(4):1S–33S.
2. Adams MA, Johnson WD, Tudor-Locke C. Steps/day translation of the moderate-to-vigorous physical activity guideline for children and adolescents. *Int J Behav Nutr Phys Act.* 2013;10:49.
3. Airaksinen O, Brox JI, Cedraschi C, et al. Chapter 4. European guidelines for the management of chronic nonspecific low back pain. *Eur Spine J.* 2006;15(Suppl 2):S192–300.
4. Aleksiev AR. Ten-year follow-up of strengthening versus flexibility exercises with or without abdominal bracing in recurrent low back pain. *Spine (Phila Pa 1976).* 2014;39(13):997–1003.
5. Almoallim H, Alwafi S, Albazli K, Alotaibi M, Bazuhair T. A simple approach of low back pain. *Intern J Clin Med.* 2014;5:1087–98.
6. American Academy of Pediatrics. Children, adolescents, and the media. *Pediatrics.* 2013;132:958–61.
7. American College of Obstetricians and Gynecologists Committee on Obstetric Practice. ACOG committee opinion. Number 267, January 2002: exercise during pregnancy and the postpartum period. *Obstet Gynecol.* 2002;99(1):171–3.
8. American College of Sports Medicine. Impact of physical activity during pregnancy and postpartum on chronic disease risk. *Med Sci Sports Exerc.* 2006;38:989–1006.
9. American College of Sports Medicine, Chodzko-Zajko WJ, Proctor DN, et al. American College of Sports Medicine position stand. Exercise and physical activity for older adults. *Med Sci Sports Exerc.* 2009;41(7):1510–30.
10. American College of Sports Medicine, Sawka MN, Burke LM, et al. American College of Sports Medicine position stand. Exercise and fluid replacement. *Med Sci Sports Exerc.* 2007;39(2):377–90.
11. Artal R, O'Toole M. Guidelines of the American College of Obstetricians and Gynecologists for exercise during pregnancy and the postpartum period. *Br J Sports Med.* 2003;37(1):6–12.
12. *Assessing Physical Performance in the Older Patient* [Internet]. Bethesda, (MD): National Institute on Aging, National Institutes of Health; 2010 [updated Jul 26]. Available from: http://www.grc.nia.nih.gov/branches/ledb/sppb/index.htm
13. Aune D, Saugstad OD, Henriksen T, Tonstad S. Physical activity and the risk of preeclampsia: a systematic review and meta-analysis. *Epidemiology.* 2014;25(3):331–43.
14. Balagué F, Mannion AF, Pellisé F, Cedraschi C. Non-specific low back pain. *Lancet.* 2012;379(9814):482–91.

15. Barakat R, Lucia A, Ruiz JR. Resistance exercise training during pregnancy and newborn's birth size: a randomised controlled trial. *Int J Obes (Lond)*. 2009;33(9):1048–57.

16. Barakat R, Ruiz JR, Stirling JR, Zakynthinaki M, Lucia A. Type of delivery is not affected by light resistance and toning exercise training during pregnancy: a randomized controlled trial. *Am J Obstet Gynecol*. 2009;201(6):590e.1–6.

17. Barbieri D, Zaccagni L. Strength training for children and adolescents: benefits and risks. *Coll Antropol*. 2013;37 Suppl 2:219–25.

18. Bar-Or O, Rowland T. *Pediatric Exercise Medicine: From Physiological Principles to Health Care Application*. Champaign (IL): Human Kinetics; 2004. 501 p.

19. Biddle SJ, Pearson N, Ross GM, Braithwaite R. Tracking of sedentary behaviours of young people: a systematic review. *Prev Med*. 2010;51(5):345–51.

20. Bonnefoy M, Jauffret M, Jusot JF. Muscle power of lower extremities in relation to functional ability and nutritional status in very elderly people. *J Nutr Health Aging*. 2007;11(3):223–8.

21. Bouwmeester W, van Enst A, van Tulder M. Quality of low back pain guidelines improved. *Spine*. 2009;34(23):2562–7.

22. Casazza BA. Diagnosis and treatment of acute low back pain. *Am Fam Physician*. 2012;85(4): 343–50.

23. Cesari M, Kritchevsky SB, Newman AB, et al. Added value of physical performance measures in predicting adverse health-related events: results from the health, aging and body composition study. *J Am Geriatr Soc*. 2009;57(2):251–9.

24. Chan BK, Marshall LM, Winters KM, Faulkner KA, Schwartz AV, Orwoll ES. Incident fall risk and physical activity and physical performance among older men: the Osteoporotic Fractures in Men Study. *Am J Epidemiol*. 2007;165(6):696–703.

25. Chou R, Qaseem A, Snow V, et al. Diagnosis and treatment of low back pain: a joint clinical practice guideline from the American College of Physicians and the American Pain Society. *Ann Intern Med*. 2007;147:478–91.

26. Clapp JF III. *Exercising through Your Pregnancy*. Omaha (NE): Addicus Books; 2002. 245 p.

27. Colley RC, Janssen I, Tremblay MS. Daily step target to measure adherence to physical activity guidelines in children. *Med Sci Sports Exerc*. 2012;44(5):977–82.

28. *Continuous Scale Physical Functional Performance: Evaluation of Functional Performance in Older Adults* [Internet]. Athens (GA): University of Georgia [cited 2016 Jun 16]. Available from: http://www.coe.uga.edu/cs-pfp/index.html

29. Cress ME, Buchner DM, Questad KA, Esselman PC, deLateur BJ, Schwartz RS. Continuous-scale physical functional performance in healthy older adults: a validation study. *Arch Phys Med Rehabil*. 1996;77(12):1243–50.

30. Daley AJ, Foster L, Long G, et al. The effectiveness of exercise for the prevention and treatment of antenatal depression: systematic review with meta-analysis. *BJOG*. 2015;122(1):57–62.

31. Daley AJ, Macarthur C, Winter H. The role of exercise in treating postpartum depression: a review of the literature. *J Midwifery Womens Health*. 2007;52(1):56–62.

32. Davarian S, Maroufi N, Ebrahimi I, Farahmand F, Parnianpour M. Trunk muscles strength and endurance in chronic low back pain patients with and without clinical instability. *J Back Musculoskelet Rehabil*. 2012;25(2):123–9.

33. Davies GA, Wolfe LA, Mottola MF, MacKinnon C, Society of Obstetricians and Gynecologists of Canada, SOGC Clinical Practice Obstetrics Committee. Joint SOGC/CSEP clinical practice guideline: exercise in pregnancy and the postpartum period. *Can J Appl Physiol*. 2003;28(3): 330–41.

34. Delitto A, George SZ, Van Dillen LR, et al. Low back pain. *J Orthop Sports Phys Ther*. 2012;42(4): A1–57.

35. Donnelly JE, Hillman CH, Castelli D, et al. Physical activity, fitness, cognitive function, and academic achievement in children: a systematic review. *Med Sci Sports Exerc*. 2016;48(6):1223–4.

36. Dugan S. The role of exercise in the prevention and management of acute low back pain. *Clin Occup Environ Med*. 2006;5(3):615–32.

37. Duque I, Parra J, Duvallet A. Aerobic fitness and limiting factors of maximal performance in chronic low back pain patients. *J Back Musculoskelet Rehabil*. 2009;22(2):113–9.

38. Expert Panel on Integrated Guidelines for Cardiovascular Health and Risk Reduction in Children and Adolescents, National Heart, Lung, and Blood Institute. Expert Panel on Integrated Guidelines for Cardiovascular Health and Risk Reduction in Children and Adolescents: summary report. *Pediatrics.* 2011;128(Suppl 5):S213–56.

39. Faigenbaum AD, Kraemer WJ, Blimkie CJ, et al. Youth resistance training: updated position statement paper from the National Strength and Conditioning Association. *J Strength Cond Res.* 2009;23(Suppl 5):S60–79.

40. Fakhouri TH, Hughes JP, Brody DJ, Kit BK, Ogden CL. Physical activity and screen-time viewing among elementary school-aged children in the United States from 2009 to 2010. *JAMA Pediatr.* 2013;167(3):223–9.

41. Federal Interagency Forum on Aging-Related Statistics. *Older Americans 2012: Key Indicators of Well-Being.* Washington (DC): Federal Interagency Forum on Aging-Related Statistics; 2012. 200 p.

42. Finestone AS, Raveh A, Mirovsky Y, Lahad A, Milgrom C. Orthopaedists' and family practitioners' knowledge of simple low back pain management. *Spine (Phila Pa 1976).* 2009;34(15):1600–3.

43. Fortin M, Macedo L. Multifidus and paraspinal muscle group cross-sectional areas of patients with low back pain and control patients: a systematic review with a focus on blinding. *Phys Ther.* 2013;93(7):873–88.

44. França FR, Burke TN, Caffaro RR, Ramos LA, Marques AP. Effects of muscular stretching and segmental stabilization on functional disability and pain in patients with chronic low back pain: a randomized, controlled trial. *J Manipulative Physiol Ther.* 2012;35(4):279–85.

45. Freeman MD, Woodham MA, Woodham AW. The role of the lumbar multifidus in chronic low back pain: a review. *PM R.* 2010;2(2):142–6.

46. Garber CE, Blissmer B, Deschenes MR, et al. American College of Sports Medicine position stand. Quantity and quality of exercise for developing and maintaining cardiorespiratory, musculoskeletal, and neuromotor fitness in apparently healthy adults: guidance for prescribing exercise. *Med Sci Sports Exerc.* 2011;43(7):1334–559.

47. Garshasbi A, Faghih Zadeh S. The effect of exercise on the intensity of low back pain in pregnant women. *Int J Gynaecol Obstet.* 2005;88(3):271–5.

48. Genest DS, Falcao S, Gutkowska J, Lavoie JL. Impact of exercise training on preeclampsia: potential preventive mechanisms. *Hypertension.* 2012;60(5):1104–9.

49. Gibbons RJ, Balady GJ, Bricker JT, et al. ACC/AHA 2002 guideline update for exercise testing: summary article: a report of the American College of Cardiology/American Heart Association Task Force on Practice Guidelines (Committee to Update the 1997 Exercise Testing Guidelines). *Circulation.* 2002;106(14):1883–92.

50. Gill TM, DiPietro L, Krumholz HM. Role of exercise stress testing and safety monitoring for older persons starting an exercise program. *JAMA.* 2000;284(3):342–9.

51. Gillespie LD, Robertson MC, Gillespie WJ, et al. Interventions for preventing falls in older people living in the community. *Cochrane Database Syst Rev.* 2012;(9):CD007146.

52. Goertz M, Thorson D, Bonsell J, et al. *Adult Acute and Subacute Low Back Pain.* Bloomington (IN): Institute for Clinical Systems Improvement; 2012. 92 p.

53. Gruther W, Wick F, Paul B, et al. Diagnostic accuracy and reliability of muscle strength and endurance measurements in patients with chronic low back pain. *J Rehabil Med.* 2009;41(8):613–9.

54. Guralnik JM, Ferrucci L, Pieper CF, et al. Lower extremity function and subsequent disability: consistency across studies, predictive models, and value of gait speed alone compared with the short physical performance battery. *J Gerontol A Biol Sci Med Sci.* 2000;55(4):M221–31.

55. Guralnik JM, Leveille S, Volpato S, Marx MS, Cohen-Mansfield J. Targeting high-risk older adults into exercise programs for disability prevention. *J Aging Phys Activ.* 2003;11(2):219–28.

56. Guralnik JM, Simonsick EM, Ferrucci L, et al. A short physical performance battery assessing lower extremity function: association with self-reported disability and prediction of mortality and nursing home admission. *J Gerontol.* 1994;49(2):M85–94.

57. Hall DC, Kauffman D. Effects of aerobic and strength conditioning on pregnancy outcomes. *Am J Obstet Gynecol.* 1987;157(5):1199–203.

58. Hasenbring MI, Hallner D, Klasen B, Streitlein-Böhme I, Willburger R, Rusche H. Pain-related avoidance versus endurance in primary care patients with subacute back pain: psychological characteristics and outcome at a 6-month follow-up. *Pain*. 2012;153(1):211–7.

59. Hasenbring M, Hallner D, Rusu A. Fear-avoidance- and endurance-related responses to pain: development and validation of the Avoidance-Endurance Questionnaire (AEQ). *Eur J Pain*. 2009;13(6):620–8.

60. Hayden J, van Tulder M, Tomlinson G. Systematic review: strategies for using exercise therapy to improve outcomes in chronic low back pain. *Ann Intern Med*. 2005;142(9):776–85.

61. Hebestreit HU, Bar-Or O. Differences between children and adults for exercise testing and prescription. In: Skinner JS, editor. *Exercise Testing and Exercise Prescription for Special Cases: Theoretical Basis and Clinical Application*. 3rd ed. Baltimore (MD): Lippincott Williams & Wilkins; 2005. p. 68–84.

62. Hegmann KT. Low back disorders. In: Hegmann KT, editor. *Occupational Medicine Practice Guidelines. Evaluation and Management of Common Health Problems and Functional Recovery in Workers*. 3rd ed. Elk Grove Village (IL): American College of Occupational and Environmental Medicine; 2011. p. 333–796.

63. Hides J, Stanton W, Mendis M, Sexton M. The relationship of transversus abdominis and lumbar multifidus clinical muscle tests in patients with chronic low back pain. *Man Ther*. 2011;16:573–7.

64. Hodselmans A, Dijkstra P, Geertzen J, van der Schans C. Exercise capacity in non-specific chronic low back pain patients: a lean body mass-based Astrand bicycle test; reliability, validity and feasibility. *J Occup Rehabil*. 2008;18(3):282–9.

65. Hopkins SA, Cutfield W. Exercise in pregnancy: weighing up the long-term impact on the next generation. *Exerc Sport Sci Rev*. 2011;39(3):120–7.

66. Huijnen IPJ. Physical functioning in low back pain: exploring different activity-related behavioural styles [dissertation]. Maastricht (The Netherlands): Universitaire Pers Maastricht; 2011. 215 p.

67. Jovanovic-Peterson L. Peterson C. Review of gestational diabetes mellitus and low-calorie diet and physical exercise as therapy. *Diabetes Metab Rev*. 1996;12(4):287–308.

68. Larson-Meyer DE. Effect of postpartum exercise on mothers and their offspring: a review of the literature. *Obes Res*. 2002;10(8):841–53.

69. Lee C, Simmonds M, Novy D, Jones S. Functional self-efficacy, perceived gait ability and perceived exertion in walking performance of individuals with low back pain. *Physiother Theory Pract*. 2002;18(4):193–203.

70. Lillegard W, Brown E, Wilson D, Henderson R, Lewis E. Efficacy of strength training in prepubescent to early postpubescent males and females: effects of gender and maturity. *Pediatr Rehabil*. 1997;1:147–57.

71. Lin CW, McAuley JH, Macedo L, Barnett DC, Smeets RJ, Verbunt JA. Relationship between physical activity and disability in low back pain: a systematic review and meta-analysis. *Pain*. 2011;152(3):607–13.

72. Louw A, Diener I, Butler DS, Puentedura EJ. The effect of neuroscience education on pain, disability, anxiety, and stress in chronic musculoskeletal pain. *Arch Phys Med Rehabil*. 2011;92(12):2041–56.

73. Majewski-Schrage T, Evans TA, Ragan B. Development of a core-stability model: a Delphi approach. *J Sport Rehabil*. 2014;23(2):95–106.

74. Mannion AF, O'Riordan D, Dvorak J, Masharawi Y. The relationship between psychological factors and performance on the Biering-Sørensen back muscle endurance test. *Spine J*. 2011;11(9):849–57.

75. Marshall PW, Desai I, Robbins DW. Core stability exercises in individuals with and without chronic nonspecific low back pain. *J Strength Cond Res*. 2011;25(12):3404–11.

76. May S, Aina A. Centralization and directional preference: a systematic review. *Man Ther*. 2012;17:497–506.

77. McGill SM, Karpowicz A. Exercises for spine stabilization: motion/motor patterns, stability progressions, and clinical technique. *Arch Phys Med Rehabil*. 2009;90(1):118–26.

78. McGregor AH, Hukins D. Lower limb involvement in spinal function and low back pain. *J Back Musculoskelet Rehabil*. 2009;22(4):219–22.

79. Melzer K, Schutz Y, Boulvain M, Kayser B. Physical activity and pregnancy: cardiovascular adaptations, recommendations and pregnancy outcomes. *Sports Med*. 2010;40(6):493–507.

80. Mørkved S, Bø K. Effect of pelvic floor muscle training during pregnancy and after childbirth on prevention and treatment of urinary incontinence: a systematic review. *Br J Sports Med.* 2014;48(4):299–310.

81. Moseley GL. Graded motor imagery is effective for long-standing complex regional pain syndrome: a randomised controlled trial. *Pain.* 2004;108(1–2):192–8.

82. Mottola MF. Exercise in the postpartum period: practical applications. *Curr Sports Med Rep.* 2002;1(6):362–8.

83. Mottola MF, Davenport MH, Brun CR, Inglis SD, Charlesworth S, Sopper MM. VO2peak prediction and exercise prescription for pregnant women. *Med Sci Sports Exerc.* 2006;38(8):1389–95.

84. Nascimento SL, Surita FG, Cecatti JG. Physical exercise during pregnancy: a systematic review. *Curr Opin Obstet Gynecol.* 2012;24(6):387–94.

85. Nelson ME, Rejeski WJ, Blair SN, et al. Physical activity and public health in older adults: recommendation from the American College of Sports Medicine and the American Heart Association. *Med Sci Sports Exerc.* 2007;39(8):1435–45.

86. O'Sullivan P. It's time for change with the management of non-specific chronic low back pain. *Br J Sports Med.* 2012;46(4):224–7.

87. Paridon SM, Alpert BS, Boas SR, et al. Clinical stress testing in the pediatric age group: a statement from the American Heart Association Council on Cardiovascular Disease in the Young, Committee on Atherosclerosis, Hypertension, and Obesity in Youth. *Circulation.* 2006;113(15):1905–20.

88. *PARmed-X for Pregnancy* [Internet]. Ottawa, Ontario (Canada): Canadian Society for Exercise Physiology; 2002 [cited 2016 Jun 16]. Available from: http://www.csep.ca/english/view.asp?x=698

89. Pelaez M, Gonzalez-Cerron S, Montejo R, Barakat R. Pelvic floor muscle training included in a pregnancy exercise program is effective in primary prevention of urinary incontinence: a randomized controlled trial. *Neurourol Urodyn.* 2014;33(1):67–71.

90. Perera S, Mody SH, Woodman RC, Studenski SA. Meaningful change and responsiveness in common physical performance measures in older adults. *J Am Geriatr Soc.* 2006;54(5):743–9.

91. Perkins C, Dewalt H. CrossFit training during pregnancy and motherhood: a new scientific frontier. *CrossFit J.* 2011:1–9.

92. Perkins CC, Pivarnik JM, Paneth N, Stein AD. Physical activity and fetal growth during pregnancy. *Obstet Gynecol.* 2007;109(1):81–7.

93. Physical Activity Guidelines Advisory Committee. *Physical Activity Guidelines Advisory Committee report, 2008* [Internet]. Washington (DC): U.S. Department of Health and Human Services; 2008 [updated Sep 24]. 683 p. Available from: http://www.health.gov/paguidelines/Report/pdf/committeereport.pdf

94. Pivarnik JM. Maternal exercise during pregnancy. *Sports Med.* 1994;18(4):215–7.

95. Plowman SA, Meredith M. *FITNESSGRAM/ACTIVITYGRAM Reference Guide.* 4th ed. Dallas (TX): The Cooper Institute; 2013. 202 p.

96. Puentedura EJ, Louw A. A neuroscience approach to managing athletes with low back pain. *Phys Ther Sport.* 2012;13(3):123–33.

97. Rainville J, Childs LA, Peña EB, et al. Quantification of walking ability in subjects with neurogenic claudication from lumbar spinal stenosis—a comparative study. *Spine J.* 2012;12(2):101–9.

98. Ratter J, Radlinger L, Lucas C. Several submaximal exercise tests are reliable, valid and acceptable in people with chronic pain, fibromyalgia or chronic fatigue: a systematic review. *J Physiother.* 2014;60(3):144–50.

99. Renkawitz T, Boluki D, Grifka J. The association of low back pain, neuromuscular imbalance, and trunk extension strength in athletes. *Spine J.* 2006;6(6):673–783.

100. Rikli RE, Jones C. Development and validation of criterion-referenced clinically relevant fitness standards for maintaining physical independence in later years. *Gerontologist.* 2013;53(2):255–67.

101. Rikli RE, Jones C. *Senior Fitness Test Manual.* Champaign (IL): Human Kinetics; 2001. 161 p.

102. Rowland T. Oxygen uptake and endurance fitness in children, revisited. *Pediatr Exerc Sci.* 2013;25(4):508–14.

103. Samanta J, Kendall J, Samanta A. 10-minute consultation: chronic low back pain. *BMJ*. 2003;326(7388):535.

104. Schoenfeld B. Resistance training during pregnancy: safe and effective program design. *Strength Cond J*. 2011;33(5):67–75.

105. Simmonds MJ, Goubert L, Moseley GL, Verbunt JA. Moving with pain. In: Flor H, Kalso E, Dostrovsky JO, editors. *Proceedings of the 11th World Congress on Pain, Sydney, Australia, August 21–26, 2005*. Seattle (WA): IASP Press; 2006. p. 799–811.

106. Singh MA. Exercise comes of age: rationale and recommendations for a geriatric exercise prescription. *J Gerontol A Biol Sci Med Sci*. 2002;57(5):M262–82.

107. Skinner JS. Aging for exercise testing and exercise prescription. In: Skinner JS, editor. *Exercise Testing and Exercise Prescription for Special Cases: Theoretical Basis and Clinical Application*. 3rd ed. Baltimore (MD): Lippincott Williams & Wilkins; 2005. p. 85–99.

108. Smeets R, van Geel K, Verbunt J. Is the fear avoidance model associated with the reduced level of aerobic fitness in patients with chronic low back pain? *Arch Phys Med Rehabil*. 2009;90(1):109–17.

109. Smeets R, Wittink H, Hidding A, Knottnerus J. Do patients with chronic low back pain have a lower level of aerobic fitness than healthy controls? Are pain, disability, fear of injury, working status, or level of leisure time activity associated with the difference in aerobic fitness level? *Spine*. 2006;31(1):90–7.

110. Strong WB, Malina RM, Blimkie CJ, et al. Evidence based physical activity for school-age youth. *J Pediatr*. 2005;146(6):732–7.

111. Sullivan M, Shoaf L, Riddle D. The relationship of lumbar flexion to disability in patients with low back pain. *Phys Ther*. 2000;80(3):240–50.

112. Tan VP, Macdonald HM, Kim S, et al. Influence of physical activity on bone strength in children and adolescents: a systematic review and narrative synthesis. *J Bone Miner Res*. 2014;29(10):2161–81.

113. Telama R. Tracking of physical activity from childhood to adulthood: a review. *Obes Facts*. 2009;2(3):187–95.

114. Toward Optimized Practice. *Guideline for the Evidence-Informed Primary Care Management of Low Back Pain*. Edmonton, Alberta (Canada): Toward Optimized Practice; 2011. p. 21.

115. Tremblay MS, LeBlanc AG, Kho ME, et al. Systematic review of sedentary behaviour and health indicators in school-aged children and youth. *Int J Behav Nutr Phys Act*. 2011;8:98.

116. Troiano RP, Berrigan D, Dodd KW, Masse LC, Tilert T, McDowell M. Physical activity in the United States measured by accelerometer. *Med Sci Sports Exerc*. 2008;40(1):181–8.

117. Tudor-Locke C, Craig CL, Beets MW, et al. How many steps/day are enough? for children and adolescents. *Int J Behav Nutr Phys Act*. 2011;8:78.

118. University of Michigan Health System. *Acute Low Back Pain*. Ann Arbor (MI): University of Michigan Health System; 2010. p. 16.

119. U.S. Department of Health and Human Services. *2008 Physical Activity Guidelines for Americans* [Internet]. Washington (DC): U.S. Department of Health and Human Services; 2008 [cited 2016 Jun 16]. Available from: http://health.gov/paguidelines/pdf/paguide.pdf

120. Van Damme BB, Stevens VK, Van Tiggelen DE, Duvigneaud NN, Neyens E, Danneels LA. Velocity of isokinetic trunk exercises influences back muscle recruitment patterns in healthy subjects. *J Electromyogr Kinesiol*. 2013;23(2):378–86.

121. Van Tulder M, Becker A, Bekkering T, et al. Chapter 3. European guidelines for the management of acute nonspecific low back pain in primary care. *Eur Spine J*. 2006;15(Suppl 2):s169–91.

122. Verbunt JA, Smeets RJ, Wittink HM. Cause or effect? Deconditioning and chronic low back pain. *Pain*. 2010;149(3):428–30.

123. Wasiak R, Kim J, Pransky G. Work disability and costs caused by recurrence of low back pain: longer and more costly than in first episodes. *Spine*. 2006;31(2):219–25.

124. Weerdesteyn V, Rijken H, Geurts AC, Smits-Engelsman BC, Mulder T, Duysens J. A five-week exercise program can reduce falls and improve obstacle avoidance in the elderly. *Gerontology*. 2006;52(3):131–41.

125. *Weight Gain During Pregnancy: Reexamining the Guideline. Report Brief* [Internet]. Washington (DC): National Academy of Sciences; 2009 [updated May 28]. Available from: http://www.iom.edu/Reports/2009/Weight-Gain-During-Pregnancy-Reexamining-the-Guidelines.aspx

126. White E, Pivarnik J, Pfeiffer K. Resistance training during pregnancy and perinatal outcomes. *J Phys Act Health*. 2014;11(6):1141–8.

127. Wolfe LA. Pregnancy. In: Skinner JS, editor. *Exercise Testing and Exercise Prescription for Special Cases: Theoretical Basis and Clinical Application*. 3rd ed. Baltimore (MD): Lippincott Williams & Wilkins; 2005. p. 377–91.

128. Work Loss Data Institute. *Low Back — Lumbar and Thoracic (Acute and Chronic)*. Encinitas (CA): Work Loss Data Institute; 2013.

129. Yahia A, Jribi S, Ghroubi S, Elleuch M, Baklouti S, Habib Elleuch M. Evaluation of the posture and muscular strength of the trunk and inferior members of patients with chronic lumbar pain. *Joint Bone Spine*. 2011;78(3):291–7.

Environmental Considerations for Exercise Prescription

EXERCISE IN HIGH-ALTITUDE ENVIRONMENTS

The progressive decrease in atmospheric pressure associated with ascent to higher altitudes reduces the partial pressure of oxygen in the inspired air, resulting in decreased arterial oxygen levels. The immediate compensatory responses to this include increased ventilation and cardiac output ($\dot{Q}$), the latter usually through elevated heart rate (HR) (27). For most individuals, the effects of altitude appear at and above 1,200 m (3,937 ft). In this section, low altitude refers to locations <1,200 m (3,937 ft), moderate altitude to locations between 1,200 and 2,400 m (3,937 and 7,874 ft), high altitude between 2,400 and 4,000 m (7,874 and 13,123 ft), and very high altitude >4,000 m (13,123 ft) (30).

Physical performance decreases with increasing altitude >1,200 m (3,937 ft). In general, the physical performance decrement will be greater as elevation, physical activity (PA) duration, and muscle mass increases but is lessened with altitude acclimatization. The most common altitude effect on physical task performance is an increased time for task completion or the need for more frequent rest breaks. With altitude exposure of ≥1 wk, significant altitude acclimatization occurs (*i.e.*, increased ventilation and arterial oxygen content and restored acid-base balance). The time to complete a task is reduced but still longer relative to sea level. The estimated percentage increases in performance time to complete tasks of various durations during initial altitude exposure and after 1 wk of altitude acclimatization are given in *Table 8.1* (19).

Medical Considerations: Altitude Illnesses

Rapid ascent to high and very high altitude increases individual susceptibility to altitude illness. The primary altitude illnesses are acute mountain sickness (AMS), high-altitude cerebral edema (HACE), and high-altitude pulmonary edema (HAPE). Additionally, many individuals develop a sore throat and bronchitis that may produce disabling, severe coughing spasms at high altitudes. Susceptibility to altitude sickness is increased in individuals with a prior history and by prolonged physical exertion and dehydration early in the altitude exposure.

TABLE 8.1								
Estimated Impact of Increasing Altitude on Time to Complete Physical Tasks at Various Altitudes (19)								
Percentage Increase in Time to Complete Physical Tasks Relative to Sea Level								
	Tasks Lasting <2 min		Tasks Lasting 2–5 min		Tasks Lasting 10–30 min		Tasks Lasting >3 h	
Altitude	Initial	>1 wk	Initial	>1 wk	Initial	>1 wk	Initial	>1 wk
Moderate	0	0	2–7	0–2	4–11	1–3	7–18	3–10
High	0–2	0	12–18	5–9	20–45	9–20	40–65	20–45
Very high	2	0	50	25	90	60	200	90

AMS is the most common form of altitude sickness. Symptoms include headache, nausea, fatigue, decreased appetite, and poor sleep, and in severe cases, poor balance and mild swelling in the hands, feet, or face. AMS develops within the first 24 h of altitude exposure. Its incidence and severity increase in direct proportion to ascent rate and altitude. The estimated incidence of AMS in unacclimatized individuals rapidly ascending directly to moderate altitudes is ≤15%; to high altitudes, 15%–70%; and to very high altitudes, 70%–85% (7). In most individuals, if ascent is stopped and physical exertion is limited, AMS symptoms peak at about 18–22 h and recovery occurs over the next 24–48 h.

HACE is a potentially fatal, although not common, illness that occurs in <2% of individuals ascending >3,658 m (12,000 ft). HACE is an exacerbation of unresolved, severe AMS. HACE most often occurs in individuals who have AMS symptoms and continue to ascend.

HAPE is a potentially fatal, although not common, illness that occurs in <10% of individuals ascending >3,658 m (12,000 ft). Individuals making repeated ascents and descents >3,658 m (12,000 ft) and who exercise strenuously early in the exposure have an increased susceptibility to HAPE. The presence of crackles and rales in the lungs and severe dyspnea may indicate increased susceptibility to developing HAPE.

Prevention and Treatment of Altitude Sickness

Altitude acclimatization is the best countermeasure to all altitude sickness. Minimizing sustained exercise/PA and maintaining adequate hydration and food intake will reduce susceptibility to altitude sickness and facilitate recovery. When moderate-to-severe symptoms and signs of an altitude-related sickness develop, the preferred treatment is to descend to a lower altitude. Descents of 305–915 m (1,000–3,000 ft) with an overnight stay are effective in prevention and recovery of all altitude sickness.

AMS may be significantly diminished or prevented with prophylactic or therapeutic use of acetazolamide (*i.e.*, Diamox). Diamox is a carbonic anhydrase inhibitor that promotes excretion of bicarbonate in the urine and production of carbon dioxide to stimulate ventilation. Headache is most effectively treated with ibuprofen. Oxygen or hyperbaric chamber therapy will usually relieve AMS symptoms and the accompanied poor sleep. Prochlorperazine (*i.e.*, Compazine) may be used to help relieve nausea and vomiting. Dexamethasone (*i.e.*, Decadron, Hexadrol) may be used if other treatments are not available or effective (23). Treatment of individuals diagnosed with HACE or HAPE includes descent, oxygen therapy, and/or hyperbaric bag therapy.

Rapid Ascent

Many unacclimatized individuals travel directly to high mountainous areas for skiing or trekking vacations. Beginning within hours after rapid ascent to a given altitude up to about 4,300 m (14,107 ft), and lasting for the first couple of days, AMS may be present, and physical and cognitive performances will be at their nadir for these individuals. During this time, voluntary PA should not be excessive, and endurance exercise training should be stopped, or its intensity greatly reduced to minimize the possibility that AMS will be exacerbated. As AMS begins to subside through developing altitude acclimatization, individuals may gradually resume normal activities and exercise training. Monitoring exercise HR provides a safe, easy, and objective means to quantify exercise intensity at altitude, as it does at sea level. For example, using any HR-based exercise prescription (Ex R_x) model at altitude (see *Table 6.2*) will provide a similar training stimulus to sea level as long as the weekly number and durations of the training sessions are also maintained. Be mindful that for the same perceived effort, jogging or running pace will be reduced at altitude relative to sea level, independent of altitude acclimatization status.

Altitude Acclimatization

With altitude acclimatization, individuals can decrease susceptibility to altitude sickness and achieve optimal physical and cognitive performance for the altitude to which they are acclimatized. Altitude acclimatization consists of physiologic adaptations that develop in a time-dependent manner during repeated or continuous exposures to moderate or high altitudes. In addition to achieving acclimatization by residing continuously at a given target altitude, at least partial altitude acclimatization can develop by living at a moderate elevation, termed *staging*, before ascending to a higher target elevation. The goal of staged ascents is to gradually promote development of altitude acclimatization while averting the adverse consequences (*e.g.*, altitude sickness) of rapid ascent to high altitudes. Breathing low concentrations of oxygen using masks, hoods, or rooms (*i.e.*, normobaric hypoxia) is not as effective as being exposed to the natural altitude environment (*i.e.*, hypobaric hypoxia) for inducing functionally useful altitude acclimatization (18).

For individuals ascending from low altitude, the first stage of all staged ascent protocols should be ≥3 d of residence at moderate altitude. At this altitude, individuals will experience small decrements in physical performance and a low

Box 8.1	Staging Guideline for Exercise at High Altitudes

The general staging guideline is as follows: For every day spent >1,200 m (3,937 ft), an individual is prepared for a subsequent rapid ascent to a higher altitude equal to the number of days at that altitude times 305 m (1,000 ft). For example, if an individual stages at 1,829 m (6,000 ft) for 6 d, physical performance will be improved, and altitude sickness will be reduced at altitudes to 3,657 m (12,000 ft). This guideline applies to altitudes up to 4,267 m (14,000 ft).

incidence of altitude sickness. At any given altitude, almost all of the acclimatization response is attained between 7 and 12 d of residence at that altitude. Short stays of 3–7 d at moderate altitudes will decrease susceptibility to altitude sickness at higher altitudes. Stays of 6–12 d are required to improve physical work performance. The magnitude of the acclimatization response is increased with additional higher staging elevations or a longer duration at a given staging elevation. The final staging elevation should be as close as possible to the target elevation. See *Box 8.1* for the staging guideline for exercise at high altitudes.

Assessing Individual Altitude Acclimatization Status

The best indices of altitude acclimatization over time at a given elevation are decline (or absence) of altitude sickness, improved physical performance, decreased HR (both resting and exercise), and an increase in percent saturation of arterial oxygen (SaO_2). The presence and severity of AMS may be evaluated by the extent of its symptoms (*i.e.,* headache, nausea, fatigue, decreased appetite, and poor sleep) and signs (*i.e.,* decreased urine output, poor balance, and mild swelling in the hands, feet, or face). The uncomplicated resolution of AMS or its absence in the first 3–4 d following ascent indicates a normal acclimatization response. After about 1–2 wk of acclimatization, physical performance improves such that most tasks can be performed for longer periods of time and with less perceived effort relative to the initial exposure to the same elevation. Another early sign of appropriate adaptation to altitude is increased urine volume, which generally occurs during the first several days at a given elevation. Urine volume will continue to increase with additional ascent and return to normal with subsequent adaptation.

Measurement of SaO_2 by noninvasive pulse oximetry is a very good indicator of acclimatization. Pulse oximetry should be performed under quiet, resting conditions. From its nadir on the first day at a given altitude, SaO_2 should progressively increase over the next 3–7 d before stabilizing. For example, with initial exposure to an altitude of 4,300 m (14,107 ft), resting SaO_2 is 81%; after a week of continuous residence at the same elevations, resting SaO_2 progressively rises to ~88% (43).

Exercise Prescription

During the first few days at high altitudes, individuals should minimize their exercise/PA to reduce susceptibility to altitude illness. After this period, if the Ex R_x specifies a target heart rate (THR), the individual should maintain the same exercise HR at higher altitudes. The personalized number of weekly training sessions and the duration of each session at altitude can remain similar to those used at sea level for a given individual. This approach reduces the risk of altitude illness and excessive physiologic strain. For example, at high altitudes, reduced speed, distance, or resistance will achieve the same THR as at lower altitudes. As altitude acclimatization develops, the THR will be achieved at a progressively higher exercise intensity.

Special Considerations

Adults and children who are acclimatized to altitude, adequately rested, nourished, and hydrated minimize their risk for developing altitude sickness and maximize their physical performance capabilities for the altitude to which they are acclimatized. The following factors should be considered to further minimize the negative effects of high altitude:

- Monitor the environment: High-altitude regions are often associated with more daily extremes of temperature, humidity, wind, and solar radiation. Follow appropriate guidelines for hot (3) and cold (2) environments.
- Modify activity at high altitudes: Consider altitude acclimatization status, physical fitness, nutrition, sleep quality and quantity, age, exercise time and intensity, and availability of fluids. Provide longer and/or more rest breaks to facilitate rest and recovery and shorten activity times. Longer duration activities are affected more by high altitude than shorter duration activities.
- Clothing: Individual clothing and equipment need to provide protection over a greater range of temperature, wind conditions, and solar radiation.
- Education: The training of participants, personal trainers, coaches, and community emergency response teams enhances the reduction, recognition, and treatment of altitude-related illnesses.

Organizational Planning

When clients exercise in high-altitude locations, physical fitness facilities and organizations should formulate a standardized management plan that includes the following procedures:

- Screening and surveillance of at-risk participants
- Using altitude acclimatization procedures to minimize the risk of altitude sickness and enhance physical performance
- Consideration of the hazards of mountainous terrain when designing exercise programs and activities
- Awareness of the signs and symptoms of altitude illness

- Develop organizational procedures for emergency medical care of altitude illnesses.
- Team physicians should consider maintaining a supply of oxygen and pharmaceuticals for preventing and treating altitude sickness.

EXERCISE IN COLD ENVIRONMENTS

Individuals exercise and work in many cold weather environments, which could include low temperature, high winds, low solar radiation, and rain/water exposure. Although unpleasant at times, cold temperatures are not necessarily a barrier to performing PA (6). Many factors, including the environment, clothing, body composition, health status, nutrition, age, and exercise intensity, interact to determine if exercising in the cold elicits additional physiologic strain and injury risk beyond that associated with the same exercise done under temperate conditions. In most cases, exercise in the cold does not increase cold injury risk. However, there are scenarios (*i.e.*, immersion, rain, and low-ambient temperature with wind) where whole body or local thermal balance cannot be maintained during exercise-related cold stress, which in turn contributes to hypothermia, frostbite, and diminished exercise capability and performance. Furthermore, exercise-related cold stress may increase the risk of morbidity and mortality in at-risk populations such as those with cardiovascular disease (CVD) and asthmatic conditions, and inhalation of cold air may also exacerbate these conditions.

Hypothermia develops when heat loss exceeds heat production, causing the body heat content to decrease (35). The environment, individual characteristics, and clothing all impact the development of hypothermia, with some specific hypothermia risk factors being immersion, rain, wet clothing, low body fat, older age (*i.e.*, ≥60 yr), and hypoglycemia (2).

Medical Considerations: Cold Injuries

Frostbite occurs when tissue temperature falls lower than 0° C (32° F) (16,28). Frostbite is most common in exposed skin (*i.e.*, nose, ears, cheeks, and exposed wrists) but also occurs in the hands and feet. Contact frostbite may occur by touching cold objects with bare skin, particularly highly conductive metal or stone that causes rapid heat loss.

The principal cold stress determinants for frostbite are air temperature, wind speed, and wetness. Wind exacerbates heat loss by facilitating convective heat loss and reducing the insulative value of clothing. The Wind Chill Temperature Index (WCT) (*Figure 8.1*) integrates wind speed and air temperature to provide an estimate of the cooling power of the environment. WCT is specific in that its correct application only estimates the danger of cooling for the exposed skin of individuals walking at 1.3 m · s^{-1} (3 mi · h^{-1}). Important information about wind and the WCT incorporates the following considerations:

- Wind does not cause an exposed object to become cooler than the ambient temperature.
- Wind speeds obtained from weather reports do not take into account manmade wind (*e.g.*, running, skiing).

Wind Speed (mph)

Air Temperature (°F)

	40	35	30	25	20	15	10	5	0	-5	-10	-15	-20	-25	-30	-35	-40	-45
5	36	31	25	19	13	7	1	-5	-11	-16	-22	-28	-34	-40	-46	-52	-57	-63
10	34	27	21	15	9	3	-4	-10	-16	-22	-28	-35	-41	-47	-53	-59	-66	-72
15	32	25	19	13	6	0	-7	-13	-19	-26	-32	-39	-45	-51	-58	-64	-71	-77
20	30	24	17	11	4	-2	-9	-15	-22	-29	-35	-42	-48	-55	-61	-68	-74	-81
25	29	23	16	9	3	-4	-11	-17	-24	-31	-37	-44	-51	-58	-64	-71	-78	-84
30	28	22	15	8	1	-5	-12	-19	-26	-33	-39	-46	-53	-60	-67	-73	-80	-87
35	28	21	14	7	0	-7	-14	-21	-27	-34	-41	-48	-55	-62	-69	-76	-82	-89
40	27	20	13	6	-1	-8	-15	-22	-29	-36	-43	-50	-57	-64	-71	-78	-84	-91
45	26	19	12	5	-2	-9	-16	-23	-30	-37	-44	-51	-58	-65	-72	-79	-86	-93
50	26	19	12	4	-3	-10	-17	-24	-31	-38	-45	-52	-60	-67	-74	-81	-88	-95
55	25	18	11	4	-3	-11	-18	-25	-32	-39	-46	-54	-61	-68	-75	-82	-89	-97
60	25	17	10	3	-4	-11	-19	-26	-33	-40	-48	-55	-62	-69	-76	-84	-91	-98

Frostbite times: ☐ Frostbite could occur in 30 min
▨ Frostbite could occur in 10 min
▨ Frostbite could occur in 5 min

Figure 8.1 Wind Chill Temperature Index and frostbite times for exposed facial skin (10,34).

- The WCT presents the relative risk of frostbite and predicted times to freezing (see *Figure 8.1*) of exposed facial skin. Facial skin was chosen because this area of the body is typically not protected.
- Frostbite cannot occur if the air temperature is >0° C (32° F).
- Wet skin exposed to the wind cools faster. If the skin is wet and exposed to wind, the ambient temperature used for the WCT table should be 10° C lower than the actual ambient temperature (9).
- The risk of frostbite is <5% when the ambient temperature is greater than −15° C (5° F), but increased safety surveillance of exercisers is warranted when the WCT falls lower than −27° C (−8° F). In those conditions, frostbite can occur in 30 min or less in exposed skin (2).

Nonfreezing cold injuries (NFCIs) typically occur when tissues are exposed to cold-wet temperatures between 0° and 15° C (32° and 60° F) for prolonged periods of time (42). These injuries may occur due to actual immersion or by the creation of a damp environment inside boots or gloves, as often seen during heavy sweating. Diagnosing NFCIs involves observation of clinical symptoms over time as different, distinct stages emerge days to months after the initial injury (42). The most common NFCIs are trench foot and chilblains, although NFCIs have also been observed in the hands.

NFCIs initially appear as swollen and edematous with a feeling of numbness. The initial color is red but soon becomes pale and cyanotic if the injury is more severe. Trench foot is accompanied by aches, increased pain, and infections, making peripheral pulses hard to detect. The exposure time needed to develop trench foot is quite variable, with estimates ranging from 12 h to 3–4 d in cold-wet environments (24,42). Most commonly, trench foot develops when wet socks and shoes are worn continuously over many days. The likelihood of trench foot in most sporting activities is low, except in winter hiking, camping, and expeditions (2).

Prevention of NFCIs can be achieved by encouraging individuals to remain active which increases blood flow to the feet and by keeping feet dry by continually changing socks. Changing socks two to three times throughout the day is highly recommended in cold-wet environments during long-term exposure. Prophylactic treatment with antiperspirants containing aluminum hydroxide may also decrease sweating in the foot. Vapor barrier boots (some hiking boots, ski boots) and liners do not allow sweat from the foot to evaporate, so sock changing becomes more important. These boots and liners should be taken off each day, wiped out, and allowed to dry. If regular boots are worn, they need time to dry to avoid getting moisture in the insulation (2).

Clothing Considerations

Cold weather clothing protects against hypothermia and frostbite by reducing heat loss through the insulation provided by the clothing and trapped air within and between clothing layers (2). Typical cold weather clothing consists of three layers: (a) an inner layer (*i.e.*, lightweight polyester or polypropylene), (b) a middle layer (*i.e.*, polyester fleece or wool) that provides the primary insulation, and (c) an outer layer designed to allow moisture transfer to the air while repelling wind and rain. Recommendations for clothing wear include the following considerations (2):

- Adjust clothing insulation to minimize sweating.
- Use clothing vents to reduce sweat accumulation.
- Do not wear an outer layer unless rainy or very windy.
- Reduce clothing insulation as exercise intensity increases.
- Do not impose a single clothing standard on an entire group of exercisers.
- Wear appropriate footwear to minimize the risks of slipping and falling in snowy or icy conditions.

Exercise Prescription

Whole body and facial cooling theoretically lower the threshold for the onset of angina during aerobic exercise. The type and intensity of exercise-related cold stress also modifies the risk for an individual with CVD. Activities that involve the upper body or increase metabolism potentially increase risk:

- Shoveling snow raises the HR to 97% maximal heart rate (HR_{max}), and systolic blood pressure increases to 200 mm Hg (17).
- Walking in snow that is either packed or soft significantly increases energy requirements and myocardial oxygen demands so that individuals with atherosclerotic CVD may have to slow their walking pace.
- Swimming in water <25° C (77° F) may be a threat to individuals with CVD because they may not be able to recognize angina symptoms and therefore may place themselves at greater risk (2).

EXERCISE IN HOT ENVIRONMENTS

Muscular contractions produce metabolic heat that is transferred from the active muscles to the blood and then to the body's core. Subsequent body temperature elevations elicit heat loss responses of increased skin blood flow and increased sweat secretion so that heat can be dissipated to the environment via evaporation (38). As a result of elevated skin blood flow, the cardiovascular system plays an essential role in temperature regulation. Heat exchange between skin and environment via sweating and dry heat exchange is governed by biophysical properties dictated by surrounding temperature, humidity and air motion, sky and ground radiation, and clothing (20). However, when the amount of metabolic heat exceeds heat loss, hyperthermia (*i.e.*, elevated internal body temperature) may develop. Sweat that drips from the body or clothing provides no cooling benefit; in fact, if secreted sweat drips from the body and is not evaporated, a higher sweating rate will be needed to achieve the evaporative cooling requirements (38). Sweat losses vary widely among individuals and depend on the amount and intensity of exercise, clothing, protective equipment, and environmental conditions (21). Other factors such as hydration state and level of aerobic fitness can alter sweat rates and ultimately fluid needs. For example, heat acclimatization results in higher and more sustained sweating rates, whereas aerobic exercise training has a modest effect on enhancing sweating rate responses (38). When properly controlled and compared, the difference in thermoregulation (*e.g.*, sweating) between men and women is minimal (13,15).

During exercise-induced heat stress, dehydration increases physiologic strain as measured by core temperature, HR, and perceived exertion responses (36). The greater the body water deficit, the greater the increase in physiologic strain for a given exercise task (29). Dehydration can exacerbate core temperature elevations during exercise in temperate (33) as well as in hot environments (41), with typical increases of 0.1° to 0.2° C (0.2° to 0.4° F) with each 1% of dehydration (37). The greater heat storage with dehydration is associated with a proportionate decrease in heat loss. Thus, decreased sweating rate (*i.e.*, evaporative heat loss) and decreased cutaneous blood flow (*i.e.*, dry heat loss) are responsible for greater heat storage observed during exercise when hypohydrated (31).

Counteracting Dehydration

Mechanisms by which dehydration might impair strength or power are presently unclear. A nonconventional analysis of the exercise performance literature revealed that the majority of studies support the concept that dehydration of ≥2% loss in body mass negatively impacts endurance exercise performance, whereas strength and power are negatively affected to a smaller degree (13). This is true whether individuals commence exercise in a dehydrated state or accumulate fluid loss during the course of exercise.

The critical water deficit (*i.e.*, >2% body mass for most individuals) and magnitude of performance decrement are likely related to environmental temperature, exercise task, and the individuals' unique biological characteristics (*e.g.*, tolerance to dehydration). Acute dehydration impairs endurance performance regardless of whole body hyperthermia or environmental temperature, and endurance capacity (*i.e.*, time to exhaustion) is reduced more in a hot environment than in a temperate or cold one (25).

Individuals have varying sweat rates, and as such, fluid needs for individuals performing similar tasks under identical conditions can be different. Determining sweat rate ($L \cdot h^{-1}$ or $q \cdot h^{-1}$) by measuring body weight before and after exercise provides a fluid replacement guide. Active individuals should drink 0.5 L (1 pint) of fluid for each pound of body weight lost. Meals can help stimulate thirst resulting in restoration of fluid balance. Snack breaks during longer training sessions can help replenish fluids and be important in replacing sodium and other electrolytes. There is presently no scientific consensus for how to best assess hydration status in a field setting. However, in most field settings, the additive use of first morning body mass measurements in combination with some measure of first morning urine concentration and gross thirst perception provides a simple and inexpensive way to dichotomize euhydration from gross dehydration resulting from sweat loss and poor fluid intakes (*Figure 8.2*) (14). When assessing first morning urine, a paler color indicates adequate hydration; a darker yellow/brown color, the greater the degree of dehydration. *Box 8.2* provides recommendations for hydration prior to, during, and following exercise or PA (3).

Overdrinking hypotonic fluid (*e.g.*, water) can lead to exercise-associated hyponatremia, a state of lower than normal blood sodium concentration (typically <135 mEq $\cdot L^{-1}$) accompanied by altered cognitive status. Hyponatremia tends

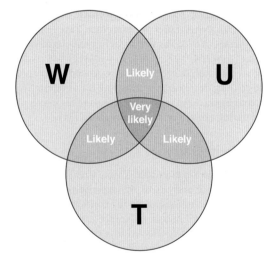

Figure 8.2 **W** stands for "weight." **U** stands for "urine." **T** stands for "thirst." When two or more simple markers are present, dehydration is likely. If all three markers are present, dehydration is very likely. Reprinted with permission from (14).

Box 8.2	Fluid Replacement Recommendations Before, During, and After Exercise	
	Fluid	**Comments**
Before exercise	Drink 5–7 mL · kg^{-1} (0.08–0.11 oz · lb^{-1}) at least 4 h before exercise (12–17 oz for 154-lb individual).	If urine is not produced or very dark, drink another 3–5 mL · kg^{-1} (0.05–0.08 oz · lb^{-1}) 2 h before exercise. Sodium-containing beverages or salted snacks will help retain fluid.
During exercise	Monitor individual body weight changes during exercise to estimate sweat loss. Composition of fluid should include 20–30 mEq · L^{-1} of sodium, 2–5 mEq · L^{-1} of potassium, and 5%–10% of carbohydrate.	Prevent a >2% loss in body weight. Amount and rate of fluid replacement depends on individual sweating rate, environment, and exercise duration.
After exercise	Consumption of normal meals and beverages will restore euhydration. If rapid recovery is needed, drink 1.5 L · kg^{-1} (23 oz · lb^{-1}) of body weight lost.	Goal is to fully replace fluid and electrolyte deficits. Consuming sodium will help recovery by stimulating thirst and fluid retention.

Adapted from (1,3).

to be more common in long duration PA and is precipitated by consumption of hypotonic fluid in excess of sweat losses (typified by body mass gains). When participating in exercise events that result in many hours of continuous or near continuous sweating, hyponatremia can be prevented by practices such as having an individualized hydration plan, not drinking in excess of sweat rate, and consuming salt-containing fluids or foods. For additional information, see the American College of Sports Medicine (ACSM) position stand on fluid replacement (3).

Medical Considerations: Exertional Heat Illnesses

Heat illnesses range from muscle cramps to life-threatening hyperthermia and are described in *Table 8.2*. Dehydration may be either a direct (*i.e.*, heat cramps and heat exhaustion) (39) or an indirect (*i.e.*, heatstroke) (12) factor in heat illness.

Heat cramps are muscle pains or spasms most often in the abdomen, arms, or legs that may occur in association with strenuous activity. Some controversy

TABLE 8.2

A Comparison of the Signs and Symptoms of Illnesses that Occur in Hot Environments (1)

Disorder	Prominent Signs and Symptoms	Mental Status Changes	Core Temperature Elevation
Exertional heatstroke	Disorientation, dizziness, irrational behavior, apathy, headache, nausea, vomiting, hyperventilation, wet skin	Marked (disoriented, unresponsive)	Marked (>40° C [>104° F])
Exertional heat exhaustion	Low blood pressure, elevated heart rate and respiratory rates, skin is wet and pale, headache, weakness, dizziness, decreased muscle coordination, chills, nausea, vomiting, diarrhea	Little or none, agitated	None to moderate (37° to 40° C [98.6° to 104° F])
Heat syncope	Heart rate and breathing rates are slow; skin is pale; patient may experience sensations of weakness, tunnel vision, vertigo, or nausea before syncope	Brief fainting episode	Little or none
Exertional heat cramps	Begins as feeble, localized, wandering spasms that may progress to debilitating cramps	None	Moderate (37° to 40° C [98.6° to 104° F])

exists regarding the etiology of exercise-induced muscle cramps; the cause is likely multifactorial and possibly unique to each athlete. Evidence suggests that muscle cramps may be more related to muscle fatigue and neuronal excitability compared to hydration status or electrolyte concentrations (40). However, water loss and significant sweat sodium have been proposed as contributing factors and may play a role in cramping in individuals identified as "heavy sweaters" or those who lose appreciable amounts of body fluid and sodium. One treatment or prevention strategy is not likely to work for every individual. However, heat cramps have been shown to respond to rest, prolonged stretching, dietary sodium chloride (*i.e.*, 1/8–1/4 tsp of table salt or one to two salt tablets added to 300–500 mL of fluid, bullion broth, or salty snacks), and, in some cases, intravenous normal saline fluid has anecdotally been reported to provide relief (22).

Heat syncope is a temporary circulatory failure caused by the pooling of blood in the peripheral veins, particularly of the lower extremities. Heat syncope tends to occur more often among physically unfit, sedentary, and nonacclimatized individuals and is caused by standing erect for a long period or at the cessation of strenuous, prolonged, upright exercise because maximal cutaneous vessel dilation results in a decline of blood pressure (BP) and insufficient oxygen delivery to the brain. Symptoms range from light-headedness to loss of consciousness; however, recovery is rapid once individuals sit or lay supine. Complete recovery of stable BP and HR may take a few hours. See the ACSM position stand on heat illness during exercise for additional information (1).

Heat exhaustion is the most common form of serious heat illness (4). It occurs during exercise/PA in the heat when the body cannot sustain the level of $\dot{Q}$ needed to support skin blood flow for thermoregulation and blood flow for metabolic requirements of exercise. It is characterized by prominent fatigue and progressive weakness without severe hyperthermia. Oral fluids are preferred for rehydration in individuals who are conscious, able to swallow, and not losing fluid (*i.e.*, vomiting and diarrhea). Intravenous fluid administration facilitates recovery in those unable to ingest oral fluids or who have severe dehydration.

Exertional heatstroke is caused by hyperthermia and is characterized by elevated body temperature ($>40°$ C or $104°$ F) (26), profound central nervous system dysfunction, and multiple organ system failure that can result in delirium, convulsions, or coma. The greatest risk for heatstroke exists during very high intensity exercise of short duration or prolonged exercise when the ambient wet-bulb globe temperature (WBGT) exceeds $28°$ C ($82°$ F). It is a life-threatening medical emergency that requires immediate and effective whole body cooling with cold water and ice water immersion therapy. Inadequate physical fitness, excess adiposity, improper clothing, protective pads, incomplete heat acclimatization, illness, and medications or dietary supplements that contain stimulants (*e.g.*, ephedra, synephrine) also increase the risk of heat exhaustion (26).

Exercise Prescription

Exercise professionals may use standards established by the National Institute for Occupational Safety and Health to define WBGT levels at which the risk of heat injury is increased, but exercise may be performed if preventive steps are taken (32), including required rest breaks between exercise periods.

If an Ex R_x specifies a THR, it will be achieved at a lower absolute workload when exercising in a warm/hot versus a cooler environment. For example, in hot or humid weather, an individual will achieve his or her THR with a reduced running speed. Reducing one's workload to maintain the same THR in the heat will help to reduce the risk of heat illness during acclimatization. As heat acclimatization develops, progressively higher exercise intensity will be required to elicit the THR. The first exercise session in the heat may last as little as 5–10 min for safety reasons but can be increased gradually as tolerated.

Special Considerations

Adults and children who are adequately rested, nourished, hydrated, and acclimatized to heat are at less risk for exertional heat illnesses. However, when clients/participants exercise in fitness or recreational settings while in hot/humid conditions, staff, coaches, trainers, educators, etc., should formulate a standardized heat stress management plan that incorporates the following considerations in order to minimize the effects of hyperthermia and dehydration, along with considering the questions in *Box 8.3* (14):

- Monitor the environment: Use the WBGT index to determine appropriate action and based on established criteria for modifying or canceling exercise/events.
- Modify activity in extreme environments: Enable access to ample fluid and bathroom facilities, provide longer and/or more rest breaks to facilitate heat dissipation and shorten or delay playing times. Perform exercise at times of the day when conditions will be cooler compared to midday (early morning, later evening). Children and older adults should modify activities in conditions of high-ambient temperatures accompanied by high humidity.

Box 8.3	Questions to Evaluate Readiness to Exercise in a Hot Environment (5)

Adults should ask the following questions to evaluate readiness to exercise in a hot environment. Corrective action should be taken if any question is answered "no."
- Have I developed a plan to avoid dehydration and hyperthermia?
- Have I acclimatized by gradually increasing exercise duration and intensity for 10–14 d?
- Do I limit intense exercise to the cooler hours of the day (early morning)?
- Do I avoid lengthy warm-up periods on hot, humid days?
- When training outdoors, do I know where fluids are available, or do I carry water bottles in a belt or a backpack?
- Do I know my sweat rate and the amount of fluid that I should drink to replace body weight loss?
- Was my body weight this morning within 1% of my average body weight?
- Is my 24-h urine volume plentiful?
- Is my urine color "pale yellow" or "straw colored"?
- When heat and humidity are high, do I reduce my expectations, my exercise pace, the distance, and/or duration of my workout or race?
- Do I wear loose-fitting, porous, lightweight clothing?
- Do I know the signs and symptoms of heat exhaustion, exertional heatstroke, heat syncope, and heat cramps (see *Table 8.2*)?
- Do I exercise with a partner and provide feedback about his or her physical appearance?
- Do I consume adequate salt in my diet?
- Do I avoid or reduce exercise in the heat if I experience sleep loss, infectious illness, fever, diarrhea, vomiting, carbohydrate depletion, some medications, alcohol, or drug abuse?

- *Optimize but do not maximize* fluid intake that (a) matches the volume of fluid consumed to the volume of sweat lost and (b) limits body weight change to <2% of body weight.
- Screen and monitor at-risk participants and establish specific emergency procedures.
- Consider heat acclimatization status, physical fitness, nutrition, sleep deprivation, previous illness (especially vomiting and/or diarrhea), and age of participants; intensity, time/duration, and time of day for exercise; availability of fluids; and playing surface heat reflection (*i.e.*, grass vs. asphalt). Allow at least 3 h, and preferably 6 h, of recovery and rehydration time between exercise sessions.
- Heat acclimatization: These adaptations include decreased rectal temperature, HR, and rating of perceived exertion (RPE); increased exercise tolerance time; increased sweating rate; and a reduction in sweat salt. Acclimatization results in the following: (a) improved heat transfer from the body's core to the external environment, (b) improved cardiovascular function, (c) more effective sweating, and (d) improved exercise performance and heat tolerance. Seasonal acclimatization will occur gradually during late spring and early summer months with sedentary exposure to the heat. However, this process can be facilitated with a structured program of moderate exercise in the heat across 10–14 d to stimulate adaptations to warmer ambient temperatures.
- Clothing: Clothes that have a high wicking capacity may assist in evaporative heat loss. Athletes should remove as much clothing and equipment (especially headgear) as possible to permit heat loss and reduce the risks of hyperthermia, especially during the initial days of acclimatization.
- Education: The training of participants, fitness specialists, coaches, and community emergency response teams enhances the reduction, recognition, and treatment of heat-related illness. Such programs should emphasize the importance of recognizing signs/symptoms of heat intolerance, being hydrated, fed, rested, and acclimatized to heat. Educating individuals about dehydration, assessing hydration state, and using a fluid replacement program can help maintain hydration.

ONLINE RESOURCES

American College of Sports Medicine Position Stand on Exertional Heat Illness during Training and Competition (1):
   http://www.acsm.org
American College of Sports Medicine Position Stand on Exercise and Fluid Replacement (3):
   http://www.acsm.org
American College of Sports Medicine Position Stand on the Prevention of Cold Injuries (2):
   http://www.acsm.org
National Athletic Trainers' Association Position Statement on Environmental Cold Injuries (11):
   http://www.nata.org/position-statements

National Athletic Trainers' Association Position Statement on Exertional Heat Illness (8):
http://www.nata.org/position-statements
United States Army Research Institute of Environmental Medicine:
http://www.usariem.army.mil

REFERENCES

1. American College of Sports Medicine, Armstrong LE, Casa DJ, et al. American College of Sports Medicine position stand. Exertional heat illness during training and competition. *Med Sci Sports Exerc.* 2007;39(3):556–72.

2. American College of Sports Medicine, Castellani JW, Young AJ, et al. American College of Sports Medicine position stand. Prevention of cold injuries during exercise. *Med Sci Sports Exerc.* 2006;38(11):2012–29.

3. American College of Sports Medicine, Sawka MN, Burke LM, et al. American College of Sports Medicine position stand. Exercise and fluid replacement. *Med Sci Sports Exerc.* 2007;39(2):377–90.

4. Armstrong LE. Classification, nomenclature, and incidence of the exertional heat illnesses. In: Armstrong LE, editor. *Exertional Heat Illnesses.* Champaign (IL): Human Kinetics; 2003. p. 17–28.

5. Armstrong LE. Heat and humidity. In: Armstrong LE, editor. *Performing in Extreme Environments.* Champaign (IL): Human Kinetics; 2000. p. 15–70.

6. Bass DE. Metabolic and energy balances of men in a cold environment. In: Horvath SM, editor. *Cold Injury.* Montpelier (VT): Capitol City Press; 1958. p. 317–38.

7. Beidleman BA, Tighiouart H, Schmid CH, Fulco CS, Muza SR. Predictive models of acute mountain sickness after rapid ascent to various altitudes. *Med Sci Sports Exerc.* 2013;45:792–800.

8. Binkley HM, Beckett J, Casa DJ, Kleiner DM, Plummer PE. National Athletic Trainers' Association position statement: exertional heat illnesses. *J Athl Train.* 2002;37(3):329–43.

9. Brajkovic D, Ducharme MB. Facial cold-induced vasodilation and skin temperature during exposure to cold wind. *Eur J Appl Physiol.* 2006;96(6):711–21.

10. *Canada's Windchill Index: Windchill Hazards and What to Do* [Internet]. Gatineau, Québec (Canada): Environment Canada; 2011 [cited 2015 Aug 18]. Available from: http://www.ec.gc.ca/meteo-weather/default.asp?lang=En&n=5FBF816A-1

11. Cappaert TA, Stone JA, Castellani JW, et al. National Athletic Trainers' Association position statement: environmental cold injuries. *J Athl Train.* 2008;43(6):640–58.

12. Carter R III, Cheuvront SN, Williams JO, et al. Epidemiology of hospitalizations and deaths from heat illness in soldiers. *Med Sci Sports Exerc.* 2005;37(8):1338–44.

13. Cheuvront SN, Kenefick RW. Dehydration: physiology, assessment and performance effects. *Compr Physiol.* 2014;4(1):257–85.

14. Cheuvront SN, Sawka MN. Hydration assessment of athletes. *Gatorade Sports Sci Exch.* 2005;18(2):1–5.

15. Cramer MN, Jay O. Selecting the correct exercise intensity for unbiased comparisons of thermoregulatory responses between groups of different mass and surface area. *J Appl Physiol (1985).* 2014;116(9):1123–32.

16. Danielsson U. Windchill and the risk of tissue freezing. *J Appl Physiol.* 1996;81(6):2666–73.

17. Franklin BA, Hogan P, Bonzheim K, et al. Cardiac demands of heavy snow shoveling. *JAMA.* 1995;273(11):880–2.

18. Fulco CS, Muza SR, Beidleman BA, et al. Effect of repeated normobaric hypoxia exposures during sleep on acute mountain sickness, exercise performance, and sleep during exposure to terrestrial altitude. *Am J Physiol Regul Integr Comp Physiol.* 2011;300(2):R428–36.

19. Fulco CS, Rock PB, Cymerman A. Maximal and submaximal exercise performance at altitude. *Aviat Space Environ Med.* 1998;69(8):793–801.

20. Gagge AP, Gonzalez RR. Mechanisms of heat exchange: biophysics and physiology. In: Fregly MJ, editor. *Handbook of Physiology/Section 4, Environmental Physiology.* Bethesda (MD): American Physiological Society; 1996. p. 45–84.

21. Gill TM, DiPietro L, Krumholz HM. Role of exercise stress testing and safety monitoring for older persons starting an exercise program. *JAMA*. 2000;284(3):342–9.

22. Givan GV, Diehl JJ. Intravenous fluid use in athletes. *Sports Health*. 2012;4(4):333–9.

23. Hackett PH, Roach RC. High-altitude illness. *N Engl J Med*. 2001;345(2):107–14.

24. Hamlet MP. Human cold injuries. In: Pandolf KB, Sawka MN, Gonzalez RR, editors. *Human Performance Physiology and Environmental Medicine at Terrestrial Extremes*. Dubuque (IA): Brown & Benchmark; 1988. p. 435–66.

25. Kenefick RW, Cheuvront SN, Palombo LJ, Ely BR, Sawka MN. Skin temperature modifies the impact of hypohydration on anaerobic performance. *J Appl Physiol*. 2010;109(1):79–86.

26. Leon LR, Kenefick RW. Pathophysiology of heat-related illnesses. In: Auerbach PS, editor. *Wilderness Medicine*. Philadelphia (PA): Elsevier; 2012. p. 215–31.

27. Mazzeo RS, Fulco CS. Physiological systems and their responses to conditions to hypoxia. In: Tipton CM, editor. *ACSM's Advanced Exercise Physiology*. Baltimore (MD): Lippincott Williams & Wilkins; 2006. p. 564–80.

28. Molnar GW, Hughes AL, Wilson O, Goldman RF. Effect of skin wetting on finger cooling and freezing. *J Appl Physiol*. 1973;35(2):205–7.

29. Montain SJ, Latzka WA, Sawka MN. Control of thermoregulatory sweating is altered by hydration level and exercise intensity. *J Appl Physiol*. 1995;79(5):1434–9.

30. Muza SR, Fulco C, Beidleman BA, Cymerman A. *Altitude Acclimatization and Illness Management*. Washington (DC): Department of the Army Technical Bulletin; 2010. 120 p.

31. Nadel ER, Fortney SM, Wenger CB. Circulatory adjustments during heat stress. In: Cerretelli P, Whipp BJ, editors. *Exercise Bioenergetics and Gas Exchange: Proceedings of the International Symposium on Exercise Bioenergetics and Gas Exchange, Held in Milan, Italy, July 7–9, 1980, a Satellite of the XXVIII International Congress of Physiological Sciences*. Amsterdam (The Netherlands): Elsevier/North-Holland Biomedical Press; 1980. p. 303–13.

32. National Institute for Occupational Safety and Health, Division of Standards Development and Technology Transfer. *Working in Hot Environments*. Cincinnati (OH): National Institute for Occupational Safety and Health; 1992. 12 p.

33. Neufer PD, Young AJ, Sawka MN. Gastric emptying during exercise: effects of heat stress and hypohydration. *Eur J Appl Physiol Occup Physiol*. 1989;58(4):433–9.

34. *NWS Windchill Chart* [Internet]. Silver Spring (MD): National Oceanic and Atmospheric Administration, National Weather Service; 2009 [cited 2015 Aug 18]. Available from: http://www.nws.noaa.gov/om/windchill/index.shtml

35. Pozos RS, Danzl DF. Human physiological responses to cold stress and hypothermia. In: Pandolf KB, editor. *Textbooks of Military Medicine: Medical Aspects of Harsh Environments*. Falls Church (VA): Office of the Surgeon General, United States Army; 2002. p. 351–82.

36. Sawka MN, Coyle EF. Influence of body water and blood volume on thermoregulation and exercise performance in the heat. *Exerc Sport Sci Rev*. 1999;27:167–218.

37. Sawka MN, Francesconi RP, Young AJ, Pandolf KB. Influence of hydration level and body fluids on exercise performance in the heat. *JAMA*. 1984;252(9):1165–9.

38. Sawka MN, Young AJ. Physiological systems and their responses to conditions of heat and cold. In: Tipton CM, American College of Sports Medicine, editors. *ACSM's Advanced Exercise Physiology*. Baltimore (MD): Lippincott Williams & Wilkins; 2006. p. 535–63.

39. Sawka MN, Young AJ, Latzka WA, Neufer PD, Quigley MD, Pandolf KB. Human tolerance to heat strain during exercise: influence of hydration. *J Appl Physiol*. 1992;73(1):368–75.

40. Schwellnus MP. Cause of exercise associated muscle cramps (EAMC) — altered neuromuscular control, dehydration or electrolyte depletion? *Br J Sports Med*. 2009;43(6):401–8.

41. Senay LC Jr. Relationship of evaporative rates to serum [Na+], [K+], and osmolarity in acute heat stress. *J Appl Physiol*. 1968;25(2):149–52.

42. Thomas JR. Oakley EHN. Nonfreezing cold injury. In: KB Pandolf RB, editor. *Textbooks of Military Medicine: Medical Aspects of Harsh Environments, Volume 1*. Falls Church (VA): Office of the Surgeon General, U. S. Army; 2002. p. 467–90.

43. Young AJ, Reeves JT. Human adaptation to high terrestrial altitude. In: Lounsbury DE, Bellamy RF, Zajtchuk R, editors. *Medical Aspects of Harsh Environments*. Washington (DC): Office of the Surgeon General, Borden Institute; 2002. p. 647–91.

Exercise Prescription for Patients with Cardiac, Peripheral, Cerebrovascular, and Pulmonary Disease

INTRODUCTION

The intent of this chapter is to describe the guidelines for developing an exercise prescription (Ex R_x) for individuals with various cardiac diseases as well as those with peripheral vascular, cerebrovascular, and pulmonary disease (*Box 9.1*). *Chapter 6* presents the general principles of Ex R_x for aerobic, resistance, and flexibility training. Refinement of the Ex R_x for patients with cardiac, peripheral, cerebrovascular, or pulmonary disease is presented in the following sections.

CARDIAC DISEASES

Individuals with cardiac disease benefit from participation in regular exercise and lifestyle change. Cardiac rehabilitation (CR) is commonly used to deliver exercise and lifestyle interventions and consists of a coordinated, multifaceted intervention designed to reduce risk, foster healthy behaviors and compliance to these behaviors, reduce disability, and promote an active lifestyle for patients with cardiovascular disease (CVD) (15). CR is typically delivered in both inpatient (previously termed *phase I CR*) and outpatient (previously termed *phase II CR*) settings and reduces the rate of mortality and morbidity in persons with various cardiac diseases by stabilizing, slowing, or even reversing the progression of the atherosclerotic process (122). The benefits provided by CR are important to the individual patient and to society as subsequent health care costs may be reduced following participation (91), with cost-effectiveness greater in patients with a higher risk for subsequent cardiac events (78). Currently, Medicare and most other commercial and private insurance companies provide CR as a benefit for those with a recent myocardial infarction (MI)/acute coronary syndrome (within the past 12 mo), coronary revascularization (coronary artery bypass graft [CABG] surgery or percutaneous coronary intervention [PCI] with or without stent placement), stable angina pectoris, heart valve repair or replacement (open surgery or transcutaneous procedure), heart failure with

Box 9.1	Manifestations of Cardiovascular Disease

- Acute coronary syndrome — the manifestation of coronary artery disease as increasing symptoms of angina pectoris, myocardial infarction, or sudden death
- Cardiovascular disease — diseases that involve the heart and/or blood vessels; includes hypertension, coronary artery disease, peripheral arterial disease; includes but not limited to atherosclerotic arterial disease
- Cerebrovascular disease — diseases of the blood vessels that supply the brain
- Coronary artery disease — disease of the arteries of the heart (usually atherosclerotic)
- Myocardial ischemia — temporary lack of adequate coronary blood flow relative to myocardial oxygen demands; often manifested as angina pectoris
- Myocardial infarction — injury/death of the muscular tissue of the heart
- Peripheral arterial disease — diseases of arterial blood vessels outside the heart and brain

reduced ejection fraction (HFrEF), and heart transplant. The following sections provide general inpatient and outpatient CR program information followed by specific exercise testing and Ex R$_x$ information on various CVDs and procedures.

Inpatient Cardiac Rehabilitation Programs

In the United States, inpatient CR refers to a brief program of early assessment and mobilization, identification of and education regarding CVD risk factors, assessment of the patient's level of readiness for physical activity (PA), and comprehensive discharge planning. It occurs during hospitalization for an acute cardiac event or procedure or other cardiac-related indication. In Europe, at least 64% of the countries provide inpatient CR in both the acute event and postevent period (21).

Following a documented physician referral, patients hospitalized after a cardiac event or procedure should begin participating in an inpatient CR program that focuses on preventive and rehabilitative services (123). Guidelines for the inpatient CR program should focus on the following (5):

- Current clinical status assessment
- Mobilization
- Identification and provision of information regarding modifiable risk factors and self-care
- Discharge planning with a home PA and activities of daily living (ADL) plan and referral to outpatient CR

Before beginning ambulation, a baseline assessment should be conducted by a competent health care provider. *Box 9.2* provides a list of adverse indications to consider prior to daily ambulation, and *Box 9.3* provides indications to discontinue an exercise session. The individual supervising an ambulatory session should possess the skills and competencies necessary to assess and document vital signs and heart

Box 9.2	American Association of Cardiovascular and Pulmonary Rehabilitation (AACVPR) Parameters for Inpatient Cardiac Rehabilitation Daily Ambulation (5)

- No new or recurrent chest pain in previous 8 h
- Stable or falling creatine kinase and troponin values
- No indication of decompensated heart failure (*e.g.*, resting dyspnea and bibasilar rales)
- Normal cardiac rhythm and stable electrocardiogram for previous 8 h

and lung sounds and provide feedback on the patient's musculoskeletal strength and flexibility. These patients should be risk stratified as early as possible following their acute cardiac event or procedure in preparation for the initiation and progression of PA. The American College of Sports Medicine (ACSM) has adopted the risk stratification system established by the American Association of Cardiovascular and Pulmonary Rehabilitation (AACVPR) for outpatients with known CVD because it considers the overall prognosis of the patient and their potential for rehabilitation (5) (see *Box 2.2*). The ACSM recommends using this system for inpatient CR.

The indications and contraindications for inpatient and outpatient CR are listed in *Box 9.4*, and exceptions to these should be considered based on the clinical judgment of the physician-in-charge or the patient's personal physician, along with the CR team. The relatively recent trend of shortened length of hospital stay after the acute event or intervention limits the time available for patient assessment and any inpatient CR intervention. Patients who undergo elective PCI might be discharged within 24 h from admission, and patients with uncomplicated events or procedures including MI, acute coronary syndrome, CABG or open valve surgery, or transluminal valve interventions (*e.g.*, transcatheter aortic valve replacement [TAVR]) are often discharged within 5 d. Activities and programs during the early recovery period will depend on the size of the MI and the occurrence of any complications while recovering. These activities should include self-care; arm and leg range of motion (ROM); postural changes; and limited, supervised ambulation (5).

Box 9.3	Adverse Responses to Inpatient Exercise Leading to Exercise Discontinuation

- Diastolic blood pressure (DBP) $\geq$110 mm Hg
- Decrease in systolic blood pressure (SBP) >10 mm Hg during exercise with increasing workload
- Significant ventricular or atrial arrhythmias with or without associated signs/symptoms
- Second- or third-degree heart block
- Signs/symptoms of exercise intolerance including angina, marked dyspnea, and electrocardiogram (ECG) changes suggestive of ischemia

Used with permission from (5).

Box 9.4	Indications and Contraindications for Inpatient and Outpatient Cardiac Rehabilitation (15)

Indications

- Medically stable postmyocardial infarction
- Stable angina
- Coronary artery bypass graft surgery
- Percutaneous transluminal coronary angioplasty
- Stable heart failure caused by either systolic or diastolic dysfunction (cardiomyopathy)
- Heart transplantation
- Valvular heart disease/surgery
- Peripheral arterial disease
- At risk for coronary artery disease with diagnoses of diabetes mellitus, dyslipidemia, hypertension, or obesity
- Other patients who may benefit from structured exercise and/or patient education based on physician referral and consensus of the rehabilitation team

Contraindications

- Unstable angina
- Uncontrolled hypertension — that is, resting systolic blood pressure >180 mm Hg and/or resting diastolic blood pressure >110 mm Hg
- Orthostatic blood pressure drop of >20 mm Hg with symptoms
- Significant aortic stenosis (aortic valve area <1.0 cm^2)
- Uncontrolled atrial or ventricular arrhythmias
- Uncontrolled sinus tachycardia (>120 beats $\cdot$ min^{-1})
- Uncompensated heart failure
- Third-degree atrioventricular block without pacemaker
- Active pericarditis or myocarditis
- Recent embolism (pulmonary or systemic)
- Acute thrombophlebitis
- Aortic dissection
- Acute systemic illness or fever
- Uncontrolled diabetes mellitus
- Severe orthopedic conditions that would prohibit exercise
- Other metabolic conditions, such as acute thyroiditis, hypokalemia, hyperkalemia, or hypovolemia (until adequately treated)
- Severe psychological disorder

Simple exposure to orthostatic or gravitational stress, such as intermittent sitting or standing, within the initial 12–24 h after an MI may prevent deterioration in exercise performance that often follows an acute cardiac event and subsequent bed rest (35,36). The optimal dose of exercise for inpatients has not been defined. Patients should progress from self-care activities (*e.g.*, sitting, toileting) to walking short-to-moderate distances with minimal or no assistance three to four times per day to independent ambulation on the hospital unit. Activity goals should be part of the overall plan of care. Other activities may include upper body movement exercises and minimal stair climbing in preparation for returning home (5). The amount of activity and rate of progression should be guided by an individual patient assessment performed daily by a qualified staff member (*e.g.*, ACSM Certified Clinical Exercise Physiologist® [CEP]). The rating of perceived exertion (RPE) can be useful in gauging exercise intensity (see *Chapter 6*). In general, the criteria for terminating an inpatient exercise session are similar to, or slightly more

■ **FITT RECOMMENDATIONS FOR INPATIENT CARDIAC REHABILITATION**[a] (5)

FITT		Aerobic	Flexibility
	Frequency	2–4 sessions · d^{-1} for the first 3 d of the hospital stay	Minimally once per day but as often as tolerated
	Intensity	Seated or standing HR$_{rest}$ +20 beats · min^{-1} for patients with an MI and +30 beats · min^{-1} for patients recovering from heart surgery Upper limit ≤120 beats · min^{-1} that corresponds to an RPE ≤13 on a scale of 6–20 (23)	Very mild stretch discomfort
	Time	Begin with intermittent walking bouts lasting 3–5 min as tolerated; progressively increase duration. The rest period may be a slower walk (or complete rest) that is shorter than the duration of the exercise bout. Attempt to achieve a 2:1 exercise/rest ratio. Progress to 10–15 min of continuous walking.	All major joints with at least 30 s per joint.
	Type	Walking. Other aerobic modes are useful in inpatient facilities that have accommodations (*e.g.*, treadmill, cycle).	Focus on ROM and dynamic movement. Pay particular attention to lower back and posterior thigh regions. Bedbound patients may benefit from passive stretching provided by an allied health care professional (*e.g.*, CEP, PT).

[a]Resistance training is not recommended in the inpatient setting.
CEP, clinical exercise physiologist; HR$_{rest}$, resting heart rate; ROM, range of motion; RPE, rating of perceived exertion; PT, physical therapist.

conservative than, those for terminating a low intensity exercise test (5). Although not all patients may be suitable candidates for inpatient exercise, virtually all will benefit from some level of inpatient intervention including the assessment of CVD risk factors (see *Table 3.1*), PA counseling, and patient and family education.

At hospital discharge, the patient should have specific instructions regarding strenuous activities (*e.g.*, heavy lifting, climbing stairs, yard work, household activities) that are permissible and those they should avoid (10). Moreover, a safe, progressive plan of exercise should be formulated before leaving the hospital. Until evaluated with an exercise test or entry into a clinically supervised outpatient CR program, the upper limit of heart rate (HR) or RPE noted during exercise should not exceed those levels observed during the inpatient program (5). Patients should be counseled to identify abnormal signs and symptoms suggesting exercise intolerance and the need for medical evaluation. All eligible patients should be strongly encouraged to participate in a clinically supervised outpatient CR program for enhancement of quality of life and functional capacity and reduction in risk of morbidity and mortality.

Outpatient Cardiac Rehabilitation

Outpatient CR/secondary prevention is a Class I recommendation (*Box 9.5*) in clinical guidelines for patients with a recent MI, acute coronary syndrome event/angina, coronary artery bypass surgery, PCI, heart failure (HF) hospitalization, heart valve repair or replacement, and heart or heart/lung transplantation (123). The goals of outpatient CR are listed in *Box 9.6*, and its components are listed in *Box 9.7*.

At the time of physician referral or program entry, the following assessments should be performed (5):

■ Medical and surgical history including the most recent cardiovascular event, comorbidities, and other pertinent medical history
■ Physical examination with an emphasis on the cardiopulmonary and musculoskeletal systems

Box 9.5	Definitions for Level of Guideline Recommendation (29)

Classification of Recommendations

Class I: conditions for which there is evidence and/or general agreement that a given procedure or treatment is useful and effective

Class II: conditions for which there is conflicting evidence and/or a divergence of opinion about the usefulness/efficacy of a procedure or treatment

Class III: conditions for which there is evidence and/or general agreement that the procedure/treatment is not useful/effective and in some cases may be harmful

Level of Evidence

Level A: data derived from multiple randomized clinical trials

Level B: data derived from a single randomized trial or nonrandomized studies

Level C: consensus opinion of experts

| Box 9.6 | Goals for Outpatient Cardiac Rehabilitation |

- Develop and assist the patient to implement a safe and effective formal exercise and lifestyle physical activity program.
- Provide appropriate supervision and monitoring to detect change in clinical status.
- Provide ongoing surveillance to the patient's health care providers in order to enhance medical management.
- Return the patient to vocational and recreational activities or modify these activities based on the patient's clinical status.
- Provide patient and spouse/partner/family education to optimize secondary prevention (e.g., risk factor modification) through aggressive lifestyle management and judicious use of cardioprotective medications.

- Review of recent cardiovascular tests and procedures including 12-lead electrocardiogram (ECG), coronary angiogram, echocardiogram, stress test (exercise or pharmacological studies), cardiac surgeries or percutaneous interventions, and pacemaker/implantable defibrillator implantation
- Current medications including dose, route of administration, and frequency
- CVD risk factors (see *Table 3.1*)

Exercise training is safe and effective for most patients with cardiac disease; however, all patients should be stratified based on their risk for occurrence of a cardiac-related event during exercise training (see *Box 2.2*). Routine assessment of risk for exercise (see *Chapters 3* and *5*) should be performed before, during, and

| Box 9.7 | Components of Outpatient Cardiac Rehabilitation |

- Cardiovascular risk factor assessment and counseling on aggressive lifestyle management
- Education and support to make healthy lifestyle changes to reduce the risk of a secondary cardiac event
- Development and implementation/supervision of a safe and effective personalized exercise plan
- Monitoring with a goal of improving blood pressure, lipids/cholesterol, and diabetes mellitus
- Psychological/stress assessment and counseling
- Communication with each patient's physician and other health care providers regarding progress and relevant medical management issues
- Return to appropriate vocational and recreational activities

after each CR session, as deemed appropriate by the qualified staff and include the following (5):

- HR
- Blood pressure (BP)
- Body weight
- Symptoms or evidence of change in clinical status not necessarily related to activity (*e.g.*, dyspnea at rest, light-headedness or dizziness, palpitations or irregular pulse, chest discomfort, sudden weight gain)
- Symptoms and evidence of exercise intolerance
- Change in medications and adherence to the prescribed medication regimen
- ECG and HR surveillance that may consist of telemetry, Bluetooth or hardwire monitoring, "quick-look" monitoring using defibrillator paddles, periodic rhythm strips depending on the risk status of the patient and the need for accurate rhythm detection, or non-ECG HR monitoring devices

Exercise Testing

The American College of Cardiology (ACC)/American Heart Association (AHA) 2002 guideline update for exercise testing (55) states exercise testing early (2–3 wk) or later (3–6 wk) after hospital discharge is useful for the development of an Ex R_x in patients who suffered from MI without (Class I recommendation) or with (Class IIa recommendation) coronary revascularization. An exercise test may also be used periodically in patients who continue to participate in supervised exercise training and CR (Class IIb recommendation). The following exercise testing considerations should be noted (5):

- The test should be symptom-limited and use standard exercise testing procedures (see *Chapter 5*).
- The test should be completed while the patient is stable on guideline-based medications. Of particular note would be the timing of a β-blocker with respect to the exercise test and exercise training participation because this could have an effect on the HR response and subsequently on the HR-based Ex R_x (5).

Because an exercise test may invoke monetary costs to the patient in the form of meeting insurance plan deductibles and co-pays, an ordering physician or mid-level provider may request that a patient participate in outpatient CR without an exercise test. The following section on Ex R_x provides methodology for guiding exercise intensity when results from an exercise test are not available.

Exercise Prescription

Prescriptive techniques for determining exercise dosage or the *F*requency, *I*ntensity, *T*ime, and *T*ype (FITT) principle of Ex R_x for the general apparently healthy population are detailed in *Chapter 6*. The Ex R_x techniques used for the apparently healthy adult population may be applied to many patients with CVD. This section provides specific considerations and modifications of the Ex R_x for patients with known CVD.

■ **FITT RECOMMENDATIONS FOR INDIVIDUALS WITH CARDIOVASCULAR DISEASE PARTICIPATING IN OUTPATIENT CARDIAC REHABILITATION** (5,50)

FITT

	Aerobic	Resistance	Flexibility
Frequency	Minimally 3 d · wk^{-1}; preferably ≥5 d · wk^{-1}	2–3 nonconsecutive d · wk^{-1}	≥2–3 d · wk^{-1} with daily being most effective
Intensity	With an exercise test, use 40%–80% of exercise capacity using HRR, $\dot{V}O_2R$, or $\dot{V}O_{2peak}$. Without an exercise test, use seated or standing HR$_{rest}$ +20 to +30 beats · min^{-1} or an RPE of 12–16 on a scale of 6–20 (23).	Perform 10–15 repetitions of each exercise without significant fatigue; RPE 11–13 on a 6–20 scale or 40%–60% of 1-RM.	To the point of feeling tightness or slight discomfort
Time	20–60 min	1–3 sets; 8–10 different exercises focused on major muscle groups.	15 s hold for static stretching; ≥4 repetitions of each exercise
Type	Arm ergometer, upper and lower (dual action) extremity ergometer, upright and recumbent cycles, recumbent stepper, rower, elliptical, stair climber, treadmill	Select equipment that is safe and comfortable for the patient to use.	Static and dynamic stretching focused on the major joints of the limbs and the lower back; consider PNF technique.

1-RM, one repetition maximum; HRR, heart rate reserve; HR$_{rest}$, resting heart rate; PNF, proprioceptive neuromuscular facilitation; RPE, rating of perceived exertion; $\dot{V}O_2R$, oxygen uptake reserve; $\dot{V}O_{2peak}$, peak oxygen uptake.

Exercise Training Considerations

- Frequency of exercise depends on several factors including baseline exercise tolerance, exercise intensity, fitness and other health goals, and types of exercise that are incorporated into the overall program.

- General guidelines for adults and older adults suggest exercise bouts of at least 10 min each (7,52). However, for patients with very limited exercise capacities, multiple shorter (*i.e.*, <10 min) daily sessions may be considered as a starting point (52). If beginning with <10 min bouts, a gradual increase in aerobic exercise time is suggested (52). This may be as little as 1–5 min per session or 10%–20% per week.

- Patients should be encouraged to perform some exercise sessions independently (*i.e.*, without direct supervision) following the recommendations outlined in this chapter.

- If a patient has an identified ischemic threshold (*i.e.*, angina and/or ≥1 mm ischemic ST-segment depression on exercise test), the exercise intensity should be prescribed at an HR and work rate below this point. If such a threshold has been determined, the upper limit of the HR-based intensity should be a minimum of 10 beats · min^{-1} below the HR at which the ischemia was initially identified (50). In addition to an exercise test, the presence of classic angina pectoris that is induced with exercise training and relieved with rest or nitroglycerin is sufficient evidence for the presence of myocardial ischemia.

- If peak HR is unknown, the RPE method should be used to guide exercise intensity using the following relationships (50):
  - <12 (<3 on CR10 Scale) is light or <40% of HRR
  - 12–13 (4–6 on CR10 Scale) is somewhat hard or 40%–59% of HRR
  - 14–16 (7–8 on CR10 Scale) is hard or 60%–80% of HRR

- It is preferable for individuals to take their prescribed medications at their usual time as recommended by their health care providers. Individuals on a β-adrenergic blocking agent (*i.e.*, β-blocker) may have an attenuated HR response to exercise and an increased or decreased maximal exercise capacity. For patients whose β-blocker dose was altered after an exercise test or during the course of CR, a new graded exercise test may be helpful (5).

- For patients who have had a β-blocker dose change but have not had an exercise test since this change, the following recommendations for guiding exercise intensity may be used: (a) Monitor signs and symptoms and (b) note the RPE and HR responses at the workload most recently used in CR. The HR and RPE observed may serve as the patient's new target for exercise intensity.

- It is recommended that an exercise test be performed any time that symptoms or clinical changes warrant (5). For example, in patients who have a change in their level of chest pain or dyspnea; or possibly for those with an ischemic etiology who have not undergone a coronary revascularization procedure, or who have been incompletely revascularized (*i.e.*, residual obstructive coronary lesions are present), or who have rhythm disturbances and desire to exercise to a higher intensity level. However, another exercise test may not be medically necessary in patients who have undergone complete coronary revascularization, who are asymptomatic, or when it is logistically impractical.

■ Patients on diuretic therapy are at an elevated risk for volume depletion, hypokalemia, or orthostatic hypotension particularly after bouts of exercise. For these patients, the BP response to exercise, symptoms of dizziness or light-headedness, and arrhythmias should be monitored while providing education regarding proper hydration (8). See *Appendix A* for other medications that may influence the hemodynamic response during and after exercise.

■ During each exercise session warm-up and cool-down activities of 5–10 min, including dynamic and static stretching, and light or very light (see *Table 6.1*) aerobic activities should be performed.

■ The aerobic exercise portion of the session should include rhythmic, large muscle group activities with an emphasis on increased caloric expenditure for maintenance of a healthy body weight and its many other associated health benefits (see *Chapters 1* and *10*).

■ To promote whole body physical fitness, conditioning that includes the upper and lower extremities and multiple forms of aerobic activities and exercise equipment should be incorporated into the exercise program.

■ High-intensity interval training (HIIT) involves alternating 3–4 min periods of exercise at 80%–90% HRR with exercise at 60%–70% HRR. Such training for approximately 40 min, three times per week has been shown to yield a greater improvement in $\dot{V}O_{2peak}$ in patients with stable coronary heart disease (73) and HF (130). HIIT has also been shown to result in greater long-term improvements in $\dot{V}O_{2peak}$ in patients after CABG (83) compared to standard continuous, moderate intensity exercise. It appears that HIIT may be both a safe and very effective method of enhancing peak aerobic fitness in those with CVD (127).

■ Safety factors that should be considered include the patient's clinical status, risk stratification category (see *Box 2.2*), exercise capacity, ischemic/angina threshold, musculoskeletal limitations, and cognitive/psychological impairment.

■ Associated factors to consider when guiding those exercising in CR include premorbid activity level, vocational and avocational goals and requirements, and personal health/fitness goals.

■ Resistance training volume can be increased in 2%–10% increments when an individual patient is able to comfortably complete one to two repetitions over the desired number of repetitions on two consecutive training days (6).

■ Avoid breath holding during resistance training and static stretching.

Continuous Electrocardiographic Monitoring

ECG monitoring during supervised exercise sessions may be helpful during the first several weeks of CR. The following recommendations for ECG monitoring are related to patient-associated risks of exercise training (50).

■ Patients with known stable CVD and low risk for complications may begin with continuous ECG monitoring and decrease to intermittent or no ECG monitoring after 6–12 sessions or sooner as deemed appropriate by the medical team.

■ Patients with known CVD and at moderate-to-high risk for cardiac complications should begin with continuous ECG monitoring and decrease to intermittent or no ECG monitoring after 12 sessions and as deemed appropriate by the medical team.

■ When considering removing or reducing ECG monitoring, the patient should understand his or her individual exercise level that is safe.

Exercise Prescription without a Preparticipation Exercise Test

With shorter hospital stays, more aggressive interventions, and greater sophistication of diagnostic procedures, it is not unusual for patients to begin CR before having an exercise test. A preparticipation exercise test may be unavailable due to extreme deconditioning of the patient, orthopedic limitations, or recent successful percutaneous intervention or revascularization surgery without residual obstructive coronary artery disease. Until an exercise test is performed, Ex R_x procedures can be based on the recommendations of these *Guidelines* and what was accomplished during the inpatient phase and home exercise activities. Use of RPE to guide exercise is recommended. The patient should be closely monitored for signs and symptoms of exercise intolerance such as excessive fatigue, dizziness or light-headedness, chronotropic incompetence, and signs or symptoms of ischemia.

Lifestyle Physical Activity

Those participating in maintenance outpatient exercise programs expend approximately 300 kcal per session (109). Thus, those who attend three times per week expend <1,000 kcals per week in exercise sessions. Based on recommendations of calorie expenditure for CVD risk reduction (see *Chapter 6*) and for weight management (see *Chapter 10*), it is important to encourage patients to perform regular PA and purposeful exercise outside of program participation. In addition to formal exercise sessions, patients should be encouraged to gradually return to general ADL such as household chores, yard work, shopping, and hobbies as evaluated and appropriately modified by the rehabilitation staff. Participation in competitive sports should be guided by the recommendations of the ACC Bethesda Conference (124). Relatively inexpensive pedometers, smartphones with stepping technology, and other wearable devices can be useful to monitor PA and may enhance adherence with walking programs (26). Many of these devices can be followed with various "apps" designed to use on smartphone or tablet technology. At this time, continued research is needed to determine if these apps appropriately assist with exercise tracking and enhanced adherence.

Patients with Heart Failure

Chronic HF is characterized by exertional dyspnea and fatigue in the setting of HFrEF (*i.e.*, systolic dysfunction), a preserved left ventricular ejection fraction (HFpEF, *i.e.*, diastolic dysfunction), or a combination of the two. Due partly to the aging of the population and to improved outcomes for acute cardiac disease, the prevalence of HF is increasing such that decompensated HF is the single most common admitting diagnosis in older Americans and results in more than 1 million hospitalizations annually (58). Twenty-five percent of patients are re-admitted within 30 d and 66% within 1 yr of their initial HF hospital admission (41,80). The number of new cases of HF annually in the United States is 825,000, and the prevalence in 2010 approached 6 million (58).

Exercise training is broadly recognized as a valuable adjunct in the ther-apeutic approach to the care of patients with stable chronic HF and is rec-ommended by the ACC and the AHA (131). The benefits of exercise training in patients with HFrEF have been previously described (71) and include im-proved clinical outcomes (*e.g.*, hospitalizations) and health-related quality of life (43,90,98,102,104). Exercise training also improves exercise capacity (10%–30%, as measured by $\dot{V}O_{2peak}$), central hemodynamic function, autonomic ner-vous system function, and peripheral vascular and skeletal muscle function in patients with HFrEF (3). In total, these adaptations allow patients to exercise to a higher peak work rate or exercise at a submaximal level with a lower HR, less perceived effort, and less dyspnea and fatigue. A meta-analysis of 57 studies that directly measured $\dot{V}O_{2peak}$ reported an average 17% improvement (116). Emerging data indicates that patients with HFpEF also benefit from exercise training, as evidenced by improved skeletal muscle function, quality of life, and exercise capacity (60).

Exercise Testing

Symptom-limited exercise testing is safe in patients with HFrEF and when com-bined with the indirect measurement of expired gases provides not only useful information pertaining to electrocardiographic and hemodynamic responses to exercise but prognostic information as well (50).

- Compared to age-matched healthy individuals, patients with HFrEF exhibit a lower peak HR, peak stroke volume, and peak cardiac output ($\dot{Q}$) response to exercise.
- Vasodilation of the large vessels (*e.g.*, brachial artery) and resistance vasculature are attenuated, limiting regional and local blood flow (45).
- Abnormalities in skeletal muscle histochemistry limit oxidative capacity of the more metabolically active cells.
- The three factors listed previously for HFrEF are also relevant and contribute to the reduced exercise capacity observed in patients with HFpEF.
- When compared to normal controls, exercise tolerance is reduced approxi-mately 30%–40% (75). Because of this limitation, an exercise protocol that starts at a lower work rate and imposes smaller increases in work rate per stage, such as the modified Naughton protocol (see *Chapter 5*), is commonly used.
- Both $\dot{V}O_{2peak}$ and the slope relationship between minute ventilation and carbon dioxide production ($\dot{V}_E$–$\dot{V}CO_2$ slope) are related to prognosis and can be used to help guide when to refer a patient to an advanced HF specialist or when to further evaluate for advanced therapies such as a continuous flow left ventricu-lar assist device (LVAD) or cardiac transplant (50).

Exercise Prescription

Because two of the main goals for exercise training in patients with HF are to reverse exercise intolerance and decrease subsequent risk for a clinical event, the principle of specificity of training dictates the use of exercise modalities that were used in trials that reported improved functional and clinical benefits. Therefore, exercise regimens should always include aerobic activities.

FITT

■	FITT RECOMMENDATIONS FOR INDIVIDUALS WITH HEART FAILURE (24,128)		
	Aerobic	**Resistance**	**Flexibility**
Frequency	3–5 d · wk^{-1}	1–2 nonconsecutive d · wk^{-1}	≥2–3 d · wk^{-1} with daily being most effective
Intensity	If HR data are available from a recent GXT, set intensity between 60% and 80% of HRR. In the absence of data from a GXT or if atrial fibrillation is present, use RPE of 11–14 on a 6–20 scale.	Begin at 40% 1-RM for upper body and 50% 1-RM for lower body exercises. Gradually increase to 70% 1-RM over several weeks to months.	Stretch to the point of feeling tightness or slight discomfort.
Time	Progressively increase to 30 min · d^{-1} and then up to 60 min · d^{-1}.	2 sets of 10–15 repetitions focusing on major muscle groups	10–30 s hold for static stretching; 2–4 repetitions of each exercise
Type	Treadmill- or free-walking and stationary cycling	Machines may be best due to loss of strength and balance.	Static, dynamic, and/or PNF stretching

1-RM, one repetition maximum; GXT, graded exercise test; HR, heart rate; HRR, heart rate reserve; PNF, proprioceptive neuromuscular facilitation; RPE, rating of perceived exertion.

Exercise Training Considerations

- In selected patients, higher intensity aerobic interval training may be considered, with training intensity up to 90% of HRR. HIIT improved $\dot{V}O_{2peak}$ by 46% in stable patients with HFrEF and was associated with reverse remodeling of the left ventricle (72,129).
- The clinician responsible for writing the Ex R$_x$ and overseeing the patient's progress needs to ensure that the volume of exercise performed each week is slowly but consistently increased over time. For most patients, the prescribed volume of exercise should approximate 3–7 MET-hr · wk^{-1} (74).

- In general, the duration and frequency of effort should be increased before exercise intensity.
- After patients have adjusted to and are tolerating aerobic training, which usually requires at least 4 wk, resistance training activities can be added.

Special Considerations

- Approximately 40% of patients with HF are compliant with prescribed exercise at the end of 1 yr, which is not different than long-term adherence for patients with established coronary artery disease (42,49,90).
- Because numerous barriers to exercise adoption and adherence exist in this population, factors amenable to interventions such as treating anxiety and depression, improving motivation, seeking additional social support, and managing logistical problems such as transportation should be addressed (see *Chapter 12*).
- Regular exercise training improves exercise tolerance and quality of life in patents with LVAD (68). The following list of special considerations is for patients with HF and an LVAD:
  - Exercise training and testing of patients that received an LVAD for either bridge-to-transplant or as a destination therapy for end-stage disease is becoming increasingly more common. These patients have a low functional capacity with a $\dot{V}O_{2peak}$ in the range of 7–23 mL · kg^{-1} · min^{-1} (69).
  - Due to the continuous flow of the LVAD (*i.e.*, lacking pulsatile flow), BP (*i.e.*, mean arterial pressure [MAP]) is measured by Doppler instead of auscultation via stethoscope. Resting mean pressure should be controlled to between 70 and 80 mm Hg (115). In general, MAP should mildly increase with increasing work rates. Studies have shown safe performance of exercise in inpatient settings with MAP maintained between 70 and 90 mm Hg (110).
  - HR during exercise increases in a manner that is generally linear with an increase in work rate.
  - LVAD typically have modest increases in flow rate (possibly as high as 10 L · min^{-1}) during progressive intensity exercise.
  - Early-onset fatigue is common with exercise. When starting an exercise training program, fatigue later in the day may be reported. If fatigue occurs, intermittent exercise may reduce the level of fatigue experienced from subsequent exercise training sessions.
  - Until more definitive information describing the relationship between HR and exercise intensity are available, using RPE of 11–13 to prescribe exercise intensity is appropriate.

Patients with a Sternotomy

The median sternotomy is the standard incision to provide optimal access for cardiovascular surgeries such as CABG or heart valve replacement.

- Although most patients heal without complications and achieve adequate sternal stability in approximately 8–10 wk, sternal instability has been observed in up to 16% of cases (14,128). Several factors such as diabetes, age, certain drugs, and obesity can predispose a patient to such a complication.

- Sternal wires are used to close the sternum after surgery in order to minimize distractive forces at the sternal edges and facilitate bone healing.
- It is common to instruct patients to restrict ROM and provide a weight load restriction for upper limb movement. The restriction of upper body movement is usually instructed during the patient's hospitalization and reinforced as an outpatient for 8–12 wk after surgery (5).
- Limitation or restriction of upper body activities usually involves activity type, load amount (*e.g.*, unloaded, restriction set at a weight limit), and allowable degrees of movement throughout a ROM (5).
- Five to 6 wk after hospital discharge in the outpatient setting, most patients have returned to pain-free, unloaded upper limb ROM.
- The instructions regarding lifting limits are usually conveyed prior to hospital discharge and might vary but are usually set at a 5- to 10-lb limit (or <50% of maximal voluntary contraction) for 10–12 wk (128).
- While in CR, certain rhythmic unloaded and low-load upper limb activities (*e.g.*, arm ergometry) should be encouraged. A general objective for patient care during 10–12 wk of CR for individuals with median sternotomy is to advance and progress through a pain-free ROM before focusing on regaining/improving muscle strength/endurance.

An important role for the exercise professional who works with patients who have undergone median sternotomy is surveillance for any early signs or symptoms indicative of sternal instability. This requires routine assessment for pain/discomfort, sternal movement/instability, and sternal clicking; if any findings are deemed to be clinically meaningful, informing the referring physician or surgeon is indicated.

Pacemaker and Implantable Cardioverter Defibrillator

Cardiac pacemakers are used to restore an optimal HR at rest and during exercise, to synchronize atrial and ventricular filling and contraction in the setting of abnormal rhythms, and to synchronize right and left ventricular contraction in the setting of left bundle-branch block (LBBB). Specific indications for pacemakers include sick sinus syndrome with symptomatic bradycardia, acquired atrioventricular (AV) block, and persistent advanced AV block after MI. The different types of pacemakers include the following:

- Rate-responsive (*i.e.*, rate-adaptive or rate-modulated) pacemakers that are programmed to increase or decrease HR to match the level of PA (*e.g.*, sitting rest or walking)
- Single-chambered pacemakers that have only one lead placed into the right atrium or the right ventricle; generally indicated for patients with chronic atrial fibrillation with concomitant symptomatic bradycardia such as seen with AV block de novo or after creation of complete heart block for definitive rate control measure

- Dual-chambered pacemakers that have two leads: one placed in the right atrium and one in the right ventricle; indicated for physiologic pacing to reestablish a normal sequence and timing of contractions between the upper and lower chambers of the heart
- Cardiac resynchronization therapy pacemakers that have three leads: one in right atrium, one in right ventricle, and one in coronary sinus or, less commonly, the left ventricular myocardium via an external surgical approach; indicated in patients with HF who have LBBB and a low functional capacity. This therapy improves functional capacity (*i.e.*, $\dot{V}O_{2peak}$ and 6-min walk test [6MWT] distance) (2).

The type of pacemaker is identified by a four-letter code as indicated in the following section:

- The first letter of the code describes the chamber paced (*e.g.*, atria [A], ventricle [V], dual [D]).
- The second letter of the code describes the chamber sensed.
- The third letter of the code describes the pacemaker's response to a sensed event (*e.g.*, triggered [T], inhibited [I], dual [D]).
- The fourth letter of the code describes the rate response capabilities of the pacemaker (*e.g.*, inhibited [I], rate responsive [R]).

For example, a VVIR code pacemaker means (a) the ventricle is paced (V) and sensed (V); (b) when the pacemaker senses a normal ventricular contraction, it is inhibited (I); and (c) the pulse generator is rate responsive (R).

Exercise testing is a Class I (see *Box 9.5*) indication for the assessment of rate-responsive pacemakers in those contemplating increase PA or competitive sports (50). In these cases, exercise testing can help to optimize the HR response and thus may increase the exercise capacity of an individual.

The implantable cardioverter defibrillator (ICD) is a device that monitors the heart rhythm and delivers an electrical shock if life-threatening rhythms are detected. ICDs are used for high-rate ventricular tachycardia or ventricular fibrillation in patients who are at risk for these conditions as a result of previous cardiac arrest, cardiomyopathy, HF, or ineffective drug therapy for abnormal heart rhythms. When ICDs detect an excessively rapid or irregular heartbeat, they may first attempt to pace the heart into a normal rate and rhythm (*i.e.*, antitachycardia pacing). If unsuccessful, they can then deliver an electrical shock (*i.e.*, cardioversion) in an attempt to reset the heart to a normal HR and electrical pattern. Thus, ICDs aim to protect against sudden cardiac death from ventricular tachycardia and ventricular fibrillation and are safe for those performing regular exercise (97).

Exercise Training Considerations

- Programmed pacemaker modes, HR limits, and ICD rhythm detection algorithms should be obtained from the patient's cardiologist prior to exercise testing or training.
- Exercise testing should be used to evaluate HR and rhythm responses prior to beginning an exercise program. Exercise training should not begin in patient's

whose HR does not increase during the exercise test. In these cases, the exercise sensing mechanism (*i.e.*, movement or respiration) needs adjustment to allow the HR to increase with PA.

- When an ICD is present, the peak heart rate (HR_{peak}) during the exercise test and exercise training program should be maintained 10–15 beats $\cdot$ min^{-1} below the programmed HR threshold for antitachycardia pacing and defibrillation.

- After the first 24 h following the device implantation, mild upper extremity ROM activities can be performed and may be useful to avoid subsequent joint complications.

- To maintain device and incision integrity, for 3–4 wk after implant, rigorous upper extremity activities such as swimming, bowling, lifting weights, elliptical machines, and golfing should be avoided. However, lower extremity activities are allowable.

- Isolated pacemaker and ICD implantation are not indications for CR. However, supervised exercise can be important for these patients, particularly those with a long history of sedentary living. Fewer supervised exercise sessions might be appropriate for those with normal cardiac function versus others with significantly reduced cardiac function and/or a history of sudden cardiac death.

Patients after Cardiac Transplantation

In patients with end-stage HF for whom expected 1-yr survival is poor and standard medical therapy fails to control symptoms, cardiac transplant may be a surgical option for those who are eligible. Approximately 4,000 such procedures are performed worldwide annually and, depending on age, 3-yr survival rates are 75%–81% (92). Following surgery, both aerobic and resistance training programs are strongly recommended to improve exercise capacity and quality of life, help restore bone mineral density, reverse sarcopenia, and help modify cardiovascular risk factors such as obesity, hypertension, and glucose intolerance (38).

In general, the improvement in exercise capacity, as measured by $\dot{V}O_{2peak}$, ranges between 15% and 30% for exercise programs between 2 and 6 mo in duration (89). Such improvement is due, in part, to improved chronotropic response and improved peripheral effects, such as oxidative capacity of the metabolically more active skeletal muscle. Additionally, resistance training leads to improved muscle strength and endurance (25). Following cardiac transplant, patients are at risk for several complications including cardiac allograft vasculopathy, graft failure, cancer, hyperlipidemia, hypertension, and diabetes mellitus (DM).

Exercise Testing

Knowledge about the denervated (*i.e.*, decentralized) heart is important to better appreciate how it responds to exercise and how to adjust the exercise protocol used for testing. Although there is some evidence of reinnervation of cardiac autonomic function a year or more after surgery, in the absence of direct cardiac sympathetic efferent innervation, peak $\dot{Q}$ is reduced 20%–35%. The skeletal muscle and peripheral abnormalities (*e.g.*, endothelial dysfunction) present before surgery are not normalized by the surgery per se and, therefore, also contribute to the reduction in exercise capacity observed in transplant patients when compared to age-matched healthy individuals (66).

- HR_{rest} is often elevated, whereas the HR response during an acute bout of exercise and at peak is attenuated. Similarly, in the absence of parasympathetic innervation, recovery HR is slow to return to preexercise levels.
- BP is often elevated at rest, with a slightly attenuated response to peak exercise.
- Given the HR and BP responses and the previously mentioned reduction in exercise capacity, a more gradual exercise testing protocol should be employed such as an incremental treadmill protocol that ramps at 1 metabolic equivalent (MET) or less every 30 s to 1 min or an incremental protocol of 1–2 METs per 2–3 min stage. The modified Naughton protocol may be appropriate (see *Chapter 5*). For stationary cycle testing, consider a ramp protocol of 10–15 W · min^{-1} or 25–30 W · 2–3 min^{-1} stage.
- Other testing issues such as test endpoints remain the same as those used for patients with other forms of CVD except for detection of angina, which is not possible due to the denervated heart.

■ FITT RECOMMENDATIONS FOR INDIVIDUALS WITH CARDIAC TRANSPLANT (70)

	Aerobic	Resistance	Flexibility
Frequency	3–5 d · wk^{-1}	1–2 nonconsecutive d · wk^{-1}	≥2–3 d · wk^{-1} with daily being most effective
Intensity	Use RPE of 11–14 on a 6–20 scale.	Slowly increase upper body activities over several weeks to months from 40% of 1-RM to 70% of 1-RM. Lower body excises should begin at 50% of 1-RM.	Stretch to the point of feeling tightness or slight discomfort.
Time	Progressively increase from 15–20 min · d^{-1} up to 30–60 min · d^{-1}	1–2 sets of 10–15 repetitions for each exercise	10–30 s hold for static stretching; 2–4 repetitions of each exercise
Type	Treadmill- or free-walking, stationary cycling, and dual action stationary bike	Weight machines are best, but dumbbells, elastic bands, and body weight can be used.	Static, dynamic, and/or PNF stretching

1-RM, one repetition maximum; PNF, proprioceptive neuromuscular facilitation; RPE, rating of perceived exertion.

Exercise Prescription

Prescribing exercise in patients having undergone cardiac transplant is, for the most part, quite similar to that of other patients with CVD. However, because of the denervated myocardium, setting an HR-based training range is not appropriate. Because of the negative effects of the immunosuppressive drug, regimen on bones and skeletal muscle resistance training should be performed and engage all major muscle groups.

Special Considerations

- Immunosuppression therapy used to prevent graft rejection can lead to bone loss, DM, and hypertension, and both regular aerobic and resistance training exercise can play an important role in helping manage these metabolic disorders.
- Higher intensity interval training has been used in patients with cardiac transplant, with intensities set at 90% of $\dot{V}O_{2peak}$ or >91% of HR_{peak} (89).
- Due to median sternotomy, ROM and the work rate of activities and exercises involving upper limbs should be restricted for up to 12 wk. See "Patients with a Sternotomy" section in this chapter.

Patients with Peripheral Artery Disease

The pathophysiologic development of peripheral artery disease (PAD) is caused by the same process as coronary artery disease in which atherosclerotic plaque leads to significant stenosis and limitations of vasodilation, resulting in the reduction of blood flow to regions distal to the area of occlusion. This reduction in blood flow creates a mismatch between oxygen supply and demand causing ischemia to develop in the affected areas (62). PAD severity can be ranked based on the presence of signs and symptoms (*Table 9.1*) or by the ankle/brachial pressure index (ABI) (*Table 9.2*) (63). The recommended treatments for PAD include an initially conservative approach of cardiovascular risk reduction and exercise training, followed by medications (*e.g.*, cilostazol) (see *Appendix A*). When there is an inadequate response to exercise or pharmacological therapy, peripheral revascularization may be indicated (63).

Intermittent claudication, the major symptom of PAD, is characterized by a reproducible aching, cramping sensation or fatigue usually affecting the muscles of the calf in one or both legs that is typically triggered by weight-bearing exercise

TABLE **9.1**	
Fontaine Classification of Peripheral Artery Disease (51)	
Stage	**Symptoms**
1	Asymptomatic
2	Intermittent claudication
2a	Distance to pain onset >200 m
2b	Distance to pain onset <200 m
3	Pain at rest
4	Gangrene, tissue loss

TABLE 9.2	
Ankle/Brachial Pressure Index Scale for Peripheral Arterial Disease (1)	
Supine, Resting ABI	**Interpretation**
>0.90	Normal
≤0.90	Threshold for PAD confirmation
Decrease of >0.15 over time	Significant PAD progression
Postexercise ABI	**Interpretation**
No change	Normal
Decrease of >30 mm HG or >20% from resting ABI	Reasonable to consider as threshold for PAD confirmation, whether ABI is normal or abnormal at rest
Decrease of >0.15 over time	Significant PAD progression

ABI, ankle-brachial index; PAD, peripheral arterial disease.

such as walking and relieved with rest (12). Depending on disease severity and lesion location, claudication may also occur in the thigh and buttock regions. On initial clinical presentation, up to 35% of individuals with PAD have typical claudication, and up to 50% have atypical leg pain that does not resolve quickly with rest (63,88). As the symptoms worsen, they may become severe enough to limit the individual from performing ADL and can greatly impact quality of life (54,63).

Symptomatic PAD prevalence increases with age with approximately 2% of those aged 50–54 yr affected, increasing to 6% in those aged ≥60 yr (88). Major risk factors for PAD include DM, hypertension, smoking, dyslipidemia, hyperhomocysteinemia, non-Caucasian race, male gender, age, inflammatory markers, and chronic renal insufficiency (88). Patients with PAD have a 20%–60% increased risk for MI and a two- to sixfold increased risk of dying from CVD compared with individuals without PAD (118).

Exercise Testing

Exercise testing can be performed in patients with PAD to determine functional capacity, to assess exercise limitations, to determine the time of onset of claudication pain and total walking time before and following therapeutic intervention, and to diagnose the presence of CVD and assess for other exercise safety factors (63):

- Medication dose and timing should be noted and repeated in an identical manner in subsequent exercise tests assessing potential therapeutic changes.
- Ankle and brachial artery systolic blood pressure (SBP) should be measured bilaterally after 5–10 min of rest in the supine position following standardized ABI procedures (61). The ABI is calculated by dividing the higher ankle SBP reading by the higher brachial artery SBP reading.
- A standardized motorized treadmill protocol should be used to ensure reproducibility of pain free maximal walking time (63). Claudication pain perception may be monitored using a numerical rating scale (see *Figure 5.3*) (126).

■ The exercise test should begin with a slow speed and have gradual increments in grade (12) (see *Chapter 5*).

■ Following the completion of the exercise test, patients should recover in the seated position.

■ The 6MWT may be used to objectively assess ambulatory functional limitations in those not amenable to treadmill testing (63).

FITT Recommendations for Individuals with Peripheral Artery Disease

Supervised exercise training is a Class IA recommendation (see *Box 9.5*) of the AHA for the treatment of lower extremity symptomatic PAD (63). Multiple studies have shown exercise training to be a safe and effective treatment for individuals with PAD. Interval exercise training leads to increases in the time and distance an individual with PAD is able to walk until the initial onset of pain and to point of maximal tolerable pain (54). Increases in pain-free walking time and distance of 106%–177% and in absolute walking ability of 64%–85% have occurred following exercise training programs (30). The following FITT principle of Ex R$_x$ is recommended for individuals with PAD.

■ **FITT RECOMMENDATIONS FOR INDIVIDUALS WITH LOWER EXTREMITY, SYMPTOMATIC PERIPHERAL ARTERIAL DISEASE** (12,63)

	Aerobic	Resistance	Flexibility
Frequency	3–5 d · wk^{-1}	At least 2 d · wk^{-1} performed on nonconsecutive days	≥2–3 d · wk^{-1} with daily being most effective
Intensity	Moderate intensity (*i.e.,* 40%–59% $\dot{V}O_2R$) to the point of moderate pain (*i.e.,* 3 out of 4 on the claudication pain scale)	60%–80% 1-RM	Stretch to the point of feeling tightness or slight discomfort.
Time	30–45 min · d^{-1} (excluding rest periods) for up to 12 wk; may progress to 60 min · d^{-1}	2–3 sets of 8–12 repetitions; 6–8 exercises targeting major muscle groups	10–30 s hold for static stretching; 2–4 repetitions of each exercise
Type	Weight-bearing (*i.e.,* free or treadmill walking) intermittent exercise with seated rest when moderate pain is reached and resumption when pain is *completely* alleviated	Whole body focusing on large muscle groups; emphasis on lower limbs if time limited.	Static, dynamic, and/or PNF stretching

1-RM, one repetition maximum; PNF, proprioceptive neuromuscular facilitation.

Exercise Training Considerations

■ Unsupervised exercise training may be beneficial but is not as well established as an effective treatment as supervised exercise training (63).

■ Some patients may need to begin the program by accumulating only 15 min · d^{-1}, gradually increasing time by 5 min · d^{-1} biweekly.

■ Weight-bearing exercise may be supplemented with non–weight-bearing exercise, such as arm and leg ergometry.

■ Cycling or other non–weight-bearing exercise modalities may be used as a warm-up but should not be the primary type of activity.

Other Considerations

■ The optimal work-to-rest ratio has not been determined for individuals with PAD and may need to be adjusted for each patient.

■ A cold environment may aggravate the symptoms of intermittent claudication; therefore, a longer warm-up may be necessary (34).

■ Encourage patients to address all CVD risk factors.

EXERCISE PRESCRIPTION FOR PATIENTS WITH A CEREBROVASCULAR ACCIDENT (STROKE)

When blood flow to a region of the brain is obstructed (*i.e.*, cerebrovascular accident, CVA, or stroke), brain function deteriorates quickly and leads to neuronal cell death. This can result in motor (functional), sensory, emotional, and cognitive impairments, the extent of which are greatly influenced by the size and location of the affected area and presence or absence of collateral blood flow. The etiology of a stroke is most often ischemic (87%, due to either thrombosis or embolism) or hemorrhagic. Each year, nearly 800,000 U.S. residents suffer a stroke, with women having a higher lifetime risk of stroke than men (58).

Physical and occupational therapy are typically utilized for up to 3–6 mo following a stroke to improve/restore functional mobility, balance, and return to ADL. The AHA/American Stroke Association recommends PA and exercise for stroke survivors across all stages of recovery (20). Loss of physical stamina, mood disturbance, and adoption of sedentary behaviors are common in stroke survivors. Although the Ex R_x is often adapted to the functional abilities of the patients, exercise training improves exercise capacity (10%–20%, as measured by $\dot{V}O_{2peak}$) and quality of life, and helps manage risk for a secondary event (95).

Exercise Testing

Compared to those who have not suffered a stroke, oxygen uptake is higher at a fixed submaximal level and reduced at peak effort among stroke survivors.

During exercise testing, both chronotropic incompetence and early-onset fatigue are common.

- Exercise testing should employ a mode of testing that accommodates a patient's physical impairment.
- Cycle ergometry (work rate increase of 5–10 W · min^{-1} or 20 W per stage) and dual action semirecumbent seated steppers may be preferred if sitting is needed to mitigate any balance deficiencies. In each case, modifications of the device (*e.g.*, pedal type, swivel seated, seated back, flip up arm rest) may be needed to facilitate patient safety and ease of use (95).
- Treadmill testing protocols should increase work rate by 0.5 to 1–2 METs · 2–3 min^{-1} stage and only be considered if patient can stand and demonstrate sufficient balance and ambulate with very minimal or no assist.

Exercise Prescription

Because the majority of patients suffering a stroke are elderly, many have comorbidities such as other CVDs, arthritis, and metabolic disorders. All comorbidities should be considered when prescribing exercise as well as any effects the medications used to treat the comorbidities have on exercise responses or exercise programming. After a patient suffers a stroke, a main objective is to restore a patient's ability to return to ADL. Subsequently, and often in tandem, aerobic, neuromuscular, and muscle-strengthening exercises can be engaged to further improve function, facilitate secondary prevention, and improve fitness.

Exercise Training Considerations

- Avoid the Valsalva maneuver during resistance training to avoid excessive elevations in BP.
- Treadmill should begin at a slow speed (0.8 mph) and provide harness apparatus for patient safety or, if needed, partially unloaded walking.

Other Considerations

- Be attentive to affective issues such as mood, motivation, frustration, and confusion. Correctly managing affective issues can favorably influence how a patient conducts, adheres to, and responds to a prescribed exercise regimen. Strategies aimed at minimizing negative influences due to these issues are helpful and include close supervision, individualized instruction until independence is established, involvement of family members, repetition of instructions, and alternate teaching methods.
- Early-onset local muscle and general fatigue are common and should be considered when setting work rates and rate of progression.

■ **FITT RECOMMENDATIONS FOR INDIVIDUALS SUFFERING A CEREBRAL VASCULAR ACCIDENT** (20)

	Aerobic	Resistance	Flexibility
Frequency	3–5 d · wk^{-1}	2 nonconsecutive d · wk^{-1}	≥2–3 d · wk^{-1} with daily being most effective
Intensity	If HR data are available from a recent GXT, use 40%–70% of HRR. In the absence of a GXT or if atrial fibrillation is present, use RPE of 11–14 on a 6–20 scale.	50%–70% of 1-RM	Stretch to the point of feeling tightness or slight discomfort.
Time	Progressively increase from 20 to 60 min · d^{-1}. Consider multiple 10-min sessions.	1–3 sets of 8–15 repetitions	10–30 s hold for static stretching; 2–4 repetitions of each exercise
Type	Cycle ergometry and semirecumbent seated steppers; may need modification based on functional and cognitive deficiencies. Treadmill walking can be considered if patient has sufficient balance and ambulation with very minimal or no assist.	Use equipment and exercises that improve safety in those with deficits (*e.g.,* strength, endurance, movement, balance): machine versus free-weight, bar versus hand-weights; seated versus standing as indicated.	Static, dynamic, and/or PNF stretching

1-RM, one repetition maximum; GXT, graded exercise test; HR, heart rate; PNF, proprioceptive neuromuscular facilitation; RPE, rating of perceived exertion.

EXERCISE TRAINING FOR RETURN TO WORK

For patients desiring to return to their previous vocation, the exercise plan should consider the musculature used and workload required to perform the required occupations tasks. A list of MET levels associated with a wide range of occupational tasks has been published and can be used to estimate the required workload (4). Specificity of training can be employed for both aerobic and resistance training in an attempt to provide an individual with the strength and endurance needed to return to his or her previous occupation. Exercise training leads to an improved

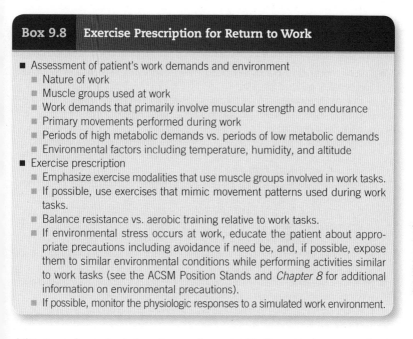

| Box 9.8 | Exercise Prescription for Return to Work |

- Assessment of patient's work demands and environment
  - Nature of work
  - Muscle groups used at work
  - Work demands that primarily involve muscular strength and endurance
  - Primary movements performed during work
  - Periods of high metabolic demands vs. periods of low metabolic demands
  - Environmental factors including temperature, humidity, and altitude
- Exercise prescription
  - Emphasize exercise modalities that use muscle groups involved in work tasks.
  - If possible, use exercises that mimic movement patterns used during work tasks.
  - Balance resistance vs. aerobic training relative to work tasks.
  - If environmental stress occurs at work, educate the patient about appropriate precautions including avoidance if need be, and, if possible, expose them to similar environmental conditions while performing activities similar to work tasks (see the ACSM Position Stands and *Chapter 8* for additional information on environmental precautions).
  - If possible, monitor the physiologic responses to a simulated work environment.

ability to perform physical work, an enhanced self-efficacy, and a greater desire and comfort level for returning to work following the illness (79,112). *Box 9.8* presents specific information regarding alterations to the standard Ex R$_x$ in preparation for return to work.

PULMONARY DISEASES

Chronic pulmonary diseases are significant causes of morbidity and mortality. There is strong evidence that pulmonary rehabilitation (PR) improves exercise tolerance, reduces symptoms, and improves quality of life. For patients with chronic obstructive pulmonary disease (COPD), evidence-based recommendations (86,117) and clinical practice guidelines (77,106) indicate that exercise training should be a mandatory component of PR. Scientific rationale supports exercise training in people with non-COPD respiratory diseases (*i.e.*, asthma, cystic fibrosis) and confirms similar benefits as those seen in COPD (107). A list of respiratory diseases in which exercise is of potential benefit is shown in *Box 9.9*.

Asthma

Asthma is a heterogeneous chronic inflammatory disorder of the airways that is characterized by a history of episodes of bronchial hyperresponsiveness; variable airflow limitation; and recurring wheeze, dyspnea, chest tightness, and coughing that occur particularly at night or early morning. These symptoms

Box 9.9	Patients with Pulmonary Disease Benefitting from Pulmonary Rehabilitation and Exercise

- Chronic obstructive pulmonary disease — a mostly irreversible airflow limitation consisting of the following:
  - Chronic bronchitis — a chronic productive cough for 3 mo in each of 2 successive years in a patient in whom other causes of productive chronic cough have been excluded
  - Emphysema — the presence of permanent enlargement of the airspaces distal to the terminal bronchioles, accompanied by destruction of their walls and without obvious fibrosis
  - Asthma — airway obstruction because of inflammation and bronchospasm that is mostly reversible
  - Cystic fibrosis — a genetic disease causing excessive, thick mucus that obstructs the airways (and other ducts) and promotes recurrent and ultimately chronic respiratory infection.
  - Bronchiectasis — abnormal chronic enlargement of the airways with impaired mucus clearance
- Restrictive lung diseases — extrapulmonary respiratory diseases that interfere with normal lung expansion. Examples include the following:
  - Interstitial lung disease/pulmonary fibrosis — scarring and thickening of the parenchyma of the lungs
  - Pneumoconiosis — long-term exposure to dusts, especially asbestos
  - Restrictive chest wall disease, (e.g., scoliosis or kyphosis)
  - Obesity-related
- Pulmonary artery hypertension — increased blood pressure in the pulmonary artery due to narrowing, blockage, or destruction
- Lung cancer — one of the deadliest cancers with cigarette smoking being a common etiology

are variable and often reversible (56). Asthma symptoms can be provoked or worsened by exercise, which may contribute to reduced participation in sports and PA and ultimately to deconditioning and lower cardiorespiratory fitness (CRF). With deconditioning, the downward cycle continues with asthma symptoms being triggered by less intense PA and subsequent worsening of exercise tolerance.

The conclusive evidence for exercise training as an effective therapy for asthma is lacking, and at present, there are no specific evidence-based guidelines for exercise training in these individuals. However, strong evidence is available for recommending regular PA because of its general health benefits (56) and reduced incidence of exacerbations (53). Some (32,47,101) but not all (94) systematic reviews and meta-analyses have suggested that exercise training can be beneficial for individuals with asthma. The data examined from these reviews are limited by small numbers of randomized controlled trials and heterogeneity of trial methods and subjects. Significant improvements in days without asthma symptoms, aerobic capacity, maximal work rate, exercise endurance, and pulmonary minute ventilation ($\dot{V}E$) have been noted. Overall, exercise training is well tolerated and should be encouraged in people with stable asthma (32,39,84).

Exercise-induced bronchoconstriction (EIB), defined as airway narrowing that occurs as a result of exercise, is experienced in a substantial proportion of people with asthma (96), but people without a diagnosis of asthma may also experience EIB. For athletes, environmental triggers such as cold or dry air and air pollution including particulate matter, allergens, and trichloramines in swimming pool areas may stimulate a bout of EIB. EIB can be successfully managed with pharmacotherapy (96). Strong recommendations have also been made for 10–15 min of vigorous intensity or variable intensity (combination of light and vigorous intensity) warm-up exercise to induce a "refractory period" in which EIB occurrence is attenuated (96,119).

Exercise Testing

- Assessment of physiologic function should include evaluations of cardiopulmonary capacity, pulmonary function (before and after exercise), and oxyhemoglobin saturation via noninvasive methods.

- Administration of an inhaled bronchodilator (*i.e.*, β_2-agonists) (see *Appendix A*) prior to testing may be indicated to prevent EIB, thus providing optimal assessment of cardiopulmonary capacity.

- Exercise testing is typically performed on a motor-driven treadmill or an electronically braked cycle ergometer. Targets for high ventilation and HRs are better achieved using the treadmill. For athletes, a sports-specific mode may be more relevant.

- The degree of EIB should be assessed using vigorous intensity exercise achieved within 2–4 min and lasting 4–6 min with the subject breathing relatively dry air. The testing should be accompanied by a spirometric evaluation of the change in forced expiratory volume in one second ($FEV_{1.0}$) from baseline and the value measured at 5, 10, 15, and 30 min following the exercise test (96). The criterion for a diagnosis of EIB varies, but many laboratories use a decrease in $FEV_{1.0}$ from baseline of $\geq 15\%$ because of its greater specificity (96).

- Appropriately trained staff should supervise exercise tests for EIB, and physician supervision is warranted when testing higher risk individuals because severe bronchoconstriction is a potential hazard following testing. Immediate administration of nebulized bronchodilators with oxygen is usually successful for relief of bronchoconstriction (40).

- Although exercise testing is considered highly specific for detecting EIB when it is unavailable or unfeasible, surrogate tests to evaluate airway's hyperresponsiveness include eucapnic voluntary hyperventilation of dry air, inhalation of hyperosmolar aerosols of 4.5% saline, dry powder mannitol, or methacholine (48). These tests should be administered by appropriately trained individuals with medical supervision.

- Procedural details for EIB diagnostic testing have been described (40,96). Although none of these surrogate tests are 100% sensitive or specific for EIB, they are useful in identifying airway hyperresponsiveness.
- Evidence of oxyhemoglobin desaturation ≤80% should be used as test termination criteria in addition to standard criteria (9).
- The 6MWT may be used in individuals with moderate-to-severe persistent asthma when other testing equipment is not available (13).

Exercise Prescription

Specific evidence-based exercise training guidelines for people with asthma are not available at this time. However, exercise training is generally well tolerated in individuals successfully managed with pharmacotherapy and when triggers to bronchoconstriction (*e.g.*, cold; dry, dusty air; inhaled pollutants) are removed to bring about symptom relief (32). As such, the general FITT recommendations for comprehensive exercise in healthy adults, adjusted to patient capabilities, are suitable (see *Chapter 6*). Position statements on exercise in asthma (84) and systematic reviews (32) support this recommendation.

■ FITT RECOMMENDATIONS FOR INDIVIDUALS WITH ASTHMA

	Aerobic	Resistance	Flexibility
Frequency	3–5 d · wk^{-1}	2–3 d · wk^{-1}	≥2–3 d · wk^{-1} with daily being most effective
Intensity	Begin with moderate intensity (40%–59% HRR or $\dot{V}O_2R$). If well tolerated, progress to 60%–70% HRR or $\dot{V}O_2R$ after 1 mo.	Strength: 60%–70% of 1-RM for beginners; ≥80% for experienced weight trainers. Endurance: <50% of 1-RM	Stretch to the point of feeling tightness or slight discomfort.
Time	Progressively increase to at least 30–40 min · d^{-1}.	Strength: 2–4 sets, 8–12 repetitions. Endurance: ≤2 sets, 15–20 repetitions	10–30 s hold for static stretching; 2–4 repetitions of each exercise
Type	Aerobic activities using large muscle groups such as walking, running, cycling, swimming, or pool exercises	Weight machines, free weight, or body weight exercises	Static, dynamic, and/or PNF stretching

1-RM, one repetition maximum; HRR, heart rate reserve; PNF, proprioceptive neuromuscular facilitation; $\dot{V}O_2R$, oxygen uptake reserve.

Special Considerations

- Caution is suggested in using HR target intensities based on prediction of maximal heart rate (HR_{max}) because of the wide variability in its association with ventilation and the potential HR effects of asthma control medications.
- Individuals experiencing exacerbations of their asthma should not exercise until symptoms and airway function have improved.
- Use of short-acting bronchodilators may be necessary before or after exercise to prevent or treat EIB (see *Appendix A*).
- Individuals on prolonged treatment with oral corticosteroids may experience peripheral muscle wasting and may benefit from resistance training.
- Exercise in cold environments or those with airborne allergens or pollutants should be limited to avoid triggering bronchoconstriction in susceptible individuals. EIB can also be triggered by prolonged exercise durations or high intensity exercise sessions.
- There is insufficient evidence supporting a clinical benefit from inspiratory muscle training (IMT) in individuals with asthma (101).
- Use of a nonchlorinated pool is preferable because this will be less likely to trigger an asthma event.
- Be aware of the possibility of asthma exacerbation shortly after exercise particularly in a high-allergen environment.

Chronic Obstructive Pulmonary Disease

COPD is the fourth leading cause of death and a major cause of chronic morbidity throughout the world (57). COPD is preventable and treatable and characterized by predisposing risk factors resulting in chronic airway inflammation chiefly due to exposure to noxious gases and particles, especially tobacco smoke and various environmental and occupational exposures. Dyspnea, chronic cough, and sputum production are common symptoms. Significant systemic effects such as weight loss, nutritional abnormalities, sarcopenia, and skeletal muscle dysfunction often accompany COPD (57). COPD encompasses chronic bronchitis and/or emphysema, and patients may be categorized according to disease severity based on pulmonary function tests and Global Initiative for Chronic Obstructive Lung Disease (GOLD) criteria (*Table 9.3*) (57).

Dyspnea or shortness of breath with exertion is a cardinal symptom of COPD resulting in PA limitations and deconditioning. Disuse muscle atrophy is common in patients with COPD because of the adverse downward spiral of increasing ventilatory limitations, shortness of breath, and further decreases in PA. This contributes to the loss of muscle strength, power, and endurance and decrements in the performance of everyday functional activities. Exercise is an effective and potent intervention that can improve symptoms, lessen the development of functional impairment and disability, and increase quality of life in all patients with COPD regardless of disease severity (86,106). The beneficial effects of exercise occur mainly through adaptations in the musculoskeletal and cardiovascular systems that in turn reduce stress on the pulmonary system during exercise (114).

TABLE 9.3		
Global Initiative for Chronic Obstructive Lung Disease Classification of Disease Severity in Patients with Chronic Obstructive Pulmonary Disease Based on the $FEV_{1.0}$ Obtained from Pulmonary Function Tests (57)		
Disease Severity	**Postbronchodilator $FEV_{1.0}$/FVC**	**Postbronchodilator $FEV_{1.0}$%**
Mild	<0.70	$FEV_{1.0} \geq 80\%$ of predicted
Moderate	<0.70	$50\% \leq FEV_{1.0} < 80\%$ of predicted
Severe	<0.70	$30\% \leq FEV_{1.0} < 50\%$ of predicted
Very Severe	<0.70	$FEV_{1.0} < 30\%$ of predicted or $FEV_{1.0} < 50\%$ of predicted with respiratory failure

$FEV_{1.0}$, forced expiratory volume in 1 s; FVC, forced vital capacity.

Exercise Testing

- Evidence-based guidelines confirm the utility of cardiopulmonary exercise testing in adults with COPD as well as other chronic lung diseases (*i.e.*, interstitial lung disease, primary pulmonary hypertension, and cystic fibrosis) in providing objective measure of exercise capacity, mechanisms of exercise intolerance, prognosis, and disease progression and treatment response (48).

- Incremental exercise tests (GXT) may be used to assess cardiopulmonary function and CRF. Modifications of traditional protocols (*e.g.*, smaller work rate increments) may be warranted depending on functional limitations and the onset of dyspnea. A test duration of 8–12 min is optimal in those with mild-to-moderate COPD (28), whereas a test duration of 5–9 min is recommended for patients with severe and very severe disease (19).

- Patients with moderate-to-severe COPD may exhibit oxyhemoglobin desaturation with exercise. Therefore, a measure of blood oxygenation, either the partial pressure of arterial oxygen (P_aO_2) or percent saturation of arterial oxygen (SaO_2), should be made during the initial GXT.

- Submaximal exercise testing may be used depending on the reason for the test and the clinical status of the patient. However, individuals with pulmonary disease may have ventilatory limitations to exercise; thus, prediction of $\dot{V}O_{2peak}$ based on age-predicted HR_{max} may not be appropriate as criteria for terminating the submaximal GXT.

- The 6MWT and shuttle walking test can assess functional exercise capacity in individuals with more severe pulmonary disease and in settings that lack exercise testing equipment (13,22,46,113,132).

- A constant work rate (CWR) test using 80%–90% of peak work rate achieved from the GXT is appealing as it assesses the type of work-related activity levels likely to be encountered in everyday life (33) particularly when performed on a treadmill.

0	No breathlessness at all
0.5	Very, very slight (just noticeable)
1	Very slight
2	Slight breathlessness
3	Moderate
4	Somewhat severe
5	Severe breathlessness
6	
7	Very severe breathlessness
8	
9	Very, very severe (almost maximal)
10	Maximal

Figure 9.1 Borg CR10 Scale modified for dyspnea. Used with Permission from (67).

- The measurement of flow volume loops during the GXT using commercially available instruments may help identify individuals with dynamic hyperinflation and increased dyspnea because of expiratory airflow limitations. Use of bronchodilator therapy may be beneficial for such individuals (117).
- Exertional dyspnea is a common symptom in people with many pulmonary diseases. The modified Borg Category-Ratio 0–10 (CR10) Scale (*Figure 9.1*) has been used extensively to measure dyspnea before, during, and after exercise (105). Patients should be given specific, standardized instructions on how to relate the wording on the scale to their level of breathlessness (13). Because dyspnea scales are subjective, some caution is advised in their interpretation as exercise intolerance may be accompanied by exaggerated dyspnea scores without corresponding physiological confirmation (37).
- In addition to standard termination criteria, exercise testing may be terminated because of severe arterial oxyhemoglobin desaturation (*i.e.*, $SaO_2 \leq 80\%$) (9).
- The exercise testing mode is typically walking or stationary cycling. Walking protocols may be more suitable for individuals with severe disease who lack the muscle strength to overcome the increasing resistance of cycle leg ergometers. Arm ergometry may result in increased dyspnea that may limit the intensity and duration of the activity.

Exercise Prescription

Presently, there are no evidence-based guidelines that describe the specific application of the FITT principle for patients with COPD, although expert reviews, official statements, and clinical practice guidelines for the components of the FITT principle have been published (77,86,106,117) and tend to be in general agreement.

Aerobic exercise training is recommended for individuals in all stages of COPD who are able to exercise (77). Pulmonary diseases and their treatments affect both the lungs and skeletal muscles (*i.e.*, limb muscle dysfunction due to atrophy and weakness) (81). Resistance training is the most potent intervention to address the muscle dysfunction seen in COPD and should be an integral part of the Ex R_x. (77,82,93,106,117). The effects of resistance training on disease outcome are not well understood. Limited evidence from a systematic review and meta-analysis on resistance training outcomes in patients with COPD demonstrated improvements in forced vital capacity (FVC) and peak minute ventilation ($\dot{V}E_{peak}$) but not $FEV_{1.0}$ COPD (120). Of growing concern is the common observation of falls in people with COPD (18,108). Because muscle weakness and gait and balance abnormalities are among the risk factors for falling (125), lower extremity strengthening and balance training are effective countermeasures.

Benefits derived from PR programs have been shown to persist for up to 12–18 mo (106). Although data suggest that exercising after PR appears to be more effective than usual care, longer term (*i.e.*, >18 mo) sustainability of benefits is not clear and requires further research; the optimal post-PR program has not been elucidated (17).

Exercise Training Considerations

- Higher intensities yield greater physiologic benefits (*e.g.*, reduced minute ventilation and HR at a given workload) and should be encouraged when appropriate (77,86).
- For patients with mild COPD, intensity guidelines for healthy older adults are appropriate (see *Chapter 7*). For those with moderate-to-severe COPD, intensities representing >60% peak work rate have been recommended (117).
- Light intensity aerobic exercise is appropriate for those with severe COPD or very deconditioned individuals. Intensity may be increased as tolerated within the target time window.
- Supervision at the outset of training allows guidance in correct execution of the exercise program, enhanced safety, and optimizing benefit (99).
- Ventilatory limitation at peak exercise in patients with severe COPD coincides with significant metabolic reserves during whole body exercise (103). This may allow these patients to tolerate relatively high work rates that approach peak levels (106) and achieve significant training effects.
- As an alternative to using peak work rate or $\dot{V}O_{2peak}$ to determine exercise intensity, dyspnea ratings of between 3 and 6 on the Borg CR10 Scale may be used (see *Figure 9.1*) (65,117). A dyspnea rating between 3 and 6 on the Borg CR10 Scale has been shown to correspond with 53% and 80% of $\dot{V}O_{2peak}$, respectively (65). Most patients with COPD can accurately and reliably produce a dyspnea rating obtained from an incremental exercise test as a target to regulate/monitor exercise intensity.
- Intensity targets based on percentage of estimated HR_{max} or HRR may be inappropriate (27). Particularly in patients with severe COPD, HR_{rest} is often elevated and ventilatory limitations as well as the effects of some medication prohibit attainment of the predicted HR_{max} and thus its use in intensity calculations.

FITT RECOMMENDATIONS FOR INDIVIDUALS WITH CHRONIC OBSTRUCTIVE PULMONARY DISEASE (76,77,86,106,117)

FITT	Aerobic	Resistance	Flexibility
Frequency	At least 3–5 d · wk^{-1}	2–3 d · wk^{-1}	≥2–3 d · wk^{-1} with daily being most effective
Intensity	Moderate-to-vigorous intensity (50%–80% peak work rate or 4–6 on the Borg CR10 Scale)	Strength: 60%–70% of 1-RM for beginners; ≥80% for experienced weight trainers Endurance: <50% of 1-RM	Stretch to the point of feeling tightness or slight discomfort.
Time	20–60 min · d^{-1} at moderate-to-high intensities as tolerated. If the 20- to 60-min durations are not achievable, accumulate ≥20 min of exercise interspersed with intermittent exercise rest periods of lower intensity work or rest.	Strength: 2–4 sets, 8–12 repetitions Endurance: ≤2 sets, 15–20 repetitions	10–30 s hold for static stretching; 2–4 repetitions of each exercise
Type	Common aerobic modes including walking (free or treadmill), stationary cycling, and upper body ergometry	Weight machines, free weight, or body weight exercises	Static, dynamic, and/or PNF stretching

1-RM, one repetition maximum; PNF, proprioceptive neuromuscular facilitation.

- The use of oximetry is recommended for the initial exercise training sessions to evaluate possible exercise-induced oxyhemoglobin desaturation and to identify the workload at which desaturation occurred.
- Flexibility exercises may help overcome the effects of postural impairments that limit thoracic mobility and therefore lung function (117).
- Regardless of the prescribed exercise intensity, the exercise professional should closely monitor initial exercise sessions and adjust intensity and duration according to individual responses and tolerance. In many cases, the presence of symptoms, particularly dyspnea/breathlessness supersedes objective methods of Ex R$_x$.

Special Considerations

- Peripheral muscle dysfunction contributes to exercise intolerance (81) and is significantly and independently related to increased use of health care resources (44), poorer prognosis (111), and mortality (121).
- Maximizing pulmonary function using bronchodilators before exercise training in those with airflow limitation can reduce dyspnea and improve exercise tolerance (117).
- Because individuals with COPD may experience greater dyspnea while performing ADL involving the upper extremities, include resistance exercises for the muscles of the upper body.
- Inspiratory muscle weakness is a contributor to exercise intolerance and dyspnea in those with COPD. In patients receiving optimal medical therapy who still present with inspiratory muscle weakness and breathlessness, IMT may prove useful in those unable to participate in exercise training (59,77,106). IMT improves inspiratory muscle strength and endurance, functional capacity, dyspnea, and quality of life which may lead to improvements in exercise tolerance (59).
- There are no clear guidelines for IMT although an intensity of the training load of ≥30% of maximal inspiratory pressure has been recommended (77).
- Supplemental oxygen is indicated for patients with a P_aO_2 ≤55 mm Hg or an SaO_2 ≤88% while breathing room air (100). This recommendation applies when considering supplemental oxygen during exercise. In patients using ambulatory supplemental oxygen, flow rates will likely need to be increased during exercise to maintain SaO_2 >88%. Although inconclusive, there is evidence to suggest the administration of supplemental oxygen to those who do not experience exercise-induced hypoxemia may lead to greater gains in exercise endurance particularly during high intensity exercise (87,106,117).
- Individuals suffering from acute exacerbations of their pulmonary disease should limit exercise until symptoms have subsided.

Exercise Training for Pulmonary Diseases Other than Chronic Obstructive Pulmonary Disease

Despite substantially less investigation into the benefits of exercise training in non-COPD chronic lung diseases, strong scientific evidence supports the inclusion of exercise training for many lung diseases other than COPD with demonstrated clinical and physiologic benefits (31,85,107). However, these programs should be modified to include disease-specific strategies. In general, the exercise programming used in patients with COPD is applicable to those with cystic fibrosis and before and after lung transplantation (107) when modifications are adapted to the individual's exercise tolerance. Exercise training recommendations have been specifically presented for patients with stable pulmonary arterial hypertension (PAH) and interstitial lung disease who are receiving optimal medical management (11,107). For these patients, the FITT guidelines are similar to those for COPD, although moderate intensity aerobic exercise should comprise the core component of the exercise program. Vigorous intensity training is inappropriate in patients with PAH due to risk of syncope consequent to rapid changes in pulmonary hemodynamics. Resistance exercise training may be added after the aerobic training is established and well tolerated. Intensities should be below those that would provoke severe dyspnea, oxygen desaturation, or hypertension (11,107). Arm ergometry, heavy resistance training, and pelvic floor exercise should be avoided to reduce the risk of a Valsalva maneuver (5). In patients with PAH, pulmonary pressures can increase suddenly and dramatically during exercise, predisposing them to right ventricular decompensation and cardiovascular collapse (16). Methods for adapting exercise training in patients with non-COPD chronic lung disease have been published (64).

ONLINE RESOURCES

American Association for Cardiovascular and Pulmonary Rehabilitation:
  http://www.aacvpr.org
American Heart Association:
  http://www.heart.org
American Lung Association:
  http://www.lungusa.org/lung-disease/copd/
Cystic Fibrosis Foundation:
  http://www.cff.org/UploadedFiles/LivingWithCF/StayingHealthy
  /LungHealth/Exercise/Day-to-Day-Exercise-and-CF.pdf
EPR3: Guidelines for the Diagnosis and Management of Asthma (Expert Panel Report 3):
  http://www.nhlbi.nih.gov/guidelines/asthma/asthgdln.htm
Global Initiative for Asthma:
  http://www.ginasthma.org
Global Initiative for Chronic Obstructive Lung Disease:
  http://www.goldcopd.org/uploads/users/files/GOLD_Report2014_Feb07.pdf
Society for Vascular Medicine:
  http://www.svmb.org

REFERENCES

1. Aboyans V, Criqui MH, Abraham P, et al. Measurement and interpretation of the ankle-brachial index: a scientific statement from the American Heart Association. *Circulation*. 2012;126:2890–909.
2. Abraham WT, Fisher WG, Smith AL. Cardiac resynchronization in chronic heart failure. *N Engl J Med*. 2002;346:1845–53.
3. Ades PA, Keteyian SJ, Balady GJ, et al. Cardiac rehabilitation exercise and self-care for chronic heart failure. *JACC Heart Fail*. 2013;1:540–7.
4. Ainsworth BE, Haskell WL, Whitt MC, et al. Compendium of physical activities: an update of activity codes and MET intensities. *Med Sci Sports Exerc*. 2000;32(9 Suppl):S498–504.
5. American Association of Cardiovascular and Pulmonary Rehabilitation. The continuum of care: from inpatient and outpatient cardiac rehabilitation to long-term secondary prevention. In: *Guidelines for Cardiac Rehabilitation and Secondary Prevention Programs*. 5th ed. Champaign (IL): Human Kinetics; 2013. p. 5–18.
6. American College of Sports Medicine. American College of Sports Medicine position stand. Progression models in resistance training for healthy adults. *Med Sci Sports Exerc*. 2009;41:687–708.

7. American College of Sports Medicine, Chodzko-Zajko WJ, Proctor DN, et al. American College of Sports Medicine position stand. Exercise and physical activity for older adults. *Med Sci Sports Exerc.* 2009;41(7):1510–30.

8. American College of Sports Medicine, Sawka MN, Burke LM, et al. American College of Sports Medicine position stand. Exercise and fluid replacement. *Med Sci Sports Exerc.* 2007;39(2):377–90.

9. American Thoracic Society, American College of Chest Physicians. ATS/ACCP Statement on cardiopulmonary exercise testing. *Am J Respir Crit Care Med.* 2003;167(2):211–77.

10. Antman EM, Anbe DT, Armstrong PW, et al. ACC/AHA guidelines for the management of patients with ST-elevation myocardial infarction: a report of the American College of Cardiology/American Heart Association Task Force on Practice Guidelines (Committee to Revise the 1999 Guidelines for the Management of Patients with Acute Myocardial Infarction). *Circulation.* 2004;110(9):e82–292.

11. Arena R. Exercise testing and training in chronic lung disease and pulmonary arterial hypertension. *Prog Cardiovasc Dis.* 2011;53(6):454–63.

12. Askew CD, Parmenter B, Leicht AS, Walker PJ, Golledge J. Exercise & Sports Science Australia (ESSA) position statement on exercise prescription for patients with peripheral arterial disease and intermittent claudication. *J Sci Med Sport.* 2014;17(6):623–9.

13. ATS Committee on Proficiency Standards for Clinical Pulmonary Function Laboratories. ATS statement: guidelines for the six-minute walk test. *Am J Respir Crit Care Med.* 2002;166(1):111–7.

14. Balachandran S, Lee A, Royse A, Denehy L, El-Ansary D. Upper limb exercise prescription following cardiac surgery via median sternotomy: a web survey. *J Cardiopulm Rehabil Prev.* 2014;34:390–5.

15. Balady GJ, Williams MA, Ades PA, et al. Core components of cardiac rehabilitation/secondary prevention programs: 2007 update: a scientific statement from the American Heart Association Exercise, Cardiac Rehabilitation, and Prevention Committee, the Council on Clinical Cardiology; the Councils on Cardiovascular Nursing, Epidemiology and Prevention, and Nutrition, Physical Activity, and Metabolism; and the American Association of Cardiovascular and Pulmonary Rehabilitation. *Circulation.* 2007;115:2675–82.

16. Barst RJ, McGoon M, Torbicki A, et al. Diagnosis and differential assessment of pulmonary arterial hypertension. *J Am Coll Cardiol.* 2004;43(12 Suppl S):40S–7S.

17. Beauchamp MK, Evans R, Janaudis-Ferreira T, Goldstein RS, Brooks D. Systematic review of supervised exercise programs after pulmonary rehabilitation in individuals with COPD. *Chest.* 2013;144:1124–33.

18. Beauchamp MK, Hill K, Goldstein RS, Janaudis-Ferreira T, Brooks D. Impairments in balance discriminate fallers from non-fallers in COPD. *Respir Med.* 2009;103:1885–91.

19. Benzo RP, Paramesh S, Patel SA, Slivka WA, Sciurba FC. Optimal protocol selection for cardiopulmonary exercise testing in severe COPD. *Chest.* 2007;132(5):1500–5.

20. Billinger SA, Arena R, Bernhardt J, et al. Physical activity and exercise recommendations for stroke survivors: a statement for healthcare professionals from the American Heart Association/American Stroke Association. *Stroke.* 2014;45:2532–53.

21. Bjarnason-Wehrens B, McGee H, Zwisler AD, et al. Cardiac rehabilitation in Europe: results from the European Cardiac Rehabilitation Inventory Survey. *Eur J Cardiovasc Prev Rehabil.* 2010;17:410–8.

22. Borel B, Pepin V, Mahler DA, Nadreau É, Maltais F. Prospective validation of the endurance shuttle walking test in the context of bronchodilation in COPD. *Eur Respir J.* 2014;44(5):1166–76.

23. Borg GA. Psychophysical bases of perceived exertion. *Med Sci Sports Exerc.* 1982;14(5):377–81.

24. Braith RW, Beck DT. Resistance exercise: training adaptations and developing a safe exercise prescription. *Heart Fail Rev.* 2008;13:69–79.

25. Braith RW, Edwards DG. Exercise following heart transplantation. *Sports Med.* 2000;30:171–92.

26. Bravata DM, Smith-Spangler C, Sundaram V, et al. Using pedometers to increase physical activity and improve health: a systematic review. *JAMA.* 2007;298(19):2296–304.

27. Brolin SE, Cecins NM, Jenkins SC. Questioning the use of heart rate and dyspnea in the prescription of exercise in subjects with chronic obstructive pulmonary disease. *J Cardiopulm Rehabil.* 2003;23(3):228–34.

28. Buchfuhrer MJ, Hansen JE, Robinson TE, Sue DY, Wasserman K, Whipp BJ. Optimizing the exercise protocol for cardiopulmonary assessment. *J Appl Physiol Respir Environ Exerc Physiol.* 1983;55(5):1558–64.

29. Budoff MJ, Achenbach S, Blumenthal RS, et al. Assessment of coronary artery disease by cardiac computed tomography: a scientific statement from the American Heart Association Committee on Cardiovascular Imaging and Intervention, Council on Cardiovascular Radiology and Intervention, and Committee on Cardiac Imaging, Council on Clinical Cardiology. *Circulation.* 2006;114(16):1761–91.

30. Bulmer AC, Coombes JS. Optimising exercise training in peripheral arterial disease. *Sports Med.* 2004;34(14):983–1003.

31. Burtin C, Hebestreit H. Rehabilitation in patients with chronic respiratory disease other than chronic obstructive pulmonary disease: exercise and physical activity interventions in cystic fibrosis and non-cystic fibrosis bronchiectasis. *Respiration.* 2015;89(3):181–9.

32. Carson KV, Chandratilleke MG, Picot J, Brinn MP, Esterman AJ, Smith BJ. Physical training for asthma. *Cochrane Database Syst Rev.* 2013;(9):CD001116.

33. Casaburi R. Factors determining constant work rate exercise tolerance in COPD and their role in dictating the minimal clinically important difference in response to interventions. *COPD.* 2005;2(1):131–6.

34. Castellani JW, Young AJ, Ducharme MB, et al. American College of Sports Medicine position stand: prevention of cold injuries during exercise. *Med Sci Sports Exerc.* 2006;38(11):2012–29.

35. Chobanian AV, Lille RD, Tercyak A, Blevins P. The metabolic and hemodynamic effects of prolonged bed rest in normal subjects. *Circulation.* 1974;49:551–9.

36. Convertino VA. Value of orthostatic stress in maintaining functional status soon after myocardial infarction or cardiac artery bypass grafting. *J Cardiovasc Nurs.* 2003;18:124–30.

37. Cooper CB, Storer TW. *Exercise Testing and Interpretation: A Practical Approach.* Cambridge (United Kingdom): Cambridge University Press; 2001. 17 p.

38. Costanzo MR, Dipchand A, Starling R, et al. The International Society of Heart and Lung Transplantation guidelines for the care of heart transplant recipients. *J Heart Lung Transplant.* 2010;29:914–56.

39. Craig TJ, Dispenza MC. Benefits of exercise in asthma. *Ann Allergy Asthma Immunol.* 2013;110(3):133–40.

40. Crapo RO, Casaburi R, Coates AL, et al. Guidelines for methacholine and exercise challenge testing-1999. This official statement of the American Thoracic Society was adopted by the ATS Board of Directors, July 1999. *Am J Respir Crit Care Med.* 2000;161(1):309–29.

41. Curtis LH, Whellan DJ, Hammill BG, et al. Incidence and prevalence of heart failure in elderly persons, 1994-2003. *Arch Intern Med.* 2008;168(4):418–24.

42. Daly J, Sindone AP, Thompson DR, Hancock K, Chang E, Davidson P. Barriers to participation in and adherence to cardiac rehabilitation programs: a critical literature review. *Prog Cardiovasc Nurs.* 2002;17:8–17.

43. Davies EJ, Moxham T, Rees K, et al. Exercise based rehabilitation for heart failure. *Cochrane Database Syst Rev.* 2010;(4):CD003331.

44. Decramer M, Gosselink R, Troosters T, Verschueren M, Evers G. Muscle weakness is related to utilization of health care resources in COPD patients. *Eur Respir J.* 1997;10:417–23.

45. Duscha BD, Schulze PC, Robbins JL, Forman DE. Implications of chronic heart failure on peripheral vasculature and skeletal muscle before and after exercise training. *Heart Failure Rev.* 2008;13:21–37.

46. Eaton T, Young P, Nicol K, Kolbe J. The endurance shuttle walking test: a responsive measure in pulmonary rehabilitation for COPD patients. *Chron Respir Dis.* 2006;3(1):3–9.

47. Eichenberger PA, Diener SN, Kofmehl R, Spengler CM. Effects of exercise training on airway hyperreactivity in asthma: a systematic review and meta-analysis. *Sports Med.* 2013;43(11):1157–70.

48. ERS Task Force, Palange P, Ward SA, et al. Recommendations on the use of exercise testing in clinical practice. *Eur Respir J.* 2007;29(1):185–209.

49. Evangelista LS, Hamilton MA, Fonarow GC, Dracup K. Is exercise adherence associated with clinical outcomes in patients with advanced heart failure? *Phys Sportsmed.* 2010;38:28–36.

50. Fletcher GF, Ades PA, Kligfield P, et al. Exercise standards for testing and training: a scientific statement from the American Heart Association. *Circulation.* 2013;128(8):873–934.

51. Fontaine R, Kim M, Kleny R. Die chirurgische Behandlung der peripheren Durchblutungssorungen (Surgical treatment of peripheral circulation disorders). *Helv Chir Acta.* 1954;21(5–6):499–533.

52. Garber CE, Blissmer B, Deschenes MR, et al. American College of Sports Medicine position stand. Quantity and quality of exercise for developing and maintaining cardiorespiratory, musculoskeletal, and neuromotor fitness in apparently healthy adults: guidance for prescribing exercise. *Med Sci Sports Exerc.* 2011;43:1334–59.

53. Garcia-Aymerich J, Varraso R, Antó JM, Camargo CA Jr. Prospective study of physical activity and risk of asthma exacerbations in older women. *Am J Respir Crit Care Med.* 2009;179(11):999–1003.

54. Gardner AW, Montgomery PS, Flinn WR, Katzel LI. The effect of exercise intensity on the response to exercise rehabilitation in patients with intermittent claudication. *J Vasc Surg.* 2005;42(4):702–9.

55. Gibbons RJ, Balady GJ, Bricker JT, et al. ACC/AHA 2002 guideline update for exercise testing: summary article. A report of the American College of Cardiology/American Heart Association Task Force on Practice Guidelines (Committee to Update the 1997 Exercise Testing Guidelines). *J Am Coll Cardiol.* 2002;40(8):1531–40.

56. Global Initiative for Asthma. *Global Strategy for Asthma Management and Prevention* [Internet]. Global Initiative for Asthma; [cited 2016 Sep 8]. Available from: http://www.ginasthma.org

57. Global Initiative for Chronic Obstructive Lung Disease. *Global Initiative for Chronic Obstructive Lung Disease Pocket Guide to COPD Diagnosis, Management, and Prevention. A Guide for Health Care Professionals: Updated 2015* [Internet]. Florence (Italy): Global Initiative for Chronic Obstructive Lung Disease; [cited 2016 Sep 8] http://www.goldcopd.it/materiale/2015/GOLD_Pocket_2015.pdf

58. Go AS, Mozaffarian D, Roger VL, et al. Heart disease and stroke statistics — 2014 update: a report from the American Heart Association. *Circulation.* 2014;129:e28–292.

59. Gosselink R, De Vos J, van den Heuvel SP, Segers J, Decramer M, Kwakkel G. Impact of inspiratory muscle training in patients with COPD: what is the evidence? *Eur Respir J.* 2011;37(2):416–25.

60. Haykowsky MJ, Kitzman DW. Exercise physiology in heart failure and preserved ejection fraction. *Heart Failure Clin.* 2014;10:445–52.

61. Hiatt WR. Medical treatment of peripheral arterial disease and claudication. *N Engl J Med.* 2001;344:1608–21.

62. Hiatt WR, Cox L, Greenwalt M, Griffin A, Schechter C. Quality of the assessment of primary and secondary endpoints in claudication and critical leg ischemia trials. *Vasc Med.* 2005;10(3):207–13.

63. Hirsch AT, Haskal ZJ, Hertzer NR, et al. ACC/AHA 2005 practice guidelines for the management of patients with peripheral arterial disease (lower extremity, renal, mesenteric, and abdominal aortic): a collaborative report from the American Association for Vascular Surgery/Society for Vascular Surgery, Society for Cardiovascular Angiography and Interventions, Society for Vascular Medicine and Biology, Society of Interventional Radiology, and the ACC/AHA Task Force on Practice Guidelines (Writing Committee to Develop Guidelines for the Management of Patients With Peripheral Arterial Disease): endorsed by the American Association of Cardiovascular and Pulmonary Rehabilitation; National Heart, Lung, and Blood Institute; Society for Vascular Nursing; TransAtlantic Inter-Society Consensus; and Vascular Disease Foundation. *Circulation.* 2006;113(11):e463–654.

64. Holland AE, Wadell K, Spruit MA. How to adapt the pulmonary rehabilitation programme to patients with chronic respiratory disease other than COPD. *Eur Respir Rev.* 2013;22(130):577–86.

65. Horowitz MB, Littenberg B, Mahler DA. Dyspnea ratings for prescribing exercise intensity in patients with COPD. *Chest.* 1996;109(5):1169–75.

66. Jendzjowsky NG, Tomczak CR, Lawrance R, et al. Impaired pulmonary oxygen uptake kinetics and reduced peak aerobic power during small muscle mass exercise in heart transplant recipients. *J Appl Physiol.* 2007;103:1722–7.

67. Kendrick KR, Baxi SC, Smith RM. Usefulness of the modified 0-10 Borg scale in assessing the degree of dyspnea in patients with COPD and asthma. *J Emerg Nurs.* 2000;26(3):216–22.

68. Kerrigan DJ, Williams CT, Ehrman JK, et al. Cardiac rehabilitation improves functional capacity and patient-reported health status in patients with continuous-flow left ventricular assist devices the Rehab-VAD randomized controlled trial. *JACC Heart Fail.* 2014;2(6):653–9.

69. Kerrigan DJ, Williams CT, Ehrman JK, et al. Muscular strength and cardiorespiratory fitness are associated with health status in patients with recently implanted continuous-flow LVADs *J Cardiopulm Rehabil Prev.* 2013;33:396–400.

70. Keteyian S, Ehrman J, Fedel F, Rhoads K. Heart rate-perceived exertion relationship during exercise in orthotopic heart transplant patients. *J Cardiopulmonary Rehabil.* 1990;10:287–93.

71. Keteyian SJ. Exercise training in congestive heart failure: risks and benefits. *Prog Cardiovasc Dis* 2011;53:419–28.

72. Keteyian SJ. High intensity interval training in patients with cardiovascular disease: a brief review of the physiologic adaptations and suggestions for future research. *J Clin Exerc Physiol*. 2013;2:12–9.

73. Keteyian SJ, Hibner BA, Bronsteen K, et al. Greater improvement in cardiorespiratory fitness using higher-intensity interval training in the standard cardiac rehabilitation setting. *J Cardiopulm Rehabil*. 2014;34:98–105.

74. Keteyian SJ, Leifer ES, Houston-Miller N, et al. Relation between volume of exercise and clinical outcomes in patients with heart failure. *J Am Coll Cardiol*. 2012;60:1899–905.

75. Kitzman DW, Little WC, Brubaker PH, et al. Pathophysiological characterization of isolated diastolic heart failure in comparison to systolic heart failure. *JAMA*. 2002;288:2144–50.

76. Kortianou EA, Nasis IG, Spetsioti ST, Daskalakis AM, Vogiatzis I. Effectiveness of interval exercise training in patients with COPD. *Cardiopulm Phys Ther J*. 2010;21(3):12–9.

77. Langer D, Hendriks E, Burtin C, et al. A clinical practice guideline for physiotherapists treating patients with chronic obstructive pulmonary disease based on a systematic review of available evidence. *Clin Rehabil*. 2009;23(5):445–62.

78. Leggett LE, Hauer T, Martin BJ, et al. Optimizing value from cardiac rehabilitation: a cost-utility analysis comparing age, sex, and clinical subgroups. *Mayo Clin Proc*. 2015;90(8):1011–20.

79. Leon AS, Franklin BA, Costa F, et al. Cardiac rehabilitation and secondary prevention of coronary heart disease: an American Heart Association scientific statement from the Council on Clinical Cardiology (Subcommittee on Exercise, Cardiac Rehabilitation, and Prevention) and the Council on Nutrition, Physical Activity, and Metabolism (Subcommittee on Physical Activity), in collaboration with the American Association of Cardiovascular and Pulmonary Rehabilitation. *Circulation*. 2005;111(3):369–76.

80. Madigan EA, Gordon NH, Fortinsky RH, Koroukian SM, Piña I, Riggs JS. Rehospitalization in a national population of home health care patients with heart failure. *Health Serv Res*. 2012;47:2316–38.

81. Maltais F, Decramer M, Casaburi R, et al. An official American Thoracic Society/European Respiratory Society statement: update on limb muscle dysfunction in chronic obstructive pulmonary disease. *Am J Respir Crit Care Med*. 2014;189(9):e15–62.

82. Marciniuk DD, Brooks D, Butcher S, et al. Optimizing pulmonary rehabilitation in chronic obstructive pulmonary disease — practical issues: a Canadian Thoracic Society Clinical Practice Guideline. *Can Respir J*. 2010;17(4):159–68.

83. Moholdt TT, Amundsen BH, Rustad LA, et al. Aerobic interval training versus continuous moderate exercise after coronary artery bypass surgery: a randomized study of cardiovascular effects and quality of life. *Am Heart J*. 2009;158(6):1031–7.

84. Morton AR, Fitch KD. Australian association for exercise and sports science position statement on exercise and asthma. *J Sci Med Sport*. 2011;14(4):312–6.

85. Naji NA, Connor MC, Donnelly SC, McDonnell TJ. Effectiveness of pulmonary rehabilitation in restrictive lung disease. *J Cardiopulm Rehabil*. 2006;26(4):237–43.

86. Nici L, Donner C, Wouters E, et al. American Thoracic Society/European Respiratory Society statement on pulmonary rehabilitation. *Am J Respir Crit Care Med*. 2006;173(12):1390–413.

87. Nonoyama M, Brooks D, Lacasse Y, Guyatt GH, Goldstein RS. Oxygen therapy during exercise training in chronic obstructive pulmonary disease. *Cochrane Database Syst Rev*. 2007;(2):CD005372.

88. Norgren L, Hiatt WR, Dormandy JA, et al. Inter-Society Consensus for the Management of Peripheral Arterial Disease (TASC II). *J Vasc Surg*. 2007;(45 Suppl S):S5–67.

89. Nytrøen K, Gullestad L. Exercise after heart transplantation: An overview. *World J Transplant*. 2013;3:78–90.

90. O'Connor CM, Whellan DJ, Lee KL, et al. Efficacy and safety of exercise training in patients with chronic heart failure: HF-ACTION randomized controlled trial. *JAMA*. 2009;301(14):1439–50.

91. Oldridge N, Furlong W, Feeny D, et al. Economic evaluation of cardiac rehabilitation soon after acute myocardial infarction. *Am J Cardiol*. 1993;72:154–61.

92. Organ Procurement and Transplantation Network Web site [Internet]. Richmond (VA): Organ Procurement and Transplantation Network; [cited 2016 Sep 8]. Available from: http://optn.transplant.hrsa.gov/

93. O'Shea SD, Taylor NF, Paratz JD. Progressive resistance exercise improves muscle strength and may improve elements of performance of daily activities for people with COPD: a systematic review. *Chest*. 2009;136(5):1269–83.

94. Pakhale S, Luks V, Burkett A, Turner L. Effect of physical training on airway inflammation in bronchial asthma: a systematic review. *BMC Pulm Med.* 2013;13:38.

95. Palmer-McLean K, Harbst K. Stroke and brain injury. In: Durstine JL, Moore GE, Painter PL, Roberts SO, editors. *ACSM's Exercise Management for Persons with Chronic Diseases and Disabilities.* Champaign (IL): Human Kinetics; 2009. p. 287–97.

96. Parsons JP, Hallstrand TS, Mastronarde JG, et al. An official American Thoracic Society clinical practice guideline: exercise-induced bronchoconstriction. *Am J Respir Crit Care Med.* 2013;187(9):1016–27.

97. Piccini JP, Hellkamp AS, Whellan DJ, et al. Exercise training and implantable cardioverter-defibrillator shocks in patients with heart failure: results from HF-ACTION (Heart Failure and A Controlled Trial Investigating Outcomes of Exercise TraiNing). *JACC Heart Fail.* 2013;1(2):142–8.

98. Piepoli MF, Davos C, Francis DP, Coats AJ, ExTraMATCH Collaborative. Exercise training meta-analysis of trials in patients with chronic heart failure (ExTraMATCH). *BMJ.* 2004;328:189.

99. Puente-Maestu L, Sánz ML, Sánz P, Cubillo JM, Mayol J, Casaburi R. Comparison of effects of supervised versus self-monitored training programmes in patients with chronic obstructive pulmonary disease. *Eur Respir J.* 2000;15(3):517–25.

100. Qaseem A, Wilt TJ, Weinberger SE, et al. Diagnosis and management of stable chronic obstructive pulmonary disease: a clinical practice guideline update from the American College of Physicians, American College of Chest Physicians, American Thoracic Society, and European Respiratory Society. *Ann Intern Med.* 2011;155:179–91.

101. Ram FS, Robinson SM, Black PN, Picot J. Physical training for asthma. *Cochrane Database Syst Rev.* 2005;(4):CD001116.

102. Rich MW, Beckham V, Wittenberg C, Leven CL, Freedland KE, Carney RM. A multidisciplinary intervention to prevent the readmission of elderly patients with congestive heart failure. *N Engl J Med.* 1995;333:1190–5.

103. Richardson RS, Sheldon J, Poole DC, Hopkins SR, Ries AL, Wagner PD. Evidence of skeletal muscle metabolic reserve during whole body exercise in patients with chronic obstructive pulmonary disease. *Am J Respir Crit Care Med.* 1999;159:881–5.

104. Riegel B, Moser DK, Anker SD, et al. State of the science: promoting self-care in persons with heart failure: a scientific statement from the American Heart Association. *Circulation.* 2009;120:1141–63.

105. Ries AL. Impact of chronic obstructive pulmonary disease on quality of life: the role of dyspnea. *Am J Med.* 2006;119(10 Suppl 1):12–20.

106. Ries AL, Bauldoff GS, Carlin BW, et al. Pulmonary Rehabilitation: joint ACCP/AACVPR Evidence-Based Clinical Practice Guidelines. *Chest.* 2007;131(5 Suppl):4S–42S.

107. Rochester CL, Fairburn C, Crouch RH. Pulmonary rehabilitation for respiratory disorders other than chronic obstructive pulmonary disease. *Clin Chest Med.* 2014;35(2):369–89.

108. Roig M, Eng JJ, MacIntyre DL, et al. Falls in people with chronic obstructive pulmonary disease: an observational cohort study. *Respir Med.* 2011;105:461–9.

109. Schairer JR, Kostelnik T, Proffitt SM, et al. Caloric expenditure during cardiac rehabilitation. *J Cardiopulm Rehabil.* 1998;18:290–4.

110. Scheiderer R, Belden C, Schwab D, Haney C, Paz J. Exercise guidelines for inpatients following ventricular assist device placement: a systematic review of the literature. *Cardiopulm Physical Ther J.* 2013;24:35.

111. Schols AM, Soeters PB, Dingemans AM, Mostert R, Frantzen PJ, Wouters EF. Prevalence and characteristics of nutritional depletion in patients with stable COPD eligible for pulmonary rehabilitation. *Am Rev Respir Dis.* 1993;147(5):1151–6.

112. Sheldahl LM, Wilke NA, Tristani FE. Evaluation and training for resumption of occupational and leisure-time physical activities in patients after a major cardiac event. *Med Exerc Nutr Health.* 1995;4:273–89.

113. Singh SJ, Morgan MD, Hardman AE, Rowe C, Bardsley PA. Comparison of oxygen uptake during a conventional treadmill test and the shuttle walking test in chronic airflow limitation. *Eur Respir J.* 1994;7(11):2016–20.

114. Skeletal muscle dysfunction in chronic obstructive pulmonary disease. A statement of the American Thoracic Society and European Respiratory Society. *Am J Respir Crit Care Med.* 1999;159(4 Pt 2):S1–40.

115. Slaughter MS, Pagani FD, Rogers JG, et al. Clinical management of continuous-flow left ventricular assist devices in advanced heart failure. *J Heart Lung Transplant.* 2010;29(4 Suppl):S1–39.

116. Smart N, Marwick T. Exercise training for patients with heart failure: a systematic review of factors that improve mortality and morbidity. *Am J Med.* 2004;116:693–706.

117. Spruit MA, Singh SJ, Garvey C, et al. An official American Thoracic Society/European Respiratory Society statement: key concepts and advances in pulmonary rehabilitation. *Am J Respir Care Med.* 2013;188:e13–64.

118. Stein R, Hrljac I, Halperin JL, Gustavson SM, Teodorescu V, Olin JW. Limitation of the resting ankle-brachial index in symptomatic patients with peripheral arterial disease. *Vasc Med.* 2006;11:29–33.

119. Stickland MK, Rowe BH, Spooner CH, Vandermeer B, Dryden DM. Effect of warm-up exercise on exercise-induced bronchoconstriction. *Med Sci Sports Exerc.* 2012;44(3):383–91.

120. Strasser B, Siebert U, Schobersberger W. Effects of resistance training on respiratory function in patients with chronic obstructive pulmonary disease: a systematic review and meta-analysis. *Sleep Breath.* 2013;17(1):217–26.

121. Swallow EB, Reyes D, Hopkinson NS, et al. Quadriceps strength predicts mortality in patients with moderate to severe chronic obstructive pulmonary disease. *Thorax.* 2007;62(2):115–20.

122. Taylor RS, Brown A, Ebrahim S, et al. Exercise-based rehabilitation for patients with coronary heart disease: systematic review and meta-analysis of randomized controlled trials. *Am J Med.* 2004;116(10):682–92.

123. Thomas RJ, King M, Lui K, et al. AACVPR/ACC/AHA 2007 performance measures on cardiac rehabilitation for referral to and delivery of cardiac rehabilitation/secondary prevention services endorsed by the American College of Chest Physicians, American College of Sports Medicine, American Physical Therapy Association, Canadian Association of Cardiac Rehabilitation, European Association for Cardiovascular Prevention and Rehabilitation, Inter-American Heart Foundation, National Association of Clinical Nurse Specialists, Preventive Cardiovascular Nurse Association, and the Society of Thoracic Surgeons. *J Am Coll Cardiol.* 2007;50:1400-33.

124. Thompson PD, Balady GJ, Chaitman BR, Clark LT, Levine BD, Myerburg RJ. Task Force 6: coronary artery disease. *J Am Coll Cardiol.* 2005;45(8):1348–53.

125. Tinetti ME, Speechley M, Ginter SF. Risk factors for falls among elderly persons living in the community. *N Engl J Med.* 1988;319(26):1701–7.

126. Treat-Jacobson D, Henly SJ, Bronas UG, Leon AS, Henly GA. The pain trajectory during treadmill testing in peripheral artery disease. *Nurs Res.* 2011;60(3 Suppl):S38–49.

127. Weston KS, Wisløff U, Coombes JS. High-intensity interval training in patients with lifestyle-induced cardiometabolic disease: a systematic review and meta-analysis. *Br J Sports Med.* 2014;48: 1227–34.

128. Williams MA, Haskell WL, Ades PA, et al. Resistance exercise in individuals with and without cardiovascular disease: 2007 update: a scientific statement from the American Heart Association Council on Clinical Cardiology and Council on Nutrition, Physical Activity, and Metabolism. *Circulation.* 2007;116(5):572–84.

129. Wisløff U, Støylen A, Loennechen JP, et al. Superior cardiovascular effect of aerobic interval training versus moderate continuous training in heart failure patients: a randomized study. *Circulation.* 2007;115(24):3086–94.

130. Womack CJ, Gardner AW. Peripheral arterial disease. In: Durstine JL, Moore GE, editors. *ACSM's Exercise Management for Persons with Chronic Diseases and Disabilities.* 2nd ed. Champaign (IL): Human Kinetics; 2003. p. 81–5.

131. Yancy CW, Jessup M, Bozkurt B, et al. 2013 ACCF/AHA guideline for the management of heart failure: a report of the American College of Cardiology Foundation/American Heart Association Task Force on Practice Guidelines. *J Am Coll Cardiol.* 2013;62:e147–239.

132. Zainuldin R, Mackey MG, Alison JA. Prescription of walking exercise intensity from the incremental shuttle walk test in people with chronic obstructive pulmonary disease. *Am J Phys Med Rehabil.* 2012;91(7):592–600.

Exercise Prescription for Individuals with Metabolic Disease and Cardiovascular Disease Risk Factors

INTRODUCTION

This chapter contains the exercise prescription (Ex R_x) guidelines and recommendations for individuals with metabolic and cardiovascular disease (CVD) risk factors. The Ex R_x guidelines and recommendations are presented using the *Frequency, Intensity, Time*, and *Type* (*FITT*) principle of Ex R_x based on the available literature. For information relating to volume and progression, exercise professionals are referred to *Chapter 6*. Information is often lacking regarding volume and progression for the chronic diseases and health conditions presented in this chapter. In these instances, the guidelines and recommendations provided in *Chapter 6* for apparently healthy populations should be adapted with good clinical judgment for the chronic disease(s) and health condition(s) being targeted.

DIABETES MELLITUS

Diabetes mellitus (DM) is a group of metabolic diseases characterized by an elevated blood glucose concentration (*i.e.*, hyperglycemia) as a result of defects in insulin secretion and/or an inability to use insulin. Sustained elevated blood glucose levels place patients at risk for microvascular and macrovascular diseases as well as neuropathies (peripheral and autonomic). According to the Centers for Disease Control and Prevention, 29 million people, or 9.3% of the U.S. population have diabetes, with 28% of those undiagnosed (20). Four types of diabetes are recognized based on etiologic origin: Type 1 diabetes mellitus (T1DM), Type 2 diabetes mellitus (T2DM), gestational (*i.e.*, diagnosed during pregnancy), and other specific origins (*i.e.*, genetic defects and drug induced); however, most patients have T2DM (90% of all cases) followed by T1DM (5%–10% of all cases) (10).

T1DM is most often caused by the autoimmune destruction of the insulin producing β cells of the pancreas, although some cases are idiopathic in origin (10). The primary characteristics of individuals with T1DM are nearly absolute insulin deficiency and a high tendency for ketoacidosis. T2DM is caused by insulin-resistant skeletal muscle, adipose tissue, and liver combined with an insulin secretory defect. A common feature of T2DM is excess body fat with fat distributed in the upper body (*i.e.*, abdominal or central obesity) (10). Assigning the type of diabetes frequently depends on the circumstances present at the time of diagnosis, with some individuals not necessarily fitting clearly into a single category (such as having T1DM or T2DM), and clinical presentation and disease progression may vary considerably between the various types of diabetes (10).

Central obesity and insulin resistance often progress to prediabetes, a condition characterized by (a) elevated blood glucose in response to dietary carbohydrate, termed *impaired glucose tolerance* (IGT), and/or (b) elevated blood glucose in the fasting state, termed *impaired fasting glucose* (IFG) (*Table 10.1*). Individuals with prediabetes are at very high risk to develop diabetes as the capacity of the β cells to hypersecrete insulin diminishes over time and becomes insufficient to restrain elevations in blood glucose.

The fundamental goal for the management of DM is glycemic control using diet, exercise, and, in many cases, medications such as insulin and oral or other hypoglycemic agents (see *Appendix A*). Intensive treatment to control blood glucose reduces the risk of progression of diabetes complications in anyone with the condition (10). Criteria for diagnosis of DM and prediabetes are presented in *Table 10.1*. Glycolated hemoglobin (HbA1C) is a blood chemistry test that reflects mean blood glucose control over the past 2–3 mo (10) (see *Chapter 3*). Both the American Diabetes Association and World Health Organization now endorse using HbA1C ≥6.5% as a diagnostic criterion for diabetes, but many diagnoses are still based on elevated fasting glucose (≥126 mg · dL^{-1} or 7.0 mmol · L^{-1}) (10).

TABLE 10.1 Diagnostic Criteria for Prediabetes and Diabetes Mellitus (10)		
Normal	**Prediabetes**	**Diabetes Mellitus**
HbA1C <5.7%	HbA1C = 5.7%–6.4%	HbA1C ≥6.5%
FPG <100 mg · dL^{-1} (5.6 mmol · L^{-1})	FPG = 100–125 mg · dL^{-1} (5.6–6.9 mmol · L^{-1}) (IFG)	FPG ≥126 mg · dL^{-1} (7.0 mmol · L^{-1})
2-h PG < 140 mg · dL^{-1} (7.8 mmol · L^{-1}) during an OGTT	2-h PG = 140–199 mg · dL^{-1} (7.8–11.0 mmol · L^{-1}) during an OGTT (IGT)	2-h PG ≥ 200 mg · dL^{-1} (11.1 mmol · L^{-1}) during an OGTT
		In a patient with classic symptoms of hyperglycemia or hyperglycemic crisis, a random PG ≥200 mg · dL^{-1} (11.1 mmol · L^{-1})

FPG, fasting plasma glucose (at least 8-h fasting); HbA1C, glycolated hemoglobin; IFG, impaired fasting glucose; IGT, impaired glucose tolerance; OGTT, oral glucose tolerance test (75 g glucose); PG, plasma glucose.

Benefits of Regular Physical Activity for Diabetes

Physical activity (PA) is a key management tool for any type of diabetes and may assist in preventing diabetes-related health complications, insulin resistance, and T2DM. Regular exercise undertaken by individuals with T2DM results in improved glucose tolerance, increased insulin sensitivity, and decreased HbA1C (95,100). Other important benefits for individuals with T1DM, T2DM, or prediabetes include improvements in CVD risk factors and well-being (29). Regular exercise participation may also prevent or delay the transition to T2DM for individuals with prediabetes at high risk for developing the disease (70).

Moderate intensity exercise totaling 150 min · wk^{-1} is associated with reduced morbidity and mortality in observational studies in all populations, including those with DM (89). Prolonged sedentary time has been found to be independently associated with deleterious health outcomes, such as T2DM and all-cause mortality; however, the deleterious outcome effects associated with sedentary time generally decrease with higher levels of PA (14). Thus, all individuals with DM or prediabetes should be encouraged to be regularly physically active, including more daily physical movement and structured exercise, to improve their health and longevity.

Exercise Testing

The following are special considerations for exercise testing in individuals with DM:

- When beginning an exercise program of light-to-moderate intensity, exercise testing is generally not necessary for individuals with DM or prediabetes who are asymptomatic for CVD and low risk (<10% risk of cardiac event over a 10-yr period using the Framingham risk calculator) (13,29,102).
- Electrocardiogram (ECG) stress testing may be indicated for individuals with DM (29,46), especially anyone who has been sedentary and desires to participate in vigorous intensity activities.
- If positive or nonspecific ECG changes in response to exercise are noted or nonspecific ST and T wave changes at rest are observed, follow-up diagnostic testing may be performed. However, the Detection of Ischemia in Asymptomatic Diabetes trial involving 1,123 individuals with T2DM and no symptoms of coronary artery disease (CAD) found that screening with adenosine-stress radionuclide myocardial perfusion imaging for myocardial ischemia over a 4.8-yr follow-up period did not alter rates of cardiac events (111). Thus, the cost-effectiveness and diagnostic value of more intensive testing remains in question.
- Silent ischemia in patients with DM often goes undetected (106); therefore, annual CVD risk factor assessments should be conducted (29).

Exercise Prescription

The FITT principle of Ex R$_x$ for healthy adults generally applies to individuals with DM (see *Chapter 6*). Participating in an exercise program confers benefits that are extremely important to individuals with T1DM and T2DM. Maximizing the cardiovascular benefits resulting from exercise is a key outcome for both types of diabetes. In nondiabetic individuals, exercise enhances sensitivity to insulin in a dose-dependent manner (39); thus, cellular uptake of glucose that facilitates improved control of blood glucose should occur in individuals with T2DM or prediabetes. For those with T1DM, greater insulin sensitivity has little impact on pancreatic function but often lowers requirements for exogenous insulin (36). Healthy weight loss and maintenance of appropriate body weight are often more pressing issues for those with T2DM and prediabetes, but excess body weight and fat can be present in those with T1DM as well, and an exercise program can be useful for either (see "Overweight and Obesity" and "Metabolic Syndrome" sections).

A recent systematic review and meta-analysis found no evidence that resistance exercise differs from aerobic exercise in impact on cardiovascular risk markers or

FITT

■ FITT RECOMMENDATIONS FOR INDIVIDUALS WITH DIABETES (29,40,41)

	Aerobic	Resistance	Flexibility
Frequency	3–7 d · wk^{-1}	A minimum of 2 nonconsecutive d · wk^{-1}, but preferably 3	≥2–3 d · wk^{-1}
Intensity	Moderate (40%–59% $\dot{V}O_2R$ or 11–12 RPE rating) to vigorous (60%–89% $\dot{V}O_2R$ or 14–17 RPE rating)	Moderate (50%–69% of 1-RM) to vigorous (70%–85% of 1-RM)	Stretch to the point of tightness or slight discomfort.
Time	T1DM: 150 min · wk^{-1} at moderate intensity or 75 min · wk^{-1} at vigorous intensity or combination T2DM: 150 min · wk^{-1} at moderate-to-vigorous intensity	At least 8–10 exercises with 1–3 sets of 10–15 repetitions to near fatigue per set early in training. Gradually progress to heavier weights using 1–3 sets of 8–10 repetitions.	Hold static stretch for 10–30 s; 2–4 repetitions of each exercise
Type	Prolonged, rhythmic activities using large muscle groups (*e.g.*, walking, cycling, swimming)	Resistance machines and free weights	Static, dynamic, and/or PNF stretching

1-RM, one repetition maximum; PNF, proprioceptive neuromuscular facilitation; RPE, rating of perceived exertion; $\dot{V}O_2R$, oxygen uptake reserve.

safety in individuals with T2DM. Therefore, selecting one modality or the other may be less important than engaging in any form of PA (109). There is some evidence that a combination of aerobic and resistance training improves blood glucose control more than either modality alone (23,36,94). Whether the added benefits are caused by a greater overall caloric expenditure (94) or are specific to the combination of aerobic and resistance training (23,36) has not yet been fully resolved.

Exercise Training Considerations

- Many people with DM have comorbid conditions; tailor the Ex Rx accordingly. Many individuals with prediabetes or DM are at high risk for or have CVD (see *Chapter 9*).

- Most individuals with T2DM and prediabetes and many with T1DM are overweight (see "Overweight and Obesity" section and the relevant American College of Sports Medicine [ACSM] position stand [37]).

- Due to low initial fitness levels, most individuals with T2DM will require at least 150 min · wk^{-1} of moderate-to-vigorous aerobic exercise to achieve optimal CVD risk reduction (29).

- Interspersing very short, high intensity intervals during moderate intensity aerobic exercise may be useful to lessen the decline in blood glucose during the early postexercise recovery period (53).

- A greater emphasis should eventually be placed on vigorous intensity aerobic exercise if cardiorespiratory fitness (CRF) is a primary goal of the exercise program and not contraindicated by complications. Better overall blood glucose control may be achieved by engaging in vigorous intensity exercise training. Both high-intensity interval training (HIIT) and continuous training are recommended forms of vigorous intensity exercise for individuals with DM (62). For T2DM, allow no more than two consecutive days without aerobic exercise to prevent a period of excessive decline of insulin action.

- Resistance training should be encouraged for individuals with DM or prediabetes in the absence of contraindications, such as uncontrolled hypertension, severe proliferative retinopathy, and recent treatments using laser surgery. Higher resistance (*i.e.*, heavier weight) may be beneficial for optimization of skeletal muscle strength, insulin action, and blood glucose control (41,108), although moderate resistance may be equally effective in previously sedentary individuals (12).

- Appropriate progression of resistance exercise is important to prevent injury because individuals with DM often have a more limited joint mobility due to the process of glycation of collagen (1). Beginning training intensity should be moderate, involving 10–15 repetitions per set, with increases in weight or resistance undertaken with a lower number of repetitions (8–10) only after the target number of repetitions per set can consistently be exceeded. This increase in resistance can be followed by a greater number of sets and lastly by increased training frequency (48).

- During combined training, completing resistance training prior to aerobic training may lower the risk of hypoglycemia in individuals with T1DM (110).

■ Although flexibility training may be desirable for individuals with all types of diabetes, it should not substitute for other recommended activities (*i.e.*, aerobic and resistance training) because flexibility training does not affect glucose control, body composition, or insulin action.

■ Potential complications may affect the appropriateness of some types of activities (*e.g.*, individuals with unhealed foot ulcers should avoid weight-bearing and aquatic activities).

Special Considerations

■ Hypoglycemia is the most common, acute concern for individuals taking insulin or certain oral hypoglycemic agents that increase insulin secretion (29) (see *Appendix A*).

   ■ Hypoglycemia, defined as a blood glucose level <70 mg $\cdot$ dL^{-1} (<3.9 mmol $\cdot$ L^{-1}), is a relative contraindication to beginning an acute bout of exercise (29).

   ■ Rapid decreases in blood glucose may occur with exercise and render individuals symptomatic even when blood glucose is well above 70 mg $\cdot$ dL^{-1}. Conversely, blood glucose levels may decrease in some individuals without generating noticeable symptoms (*i.e.*, *hypoglycemic unawareness*).

   ■ Common adrenergic symptoms associated with hypoglycemia include shakiness, weakness, abnormal sweating, nervousness, anxiety, tingling of the mouth and fingers, and hunger. More severe neuroglycopenic symptoms may include headache, visual disturbances, mental dullness, confusion, amnesia, seizures, and coma.

■ Individuals with DM who take insulin or medications that increase insulin secretion should monitor blood glucose levels before, occasionally during, and after exercise and compensate with appropriate dietary and/or medication regimen changes (in consultation with their health care provider) as needed to maintain euglycemia (29) (see [30]).

■ Hypoglycemia risk is higher during and immediately following exercise but can occur up to 12 h or more postexercise, making food and/or medication adjustments necessary, mostly in insulin users (79). Frequent blood glucose monitoring is the key to detecting and preventing later onset hypoglycemia.

■ Sulfonylurea drugs and other compounds that enhance insulin secretion (*e.g.*, glyburide, glipizide, glimepiride, nateglinide, and repaglinide) increase the risk of hypoglycemia because the effects of insulin and muscle contraction on blood glucose uptake are additive (47,66). Blood glucose monitoring is recommended when beginning a program of regular exercise to assess whether changes in these medication doses are necessary.

■ The timing of exercise is particularly important in individuals taking insulin. Changing insulin timing, reducing insulin doses, and/or increasing carbohydrate intake are effective strategies to prevent hypoglycemia and hyperglycemia during and after exercise (22). Early morning exercise, in particular, may result in elevations in blood glucose levels instead of the usual decrease with moderate activity (91).

- Most insulin users will need to consume carbohydrates (up to 15 g) prior to exercise participation when starting blood glucose levels are ≤100 mg · dL^{-1} (29).

- Prior to planned exercise, rapid- or short-acting insulin doses will likely have to be reduced to prevent hypoglycemia, particularly if exercise occurs during peak insulin times (usually within 2–3 h). Synthetic, rapid-acting insulin analogs (*i.e.*, lispro, aspart, and glulisine) induce more rapid decreases in blood glucose than regular human insulin.

- Longer acting basal insulins (*e.g.*, glargine, detemir, and neutral protamine hagedorn [NPH]) are less likely to cause exercise-induced hypoglycemia (90), although overall doses may need to be reduced to accommodate regular training.

- For individuals with T1DM using insulin pumps, insulin delivery during exercise can be markedly reduced by decreasing the basal rate or disconnecting the pump for short durations, depending on the intensity and duration of exercise. Reducing basal insulin delivery rates for up to 12-h postexercise may be necessary to avoid later onset hypoglycemia.

- Continuous glucose monitors can be very useful in detecting patterns in blood glucose across multiple days and evaluating both the immediate and delayed effects of exercise (5).

- Individuals with DM who have experienced exercise-induced hypoglycemia should ideally exercise with a partner or under supervision to reduce the risk of problems associated with hypoglycemic events. During exercise, carrying medical ID identifying diabetes, a cell phone, and glucose tablets or other rapid carbohydrate treatment for hypoglycemia is recommended.

- Diabetic autonomic neuropathy, long-duration T1DM, and recent antecedent hypoglycemia or exercise contribute to impaired epinephrine and other hormonal responses and hypoglycemia unawareness (45), so frequent blood glucose monitoring is warranted. In older patients with T2DM, the joint occurrence of hypoglycemia unawareness and deteriorated cognitive function is a critical factor that needs to be considered in their exercise blood glucose management (16).

- Hyperglycemia with or without ketosis is a concern for individuals with T1DM who are not in adequate glycemic control. Common symptoms associated with hyperglycemia include polyuria, fatigue, weakness, increased thirst, and acetone breath. Individuals who present with hyperglycemia (*i.e.*, blood glucose ≥300 mg · dL^{-1} or 16.7 mmol · L^{-1}), provided they feel well and have no ketones present when testing either blood or urine, may exercise up to a moderate intensity; however, they should test blood glucose frequently, refrain from vigorous intensity exercise until glucose levels are declining, and ensure adequate hydration (29).

- Exercise should be postponed when both hyperglycemia and ketones are evident. It is recommended that individuals with T1DM check for urine ketones when blood glucose levels are ≥250 mg · dL^{-1} (13.9 mmol · L^{-1}) before starting to exercise (69).

- If blood glucose has been elevated for <2–3 h following a meal, individuals with T2DM will likely experience a reduction in blood glucose during aerobic exercise because endogenous insulin levels will be high (47,77). Those with T1DM may experience similar declines in blood glucose levels if injected or pumped levels of insulin are higher during postprandial exercise.

- Regardless of initial blood glucose levels, vigorous activity of any type may cause elevations in glucose due to an exaggerated release of counterregulatory hormones like epinephrine and glucagon (93). In such cases, individuals with T1DM may need small doses of supplemental insulin to lower postexercise hyperglycemia.

- Dehydration resulting from polyuria secondary to hyperglycemia may contribute to a compromised thermoregulatory response (17). Dehydration may also contribute to elevations in blood glucose levels. Anyone with hyperglycemia has an elevated risk for heat illness and should frequently monitor for signs and symptoms (see *Chapter 8* and other relevant ACSM positions stands [7,9]).

- Given the likelihood that thermoregulation in hot and cold environments is impaired, additional precautions for heat and cold illness are warranted (see *Chapter 8* and other relevant ACSM positions stands [7,9,18]).

- Individuals with DM and retinopathy are at risk for vitreous hemorrhage. However, risk may be minimized by avoiding activities that dramatically elevate blood pressure (BP). Anyone with severe nonproliferative and proliferative diabetic retinopathy should avoid vigorous intensity aerobic and resistance exercise, jumping, jarring, and head-down activities and the Valsalva maneuver (29).

- During exercise, autonomic neuropathy may cause chronotropic incompetence (*i.e.*, a blunted heart rate [HR] response), attenuated volume of oxygen consumed per unit of time ($\dot{V}O_2$) kinetics, and anhydrosis (*i.e.*, water deprivation) (29). In the presence of autonomic neuropathy, the following should be considered:
  - Monitor for signs and symptoms of silent ischemia, such as unusual shortness of breath or back pain, because of the inability to perceive angina.
  - Monitor BP before and after exercise to manage hypotension and hypertension associated with vigorous intensity exercise (see "Hypertension" section).
  - HR and BP responses to exercise may be blunted secondary to autonomic dysfunction. RPE should be used to assess exercise intensity (31).

- For individuals with peripheral neuropathy, proper care of the feet is needed to prevent foot ulcers and lower the risk of amputation (29). Special precautions should be taken to prevent blisters on the feet. Feet should be kept dry and silica gel or air midsoles as well as polyester or blend socks should be used. All individuals should closely examine their feet on a daily basis to detect and treat sores or ulcers early.

- For individuals with nephropathy, exercise does not appear to accelerate progression of kidney disease even though protein excretion acutely increases after exercise (11,29). Both aerobic and resistance training improve physical function and quality of life in individuals with kidney disease, and individuals should be encouraged to be active. Exercise should begin at a low intensity and volume if aerobic capacity and muscle function are substantially reduced (105).

ONLINE RESOURCES

American College of Sports Medicine Position Stand on Exercise and Type 2
 Diabetes Mellitus:
 http://www.acsm.org
American Diabetes Association:
 http://www.diabetes.org
Diabetes Motion (for information about exercising safely with diabetes):
 http://www.diabetesmotion.com
National Institute of Diabetes and Digestive and Kidney Diseases:
 https://www.niddk.nih.gov/

DYSLIPIDEMIA

Dyslipidemia is an abnormal amount of lipids (*e.g.*, cholesterol) in the blood. It is
further defined by the presence of elevated levels of total cholesterol or low-density
lipoprotein (LDL-C), elevated levels of triglycerides (TG), or low levels of
high-density lipoprotein (HDL-C). Current definitions for dyslipidemia are found
in *Table 3.3*. Nearly 30% of people in the United States have dyslipidemia (50), a
major risk factor for atherosclerotic CVD.

 There are many causes of dyslipidemia. The most common contributing cause
is poor dietary and lifestyle choices; however, genetics often play a prominent contributing role, and very high levels of cholesterol often cluster within families (both
pure familial hypercholesterolemia as well as familial combined hyperlipidemia)
(57). Various disease states can also alter blood lipid levels. LDL-C levels are often
increased in patients with hypothyroidism and the nephrotic syndrome. Very high
levels of TG are often found in patients with obesity, insulin resistance, or diabetes. Metabolic syndrome (Metsyn) is partially defined by the presence of high TG
levels. Additionally, the use of oral anabolic steroids has been associated with a
20%–70% reduction in HDL-C levels (2).

 Lifestyle changes are the foundation for the treatment of dyslipidemia even for
patients who may eventually require medications to treat their dyslipidemia. Exercise is useful to improve dyslipidemia, although the magnitude of effect is often
small. Aerobic exercise training consistently reduces LDL-C by 3–6 mg · dL^{-1}
(0.17–0.33 mmol · L^{-1}) but does not appear to have a consistent effect on HDL-C
or TG blood levels (43). Resistance training appears to reduce LDL-C and TG
concentrations by 6–9 mg · dL^{-1} (0.33–0.5 mmol · L^{-1}), but results have been
less consistent as compared to aerobic exercise (43). Additionally, dietary improvements and weight loss appear to have important beneficial effects on improving
dyslipidemia and should be encouraged (34,98).

 Statin drugs, also known as hydroxymethylglutaryl-CoA (HMG-CoA) reductase inhibitors, are very effective for the treatment of dyslipidemia (96). When used
appropriately, statin therapy consistently improves survival by preventing myocardial infarction and stroke. The four most important groups of people who benefit

from statins are (a) patients with established CVD, (b) patients with LDL-C levels >190 mg · dL^{-1}, (c) patients with diabetes who are ≥40 yr, and (d) patients with an estimated 10-yr risk for CVD of ≥7.5%. The 10-yr risk score is based on the presence and severity of risk markers for heart disease and can be calculated using readily available online calculators (see "Online Resources" at end of this section). Current guidelines for risk stratification for the determination of drug treatment of dyslipidemia are available in the 2013 ACC/AHA reports on the Assessment of Cardiovascular Risk and on the Treatment of Blood Cholesterol to Reduce Cardiovascular Risk in Adults (43,51,96). When considering treatment with medication, the use of evidence-based prescribing guidelines and personalized assessment and decision making are strongly recommended in conjunction with the person's health care provider.

Overall, the population's blood lipid levels are improving (63). This improvement is attributed to improved cholesterol awareness, changes in dietary eating patterns, reduced trans-fat consumption, and increased use of medications (63). However, substantial numbers of people throughout the United States and the world still have uncontrolled dyslipidemia, and in the past decade, the population rate of improvement in dyslipidemia appears to have slowed (63).

The ACSM makes the following recommendations regarding exercise testing and training of individuals with dyslipidemia.

Exercise Testing

■ In general, an exercise test is not required for asymptomatic patients prior to beginning an exercise training program at a light to moderate intensity.
■ Standard exercise testing methods and protocols are appropriate for use with individuals with dyslipidemia cleared for exercise testing (see *Chapter 5*).
■ Use caution when testing individuals with dyslipidemia because undetected underlying CVD may be present.
■ Special consideration should be given to the presence of other chronic diseases and health conditions (*e.g.*, Metsyn, obesity, hypertension) that may require modifications to standard exercise testing protocols and modalities (see the sections of this chapter and other relevant ACSM positions stands on these chronic diseases and health conditions [37,87]).

Exercise Prescription

The FITT principle of Ex R$_x$ for individuals with dyslipidemia without comorbidities is very similar to the Ex R$_x$ for healthy adults (48,55) (see *Chapter 6*). However, an important difference in the FITT principle of Ex R$_x$ for individuals with dyslipidemia compared to healthy adults is that healthy weight maintenance should be highly emphasized. Accordingly, aerobic exercise for the purpose of maximizing energy expenditure (EE) for weight loss becomes the foundation of the Ex R$_x$, and the FITT recommendations are consistent with the recommendations for healthy weight loss and maintenance of 250–300 min · wk^{-1} (see "Overweight and Obesity" section and the relevant ACSM position stand [37]). Although beneficial for general health, resistance and flexibility exercises should be considered adjuncts to an aerobic training program because these modes of exercise have less consistent beneficial effects in patients with dyslipidemia (15,65). Flexibility training is recommended for general health benefits only.

■ **FITT RECOMMENDATIONS FOR INDIVIDUALS WITH DYSLIPIDEMIA** (15,37,48)

	Aerobic	Resistance	Flexibility
Frequency	≥5 d · wk^{-1} to maximize caloric expenditure	2–3 d · wk^{-1}	≥2–3 d · wk^{-1}
Intensity	40%–75% $\dot{V}O_2R$ or HRR	Moderate (50%–69% of 1-RM) to vigorous (70%–85% of 1-RM) to improve strength; <50% 1-RM to improve muscle endurance	Stretch to the point of tightness or slight discomfort.
Time	30–60 min · d^{-1}. To promote or maintain weight loss, 50–60 min · d^{-1} or more of daily exercise is recommended.	2–4 sets, 8–12 repetitions for strength; ≤2 sets, 12–20 repetitions for muscular endurance	Hold static stretch for 10–30 s; 2–4 repetitions of each exercise
Type	Prolonged, rhythmic activities using large muscle groups (*e.g.*, walking, cycling, swimming)	Resistance machines, free weights and/or body weight	Static, dynamic, and/or PNF stretching

1-RM, one repetition maximum; HRR, heart rate reserve; PNF, proprioceptive neuromuscular facilitation; $\dot{V}O_2R$, oxygen uptake reserve.

Exercise Training Considerations

■ The FITT principle of Ex R$_x$ may need to be modified should the individuals with dyslipidemia present with other chronic diseases and health conditions such as Metsyn, obesity, and hypertension (see "Metabolic Syndrome," "Overweight and Obesity," and "Hypertension" sections and other relevant ACSM position stands on these chronic diseases and health conditions [37,87]).

■ Adults over age 65 yr and with dyslipidemia should follow the ACSM exercise guidelines for older adults (8).

- Performance of intermittent aerobic exercise of at least 10 min in duration to accumulate the duration recommendations appears to be an effective alternative to continuous exercise but should only be performed by those who cannot accumulate 30–60 min of continuous exercise (6).

Special Consideration

- Individuals taking lipid-lowering medications (*i.e.*, statins and fibric acid) may experience muscle weakness and soreness termed *myalgia* (see *Appendix A*). Although rare, these medicines can cause direct and severe muscle injury. A health care provider should be consulted if an individual experiences unusual or persistent muscle soreness when exercising while taking these medications.

ONLINE RESOURCES

American Heart Association:
   http://my.americanheart.org/professional/ScienceNews/Clinical-Practice
   -Guidelines-for-Prevention_UCM_457211_Article.jsp
ASCVD Risk Estimator:
   http://tools.cardiosource.org/ASCVD-Risk-Estimator/

HYPERTENSION

Chronic primary (essential) hypertension is defined by the Seventh Report of the Joint National Committee (JNC7) on the Prevention, Detection, Evaluation, and Treatment of High Blood Pressure as having a resting systolic blood pressure (SBP) $\geq$140 mm Hg and/or a resting diastolic blood pressure (DBP) $\geq$90 mm Hg, confirmed by a minimum of two measures taken on at least two separate days, or taking antihypertensive medication for the purpose of BP control (21). Primary hypertension accounts for 95% of all cases and is a risk factor for the development of CVD and premature mortality (21,92). The known contributors of primary hypertension include genetic and lifestyle factors such as high-fat and high-salt diets and physical inactivity (21,92). Secondary hypertension accounts for the remaining 5%. The principal causes of secondary hypertension are chronic kidney disease, renal artery stenosis, pheochromocytoma, excessive aldosterone secretion, and sleep apnea (21,49,92). An estimated 77.9 million U.S. adults $\geq$20 yr of age and more than 1 billion people worldwide have hypertension (49,64).

Approximately 42 million men and 28 million women (37% of the adult U.S. population) have prehypertension (see *Table 3.2* for all levels of hypertension classification), a frequent precursor of hypertension (49). The 4-yr incidence rate of progression to hypertension is estimated to be 26%–50% among individuals $\geq$65 yr of age (104). Although the rate of progression from prehypertension to hypertension is positively associated with age, baseline BP, and comorbidities (54), hypertension does not appear to be a fundamental feature of human aging but the outcome of lifestyle factors (*i.e.*, diets high in salt and fat, excess body weight, and physical inactivity) (54,71).

A variety of medications are available in the treatment of hypertension. Current guidelines for the management of hypertension provide specific instructions on the implementation of pharmacologic therapies (60). Most patients treated with medication require more than one medication to achieve their targeted BP. Some antihypertensive medications may affect the physiological response to exercise and therefore must be taken into consideration during exercise testing and when prescribing exercise (see *Appendix A*) (87).

Guidelines for the management of hypertension also emphasize lifestyle modifications that include habitual PA as initial therapy to lower BP and to prevent or attenuate progression to hypertension in individuals with prehypertension (21,60,87,92). Other recommended lifestyle changes include smoking cessation, weight management, reduced sodium intake, moderation of alcohol consumption, and an overall health dietary pattern consistent with the Dietary Approaches to Stop Hypertension diet (21,92).

Exercise Testing

Although hypertension is not an indication for exercise testing, the test may be useful to evaluate the BP response to exercise which may be useful to guide Ex R$_x$ (46). Individuals with hypertension may have an exaggerated BP response to exercise, even if resting BP is controlled (71). Some individuals with prehypertension may also have a similar response (73).

Recommendations regarding exercise testing for individuals with hypertension vary depending on their BP level and the presence of other CVD risk factors (see *Table 3.1*), target organ disease, or clinical CVD (46,87). For most asymptomatic individuals with hypertension and prehypertension adequate BP management prior to engaging in light-to-moderate intensity exercise programs such as walking is sufficient with no need for medical evaluation or exercise testing (46).

Recommendations include the following:

- Individuals with hypertension whose BP is not controlled (*i.e.*, resting SBP ≥140 mm Hg and/or DBP ≥90 mm Hg) should consult with their physician prior to initiating an exercise program to determine if an exercise test is needed.
- Individuals with stage 2 hypertension (SBP ≥160 mm Hg or DBP ≥100 mm Hg) or with target organ disease (*e.g.*, left ventricular hypertrophy, retinopathy) must not engage in any exercise, including exercise testing, prior to a medical evaluation and adequate BP management. A medically supervised symptom-limited exercise test is recommended prior to engaging in an exercise program for these individuals. Additional evaluations may ensue and vary depending on findings of the exercise test and the clinical status of the individual.
- When exercise testing is performed for the specific purpose of designing the Ex R$_x$, it is preferred that individuals take their usual antihypertensive medications as recommended (46).
- Individuals on β-blocker therapy are likely to have an attenuated HR response to exercise and reduced maximal exercise capacity. Individuals on diuretic therapy may experience hypokalemia and other electrolyte imbalances, cardiac dysrhythmias, or potentially a false-positive exercise test (see *Appendix A*).

Exercise Prescription

Chronic aerobic exercise of adequate intensity, duration, and volume that promotes an increased exercise capacity leads to reductions in resting SBP and DBP of 5–7 mm Hg and reductions in exercise SBP at submaximal workloads in individuals with hypertension (71,87). Regression of cardiac wall thickness and left ventricular mass in individuals with hypertension who participate in regular aerobic exercise training (56,73) and a lower left ventricular mass in individuals with prehypertension and a moderate-to-high physical fitness status have also been reported (72). Emphasis should be placed on aerobic activities; however, these may be supplemented with moderate intensity resistance training. Some support exists that resistance exercise alone can lower BP, although the evidence is inconsistent (43). Flexibility exercise should be performed after a thorough warm-up or during the cool-down period following the guidelines for healthy adults (see *Chapter 6*).

■ **FITT RECOMMENDATIONS FOR INDIVIDUALS WITH HYPERTENSION** (43,48,88)

FITT	Aerobic	Resistance	Flexibility
Frequency	5–7 d · wk^{-1}	2–3 d · wk^{-1}	≥2–3 d · wk^{-1}
Intensity	Moderate intensity (*i.e.*, 40%–59% $\dot{V}O_2R$ or HRR; RPE 12–13 on a 6–20 scale)	60%–70% 1-RM; may progress to 80% 1-RM. For older individuals and novice exercisers, begin with 40%–50% 1-RM.	Stretch to the point of feeling tightness or slight discomfort.
Time	≥30 min · d^{-1} of continuous or accumulated exercise. If intermittent exercise performed, begin with a minimum of 10 min bouts.	2–4 sets of 8–12 repetitions for each of the major muscle groups	Hold static stretch for 10–30 s; 2–4 repetitions of each exercise
Type	Prolonged, rhythmic activities using large muscle groups (*e.g.*, walking, cycling, swimming)	Resistance machines, free weights, and/or body weight	Static, dynamic, and/or PNF stretching

1-RM, one repetition maximum; HRR, heart rate reserve; PNF, proprioceptive neuromuscular facilitation; RPE, rating of perceived exertion; $\dot{V}O_2R$, oxygen uptake reserve.

Exercise Training Considerations

■ Consideration should be given to the level of BP control, recent changes in antihypertensive drug therapy, medication-related adverse effects, the presence of target organ disease, other comorbidities, and age. Adjustments to the Ex R_x should be made accordingly. In general, progression should be gradual, avoiding large increases in any of the FITT components of the Ex R_x, especially intensity for most individuals with hypertension.

■ An exaggerated BP response to relatively low exercise intensities and at HR levels <85% of the age-predicted maximal heart rate (HR_{max}) is likely to occur in some individuals, even after resting BP is controlled with antihypertensive medication. In some cases, an exercise test may be beneficial to establish the exercise HR corresponding to the exaggerated BP in these individuals.

■ It is prudent to maintain SBP ≤220 mm Hg and/or DBP ≤105 mm Hg when exercising (87).

■ Although vigorous intensity aerobic exercise (*i.e.*, ≥60% $\dot{V}O_2R$) is not necessarily contraindicated in patients with hypertension, moderate intensity aerobic exercise (*i.e.*, 40%–59% $\dot{V}O_2R$) is generally recommended to optimize the benefit-to-risk ratio.

■ Individuals with hypertension are often overweight or obese. Ex R_x should focus on increasing caloric expenditure coupled with reducing caloric intake to facilitate weight reduction (see "Overweight and Obesity" section and the relevant ACSM position stand [37]).

■ Inhaling and breath-holding while engaging in the actual lifting of a weight (*i.e.*, Valsalva maneuver) can result in extremely high BP responses, dizziness, and even fainting. Thus, such practice should be avoided during resistance training.

Special Considerations

■ Exercise testing and vigorous intensity exercise training for individuals with hypertension at moderate-to-high risk for cardiac complications should be medically supervised until the safety of the prescribed activity has been established (46).

■ β-Blockers and diuretics may adversely affect thermoregulatory function. β-Blockers may also increase the predisposition to hypoglycemia in certain individuals (especially patients with DM who take insulin or insulin secretagogue medication that increases pancreas insulin secretion) and mask some of the manifestations of hypoglycemia (particularly tachycardia). In these situations, educate patients about the signs and symptoms of heat intolerance and hypoglycemia and the precautions that should be taken to avoid these situations (see "Diabetes Mellitus" section and *Appendix A*).

■ β-Blockers, particularly the nonselective types, may reduce submaximal and maximal exercise capacity primarily in patients without myocardial ischemia (see *Appendix A*). The peak exercise HR achieved during a standardized exercise stress test should then be used to establish the exercise training intensity. If the peak exercise HR is not available, RPE should be used.

- Antihypertensive medications such as α-blockers, calcium channel blockers, and vasodilators may lead to sudden excessive reductions in postexercise BP. Therefore, termination of the exercise should be gradual, and the cool-down period should be extended and carefully monitored until BP and HR return to near resting levels.

- A majority of older individuals are likely to have hypertension. The exercise-related BP reduction is independent of age. Therefore, older individuals experience similar exercise induced BP reductions as younger individuals (see *Chapter 7* and the relevant ACSM/AHA recommendations [83]).

- The BP-lowering effects of aerobic exercise are immediate, a physiologic response referred to as *postexercise hypotension*. Patients should be made aware of postexercise hypotension and instructed how to modulate its effects (*e.g.*, continued very light intensity exercise such as slow walking).

- If an individual with hypertension has ischemia during exercise, the Ex R_x recommendations for those with CVD with ischemia should be utilized. See *Chapter 9* for more information.

ONLINE RESOURCES

American College of Sports Medicine Position Stand on Exercise and
    Hypertension:
    http://www.acsm.org
American Heart Association:
    http://www.heart.org/HEARTORG/Conditions/HighBloodPressure
    /PreventionTreatmentofHighBloodPressure/Physical-Activity-and-Blood
    -Pressure_UCM_301882_Article.jsp
American Society of Hypertension:
    http://www.ash-us.org/ASH-Patient-Portal/Get-in-Control/Make-Physical
    -Activity-Part-of-Your-Day.aspx

METABOLIC SYNDROME

The Metsyn is characterized by a clustering of risk factors associated with an increased incidence of CVD, DM, and stroke (26). Uncertainty exists as to whether Metsyn is a distinct pathophysiological entity or simply a clinical marker of future untoward events, particularly CVD mortality. Observational research shows a greater risk of CVD death in individuals with Metsyn compared to those without Metsyn (58), yet no evidence exits from prospective studies to confirm these findings.

Until recently, the criteria for defining Metsyn varied by organization (24) and yielded a prevalence rate of 34% and 39% in U.S. adults (3,80). A consensus definition now exists (3), in which each organization includes hyperglycemia (or current blood glucose medication use), elevated BP (or current hypertension medication use), dyslipidemia (or current lipid-lowering medication use), and national or regional cutpoints for central adiposity based on waist circumference; however, differences in specific value within these criteria remain (*Table 10.2*). It is further agreed that an individual is categorized as having Metsyn when he or she displays at least three of the defining risk factors.

The treatment guidelines for Metsyn recommended by National Cholesterol Education Program (NCEP) Adult Treatment Panel III (ATP III) focus on three interventions including weight control, PA, and treatment of the associated CVD risk factors that may include pharmacotherapy (82). The International Diabetes Federation (IDF) *Guidelines* for primary intervention include (a) moderate restriction in energy intake (EI) to achieve a 5%–10% weight loss within 1 yr, (b) moderate increases in PA consistent with the consensus public health recommendations of 30 min of moderate intensity PA on most days of the week (55), and (c) change in dietary intake composition consistent with modifying specified CVD risk factors (*i.e.*, decreased simple carbohydrates, increased lean protein, reduced saturated fat) (99). The IDF secondary intervention includes pharmacotherapy for associated CVD risk factors (35,99).

Exercise Testing

- The presence of Metsyn does not result in the requirement of an exercise test prior to beginning a low-to-moderate intensity exercise program.
- If an exercise test is performed, the general recommendations can be followed (see *Chapter 5*), with particular consideration for dyslipidemia, hypertension, or hyperglycemia when present.
- Because many individuals with the Metsyn are either overweight or obese, exercise testing considerations specific to those individuals should be followed (see "Overweight and Obesity" section and the relevant ACSM position stand [37]).
- The potential for low exercise capacity in individuals who are overweight or obese may necessitate a low initial workload (*i.e.*, 2–3 metabolic equivalents [METs]) and small increments per testing stage (0.5–1.0 MET) (see *Chapter 5*).
- Because of the potential presence of elevated BP, strict adherence to protocols for assessing BP before and during exercise testing should be followed (86) (see *Chapters 3* and *5*).

Exercise Prescription/Special Considerations

The FITT principle of Ex R$_x$ in Metsyn is generally consistent with the recommendations for healthy adults regarding aerobic, resistance, and flexibility exercise (see *Chapter 6*). Similarly, the minimal dose of PA to improve health/fitness outcomes is consistent with the consensus public health recommendations of 150 min · wk^{-1} or 30 min of moderate intensity PA on most days of the week (55,89). However, due to the clustering of CVD and DM risk factors, along with the likely presence

TABLE 10.2			
Metabolic Syndrome Criteria: NCEP/ATP III, IDF, and WHO			
Criteria	**NCEP/ATP III (52)**	**IDF (99)**	**WHO (4)**[a]
Body Weight	Waist circumference[a,b]	Waist circumference[c]	Waist-to-hip ratio (males >0.90; females >0.85) and/or BMI of >30 kg · m^{-2}
Men	>102 cm (>40 in)	≥94 cm (≥37 in)	>0.9 ratio
Women	>88 cm (>35 in)	≥80 cm (≥31.5 in)	>0.85 ratio
Insulin resistance/ glucose	≥100 mg · dL^{-1d} or on drug treatment for elevated blood glucose	≥100 mg · dL^{-1} or previously diagnosed Type 2 diabetes	See footnote[e]
Dyslipidemia			
HDL	Men: <40 mg · dL^{-1} Women: <50 mg · dL^{-1} Anyone on drug treatment for reduced HDL-C	Men: <40 mg · dL^{-1} Women: <50 mg · dL^{-1} Anyone on drug treatment for reduced HDL-C	Men: <35 mg · dL^{-1} Women: <39 mg · dL^{-1f}
Triglycerides	≥150 mg · dL^{-1} or on drug treatment for high triglycerides	≥150 mg · dL^{-1} or on drug treatment for high triglycerides	≥150 mg · dL^{-1} or on drug treatment for high triglycerides
Elevated blood pressure	≥130 or ≥85 mm Hg or on drug treatment for hypertension	≥130 or ≥85 mm Hg or treatment of previously diagnosed hypertension	Antihypertensive medication and/or a BP of ≥140 or ≥90 mm Hg
Other	N/A	N/A	Urinary albumin excretion rate ≥20 μg · min^{-1} or albumin: creatinine ratio ≥30 mg · g^{-1}

[a]Overweight and obesity are associated with insulin resistance and the metabolic syndrome (Metsyn). However, the presence of abdominal obesity is more highly correlated with these metabolic risk factors than is elevated BMI. Therefore, the simple measure of waist circumference is recommended to identify the body weight component of the Metsyn.

[b]Some men develop multiple metabolic risk factors when the waist circumference is only marginally increased (94–102 cm [37–39 in]). Such patients may have a strong genetic contribution to insulin resistance. They should benefit from changes in life habits, similarly to men with categorical increases in waist circumference.

[c]A required criterion defined as waist circumference ≥94 cm (≥37 in) for Europid men and ≥80 cm (≥31.2 in) for Europid women, with ethnicity-specific values for other groups.

[d]The American Diabetes Association has established a cutpoint of ≥100 mg · dL^{-1}, above which individuals have either prediabetes (impaired fasting glucose) or diabetes mellitus (10). This cutpoint should be applicable for identifying the lower boundary to define an elevated glucose as one criterion for metabolic syndrome.

[e]A required criterion is one of the following: Type 2 diabetes mellitus, impaired fasting glucose, impaired glucose tolerance, or for those with normal fasting glucose levels (<100 mg · dL^{-1}), glucose uptake below the lowest quartile for background populations under investigation under hyperinsulinemic and euglycemic conditions. Note this value has been updated to be consistent with current ADA recommendations regarding normal fasting plasma glucose levels (10).

[f]These values have been updated from those originally presented to ensure consistence with ATP III cutpoints.

NOTE: To convert glucose from mg · dL^{-1} to mmol · L^{-1}, multiply by 0.0555. To convert HDL from mg · dL^{-1} to mmol · L^{-1}, multiply by 0.0259. To convert triglycerides from mg · dL^{-1} to mmol · L^{-1}, multiply by 0.0113.

ATP III, Adult Treatment Panel III; BMI, body mass index; BP, blood pressure; HDL-C, high-density lipoprotein cholesterol; IDF, International Diabetes Federation; NCEP, National Cholesterol Education Program; WHO, World Health Organization.

of chronic diseases and health conditions that accompany Metsyn, the following Ex R$_x$ special considerations are suggested:

■ When developing the Ex R$_x$ for Metsyn, attention should be given to each risk factor/condition present, with the most conservative criteria used to set initial workloads (see other sections of this chapter on the FITT principle Ex R$_x$ for these other chronic diseases and health conditions as well as relevant ACSM position stands [29,37,87]). Over time and as tolerated, longer duration and higher intensities may be necessary to achieve significant health and fitness outcomes.

■ To reduce the impact of the Metsyn, variables that are considered risk factors for CVD and DM, initial exercise training should be performed at a moderate intensity (*i.e.*, 40%–59% $\dot{V}O_2R$ or HRR) totaling a minimum of 150 min · wk^{-1} or 30 min · d^{-1} most days of the week to allow for optimal health/fitness improvements. When appropriate, progress to a more vigorous intensity (*i.e.*, ≥60% $\dot{V}O_2R$ or HRR).

■ Reduction of body weight is an important goal for individuals with Metsyn (52); therefore, gradually increasing PA levels to approximately 250–300 min · wk^{-1} or 50–60 min on 5 d · wk^{-1} may be necessary when appropriate (37). Daily and weekly amounts of PA may be accumulated in multiple shorter bouts (≥10 min in duration) and can include various forms of moderate intensity lifestyle PAs. For some individuals, progression to 60–90 min · d^{-1} of PA may be necessary to promote or maintain weight loss (see the Ex R$_x$ recommendations for those with overweight and obesity in this chapter and the relevant ACSM position stand [37]).

■ Resistance training, when combined with aerobic training, can produce greater decreases in Metsyn prevalence than that of aerobic training alone (42,78). Reported participation in ≥2 d · wk^{-1} of muscle strengthening activity reduces the risk of acquiring dyslipidemia, IFG, prehypertension, and increased waist circumference, all part of the Metsyn cluster (25) (see *Chapter 6* for resistance training guidelines).

ONLINE RESOURCES

American College of Sports Medicine Position Stand on Exercise and Hypertension:
http://www.acsm.org
American Heart Association, Metabolic Syndrome:
http://www.heart.org/HEARTORG/Conditions/More/MetabolicSyndrome/Metabolic-Syndrome_UCM_002080_SubHomePage.jsp
Mayo Clinic Diseases and Conditions, Metabolic Syndrome:
http://www.mayoclinic.org/diseases-conditions/metabolic-syndrome/basic/definition/con-20027243
National Heart Lung and Blood Institute. What Is Metabolic Syndrome?:
http://www.nhlbi.nih.gov/health/health-topics/topics/ms

OVERWEIGHT AND OBESITY

Overweight and *obesity* are defined by a body mass index (BMI) of 25–29.9 kg · m^{-2} and 30 kg · m^{-2} or greater, respectively. Recent estimates indicate that 68% of U.S. adults are classified as either overweight or obese (BMI ≥25 kg · m^{-2}), with 34% obese (BMI ≥30 kg · m^{-2}), and 6% extremely obese (BMI ≥40 kg · m^{-2}) (84). Obesity rates are highest in certain ethnic and gender groups. For example, non-Hispanic Black women have age-adjusted overweight/obesity rates of 82%, followed closely by Hispanic men (78.6%) (84). Although the prevalence of obesity has steadily risen over the last three decades, recent data indicate a plateau in the overall prevalence of obesity (84).

Statistics relating to youth indicate that 32% of children and adolescents are overweight or obese (84). In the United States, the percentage of children 6–11 yr of age who are considered obese increased from 7% in 1980 to 18% in 2012; the percentage of adolescents (12–19 yr of age) who are obese increased from 5% to 21% during the same time period (84). The troubling data on overweight/obesity prevalence among the adult and pediatric populations and its health implications have precipitated an increased awareness in the value of identifying and treating individuals with excess body weight (33,37,74,103).

For all ages and ethnicities, overweight and obesity are linked to an increased risk of the development of numerous chronic diseases including CVD, DM, some forms of cancer, and musculoskeletal problems (27). It is estimated obesity-related conditions account for more than 7% of total health care costs in the United States, and the direct and indirect costs of obesity are in excess of $190 billion annually (19).

The management of body weight is dependent on energy balance that is determined by EI and EE. For an individual who is overweight or obese to reduce body weight, EE must exceed EI. Sustained weight loss of 3%–5% is likely to result in clinically meaningful reductions in several CVD risk factors, including TG, blood glucose, and HbA1C levels, and the risk of developing T2DM (61). There is evidence that as little as 2%–3% loss can result in similar CVD risk factor improvement (37). These benefits are more likely to be sustained through the maintenance of weight loss, but maintenance is challenging with weight regain averaging approximately 33%–50% of initial weight loss within 1 yr of terminating treatment (97).

Lifestyle interventions for weight loss that combine reductions in EI with increases in EE through exercise and other forms of PA often result in an initial 5%–10% reduction in body weight (107). PA appears to have a modest impact on the magnitude of weight loss observed across the initial weight loss intervention compared with reductions in EI (27). A review of weight loss interventions found that programs which combined diet and exercise resulted in a 20% (~3 kg) greater weight loss versus diet restriction alone (32); however, this effect is lost when EI is severely reduced (37). PA and diet restriction will provide comparable weight loss if they provide similar levels of negative energy balance (37). Due to low levels of fitness, it may be difficult for overweight/obese individuals to perform a volume of PA required to achieve clinically meaningful weight loss. Therefore, the combination of moderate reductions in EI with adequate levels of PA maximizes weight loss in individuals with overweight and obesity.

There is a dose-response relationship between PA levels and the magnitude of weight loss. The ACSM's position stand on PA and weight loss concluded that (a) <150 min · wk^{-1} of PA promotes minimal weight loss, (b) >150 min · wk^{-1} of PA results in modest weight loss of ~2–3 kg, and (c) >225–420 min · wk^{-1} of PA results in a 5- to 7.5-kg weight loss (37).

PA appears necessary for most individuals to prevent weight regain, but there are no correctly designed, adequately powered, energy balance studies to provide evidence for the amount of PA needed to prevent weight regain after weight loss (37). However, there is literature that suggests it may take more than the consensus public health recommendation for PA of 150 min · wk^{-1} or 30 min of PA on most days of the week (37,55,101). Some studies support the value of ~200–300 min · wk^{-1} of PA during weight maintenance to reduce weight regain after weight loss, and it seems that "more is better" (37).

Based on the existing scientific evidence and practical clinical guidelines (37), the ACSM makes the following recommendations regarding exercise testing and training for individuals with overweight and obesity.

Exercise Testing

- An exercise test is often not necessary in the overweight/obese population prior to beginning a low-to-moderate intensity exercise program.
- Overweight and obese individuals are at risk for other comorbidities (*e.g.*, dyslipidemia, hypertension, hyperinsulinemia, hyperglycemia), which are associated with CVD risk.
- The timing of medications to treat comorbidities relative to exercise testing should be considered, particularly in those take β-blockers and antidiabetic medications.
- The presence of musculoskeletal and/or orthopedic conditions may necessitate the need for using leg or arm ergometry.
- The potential for low exercise capacity in individuals with overweight and obesity may necessitate a low initial workload (*i.e.*, 2–3 METs) and small increments per testing stage of 0.5–1.0 MET. See *Chapter 5* for protocol examples.
- Exercise equipment must be adequate to meet the weight specification of individuals with overweight and obesity for safety and calibration purposes.
- The appropriate cuff size should be used to measure BP in individuals who are overweight and obese to minimize the potential for inaccurate measurement.

Exercise Prescription

The goals of exercise during the active weight loss phase are to (a) maximize the amount of caloric expenditure to enhance the amount of weight loss and (b) integrate exercise into the individual's lifestyle to prepare them for a successful weight loss maintenance phase.

■ **FITT RECOMMENDATIONS FOR INDIVIDUALS WITH OVERWEIGHT AND OBESITY** (37,85)

	Aerobic	Resistance	Flexibility
Frequency	≥ 5 d · wk^{-1}	2–3 d · wk^{-1}	$\geq$2–3 d · wk^{-1}
Intensity	Initial intensity should be moderate (40%–59% $\dot{V}O_2R$ or HRR); progress to vigorous ($\geq$60% $\dot{V}O_2R$ or HRR) for greater health benefits.	60%–70% of 1-RM; gradually increase to enhance strength and muscle mass.	Stretch to the point of feeling tightness or slight discomfort.
Time	30 min · d^{-1} (150 min · wk^{-1}); increase to 60 min · d^{-1} or more (250–300 min · wk^{-1}).	2–4 sets of 8–12 repetitions for each of the major muscle groups	Hold static stretch for 10–30 s; 2–4 repetitions of each exercise
Type	Prolonged, rhythmic activities using large muscle groups (*e.g.*, walking, cycling, swimming)	Resistance machines and/or free weights	Static, dynamic, and/ or PNF

1-RM, one repetition maximum; HRR, heart rate reserve; PNF, proprioceptive neuromuscular facilitation; $\dot{V}O_2R$, oxygen uptake reserve.

Exercise Training Considerations

◀ The duration of moderate-to-vigorous intensity PA should initially progress to at least 30 min · d^{-1} (55,101).

◀ To promote long-term weight loss maintenance, individuals should progress to at least 250 min · wk^{-1} ($\geq$2,000 kcal · wk^{-1}) of moderate-to-vigorous exercise. To achieve the weekly maintenance activity goal of $\geq$250 min · wk^{-1}, exercise and PA should be performed on 5–7 d · wk^{-1}.

◀ Individuals with overweight and obesity may accumulate this amount of PA in multiple daily bouts of at least 10 min in duration or through increases in other forms of moderate intensity lifestyle PA. Accumulation of intermittent exercise may increase the volume of PA achieved by previously sedentary individuals and may enhance the likelihood of adoption and maintenance of PA (76).

◀ Resistance training does not result in clinically significant weight loss (37). The addition of resistance exercise to energy restriction does not appear to prevent the loss of fat-free mass or the observed reduction in resting EE (38).

◀ Resistance exercise may enhance muscular strength and physical function in individuals who are overweight or obese. Moreover, there may be additional health benefits of participating in resistance exercise such as improvements in CVD and DM risk factors and other chronic disease risk factors (38).

Special Considerations (37,59)

- Utilize goal setting to target short- and long-term weight loss. Target a minimal reduction in body weight of at least 3%–10% of initial body weight over 3–6 mo.
- Target reducing current EI to achieve weight loss. A reduction of 500–1,000 kcal · d^{-1} is adequate to elicit a weight loss of 1–2 lb · wk^{-1} (0.5–0.9 kg · wk^{-1}). This reduced EI should be combined with a reduction in dietary fat intake.
- Weight loss beyond 5%–10% may require more aggressive nutrition, exercise, and behavioral intervention (see *Chapter 12*). For those who do not respond to any degree of lifestyle intervention, medical treatments such as medications or surgery may be appropriate.
- Medically indicated very low calorie diets with energy restrictions of up to 1,500 kcal · d^{-1} can result in greater initial weight loss amounts compared to more conservative EI reductions. These medically managed meal plans are typically only used for selected individuals and for short periods of time.
- Incorporate opportunities to enhance communication between health care professionals, registered dietitian nutritionists, and exercise professionals and individuals with overweight and obesity following the initial weight loss period.
- Target changing eating and exercise behaviors because sustained changes in both behaviors result in significant long-term weight loss and maintenance. Assist clients with achieving evidence-based recommendations for aerobic exercise during both the weight loss and weight loss maintenance phases.

Bariatric Surgery

Surgery for weight loss may be indicated for individuals with a BMI ≥40 kg · m^{-2} or those with comorbid risk factors and BMI ≥35 kg · m^{-2}. Comprehensive treatment following surgery includes exercise as there is evidence for enhanced weight loss (44,81); however, this has not been studied systematically. Exercise will likely facilitate the achievement and maintenance of energy balance postsurgery, and there is evidence that exercise improves insulin sensitivity and CRF following surgery (28). A multicenter National Institutes of Health–sponsored trial is underway (*i.e.*, or Longitudinal Assessment of Bariatric Surgery [LABS]) (75). When the results are published, they will provide the most comprehensive findings for exercise and bariatric surgery to date (67). Preliminary data from the LABS trial reported that the majority of those undergoing bariatric surgery increased their PA levels postsurgery, but 24%–29% were less active than prior to surgery (68).

Once individuals are cleared for exercise by their physician after surgery, a progressive exercise program for all individuals should follow the FITT principle of Ex R_x for weight loss and maintenance for overweight and obese individuals as listed previously in this section. Those with a prior history of orthopedic injuries should be assessed to reduce the risk of aggravation by weight-bearing exercise. In those for whom excessive body weight may limit the ability to engage in weight-bearing exercise or continuous exercise, intermittent exercise and non–weight-bearing alternatives should be considered. Subsequently, continuous exercise and weight-bearing exercise such as walking may be slowly introduced to make up a greater portion of the exercise program.

ONLINE RESOURCES

American College of Sports Medicine Position Stand on Overweight and Obesity: http://www.acsm.org

National Heart, Lung, and Blood Institute. Clinical Guidelines on the Identification, Evaluation, and Treatment of Overweight and Obesity in Adults: The Evidence Report:
http://www.nhlbi.nih.gov/health-pro/guidelines/archive/clinical-guidelines -obesity-adults-evidence-report

REFERENCES

1. Abate M, Schiavone C, Pelotti P, Salini V. Limited joint mobility (LJM) in elderly subjects with type II diabetes mellitus. *Arch Gerontol Geriatr*. 2011;53(2):135–40.
2. Achar S, Rostamian A, Narayan SM. Cardiac and metabolic effects of anabolic-androgenic steroid abuse on lipids, blood pressure, left ventricular dimensions, and rhythm. *Am J Cardiol*. 2010;106(6):893–901.
3. Alberti KG, Eckel RH, Grundy SM, et al. Harmonizing the metabolic syndrome. A joint interim statement of the International Diabetes Federation Task Force on Epidemiology and Prevention; National Heart, Lung, and Blood Institute; American Heart Association; World Heart Federation; International Atherosclerosis Society; and International Association for the Study of Obesity. *Circulation*. 2009;120:1640–5.
4. Alberti KG, Zimmet PZ. Definition, diagnosis and classification of diabetes mellitus and its complications. Part 1: diagnosis and classification of diabetes mellitus provisional report of a WHO consultation. *Diabet Med*. 1998:15(7):539–53.
5. Allen NA, Fain JA, Braun B, Chipkin SR. Continuous glucose monitoring counseling improves physical activity behaviors of individuals with type 2 diabetes: a randomized clinical trial. *Diabetes Res Clin Pract*. 2008;80(3):371–9.
6. Altena TS, Michaelson JL, Ball SD, Guilford BL, Thomas TR. Lipoprotein subfraction changes after continuous or intermittent exercise training. *Med Sci Sports Exerc*. 2006;38(2):367–72.
7. American College of Sports Medicine, Armstrong LE, Casa DJ, et al. American College of Sports Medicine position stand. Exertional heat illness during training and competition. *Med Sci Sports Exerc*. 2007;39(3):556–72.
8. American College of Sports Medicine, Chodzko-Zajko WJ, Proctor DN, et al. American College of Sports Medicine position stand. Exercise and physical activity for older adults. *Med Sci Sports Exerc*. 2009;41(7):1510–30.
9. American College of Sports Medicine, Sawka MN, Burke LM, et al. American College of Sports Medicine position stand. Exercise and fluid replacement. *Med Sci Sports Exerc*. 2007;39(2): 377–90.
10. American Diabetes Association. Section 2: classification and diagnosis of diabetes. *Diabetes Care*. 2015;38(1 Suppl):S8–16.
11. American Diabetes Association. Section 4: foundations of care: education, nutrition, physical activity, smoking cessation, psychosocial care, and immunization. *Diabetes Care*. 2015;38 (1 Suppl):S20–30.

12. Balducci S, Zanuso S, Cardelli P, et al. Effect of high- versus low-intensity supervised aerobic and resistance training on modifiable cardiovascular risk factors in type 2 diabetes; the Italian Diabetes and Exercise Study (IDES). *PLoS One*. 2012;7(11):e49297.

13. Bax JJ, Young LH, Frye RL, et al. Screening for coronary artery disease in patients with diabetes. *Diabetes Care*. 2007;30:2729–36.

14. Biswas A, Oh PI, Faulkner GE, et al. Sedentary time and its association with risk for disease incidence, mortality, and hospitalization in adults: a systematic review and meta-analysis. *Ann Intern Med*. 2015;162(2):123–32.

15. Braith RW, Stewart K. Resistance exercise training: its role in the prevention of cardiovascular disease. *Circulation*. 2006;113:2642–50.

16. Bremer JP, Jauch-Chara K, Hallschmid M, Schmid S, Schultes B. Hypoglycemia unawareness in older compared with middle-aged patients with type 2 diabetes. *Diabetes Care*. 2009;32(8):1513–7.

17. Burge MR, Garcia N, Qualls CR, Schade DS. Differential effects of fasting and dehydration in the pathogenesis of diabetic ketoacidosis. *Metabolism*. 2001;50(2):171–7.

18. Castellani JW, Young AJ, Ducharme MB, et al. American College of Sports Medicine position stand: prevention of cold injuries during exercise. *Med Sci Sports Exerc*. 2006;38(11):2012–29.

19. Cawley J, Meyerhoefer C. The medical care costs of obesity: an instrumental variables approach. *J Health Econ*. 2012;31:219–30.

20. Centers for Disease Control and Prevention. *National Diabetes Statistics Report, 2014* [Internet]. Atlanta (GA): U.S. Department of Health and Human Services; [cited 2014 Jan 14]. Available from: http://www.cdc.gov/diabetes/pubs/statsreport14/national-diabetes-report-web.pdf

21. Chobanian AV, Bakris GL, Black HR, et al. The Seventh Report of the Joint National Committee on Prevention, Detection, Evaluation, and Treatment of High Blood Pressure: the JNC 7 report. *JAMA*. 2003;289(19):2560–72.

22. Chu L, Hamilton J, Riddell MC. Clinical management of the physically active patient with type 1 diabetes. *Phys Sportsmed*. 2011;39(2):64–77.

23. Church TS, Blair SN, Cocreham S, et al. Effects of aerobic and resistance training on hemoglobin A1c levels in patients with type 2 diabetes: a randomized controlled trial. *JAMA*. 2010;304(20):2253–62.

24. Churilla JR, Fitzhugh EC, Thompson DL. The metabolic syndrome: how definition impacts the prevalence and risk in U.S. adults: 1999–2004 NHANES. *Metab Syndr Relat Disord*. 2007;5(4):331–42.

25. Churilla JR, Magyari PM, Ford ES, Fitzhugh EC, Johnson TM. Muscular strengthening activity patterns and metabolic health risk among US adults. *J Diabetes*. 2012;4:77–84.

26. Churilla JR, Zoeller R. Physical activity: physical activity and the metabolic syndrome: a review of the evidence. *Am J Lifestyle Med*. 2008;2:118–25.

27. Clinical guidelines on the identification, evaluation, and treatment of overweight and obesity in adults — the evidence report. National Institutes of Health. *Obes Res*. 1998;(6 Suppl 2):51S–209S.

28. Coen PM, Tanner CJ, Helbling NL, et al. Clinical trial demonstrates exercise following bariatric surgery improves insulin sensitivity. *J Clin Invest*. 2015;125(1):248–57.

29. Colberg SR, Albright AL, Blissmer BJ, et al. Exercise and type 2 diabetes: American College of Sports Medicine and the American Diabetes Association: joint position statement. Exercise and type 2 diabetes. *Med Sci Sports Exerc*. 2010;42(12):2282–303.

30. Colberg SR, Riddell MC. Physical activity: regulation of glucose metabolism, clinical management strategies and weight control. In: Peters A, Laffel L, editors. *American Diabetes Association/JDRF Type 1 Diabetes Sourcebook*. Alexandria (VA): American Diabetes Association; 2013. p. 249–92.

31. Colberg SR, Swain DP, Vinik AI. Use of heart rate reserve and rating of perceived exertion to prescribe exercise intensity in diabetic autonomic neuropathy. *Diabetes Care*. 2003;26(4):986–90.

32. Curioni CC, Lourenço PM. Long-term weight loss after diet and exercise: a systematic review. *Int J Obes*. 2005;29:1168–74.

33. Daniels SR, Jacobson MS, McCrindle BW, Eckel RH, Sanner BM. American Heart Association Childhood Obesity Research Summit Report. *Circulation*. 2009;119(15):e489–517.

34. Dattilo AM, Kris-Etherton PM. Effects of weight reduction on blood lipids and lipoproteins: a meta-analysis. *Am J Clin Nutr*. 1992;56(2):320–8.

35. Dela F, Larsen JJ, Mikines KJ, Ploug T, Petersen LN, Galbo H. Insulin-stimulated muscle glucose clearance in patients with NIDDM. Effects of one-legged physical training. *Diabetes*. 1995;44(9):1010–20.

36. D'hooge R, Hellinckx T, Van Laethem C, et al. Influence of combined aerobic and resistance training on metabolic control, cardiovascular fitness and quality of life in adolescents with type 1 diabetes: a randomized controlled trial. *Clin Rehabil*. 2011;25(4):349–59.

37. Donnelly JE, Blair SN, Jakicic JM, et al. American College of Sports Medicine position stand. Appropriate physical activity intervention strategies for weight loss and prevention of weight regain for adults. *Med Sci Sports Exerc*. 2009;41(2):459–71.

38. Donnelly JE, Jakicic JM, Pronk NP, et al. Is resistance exercise effective for weight management? *Evid Based Prev Med*. 2004;1(1):21–9.

39. Dubé JJ, Allison KF, Rousson V, Goodpaster BH, Amati F. Exercise dose and insulin sensitivity: relevance for diabetes prevention. *Med Sci Sports Exerc*. 2012;44(5):793–9.

40. Dunstan DW, Daly RM, Owen N, et al. High-intensity resistance training improves glycemic control in older patients with type 2 diabetes. *Diabetes Care*. 2002;25(10):1729–36.

41. Dunstan DW, Daly RM, Owen N, et al. Home-based resistance training is not sufficient to maintain improved glycemic control following supervised training in older individuals with type 2 diabetes. *Diabetes Care*. 2005;28(1):3–9.

42. Earnest CP, Johannsen NM, Swift DL, et al. Aerobic and strength training in concomitant metabolic syndrome and type 2 diabetes. *Med Sci Sports Exerc*. 2014;46(7):1293–301.

43. Eckel RH, Jakicic JM, Ard JD, et al. 2013 AHA/ACC guideline on lifestyle management to reduce cardiovascular risk: a report of the American College of Cardiology/American Heart Association Task Force on Practice Guidelines. *Circulation*. 2014;129(25 Suppl 2):S76–99.

44. Egberts K, Brown WA, Brennan L, O'Brien PE. Does exercise improve weight loss after bariatric surgery? A systematic review. *Obes Surg*. 2012;22:335–41.

45. Fanelli C, Pampanelli S, Lalli C, et al. Long-term intensive therapy of IDDM patients with clinically overt autonomic neuropathy: effects on hypoglycemia awareness and counterregulation. *Diabetes*. 1997;46(7):1172–81.

46. Fletcher GF, Ades PA, Kligfield P, et al. Exercise standards for testing and training: a scientific statement from the American Heart Association. *Circulation*. 2013;128(8):873–934.

47. Galbo H, Tobin L, van Loon LJ. Responses to acute exercise in type 2 diabetes, with an emphasis on metabolism and interaction with oral hypoglycemic agents and food intake. *Appl Physiol Nutr Metab*. 2007;32(3):567–75.

48. Garber CE, Blissmer B, Deschenes MR, et al. American College of Sports Medicine position stand. Quantity and quality of exercise for developing and maintaining cardiorespiratory, musculoskeletal, and neuromotor fitness in apparently healthy adults: guidance for prescribing exercise. *Med Sci Sports Exerc*. 2011;43(7):1334–59.

49. Go AS, Mozaffarian D, Roger VL, et al. Heart disease and stroke statistics—2014 update: a report from the American Heart Association. *Circulation*. 2014;129:e28–292.

50. Goff DC Jr, Bertoni AG, Kramer H, et al. Dyslipidemia prevalence, treatment, and control in the Multi-Ethnic Study of Atherosclerosis (MESA): gender, ethnicity, and coronary artery calcium. *Circulation*. 2006;113(5):647–56.

51. Goff DC Jr, Lloyd-Jones DM, Bennett G, et al. 2013 ACC/AHA guideline on the assessment of cardiovascular risk: a report of the American College of Cardiology/American Heart Association Task Force on Practice Guidelines. *Circulation*. 2014;129(25 Suppl 2):S49–73.

52. Grundy SM, Cleeman JI, Daniels SR, et al. Diagnosis and management of the metabolic syndrome: an American Heart Association/National Heart, Lung, and Blood Institute Scientific Statement. *Circulation*. 2005;112(17):2735–52.

53. Guelfi KJ, Ratnam N, Smythe GA, Jones TW, Fournier PA. Effect of intermittent high-intensity compared with continuous moderate exercise on glucose production and utilization in individuals with type 1 diabetes. *Am J Physiol Endocrinol Metab*. 2007;292(3):E865–70.

54. Gurven M, Blackwell AD, Rodríguez DE, Stieglitz J, Kaplan H. Does blood pressure inevitably rise with age? Longitudinal evidence among forager-horticulturalists. *Hypertension*. 2012;60:25–33.

55. Haskell WL, Lee IM, Pate RR, et al. Physical activity and public health: updated recommendation for adults from the American College of Sports Medicine and the American Heart Association. *Med Sci Sports Exerc*. 2007;39(8):1423–34.

56. Hinderliter A, Sherwood A, Gullette EC, et al. Reduction of left ventricular hypertrophy after exercise and weight loss in overweight patients with mild hypertension. *Arch Intern Med.* 2002;162:1333–9.
57. Hopkins PN, Toth PP, Ballantyne CM, Rader DJ, National Lipid Association Expert Panel on Familial Hypercholesterolemia. Familial hypercholesterolemias: prevalence, genetics, diagnosis and screening recommendations from the National Lipid Association Expert Panel on Familial Hypercholesterolemia. *J Clin Lipidol.* 2011;5(3 Suppl):S9–17.
58. Isomaa B, Almgren P, Tuomi T, et al. Cardiovascular morbidity and mortality associated with the metabolic syndrome. *Diabetes Care.* 2001;24(4):683–9.
59. Jakicic JM, Clark K, Coleman E, et al. American College of Sports Medicine position stand. Appropriate intervention strategies for weight loss and prevention of weight regain for adults. *Med Sci Sports Exerc.* 2001;33(12):2145–56.
60. James PA, Oparil S, Carter BL, et al. 2014 evidence-based guideline for the management of high blood pressure in adults: report from the panel members appointed to the Eighth Joint National Committee (JNC 8). *JAMA.* 2014;311(5):507–20.
61. Jensen MD, Ryan DH, Apovian CM, et al. 2013 AHA/ACC/TOS guideline for the management of overweight and obesity in adults: a report of the American College of Cardiology/American Heart Association Task Force on Practice Guidelines and The Obesity Society. *J Am Coll Cardiol.* 2014;63:25.
62. Karstoft K, Winding K, Knudsen SH, et al. Mechanisms behind the superior effects of interval vs continuous training on glycaemic control in individuals with type 2 diabetes: a randomised controlled trial. *Diabetologia.* 2014;57(10):2081–93.
63. Kaufman HW, Blatt AJ, Huang X, Odeh MA, Superko HR. Blood cholesterol trends 2001–2011 in the United States: analysis of 105 million patient records. *PloS One.* 2013;8(5):e63416.
64. Kearney PM, Whelton M, Reynolds K, Muntner P, Whelton PK, He J. Global burden of hypertension: analysis of worldwide data. *Lancet.* 2005;365(9455):217–23.
65. Kelley GA, Kelley KS. Impact of progressive resistance training on lipids and lipoproteins in adults: another look at a meta-analysis using prediction intervals. *Prev Med.* 2009;49(6):473–5.
66. Khayat ZA, Patel N, Klip A. Exercise- and insulin-stimulated muscle glucose transport: distinct mechanisms of regulation. *Can J Appl Physiol.* 2002;27(2):129–51.
67. King WC, Belle SH, Eid GM, et al. Physical activity levels of patients undergoing bariatric surgery in the Longitudinal Assessment of Bariatric Surgery study. *Surg Obes Relat Dis.* 2008;4(6):721–8.
68. King WC, Hsu JY, Belle SH, et al. Pre- to postoperative changes in physical activity: report from the Longitudinal Assessment of Bariatric Surgery-2 (LABS-2). *Surg Obes Relat Dis.* 2012;8(5):522–32.
69. Kitabchi AE, Umpierrez GE, Murphy MB, et al. Hyperglycemic crises in diabetes. *Diabetes Care.* 2004;27(Suppl 1):S94–102.
70. Knowler WC, Barrett-Connor E, Fowler SE, et al. Reduction in the incidence of type 2 diabetes with lifestyle intervention or metformin. *N Engl J Med.* 2002;346(6):393–403.
71. Kokkinos P. Cardiorespiratory fitness, exercise, and blood pressure. *Hypertension.* 2014;64:1160–4.
72. Kokkinos P, Pittaras A, Narayan P, Faselis C, Singh S, Manolis A. Exercise capacity and blood pressure associations with left ventricular mass in prehypertensive individuals. *Hypertension.* 2007;49:55–61.
73. Kokkinos PF, Narayan P, Colleran JA, et al. Effects of regular exercise on blood pressure and left ventricular hypertrophy in African-American men with severe hypertension. *N Engl J Med.* 1995;333:1462–7.
74. Kumanyika SK, Obarzanek E, Stettler N, et al. Population-based prevention of obesity: the need for comprehensive promotion of healthful eating, physical activity, and energy balance: a scientific statement from American Heart Association Council on Epidemiology and Prevention Interdisciplinary Committee for Prevention (formerly the Expert Panel on Population and Prevention Science). *Circulation.* 2008;118(4):428–64.
75. *Longitudinal Assessment of Bariatric Surgery* [Internet]. Pittsburgh (PA): University of Pittsburgh Epidemiology Data Center; [cited 2014 Dec 5]. Available from: http://www.edc.gsph.pitt.edu/labs/
76. Macfarlane DJ, Taylor LH, Cuddihy TF. Very short intermittent vs continuous bouts of activity in sedentary adults. *Prev Med.* 2006;43(4):332–6.
77. MacLeod SF, Terada T, Chahal BS, Boulé NG. Exercise lowers postprandial glucose but not fasting glucose in type 2 diabetes: a meta-analysis of studies using continuous glucose monitoring. *Diabetes Metab Res Rev.* 2013;29(8):593–603.

78. Mann S, Beedie C, Balducci S, et al. Changes in insulin sensitivity in response to different modalities of exercise: a review of the evidence. *Diabetes Metab Res Rev*. 2014;30:257–68.

79. McMahon SK, Ferreira LD, Ratnam N, et al. Glucose requirements to maintain euglycemia after moderate-intensity afternoon exercise in adolescents with type 1 diabetes are increased in a biphasic manner. *J Clin Endocrinol Metab*. 2007;92(3):963–8.

80. Mozumdar A, Liguori G. Persistent increase of prevalence of metabolic syndrome among U.S. adults: NHANES III to NHANES 1999–2006. *Diabetes Care*. 2011;34(1):216–9.

81. Mundi MS, Lorentz PA, Swain J, Grothe K, Collazo-Clavell M. Moderate physical activity as predictor of weight loss after bariatric surgery. *Obes Surg*. 2013;23:1645–9.

82. National Cholesterol Education Program (NCEP) Expert Panel on Detection, Evaluation, and Treatment of High Blood Cholesterol in Adults (Adult Treatment Panel III). Third Report of the National Cholesterol Education Program (NCEP) Expert Panel on Detection, Evaluation, and Treatment of High Blood Cholesterol in Adults (Adult Treatment Panel III) final report. *Circulation*. 2002;106(25):3143–421.

83. Nelson ME, Rejeski WJ, Blair SN, et al. Physical activity and public health in older adults: recommendation from the American College of Sports Medicine and the American Heart Association. *Circulation*. 2007;116:1094–105.

84. Ogden CL, Carroll MD, Kit BK, Flegal KM. Prevalence of childhood and adult obesity in the United States, 2011–2012. *JAMA*. 2014;311(8):806–14.

85. Pate RR, Pratt M, Blair SN, et al. Physical activity and public health. A recommendation from the Centers for Disease Control and Prevention and the American College of Sports Medicine. *JAMA*. 1995;273(5):402–7.

86. Perri MG, Anton SD, Durning PE, et al. Adherence to exercise prescriptions: effects of prescribing moderate versus higher levels of intensity and frequency. *Health Psychol*. 2002;21(5):452–8.

87. Pescatello LS, Franklin BA, Fagard R, et al. American College of Sports Medicine position stand. Exercise and hypertension. *Med Sci Sports Exerc*. 2004;36(3):533–53.

88. Pescatello LS, MacDonald HV, Ash GI, et al. Assessing the existing professional exercise recommendations for hypertension: a review and recommendations for future research priorities. *Mayo Clin Proc*. 2015;90(6):801–12.

89. Physical Activity Guidelines Advisory Committee. *Physical Activity Guidelines Advisory Committee Report, 2008* [Internet]. Washington (DC): U.S. Department of Health and Human Services; [cited 2016 Jan 18]. 683 p. Available from: http://www.health.gov/paguidelines/Report/pdf/CommitteeReport.pdf

90. Plöckinger U, Topuz M, Riese B, Reuter T. Risk of exercise-induced hypoglycaemia in patients with type 2 diabetes on intensive insulin therapy: comparison of insulin glargine with NPH insulin as basal insulin supplement. *Diabetes Res Clin Pract*. 2008;81(3):290–5.

91. Poirier P, Mawhinney S, Grondin L, et al. Prior meal enhances the plasma glucose lowering effect of exercise in type 2 diabetes. *Med Sci Sports Exerc*. 2001;33(8):1259–64.

92. Rosendorff C, Black HR, Cannon CP, et al. Treatment of hypertension in the prevention and management of ischemic heart disease: a scientific statement from the American Heart Association Council for High Blood Pressure Research and the Councils on Clinical Cardiology and Epidemiology and Prevention. *Circulation*. 2007;115(21):2761–88.

93. Sigal RJ, Fisher SJ, Halter JB, Vranic M, Marliss EB. Glucoregulation during and after intense exercise: effects of beta-adrenergic blockade in subjects with type 1 diabetes mellitus. *J Clin Endocrinol Metab*. 1999;84(11):3961–71.

94. Sigal RJ, Kenny GP, Boulé NG, et al. Effects of aerobic training, resistance training, or both on glycemic control in type 2 diabetes: a randomized trial. *Ann Intern Med*. 2007;147(6):357–69.

95. Snowling NJ, Hopkins WG. Effects of different modes of exercise training on glucose control and risk factors for complications in type 2 diabetic patients: a meta-analysis. *Diabetes Care*. 2006;29(11):2518–27.

96. Stone NJ, Robinson JG, Lichtenstein AH, et al. 2013 ACC/AHA guideline on the treatment of blood cholesterol to reduce atherosclerotic cardiovascular risk in adults: a report of the American College of Cardiology/American Heart Association Task Force on Practice Guidelines. *Circulation*. 2014;129(25 Suppl 2):S1–45.

97. Svien LR, Berg P, Stephenson C. Issues in aging with cerebral palsy. *Top Geriatr Rehabil*. 2008;24(1):26–40.

98. Tang JL, Armitage JM, Lancaster T, Silagy CA, Fowler GH, Neil HA. Systematic review of dietary intervention trials to lower blood total cholesterol in free-living subjects. *BMJ*. 1998;316(7139):1213–20.

99. *The IDF Consensus Worldwide Definition of the Metabolic Syndrome* [Internet]. Brussels (Belgium): International Diabetes Federation; [cited 2016 Jan 18]. Available from: http://www.idf.org/webdata/docs/IDF_Meta_def_final.pdf

100. Umpierre D, Ribeiro PA, Kramer CK, et al. Physical activity advice only or structured exercise training and association with HbA1c levels in type 2 diabetes: a systematic review and meta-analysis. *JAMA*. 2011;305(17):1790–9.

101. Unnithan VB, Clifford C, Bar-Or O. Evaluation by exercise testing of the child with cerebral palsy. *Sports Med*. 1998;26(4):239–51.

102. U.S. Preventive Services Task Force. Screening for coronary heart disease: recommendation statement. *Ann Intern Med*. 2004;140(7):569–72.

103. U.S. Preventive Services Task Force, Barton M. Screening for obesity in children and adolescents: U.S. Preventive Services Task Force recommendation statement. *Pediatrics*. 2010;125(2):361–7.

104. Vasan RS, Larson MG, Leip EP, Kannel WB, Levy D. Assessment of frequency of progression to hypertension in non-hypertensive participants in the Framingham Heart Study: a cohort study. *Lancet*. 2001;358:1682–6.

105. Violan MA, Pomes T, Maldonado S, et al. Exercise capacity in hemodialysis and renal transplant patients. *Transplant Proc*. 2002;34(1):417–8.

106. Wackers FJ, Young LH, Inzucchi SE, et al. Detection of silent myocardial ischemia in asymptomatic diabetic subjects: the DIAD study. *Diabetes Care*. 2004;27(8):1954–61.

107. White LJ, McCoy SC, Castellano V, et al. Resistance training improves strength and functional capacity in persons with multiple sclerosis. *Mult Scler*. 2004;10(6):668–74.

108. Willey KA, Singh MA. Battling insulin resistance in elderly obese people with type 2 diabetes: bring on the heavy weights. *Diabetes Care*. 2003;26:1580–8.

109. Yang Z, Scott CA, Mao C, Tang J, Farmer AJ. Resistance exercise versus aerobic exercise for type 2 diabetes: a systematic review and meta-analysis. *Sports Med*. 2014;44(4):487–99.

110. Yardley JE, Kenny GP, Perkins BA, et al. Effects of performing resistance exercise before versus after aerobic exercise on glycemia in type 1 diabetes. *Diabetes Care*. 2012;35(4):669–75.

111. Young LH, Wackers FJ, Chyun DA, et al. Cardiac outcomes after screening for asymptomatic coronary artery disease in patients with type 2 diabetes: the DIAD study: a randomized controlled trial. *JAMA*. 2009;301(15):1547–55.

Exercise Testing and Prescription for Populations with Other Chronic Diseases and Health Conditions

INTRODUCTION

This chapter contains the exercise testing and exercise prescription (Ex R$_x$) guidelines and recommendations for individuals with chronic diseases and other health conditions not addressed in *Chapters 9* (cardiovascular and pulmonary) and *10* (metabolic). As with the other chapters, the Ex R$_x$ guidelines and recommendations are presented using the Frequency, Intensity, Time, and Type (*FITT*) principle of Ex R$_x$ based on the available professional society position papers and scientific statements or using other literature. The general principles of exercise testing are presented in *Chapter 5* and Ex R$_x$ in *Chapter 6*. In many instances, exercise training can be performed without a prior clinical exercise test. However, if an exercise test is to be performed, this chapter presents specific recommendations for individuals with various chronic diseases and health conditions. Note that information is often lacking regarding volume and progression of exercise training for the chronic diseases and health conditions presented in this chapter. In these instances, the guidelines and recommendations provided in *Chapter 6* for apparently healthy populations should be adapted with good clinical judgment for the chronic disease(s) and health condition(s) being targeted.

ARTHRITIS

Arthritis and other rheumatic diseases are the leading cause of disability in the United States (42), and worldwide, the burden of these musculoskeletal conditions is rapidly increasing (191). Among adults (≥18 years) in the United States, approximately 23% (52.5 million) report having a doctor's diagnosis of arthritis, of which around 43% (22.7 million) complain of arthritis-related physical activity (PA) limitations (44). Arthritis is characterized by pain, impaired physical function, fatigue, and adverse changes in body composition (*i.e.*, muscle loss and increased adiposity), with 66% of afflicted individuals either overweight or obese (264). Due to the aging population and high rate of obesity, the prevalence of physician-diagnosed arthritis is expected to increase to an estimated 67 million Americans by 2030 (130).

There are over 100 rheumatic diseases — two of the most common being osteoarthritis and rheumatoid arthritis. *Osteoarthritis* (OA) is a progressive local degenerative joint disease affecting one or multiple joints (*i.e.*, most commonly, the hands, hips, spine, and knees) and is associated with risk factors including overweight/obesity, history of joint injury or surgery, genetic predisposition, and aging. *Rheumatoid arthritis* (RA) is a chronic, systemic, inflammatory autoimmune disease of unknown etiology, in which the inflammatory response locally causes inflammation of the joint lining (synovitis); bony erosions; and, systemically, muscle loss, fat gain, and accelerated atherosclerosis (181). Other common rheumatic diseases include fibromyalgia (discussed later in this chapter), gout, spondyloarthropathies (*e.g.*, ankylosing spondylitis [AS], psoriatic arthritis, reactive arthritis, and enteropathic arthritis), and specific connective tissue diseases (*e.g.*, systemic lupus erythematosus, systemic sclerosis [scleroderma], and dermatomyositis).

Pharmaceutical treatment of arthritis primarily involves analgesics, glucocorticoids, nonsteroidal anti-inflammatory drugs (NSAIDs), and for RA, disease-modifying antirheumatic drugs (DMARDs). Optimal treatment of arthritis features a multidisciplinary approach involving patient education in self-management, occupational therapy, and exercise (63,125). When joint damage and loss of mobility is severe and restoration of a reasonable level of function and control of pain is no longer achievable by pharmacological and conservative management (*i.e.*, "end-stage" disease), total joint replacement and other surgeries are increasingly routine options.

Although pain and functional limitations can present challenges to PA among individuals with arthritis, regular exercise is essential for managing these conditions. For instance, due to reduced PA and the disease process itself, individuals with arthritis are more likely to have muscle wasting and be overweight than healthy individuals of the same age and sex (281). Exercise maintains or improves strength and aerobic capacity, thereby minimizing or preventing functional decline; attenuates pain and joint stiffness; aids in weight control and achieving a healthy body composition; reduces comorbidities such as cardiovascular disease (CVD), Type 2 diabetes mellitus (T2DM), metabolic syndrome (Metsyn), and osteoporosis; and improves mental health and quality of life (31,58,90,91,134,181).

Exercise Testing

Most individuals with arthritis tolerate symptom-limited exercise testing consistent with recommendations for apparently healthy adults (see *Chapters 4* and *5*). The following are special considerations for individuals with arthritis:

- High intensity exercise, as during a maximal stress test, is contraindicated when there is acute inflammation (*i.e.*, hot, swollen, and painful joints). If individuals are experiencing acute inflammation, exercise testing should be postponed until the flare-up has subsided.
- Although most individuals with arthritis tolerate treadmill walking, use of cycle leg ergometry or arm ergometry may be less painful for some and allow better

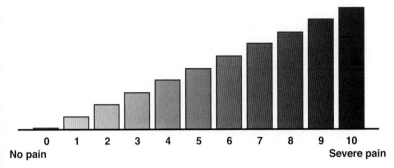

0 **1** **2** **3** **4** **5** **6** **7** **8** **9** **10**
No pain   **Severe pain**

Figure 11.1 Visual numeric pain scale. Reprinted with permission from (242).

assessment of cardiorespiratory function. The mode of exercise chosen should be that which is least painful for the individual being tested.

- Allow time for individuals to warm up (at a very light or light intensity level) according to each individual's functional status prior to beginning the graded exercise test (GXT).
- Monitor pain levels during testing using a validated pain scale such as the Borg CR10 Scale (see *Figure 5.2*) (28) and the visual numeric scale (*Figure 11.1*) (242).
- Muscle strength and endurance can be measured using standard protocols (see *Chapter 4*). However, the tester should be aware that pain may impair maximum voluntary muscle contraction in affected joints.

Exercise Prescription

A major barrier to individuals with arthritis starting an exercise program is a belief that exercise, particularly weight-bearing exercise, will exacerbate joint damage and symptoms such as pain and fatigue. This fear is prevalent not only among persons with arthritis but also among physicians and allied health professionals overseeing their disease management (190). Thus, individuals with arthritis need to be reassured that exercise is not only safe but is also generally reported to reduce pain, fatigue, inflammation, and disease activity (12,31,58,64,90,91,134). Those with arthritis, particularly those with pain and those who are deconditioned, should gradually progress to exercise intensities and volumes that provide clinically significant health benefits. In general, recommendations for Ex R_x are consistent with those for apparently healthy adults (see *Chapter 6*) with observance of FITT recommendations and additional consideration of an individual's disease activity, pain, functional limitations, and personal exercise/PA preferences. Although these recommendations will likely be appropriate for most persons with arthritis for both aerobic and resistance training, a patient's personal intensity preference needs to be considered to optimize adoption and adherence to exercise.

■ **FITT RECOMMENDATIONS FOR INDIVIDUALS WITH ARTHRITIS** (64,65,109,111,165,190,299)

FITT

	Aerobic	Resistance	Flexibility
Frequency	3–5 d · wk^{-1}	2–3 d · wk^{-1}	Daily
Intensity	Moderate (40%–59% $\dot{V}O_2R$ or HRR) to vigorous (≥60% $\dot{V}O_2R$ or HRR)	60%–80% 1-RM. Initial intensity should be lower (*i.e.*, 50%–60% 1-RM) for those unaccustomed to resistance training.	Move through ROM feeling tightness/stretch without pain. Progress ROM of each exercise only when there is very little or no joint pain.
Time	150 min · wk^{-1} of moderate intensity, 75 min · wk^{-1} of vigorous intensity, or an equivalent combination of the two	Use healthy adult values and adjust accordingly (*i.e.*, 8–12 repetitions for 2–4 sets); include all major muscle groups.	Up to 10 repetitions for dynamic movements; hold static stretched for 10–30 s.
Type	Activities with low joint stress, such as walking, cycling, swimming, or aquatic exercise	Machine or free weights. Body weight exercises might also be appropriate for select individuals.	A combination of dynamic and static stretching focused on all major joints

1-RM, one repetition maximum; HRR, heart rate reserve; ROM, range of motion; $\dot{V}O_2R$, oxygen uptake reserve.

Exercise Training Considerations

■ The goal of aerobic exercise training is to improve cardiorespiratory fitness (CRF) with little to no joint pain or damage. There is no clear evidence that persons with arthritis cannot engage in high-impact activities, such as running, stair climbing, and those with stop and go actions. But, because persons with arthritis often have lower levels of CRF and muscle strength, prior to engaging in high-impact activities, they should train carefully to minimize the chance of associated injuries and/or exacerbation of joint symptoms.

■ Long continuous bouts of aerobic exercise may initially be difficult for those who are very deconditioned and restricted by pain and joint mobility. It is appropriate to start with short bouts of 10 min (or less if needed).

■ In addition to improving muscular strength and endurance, resistance training may reduce pain and improve physical function.

- Flexibility training is important to enhance range of motion (ROM) and to avoid the negative effects of arthritis on joints.
- Adequate warm-up and cool-down periods (5–10 min) are critical for minimizing pain. Warm-up and cool-down activities should involve controlled movement of joints through their full ROM and very light or light intensity aerobic exercise.
- Individuals with significant pain and functional limitation may need interim goals shorter than the recommended duration of aerobic exercise and should be encouraged to undertake and maintain any amount of PA that they are able to perform. In the absence of specific recommendations for people with arthritis, the general population recommendation of increasing duration by 5–10 min every 1–2 wk over the first 4–6 wk of an exercise training program can be applied.

Special Considerations (180,183)

- Avoid strenuous exercises during acute flare-ups. However, it is appropriate to gently move joints through their full ROM during these periods.
- Inform individuals with arthritis that a small amount of discomfort in the muscles or joints during or immediately after exercise is common following performance of unfamiliar exercise and hence does not necessarily mean joints are being further damaged. However, if the patient's pain rating 2 h after exercising is higher than it was prior to exercise, the duration and/or intensity of exercise should be reduced in future sessions. Higher pain ratings 48–72 h after exercise may be due to delayed onset muscle soreness (DOMS), especially in those who are new to exercise.
- If specific exercises exacerbate joint pain, alternative exercises that work the same muscle groups and energy systems should be substituted.
- Encourage individuals with arthritis to exercise during the time of day when pain is typically least severe and/or in conjunction with peak activity of pain medications.
- Appropriate shoes that provide good shock absorption and stability are particularly important for individuals with arthritis. Shoe specialists can provide recommendations appropriate for an individual's biomechanics.
- Incorporate functional exercises such as the sit-to-stand, step-ups, stair climbing, and carrying to improve neuromuscular control, balance, and ability to perform activities of daily living (ADL).
- For pool-based exercise, a water temperature of 83° to 88° F (28° to 31° C) aids in relaxing and increasing the compliance of muscles and reducing pain.

ONLINE RESOURCES

Arthritis Foundation:
    http://www.arthritis.org
American College of Rheumatology:
    http://www.rheumatology.org

CANCER

Cancer is a group of nearly 200 diseases characterized by the uncontrolled growth and spread of abnormal cells resulting from damage to deoxyribonucleic acid (DNA) by internal factors (*e.g.,* inherited mutations) and environmental exposures (*e.g.,* tobacco smoke). Most cancers are classified according to the cell type from which they originate. Carcinomas develop from the epithelial cells of organs and compose at least 80% of all cancers. Other cancers arise from the cells of the blood (leukemia), immune system (lymphoma), and connective tissues (sarcoma). The lifetime prevalence of cancer is one in two for men and one in three for women (4). Cancer affects all ages but is most common in older adults. About 78% of all cancers are diagnosed in individuals ≥55 yr (4); hence, there is a strong likelihood that individuals diagnosed with cancer will have other chronic diseases (*e.g.,* cardiopulmonary disease, diabetes mellitus [DM], osteoporosis, arthritis) (23,33,54,56). Adding to the likelihood of the development of other chronic conditions is the fact that for many cancers, life expectancy is lengthening following diagnosis and treatment.

Treatment for cancer may involve surgery, radiation, chemotherapy, hormones, and immunotherapy. In the process of destroying cancer cells, some treatments also damage healthy tissue. Patients may experience side effects that limit their ability to exercise during treatment and afterward. These long-term and late effects of cancer treatment are described elsewhere (178). Furthermore, overall physical function is generally diminished (145,222). Even among cancer survivors who are 5 yr or more posttreatment, more than half report physical performance limitations for activities such as crouching/kneeling, standing for 2 h, lifting/carrying 10 lb (4.5 kg), and walking 0.25 mi (0.4 km) (201). In the following sections, we use the National Coalition for Cancer Survivorship definition of cancer survivor; that is, from the time of diagnosis to the rest of life, including cancer treatment (193).

Exercise Testing

A diagnosis of cancer and curative cancer treatments pose challenges for multiple body systems involved in performing exercise or affected by exercise. For example, survivors of breast cancer who have had lymph nodes removed may respond differently to inflammation and injury on the side of the body that underwent surgery, having implications for exercise testing and Ex R$_x$. Cancer and cancer therapy have the potential to affect the health-related components of physical fitness (*i.e.,* CRF, muscular strength and endurance, body composition, and flexibility) as well as neuromotor function.

Understanding how an individual has been affected by his or her cancer experience is important prior to exercise testing and designing the Ex R$_x$ for survivors of cancer during and after treatment (167). Every individual with cancer can have a unique experience and response. Because of the diversity in this patient population, the safety guidance for preexercise evaluations of cancer survivors focuses on general as well as cancer site–specific recommendations of the medical assessments (*Table 11.1*) (258).

TABLE 11.1

Preexercise Medical Assessments for Individuals with Cancer

Cancer Site	Breast	Prostate	Colon	Adult Hematologic (No HSCT)	Adult HSCT	Gynecologic
General medical assessments recommended prior to exercise	Recommend evaluation for peripheral neuropathies and musculoskeletal morbidities secondary to treatment regardless of time since treatment. If there has been hormonal therapy, recommend evaluation of fracture risk. Individuals with known metastatic disease to the bone will require evaluation to discern what is safe prior to starting exercise. Individuals with known cardiac conditions (secondary to cancer or not) require medical assessment of the safety of exercise prior to starting. There is always a risk that metastasis to the bone or cardiac toxicity secondary to cancer treatments will be undetected. This risk will vary widely across the population of survivors. Fitness professionals may want to consult with the patient's medical team to discern this likelihood. However, requiring medical assessment for metastatic disease and cardiotoxicity for all survivors prior to exercise is not recommended, as this would create an unnecessary barrier to obtaining the well-established health benefits of exercise for the majority of survivors, for whom metastasis and cardiotoxicity are unlikely to occur.					
Cancer site specific medical assessments recommended prior to starting an exercise program	Recommend evaluation for arm/shoulder morbidity prior to upper body exercise.	Evaluation of muscle strength & wasting.	Patient should be evaluated as having established consistent and proactive infection prevention behaviors for an existing ostomy prior to engaging in exercise training more vigorous than a walking program.	None	None	Patients with morbid obesity may require additional medical assessment for the safety of activity beyond cancer-specific risk. Recommend evaluation for lower extremity lymphedema prior to vigorous aerobic exercise or resistance training.

HSCT, hematopoietic stem cell transplantation.

Reprinted with permission from (259).

Standard exercise testing methods are generally appropriate for patients with cancer who have been medically cleared for exercise with the following considerations:

■ Ideally, patients with cancer should receive a comprehensive assessment of all components of health-related physical fitness (see *Chapter 4*). However, requiring a comprehensive physical fitness assessment prior to starting exercise may create an unnecessary barrier to starting activity. For this reason, no assessments are required to start a light intensity walking, progressive strength training, or flexibility program in most survivors.

■ Be aware of a survivor's health history, comorbid chronic diseases and health conditions, and any exercise contraindications before commencing health-related fitness assessments or designing the Ex R_x (*Figure 11.2*) (194).

■ Health-related fitness assessments may be valuable for evaluating the degree to which musculoskeletal strength and endurance or CRF have been affected by cancer-related fatigue or other commonly experienced symptoms that impact function (176).

■ There is no evidence the level of medical supervision required for symptom-limited or maximal exercise testing needs to be different for patients with cancer than for other populations (see *Chapter 5*).

■ It is important for exercise professionals to understand the most common toxicities associated with cancer treatments including increased risk for fractures, cardiovascular events, and neuropathies related to specific types of treatment and musculoskeletal morbidities secondary to treatment (178,194). The evidence-based literature indicates one repetition maximum (1-RM) testing is safe among survivors of breast cancer (258).

Exercise Prescription

Survivors of cancer should avoid physical inactivity during and after treatment. A single, precise recommendation regarding the FITT principle of Ex R_x is not possible, given the diversity of the population affected by cancer. The American College of Sports Medicine (ACSM) expert panel on guidelines for exercise in adult survivors of cancer concluded there is ample evidence exercise is safe both during and after treatment for all types of cancer reviewed (*i.e.*, breast, prostate, colon, hematologic, and gynecologic cancers) (258). Overall recommendations for survivors of cancer are consistent with the guidelines provided in *Chapter 6* and with the ACSM, National Comprehensive Cancer Network, and American Cancer Society's recommendation of 30–60 min of moderate-to-vigorous intensity PA at least 5 d · wk^{-1} (194,244). It is important to note, however, that the FITT principle of Ex R_x recommendations for individuals with cancer that follow are based on limited literature. The appropriate FITT recommendations will vary across the cancer experience and require individualization of the Ex R_x. Special considerations needed to ensure the safety of this potentially vulnerable population are in *Table 11.2* (258). To date, there is no evidence base from which to make recommendations regarding the supervision of exercise across the continuum of survivorship or in various exercise settings (*e.g.,* home, health/fitness, clinical). Exercise professionals should use good judgment in deciding the level of exercise supervision needed on an individual basis.

■ FITT RECOMMENDATIONS FOR INDIVIDUALS WITH CANCER
(194,196,258,259)

FITT	Aerobic	Resistance	Flexibility
Frequency	3–5 d · wk^{-1}	2–3 d · wk^{-1}	≥2–3 d · wk^{-1} with daily being most effective
Intensity	Moderate (40%–59% $\dot{V}O_2R$; 64%–75% HR_{max}; RPE of 12–13) to vigorous (60%–89% $\dot{V}O_2R$; 76%–95% HR_{max}; RPE of 14–17)	Start with low resistance (*e.g.,* <30% 1-RM) and progress with smallest increments possible.	Move through ROM as tolerated.
Time	75 min · wk^{-1} of vigorous intensity or 150 min · wk^{-1} of moderate intensity activity or an equivalent combination of the two	At least 1 set of 8–12 repetitions	10–30 s hold for static stretching
Type	Prolonged, rhythmic activities using large muscle groups (*e.g.,* walking, cycling, swimming)	Free weights, resistance machines, or weight-bearing functional tasks (*e.g.,* sit-to-stand) targeting all major muscle groups	Stretching or ROM exercises for all major muscle groups. Address specific areas of joint or muscle restriction that may have resulted from treatment with steroids, radiation, or surgery.

1-RM, one repetition maximum; HR_{max}, maximal heart rate; HRR, heart rate reserve; ROM, range of motion; RPE, rating of perceived exertion; $\dot{V}O_2R$, oxygen uptake reserve.

PHYSICAL ACTIVITY ASSESSMENT

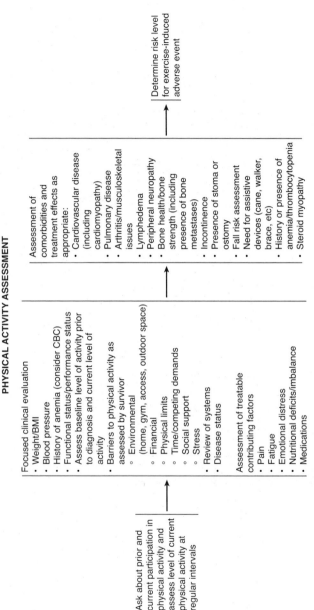

Ask about prior and current participation in physical activity and assess level of current physical activity at regular intervals

→

Focused clinical evaluation
- Weight/BMI
- Blood pressure
- History of anemia (consider CBC)
- Functional status/performance status
- Assess baseline level of activity prior to diagnosis and current level of activity
- Barriers to physical activity as assessed by survivor
  ○ Environmental (home, gym, access, outdoor space)
  ○ Financial
  ○ Physical limits
  ○ Time/competing demands
  ○ Social support
  ○ Stress
- Review of systems
- Disease status

Assessment of treatable contributing factors
- Pain
- Fatigue
- Emotional distress
- Nutritional deficits/imbalance
- Medications

→

Assessment of comorbidities and treatment effects as appropriate:
- Cardiovascular disease (including cardiomyopathy)
- Pulmonary disease
- Arthritis/musculoskeletal issues
- Lymphedema
- Peripheral neuropathy
- Bone health/bone strength (including presence of bone metastases)
- Incontinence
- Presence of stoma or ostomy
- Fall risk assessment
- Need for assistive devices (cane, walker, brace, etc)
- History or presence of anemia/thrombocytopenia
- Steroid myopathy

→

Determine risk level for exercise-induced adverse event

Figure 11.2 Recommendations for assessments prior to exercise among participants with a history of cancer. Reproduced with permission from (194). BMI, body mass index; CBC, complete blood count.

TABLE 11.2

Review of U.S. DHHS Physical Activity Guidelines (PAGs) for Americans and Alterations Needed for Cancer Survivors

	Breast	Prostate	Colon	Adult Hematologic (No HSCT)	Adult HSCT	Gynecologic
General Statement	Avoid inactivity, return to normal daily activities as quickly as possible after surgery. Continue normal daily activities and exercise as much as possible during and after non-surgical treatments. Individuals with known metastatic bone disease will require modifications to avoid fractures. Individuals with cardiac conditions (secondary to cancer or not) may require modifications and may require greater supervision for safety.					
Aerobic exercise training (volume, intensity, progression)	Recommendations are the same as age appropriate guidelines from the PAGs for Americans.				Ok to exercise every day, lighter intensity and lower progression of intensity recommended.	Recommendations are the same as age appropriate guidelines from the PAGs for Americans. Women with morbid obesity may require additional supervision and altered programming.
Cancer site specific comments on aerobic exercise training prescriptions	Be aware of fracture risk.	Be aware of increased potential for fracture.	Physician permission recommended for patients with an ostomy prior to participation in contact sports (risk of blow).	None	Care should be taken to avoiding overtraining given immune effects of vigorous exercise.	If peripheral neuropathy is present, a stationary bike might be preferable over weight bearing exercise.

(continued)

TABLE 11.2

Review of U.S. DHHS Physical Activity Guidelines (PAGs) for Americans and Alterations Needed for Cancer Survivors (Continued)

	Breast	Prostate	Colon	Adult Hematologic (No HSCT)	Adult HSCT	Gynecologic
Resistance training (volume, intensity, progression)	Altered recommendations. See below.	Recommendations same as age appropriate PAGs.	Altered recommendations. See below.	Recommendations same as age appropriate PAGs.	Recommendations same as age appropriate PAGs.	Altered recommendations. See below.
Cancer site specific comments on resistance training prescription	Start with a supervised program of at least 16 sessions and very low resistance, progress resistance at small increments. No upper limit on the amount of weight to which survivors can progress. Watch for arm/shoulder symptoms, including lymphedema, and reduce resistance or stop specific exercises according to symptom response. If a break is taken, lower the level of resistance by 2 wk worth for every wk of no exercise (e.g., a 2 wk exercise vacation = lower to the resistance used 4 wk ago). Be aware of risk for fracture in this population.	Add pelvic floor exercises for those who undergo radical prostatectomy. Be aware of risk for fracture.	Recommendations same as age-appropriate PAGs. For patients with a stoma, start with low resistance and progress resistance slowly to avoid herniation at the stoma.	None	Resistance training might be more important than aerobic exercise in BMT patients. See text for further discussion on this point.	There is no data on the safety of resistance training in women with lower limb lymphedema secondary to gynecologic cancer. This condition is very complex to manage. It may not be possible to extrapolate from the findings on upper limb lymphedema. Proceed with caution if the patient has had lymph node removal and/or radiation to lymph nodes in the groin.

Flexibility training (volume, intensity, progression)	Recommendations are the same as age appropriate PAGs for Americans.	Research gap.	Recommendations same as age appropriate PAGs, with care to avoid excessive intraabdominal pressure for patients with ostomies.	Recommendations are the same as age appropriate PAGs for Americans.	
Exercises with special considerations (e.g., yoga, organized sports, and Pilates)	Yoga appears safe as long as arm and shoulder morbidities are taken into consideration. Dragon boat racing not empirically tested, but the volume of participants provides face validity of safety for this activity. No evidence on organized sport or Pilates.	Research gap.	If an ostomy is present, modifications will be needed for swimming or contact sports. Research gap.	Research gap.	Research gap.

BMT, bone marrow transplantation; HSCT, hematopoietic stem cell transplantation; U.S. DHHS, U.S. Department of Health and Human Services.

Exercise Prescription Considerations

- Awareness of the highly variable impact of exercise on symptoms in those undergoing treatment is needed (259).
- Slower progression may be needed compared to healthy adults. If exercise progression leads to an increase in fatigue or other common adverse symptoms as a result of prescribed exercise, the FITT principle of Ex R$_x$ should be reduced to a level that is better tolerated.
- Survivors who have completed treatment can gradually increase exercise duration when tolerated and without exacerbation of symptoms or side effects for all activities. The frequency of aerobic exercise should be increased gradually from the current PA level to 3–5 d · wk^{-1}.
- If tolerated without adverse effects of symptoms or side effects, the Ex R$_x$ need not differ from healthy populations.
- There is a recent indication that heart rate reserve (HRR) may be less reliable for monitoring aerobic exercise intensity for cancer survivors currently undergoing treatment or early posttreatment due to differences in resting and maximal heart rate (HR) values; educating survivors to use perceived exertion to monitor intensity or using a percentage of maximal heart rate (HR$_{max}$) may be advisable (254).
- Individuals with lymphedema should wear a compression sleeve during resistance training activity (194,196).
- Survivors of breast and gynecologic cancer should consider beginning a supervised resistance training program (48).
- Flexibility exercise can be implemented even during active treatment. Focus on joints in which a loss of ROM occurred because of surgery, corticosteroid use, and/or radiation therapy (177).
- Evidence indicates even those currently undergoing systemic cancer treatments can increase daily PA sessions over the course of 1 mo (258).
- Several short bouts per day rather than a single bout may be useful, particularly during active treatment.

Special Considerations

- Up to 90% of all survivors of cancer will experience cancer-related fatigue at some point (280). Cancer-related fatigue is prevalent in patients receiving chemotherapy and radiation and may prevent or restrict the ability to exercise. In some cases, fatigue may persist for months or years after treatment completion. However, survivors are advised to avoid physical inactivity, even during treatment, given evidence that aerobic exercise improves fatigue (32).
- Bone is a common site of metastases in many cancers, particularly breast, prostate, lung cancer, and multiple myeloma. Survivors with metastatic disease to the bone will require modification of their exercise program (*e.g.*, reduced impact, intensity, volume) given the increased risk of bone fragility and fractures (194).
- Cachexia or muscle wasting is prevalent in individuals with advanced gastrointestinal cancers and may limit exercise capacity, depending on the extent of muscle wasting.

■ Identify when a patient/client is in an immune suppressed state (*e.g.*, taking immunosuppressive medications after a bone marrow transplant or those undergoing chemotherapy or radiation therapy). There may be times when exercising at home or a medical setting would be more advisable than exercising in a public fitness facility.

■ Swimming should not be prescribed for patients with indwelling catheters or central lines and feeding tubes, those with ostomies, those in an immune suppressed state, or those receiving radiation.

■ Patients receiving chemotherapy may experience fluctuating periods of sickness and fatigue during treatment cycles that require frequent modifications to the Ex R$_x$ such as periodically reducing the intensity and/or time (duration) of the exercise session during symptomatic periods.

■ Safety considerations for exercise training for patients with cancer are presented in *Table 11.3*. More information on safety considerations for patients with cancer can be found elsewhere (194,196). In general, exercise should not be performed immediately following surgery among those with severe anemia, a worsening condition, or an active infection (258). As with other populations, the risks associated with PA must be balanced against the risks of physical inactivity for survivors of cancer. As with other populations, exercise should be stopped if unusual symptoms are experienced (*e.g.*, dizziness, nausea, chest pain).

ONLINE RESOURCES

American Cancer Society:
http://www.cancer.org
American College of Sports Medicine Expert Panel Report on Exercise and Cancer:
http://www.acsm.org
National Academies Press (*From Cancer Patient to Survivor*, 2011):
http://www.nap.edu/catalog.php?record_id=11468#toc
National Comprehensive Cancer Network:
http://www.nccn.org/professionals/physician_gls/f_guidelines.asp#supportive

CEREBRAL PALSY

Cerebral palsy (CP) is a nonprogressive lesion of the brain occurring before, at, or soon after birth that interferes with normal brain development. CP is caused by damage to areas of the brain that control and coordinate muscle tone, reflexes, posture, and movement. The resulting impact on muscle tone and reflexes depends on the location and extent of the injury within the brain. Consequently, the type and severity of dysfunction vary considerably among individuals with CP. In developed countries, the incidence of CP is reported to be between 1.5 and 5 per 1,000 live births.

Despite its diverse manifestations, CP predominantly exists in two forms: spastic (70% of those with CP) (169) and athetoid (293). *Spastic CP* is characterized by an increased muscle tone typically involving the flexor muscle groups of the upper

TABLE 11.3

Contraindications for Starting Exercise, Stopping Exercise, and Injury Risk for Cancer Survivors

	Breast	Prostate	Colon	Adult Hematologic (No HSCT)	Adult HSCT	Gynecologic
General contraindications for starting an exercise program common across all cancer sites	Allow adequate time to heal after surgery. The number of weeks required for surgical recovery may be as high as 8. Do not exercise individuals who are experiencing fever, extreme fatigue, significant anemia, or ataxia. Follow *ACSM Guidelines* for exercise prescription with regard to cardiovascular and pulmonary contraindications for starting an exercise program. However, the potential for an adverse cardiopulmonary event might be higher among cancer survivors than age matched comparisons given the toxicity of radiotherapy and chemotherapy and long term/late effects of cancer surgery.					
Cancer specific contraindications for starting an exercise program	Women with acute arm or shoulder problems secondary to breast cancer treatment should seek medical care to resolve those issues prior to exercise training with the upper body.	None	Physician permission recommended for patients with an ostomy prior to participation in contact sports (risk of blow), weight training (risk of hernia).	None	None	Women with swelling or inflammation in the abdomen, groin, or lower extremity should seek medical care to resolve these issues prior to exercise training with the lower body.
Cancer specific reasons for stopping an exercise program. (Note: General *ACSM Guidelines* for stopping exercise remain in place for this population.)	Changes in arm/shoulder symptoms or swelling should result in reductions or avoidance of upper body exercise until after appropriate medical evaluation and treatment resolves the issue.	None	Hernia, ostomy related systemic infection.	None	None	Changes in swelling or inflammation of the abdomen, groin, or lower extremities should result in reductions or avoidance of lower body exercise until after appropriate medical evaluation and treatment resolves the issue.

General injury risk issues in common across cancer sites	Patients with bone metastases may need to alter their exercise program with regard to intensity, duration, and mode given increased risk for skeletal fractures. Infection risk is higher for patients that are currently undergoing chemotherapy or radiation treatment or have compromised immune function after treatment. Care should be taken to reduce infection risk in fitness centers frequented by cancer survivors. Patients currently in treatment and immediately following treatment may vary from exercise session to exercise session with regard to exercise tolerance, depending on their treatment schedule. Individuals with known metastatic disease to the bone will require modifications and increased supervision to avoid fractures. Individuals with cardiac conditions (secondary to cancer or not) will require modifications and may require increased supervision for safety.					
Cancer specific risk of injury, emergency procedures	The arms/shoulders should be exercised, but proactive injury prevention approaches are encouraged, given the high incidence of arm/shoulder morbidity in breast cancer survivors. Women with lymphedema should wear a well-fitting compression garment during exercise. Be aware of risk for fracture among those treated with hormonal therapy, a diagnosis of osteoporosis, or bony metastases.	Be aware of risk for fracture among patients treated with ADT, a diagnosis of osteoporosis or bony metastases	Advisable to avoid excessive intra-abdominal pressures for patients with an ostomy.	Multiple myeloma patients should be treated as if they are osteoporotic.	None	The lower body should be exercised, but proactive injury prevention approaches are encouraged, given the potential for lower extremity swelling or inflammation in this population. Women with lymphedema should wear a well-fitting compression garment during exercise. Be aware of risk for fractures among those treated with hormonal therapies, with diagnosed osteoporosis, or with bony metastases.

ACSM, American College of Sports Medicine; ADT, androgen deprivation therapy; HSCT, hematopoietic stem cell transplantation. Reprinted with permission from (258).

extremity (*e.g.*, biceps brachii, brachialis, pronator teres) and extensor muscle groups of the lower extremities (*e.g.*, quadriceps, triceps surae). The antagonistic muscles of the hypertonic muscles are usually weak. *Spasticity* is a dynamic condition that decreases with slow stretching, warm external temperature, and good positioning. However, quick movements, cold external temperature, fatigue, or emotional stress increases hypertonicity. It is important to note that hypertonicity is observed in the extremities, and hypotonicity is commonly found in the head, neck, and trunk. *Athetoid CP* is characterized by involuntary and/or uncontrolled movement that occurs primarily in the extremities. These extraneous movements may increase with effort and emotional stress.

CP can further be categorized topographically (*e.g.*, quadriplegia, diplegia, hemiplegia). Although its usage is now limited in sport, the Cerebral Palsy International Sport and Recreation Association (CPISRA) functional classification may be relevant to Ex R$_x$ (*Table 11.4*) (46). The table moves from those with the most severe spasticity and athetoid effects to the least amount. Functionally, classes 1 through 4 are used to describe those who are wheelchair users, and classes 5 through 8 are for those who remain ambulatory (46).

The variability in motor control pattern in CP is large and becomes even more complex because of the persistence of primitive reflexes. In normal motor development, reflexes appear, mature, and become integrated into normal movement

---

TABLE 11.4

Cerebral Palsy International Sports and Recreation Association (CPISRA) Functional Classification System (46)

Class	Functional Ability
1	Severe involvement in all four limbs; limited trunk control; unable to grasp; poor functional strength in upper extremities, often necessitating the use of an electric wheelchair for independence
2	Severe-to-moderate quadriplegic, normally able to propel a wheelchair very slowly with arms or by pushing with feet; poor functional strength and severe control problems in the upper extremities
3	Moderate quadriplegia, fair functional strength and moderate control problems in upper extremities and torso; uses wheelchair
4	Lower limbs have moderate-to-severe involvement; good functional strength and minimal control problem in upper extremities and torso; uses wheelchair
5	Good functional strength and minimal control problems in upper extremities; may walk with or without assistive devices for ambulatory support
6	Moderate-to-severe quadriplegia; ambulates without walking aids; less coordination; balance problems when running or throwing; has greater upper extremity involvement
7	Moderate-to-minimal hemiplegia; good functional ability in nonaffected side; walks/runs with noted limp
8	Minimally affected; may have minimal coordination problems; able to run and jump freely; has good balance

pattern, whereas other reflexes become controlled or mediated at a higher level (*i.e.*, the cortex). In CP, primitive reflexes (*e.g.*, the palmar and tonic labyrinthine reflexes) may persist, and higher level reflex activity (*i.e.*, postural reflexes) may be delayed or absent. Severely involved individuals with CP may primarily move in reflex patterns, whereas those with mild involvement may be only hindered by reflexes during extreme effort or emotional stress (169).

Exercise Testing

The hallmark of CP is disordered motor control; however, CP is often associated with other sensory (*e.g.*, vision, hearing impairment) or cognitive (*e.g.*, intellectual disability, perceptual motor disorder) disabilities that may limit participation as much as or perhaps more than the motor limitations (59). Associated conditions such as convulsive seizures (*i.e.*, epilepsy) may significantly interfere with exercise testing and programming. Exercise testing may be done in individuals with CP to uncover challenges or barriers to regular PA, to identify risk factors for secondary health conditions, to determine the functional capacity of the individual, and to prescribe the appropriate exercise intensity for aerobic and strengthening exercises. However, symptom-limited graded exercise testing is not required for those with CP to begin an exercise training program.

Exercise Testing Considerations

- Initially, a functional assessment should be taken of the trunk and upper and lower extremity involvement that includes measures of functional ROM, strength, flexibility, and balance. This assessment will facilitate the choice of exercise testing equipment, protocols, and adaptations. Medical clearance should be sought before any physical fitness testing.
- All testing should be conducted using appropriate, and if necessary, adaptive equipment such as straps and holding gloves, and guarantee safety and optimal testing conditions for mechanical efficiency.
- Consider patient positioning and level of comfort, particularly when using adaptive equipment, to avoid unintended increases in muscle tone or facilitation of primitive reflexes.
- The testing mode used to assess CRF is dependent on the functional capacity and ambulatory ability of the individual and — if an athlete with CP — the desired sport. In general,
  - Arm and leg ergometry are preferred for individuals with athetoid CP because of the benefit of moving in a closed chain. Weight bearing and symmetrical/ rhythmical movement will facilitate a decrease in the extent of athetosis.
  - In individuals with significant limitation (classes 1 and 2), minimal efforts may result in work levels that are above the anaerobic threshold and in some instances may be maximal efforts.
  - Wheelchair ergometry is recommended for individuals with moderate limitation (classes 3 and 4) with good functional strength and minimal coordination problems in the upper extremities and trunk.

- In highly functioning individuals (classes 5 through 8) who are ambulatory, treadmill testing may be recommended, but care should be taken at the final stages of the protocol when fatigue occurs, and the individual's walking or running skill may deteriorate as there may be a significant risk of falling.
- Because of the heterogeneity of the CP population, a maximal exercise test protocol cannot be generalized. It is recommended to test new participants at two or three submaximal levels, starting with a minimal power output assessment before determining the maximal exercise test protocol.
- When maximal testing is appropriate and needed to identify performance limiting factors to exercise capacity, the 10-m shuttle run test (SRT-I and SRT-II), the McMaster all-out protocol cycle test, the McMaster all-out protocol arm-cranking test, and the 7.5-m SRT (SRT-II) have been identified for use in this population (304).
- Because of poor economy of movement, true maximal CRF testing may not be appropriate or accurate. In this case, CRF testing should involve submaximal steady-state workloads at levels comparable with sporting conditions. Movement during these submaximal workloads should be controlled to optimize economy of movement (*i.e.*, mechanical efficiency). For example, with cycle leg ergometry, the choice of resistance or gearing is extremely important in individuals with CP. Some individuals will benefit from a combination of low resistance and high segmental velocity, whereas others will have optimal economy of movement with a high-resistance, low segmental velocity combination.
- For submaximal exercise tests to determine exercise tolerance, the 6-min walk test (6-MWT) can be used as a field-based test and corresponds well to functional activities used in daily living (206,304). However, this test may be more suitable as a measure of walking ability, and thus, it is critical that individuals be allowed to use their typical assistive device (172,273). Practice tests may improve consistency in distance covered. HR and rating of perceived exertion (RPE) should be monitored during the test.
- An arm-cranking protocol performed in a laboratory setting may be appropriate for some individuals to determine submaximal exercise tolerance, particularly those who are wheelchair-bound (304).
- Progressive maximal cycle ergometer tests have been found reliable when utilized to assess peak oxygen consumption ($\dot{V}O_{2peak}$) in high-functioning adults and children with CP and can detect changes in CRF (30,251).
- In individuals with moderate or severe CP, motion is considered a series of discrete bursts of activity. Hence, the assessment of anaerobic power derived from the Wingate anaerobic test (cycle or arm crank) gives a good indication of the performance potential of the individual (304).
- The muscle power sprint test and the 10 × 5 sprint test can also be utilized to assess anaerobic performance and agility (306).
- In individuals with athetoid CP, strength tests should be performed through movement in a closed chain.

- For athletes with CP, sport-specific fitness testing may be effective in determining fitness/performance areas for improvement and in planning a fitness-related intervention program for addressing the specific sports-specific goals of the athlete (152).
- Results from any exercise test in the same individual with CP may vary considerably from day to day because of fluctuations in muscle tone.

Exercise Prescription

Individuals with CP have decreased physical fitness levels compared with their peers without disability (305). However, investigation in this area is limited, focusing almost entirely on children and adolescents and comprising primarily individuals with minimal or moderate involvement (*i.e.*, those who are ambulatory) (60,69,224). CP is a nonprogressive condition, but as a result of the clinical symptoms and secondary conditions that result, it often leads to functional declines that are often exacerbated by the aging process as well as environmental, social, economic, and access-related consequences. As they age, adolescents with CP may show a decline in gross motor capacity related to loss of ROM, postural changes, or pain as well as reduced aerobic capacity. There are several documented disability-related changes in older adults with CP such as greater physical fatigue, impaired motion/problematic joint contractures, and loss of mobility, which would impact the overall fitness level of the older adult with CP (284). In fact, 25% of adults with CP report a mobility decline with age that is associated with higher levels of pain and fatigue (185). Adults with CP should maintain a high level of physical fitness to offset its decline associated with both aging and the effects of CP. PA may improve muscle strength in the legs. Poor leg strength is considered a limiting factor in anaerobic and aerobic activities involving the lower limbs for individuals with CP (62). Therefore, training to develop muscular strength and endurance could be valuable in hindering the functional deterioration and the associated physical dependence adults with CP experience (128).

Generally, the FITT principle of Ex R_x recommendations for the general population should be applied to individuals with CP (see *Chapter 6*) (95,116). It is important to note, however, that the FITT principle of Ex R_x recommendations for individuals with CP is based on very limited literature. For this reason and because of the impact of CP on neuromotor function, recommendations regarding the FITT principle of Ex R_x are included in the following "Special Considerations" section.

Special Considerations

- The FITT principle of Ex R_x needed to elicit health/fitness benefits in individuals with CP is unclear. Even though the design of exercise training programs to enhance health/fitness benefits should be based on the same principles as the general population, modifications to the training protocol may have to be made based on the individual's functional mobility level, number and type of associated conditions, and degree of involvement of each limb (240).
- Because of altered movement control, energy expenditure (EE) is high even at low power output levels. In individuals with severe involvement (classes 1

and 2), aerobic exercise programs should start with frequent but short bouts at moderate intensity (*i.e.*, 40%–50% oxygen uptake reserve [$\dot{V}O_2R$] or HRR or RPE of 12–13 on a scale of 6–20). Recovery periods should begin each time this intensity level is exceeded. Exercise bouts should be progressively increased to reach an intensity of 50%–85% $\dot{V}O_2R$ for 20 min. Because of poor economy of movement, shorter durations that can be accumulated should be considered.

- If balance deficits during exercise are an issue, leg ergometry with a tricycle or recumbent stationary bicycle (88) for the lower extremities and hand cycling for the upper extremities are recommended because (a) they allow for a wide range of power output, (b) movements occur in a closed chain, (c) muscle contraction velocity can be changed without changing the power output through the use of resistance or gears, and (d) there is minimal risk for injuries caused by lack of movement or balance control.

- Recumbent stepping is feasible and safe for individuals with CP who have significant motor impairment (221). This type of progressive aerobic activity can often be performed without significant postexercise pain.

- Individuals with CP fatigue easily because of poor economy of movement. Fatigue can deteriorate the voluntary movement patterns of hypertonic muscles. Training sessions can be more effective, particularly for individuals with high muscle tone, if (a) several short training sessions are conducted rather than one longer session, (b) relaxation and stretching routines are included throughout the session, and (c) new skills are introduced early in the session (39,245).

- The impact of CP on health-related physical fitness results in a reduction of muscular strength and muscular endurance (128).

- Children often have reduced aerobic and anaerobic exercise responses as compared to a typically developing child (11).

- Resistance training increases strength in individuals with CP without an adverse effect on muscle tone (69,217). However, the effects of resistance training on functional outcome measures and mobility in this population are inconclusive (184,260). Emphasize the role of flexibility training in conjunction with any resistance training program designed for individuals with CP.

- Resistance exercises designed to target weak muscle groups that oppose hypertonic muscle groups improve the strength of the weak muscle group and normalize the tone in the opposing hypertonic muscle group through reciprocal inhibition. Other techniques, such as neuromuscular electrical stimulation (217) and whole body vibration (2), increase muscle strength without negative effects on spasticity. Dynamic strengthening exercises over the full ROM that are executed at slow contraction speeds to avoid stretch reflex activity in the opposing muscles are recommended.

- Before initiating open kinetic chain strengthening exercises (*e.g.*, dumbbells, barbells, other free weights), always check the impact of primitive reflexes on performance (*i.e.*, position of head, trunk, and proximal joints of the extremities) and whether the individual has adequate neuromotor control to exercise with free weights.

- In children with CP, eccentric strength training increases eccentric torque production throughout the ROM while decreasing electromyographic (EMG) activity in the exercising muscle. Eccentric training may decrease cocontraction and improve net torque development in muscles exhibiting increased tone (236).

- Hypertonic muscles should be stretched slowly to their limits throughout the workout program to maintain length. Stretching for 30 s improves muscle activation of the antagonistic muscle group, whereas sustained stretching for 30 min is effective in temporarily reducing spasticity in the muscle being stretched (313). Ballistic stretching should be avoided.

- Generally, the focus for children with CP is on inhibiting abnormal reflex activity, normalizing muscle tone, and developing reactions to increase equilibrium. The focus with adolescents and adults is more likely to be on functional outcomes and performance.

- During growth, hypertonicity in the muscles — and consequently, muscle balance around the joints — may change significantly because of inadequate adaptations in muscle length. Training programs should be adapted continuously to accommodate these changing conditions (217).

- Medical interventions such as botulinum toxin (Botox) injections, a medication which decreases spasticity, may drastically change the functional potential of the individual. Little information is available to guide exercise during the time between injections. Spasticity reductions may last for several months following injection and may provide a period for effective exercise training.

- Good positioning of the head, trunk, and proximal joints of extremities to control persistent primitive reflexes is preferred to strapping. Inexpensive modifications that enable good position such as Velcro gloves to attach the hands to the equipment should be used whenever needed.

- Individuals with CP are more susceptible to overuse injuries because of their higher incidence of inactivity and associated conditions (*i.e.*, hypertonicity, contractures, and joint pain) (2).

- Studies of elite athletes with CP are sparse, and general assumptions are still unclear. Strong support for sport participation is suggested because elite athletes with CP do not show associated lower neuromuscular fatigue (249).

ONLINE RESOURCES

National Institutes of Neurological Disorders and Stroke:
    http://www.ninds.nih.gov/disorders/cerebral_palsy/cerebral_palsy.htm
Centers for Disease Control and Prevention: Increasing Physical Activity among Adults with Disabilities:
    http://www.cdc.gov/ncbddd/disabilityandhealth/pa.html
Peter Harrison Centre for Disability Sport:
    http://www.lboro.ac.uk/research/phc/educational-toolkit/

FIBROMYALGIA

Fibromyalgia is a syndrome characterized by chronic widespread nonarticular pain, generalized sensory hypersensitivity, diffuse multiple tender points, fatigue, poor sleep, morning stiffness, memory impairment (*e.g.*, confusion or forgetfulness), and psychological distress (15,51,314). Fibromyalgia affects approximately 1%–4% of the population in Canada, Europe, and the United States, and women are affected more often than men (29,163,314). The prevalence of fibromyalgia in the general population increases with age, peaking between the fifth and eighth decade of life (29,163,314).

Individuals with fibromyalgia do not show signs of acute inflammation or muscle tissue abnormalities and do not develop joint deformities or joint disease. Therefore, fibromyalgia is not considered a true form of arthritis but is instead thought to be the result of aberrant central pain and sensory processing (51). Pain is typically present for many years but with no specific pattern (*i.e.*, fibromyalgia pain can intensify and subside and present in different areas of the body at different times) (15). Fatigue affects 78%–94% of individuals with fibromyalgia and often is linked to poor nonrestorative sleep (205). However, treatment for specific sleep disorders has not generally been found effective in alleviating fibromyalgia symptoms (see *Box 11.1* for a complete listing of signs and symptoms) (51). The condition is frequently associated with other disorders such as irritable bowel syndrome, interstitial cystitis, temporomandibular disorder, and chronic fatigue syndrome (15,51).

Because of the nature of fibromyalgia, a confirmed diagnosis can be difficult. The 2013 alternative diagnostic criteria (17) include determining the number of locations where the individual has pain and the severity of symptoms over the last 7 d. Specific areas of the body where pain is assessed are the neck, upper and lower

---

Box 11.1	Signs and Symptoms[a] of Fibromyalgia

Widespread pain
Fatigue
Nonrestorative sleep
Environmental sensitivity (cold, lights, noise, odor)
Paresthesias (sensations of burning, prickling, tingling, or itching of skin with no apparent physical cause)
Weakness
Feelings of swelling in hands or feet
Headaches
Restless legs
Anxiety
Depression

[a]Symptoms may worsen with emotional stress, poor sleep, injury or surgery, high humidity, physical inactivity, or excessive physical activity.

back, front of chest, jaw, shoulder, arm, wrist, hand, hip, thigh, knee, ankle, and foot. Level of severity is determined for 10 symptoms: pain, energy, stiffness, sleep, depression, memory, anxiety, tenderness, balance, and environmental sensitivity.

Individuals with fibromyalgia have reduced aerobic capacity and muscle function (*i.e.*, strength and endurance) as well as overall reductions in PA, functional performance (*e.g.*, walking, stair climbing), and physical fitness (37,85,142). In general, these reductions are caused by the chronic widespread pain that limits the individual's abilities to complete his or her everyday activities, ultimately resulting in continued deconditioning and a loss of physiologic reserve.

Treatment for individuals with fibromyalgia includes medications for pain, sleep, and mood as well as educational programs, cognitive behavioral therapy, and exercise. However, there is a great deal of heterogeneity among individuals with fibromyalgia. Thus, although able to progress exercise to levels sufficient to improve physical fitness (37), the response to treatment may depend on the unique physical and psychosocial characteristics of the individual (37,126,174,290). In general, exercise improves flexibility, neuromuscular function, cardiorespiratory function, functional performance, PA levels, pain, and other symptoms of fibromyalgia as well as self-efficacy, depression, anxiety, and quality of life (21,37,110, 143,144,157,248,295,296). Additionally, even small increases in lifestyle PA lead to improvements in physical function, pain, and mood.

Based on the potential for pain and exacerbation of symptoms, an individual's medical history and current health status must be reviewed prior to conducting exercise tests or prescribing an exercise program. Objectively assessing physiologic and functional limitations will allow for the proper exercise testing and most optimal exercise training.

Exercise Testing

When indicated, individuals with fibromyalgia can generally participate in symptom-limited exercise testing as described in *Chapter 5*. Clinical judgment regarding individual tolerance for continuing the exercise test with subjective reports of increased pain or fatigue will be required. In this population, the 6-min walk test is also frequently used to measure aerobic performance (36). However, some special precautions should be considered when conducting exercise testing among those with fibromyalgia.

- Review symptoms prior to testing to determine the severity and location of pain and the individual's level of fatigue. The revised version of the Fibromyalgia Impact Questionnaire is most often used to assess physical function, overall impact of fibromyalgia, and fibromyalgia-related symptoms (16).
- Assess previous and current exercise experience to determine the probability of the individual having an increase in symptoms after testing as well as testing mode preference.
- Provide high levels of motivation using constant verbal encouragement to have the individual perform to a peak level during testing.
- For individuals with cognitive dysfunction, determine their level of understanding when following through with verbal and written testing and training directions.

- The appropriate testing protocol (see *Chapters 4* and *5*) should be selected based on an individual's symptomatology. Individualize test protocols as needed.
- The order of testing must be considered to allow for adequate rest and recovery of different physiologic systems and/or muscle groups. For example, depending on the most prevalent symptoms (*e.g.*, pain, fatigue) and their locations on the day of testing, endurance testing may be completed before strength testing and alternate between upper and lower extremities.
- Monitor pain and fatigue levels continuously throughout the tests. Numerical rating scales are available for these symptoms and are easy to administer during exercise (see *Figure 11.1*).
- Care should be taken to position the individual correctly on the testing or training equipment to allow for the most pain-free exercise possible. This accommodation may require modification to equipment such as adjusting the seat height and types of pedals on a cycle leg ergometer, raising an exercise bench to limit the amount of joint (*e.g.*, hip, knee, back) flexion or extension when getting on or off the equipment, or providing smaller weight increments on standard weight machines.
- If the individual has pain in the lower extremities prior to testing, consider a non–weight-bearing type of exercise (*e.g.*, leg ergometry) to achieve a more accurate measurement of CRF, thereby allowing the individual to perform to a higher intensity prior to stopping because of pain.
- Prior to exercise testing and training, educate the individual on the differences between postexercise soreness and fatigue and normal fluctuations in pain and fatigue experienced as a result of fibromyalgia.

Exercise Prescription

It is important to note that the FITT principle of Ex R_x recommendations for individuals with fibromyalgia is based on very limited literature and there is no evidence-based statement available. For this reason, the FITT principle of Ex R_x is generally consistent with the Ex R_x for apparently healthy adults (see *Chapter 6*) with the following considerations.

Exercise Training Considerations

- Although positive changes are noted with a frequency of 1–2 d · wk^{-1}, symptom reduction is greater when the frequency is increased to 3 d · wk^{-1} (21).
- Give adequate recovery time between exercises within a session and between days of exercise. Exercises should be alternated between different parts of the body or different systems (*e.g.*, musculoskeletal vs. cardiorespiratory).
- If a single bout of 30 min of continuous aerobic exercise is not initially tolerated, it may be performed in a series of bouts of ≥10 min each. Additional support and encouragement may be required to maintain adherence.
- The rate of progression of the FITT principle of Ex R_x for individuals with fibromyalgia will depend entirely on their symptoms. They should be educated on how to reduce intensity or duration of exercises when their symptoms are exacerbated. Individuals with fibromyalgia should be advised to attempt low

FITT

FITT RECOMMENDATIONS FOR INDIVIDUALS WITH FIBROMYALGIA (21,36,38,85,98,110,143,144,157,174,248,295,296)

	Aerobic	Resistance	Flexibility
Frequency	Begin with 1–2 d · wk^{-1} and gradually progress to 2–3 d · wk^{-1}.	2–3 d · wk^{-1} with a minimum of 48 h between sessions	Begin with 1–3 d · wk^{-1} and progress to 5 d · wk^{-1}.
Intensity	Begin at very light intensity (<30% $\dot{V}O_2R$ or HRR). Gradually progress to moderate intensity (40%–59% $\dot{V}O_2R$ or HRR).	40%–80% 1-RM. Gradually increase to 60%–80% 1-RM for strength. For muscle endurance, use ≤50% 1-RM.	Active and gentle ROM stretches for all muscle tendon groups in the pain-free range. Stretch to the point of tightness or slight discomfort.
Time	Begin with 10 min · d^{-1} and gradually progress to a total of 30–60 min · d^{-1}.	Strength: Gradually progress from 4–5 to 8–12 repetitions, increasing to 2–4 sets per muscle group with at least 2–3 min between sets. Endurance: 15–25 repetitions, increasing to 2 sets with a shorter rest interval	Initially hold the stretch for 10–30 s. Progress to holding each stretch for up to 60 s.
Type	Low-impact/non–weight-bearing exercise (e.g., water exercise, cycling, walking, swimming) initially to minimize pain that may be caused by exercise	Elastic bands, dumbbells, cuff/ankle weights, weight machines, or body weight exercises	Elastic bands and unloaded (non–weight-bearing) stretching

1-RM, one repetition maximum; HRR, heart rate reserve; ROM, range of motion; $\dot{V}O_2R$, oxygen uptake reserve.

levels of exercise during flare-ups but should be cognizant of their symptoms in order to minimize the chance of injury.

- Minimize the eccentric component of dynamic resistance exercises to lessen exercise-induced muscle microtrauma, particularly during a symptom flare-up (144).
- Decrease exercise volume if symptoms increase during or after exercise. It may be better to initially decrease intensity or duration prior to reducing frequency to maintain a pattern of regular PA (144,173).

Special Considerations

- Individuals with fibromyalgia are commonly physically inactive because of their symptoms. Prescribe exercise, especially at the beginning, at a physical exertion level that the individual will be able to do without undue pain and progress slowly to allow for physiologic adaptation without an increase in symptoms. Monitor pain level and location (28,36,37,57,85,117,173,287).
- Select an exercise program that minimizes barriers to adherence and takes into account individual preferences. Exercise adherence in those with fibromyalgia may be improved if exercise is performed in a longer, continuous bout as opposed to two shorter sessions (253). Supervised or group exercise should be encouraged, especially early, to provide a social support system for reducing physical and emotional stress and promote adherence (37,247,253,287).
- For individuals with symptoms such as pain and fatigue, functional activities (*e.g.*, walking, stair climbing, rising from a chair, dancing) are recommended to allow for maintenance of light-to-moderate intensity PA even when symptomatic.
- Teach and have individuals with fibromyalgia demonstrate the correct mechanics for performing each exercise to reduce the potential for injury.
- Individuals with fibromyalgia should consider exercising in a temperature- and humidity-controlled room if this minimizes exacerbation of symptoms.
- Both land- and water-based aerobic exercise are beneficial for improving physical function and overall well-being in individuals with fibromyalgia (21,36,37, 117,287).
- Consider including complementary therapies such as tai chi (263) and yoga because they have been shown to reduce symptoms in individuals with fibromyalgia.
- Assist individuals with fibromyalgia to set realistic goals. Improvement in pain and function may take more than 7 wk after initiating an exercise program to be clinically relevant (21,263).

ONLINE RESOURCES

Arthritis Foundation:
    http://www.arthritistoday.org/about-arthritis/types-of-arthritis/fibromyalgia/
National Fibromyalgia Association:
    http://www.fmaware.org

HUMAN IMMUNODEFICIENCY VIRUS

Broad use of antiretroviral therapy (ART) by industrialized countries to reduce the viral load of human immunodeficiency virus (HIV) has significantly increased life expectancy following diagnosis of HIV infection (75,303). As a result, we have begun to experience more and more individuals living beyond 50 yr of age with HIV. Recent investigations have even indicated that most individuals who are HIV-positive can expect to live just as long as someone without HIV (192). ART dramatically reduces the prevalence of the wasting syndrome and immunosuppression. However, certain ART drugs are associated with metabolic and anthropomorphic health conditions including dyslipidemia, abnormal distribution of body fat (*i.e.*, abdominal obesity and subcutaneous fat loss), and insulin resistance (8). More specifically, protease inhibitors are known to be associated with insulin resistance and increasing the risk of developing T2DM. Emerging data suggest an association of HIV infection, cardiac dysfunction, and an increased risk of CVD among individuals living with HIV. Over the last two decades, rates of new HIV infection have been among predominantly minority and lower socioeconomic classes; therefore, individuals with HIV are now beginning therapy with higher body mass index (BMI) and reduced muscle strength and mass. They are also more likely to have personal and environmental conditions that predispose them to high visceral fat and obesity (200,267). It is unclear how the aging process will interact with HIV status, sociodemographic characteristics, chronic disease risk, and the extended life expectancy associated with ART use. However, in older men, evidence suggests that low CRF is associated with the presence of additional comorbidities but not CD4 cell count or viral load (209). PA and dietary counseling should be evaluated as viable treatment options in conjunction with ART for individuals with HIV. Additional treatment options have included anabolic steroids, growth hormone, and growth factors for those with muscle wasting (316).

Aerobic and resistance exercise provide important health benefits for individuals with HIV/acquired immunodeficiency syndrome (AIDS) (97,114,135,136,208,289). Exercise training enhances functional aerobic capacity, cardiorespiratory and muscular endurance, and general well-being. Additionally, PA can reduce body fat and indices of metabolic dysfunction. Although there are less data on effects of resistance training, progressive resistance exercise increases lean tissue mass and improves muscular strength. People living with AIDS/HIV are at risk for osteopenia likely because of long-term ART. Long-term progressive resistance exercise may improve or sustain bone mineral density (BMD) in the population without HIV/AIDS and therefore could potentially be effective in delaying the onset of osteopenia among people living with HIV/AIDS. There is also evidence of enhanced mood and psychological status with regular exercise training (135). Of importance, there is no evidence to suggest regular participation in an exercise program of moderate intensity will suppress immune function of asymptomatic or symptomatic individuals with HIV (114,115).

Exercise Testing

Not all persons with HIV/AIDS require a preparticipation exercise test. However, if an exercise test is to be performed, the increased prevalence of cardiovascular pathophysiology, metabolic disorders, T2DM, hyperlipidemia, and the complex medication routines of individuals with HIV/AIDS require specialized provider consultation before exercise testing. This consultation should be completed by an infectious disease expert, or at minimum, a health care professional with extensive knowledge of HIV-related pharmacological regimens. Besides the usual considerations prior to exercise testing, the following list of issues should be considered with exercise testing:

- Exercise testing should be postponed in individuals with acute infections.
- Variability of exercise test results will be higher for individuals with HIV than in a healthy population. It is common for this population to have a significantly lower $\dot{V}O_{2peak}$ when compared to someone of the same age without HIV (210,276).
- When conducting cardiopulmonary exercise tests, infection control measures should be employed for persons being tested as well as those performing the test (149). Although HIV is not transmitted through saliva, a high rate of oral infections and possible presence of blood within the mouth or gums necessitates thorough sterilization of reusable equipment and supplies when disposables are not available. Consider the use of disposable mouth pieces, proper sterilization of all nondisposable equipment used after each test, yearly flu vaccinations, and tuberculosis testing for all facility staff and personnel.
- The increased prevalence of cardiovascular impairments and particularly cardiac arrhythmias requires monitoring of blood pressure (BP) and the electrocardiogram (ECG).
- Because of the higher prevalence of peripheral neuropathies, testing mode should be altered, if necessary, to the appropriate exercise type, intensity, and ROM.
- Typical limitations to stress testing by stage of disease include the following:
  - Asymptomatic — normal exercise test with reduced exercise capacity
  - Symptomatic — reduced exercise time, $\dot{V}O_{2peak}$, and ventilatory threshold (VT)
  - AIDS will dramatically reduce exercise time and $\dot{V}O_{2peak}$. Reduced exercise time will likely preclude reaching VT, and achieving >85% of age-predicted HR_{max} will potentially produce abnormal nervous and endocrine responses.

Exercise Prescription

The chronic disease and health conditions associated with HIV infection suggest health benefits would be gained by regular participation in a program of combined aerobic and resistance exercise. Indeed, numerous clinical studies have shown participation in habitual PA results in physical and mental health benefits among this population (97,113,114,135,136,208,289). The varied presentation of individuals with HIV requires a flexible approach. Notably, no clinical study of the effects of

PA on symptomatology of HIV infection has shown an immunosuppressive effect. Furthermore, data indicate individuals living with HIV adapt readily to exercise training, with some studies showing more robust responses than would be expected in a healthy population (97,115,135,136,208,289). There is little data available to specifically guide exercise training in the HIV population (102). Therefore, the general FITT principle of Ex R_x is consistent with that for apparently healthy adults (see *Chapter 6*) or older adults (see *Chapter 7*), but the management of CVD risk should be emphasized. However, exercise professionals should be mindful of the potentially rapid change in health status of this population, particularly the high incidence of acute infections, and should adjust the FITT principle of Ex R_x accordingly.

■ FITT RECOMMENDATIONS FOR INDIVIDUALS WITH HUMAN IMMUNODEFICIENCY VIRUS

	Aerobic	Resistance	Flexibility
Frequency	3–5 d · wk^{-1}	2–3 d · wk^{-1}	≥2–3 d · wk^{-1}
Intensity	Begin at light intensity (30%–39% $\dot{V}O_2R$ or HRR). Gradually progress to moderate intensity (40%–59% $\dot{V}O_2R$ or HRR).	Begin a light intensity with goal of gradual progression to 60% 1-RM.	Stretch to the point of tightness or slight discomfort.
Time	Begin with 10 min and progress to 30–60 min · d^{-1}.	1–2 sets, with gradual progression to 3 sets of 8–10 repetitions	Hold static stretch for 10–30 s; 2–4 repetitions of each exercise
Type	Modality will vary with the health status and interests of the individual. Presence of osteopenia will require weight-bearing physical activities.	Machine weights are safe and effective without supervision; free weights can be used for experienced lifters and/or under supervision.	Static, dynamic, and/or PNF stretching

1-RM, one repetition maximum; HRR, heart rate reserve; PNF, proprioceptive neuromuscular facilitation; $\dot{V}O_2R$, oxygen uptake reserve.

Exercise Training Considerations

■ Contact and high-risk (*e.g.*, skateboarding, rock climbing) sports are not recommended because of risk of bleeding.

■ Because of virus and drug side effects, progression will likely occur at a slower rate than in healthy populations. However, the long-term goals for asymptomatic individuals with HIV/AIDS should be to achieve the ACSM FITT principle of Ex R_x recommendations for aerobic and resistance exercise for healthy adults with appropriate modifications for symptomatic individuals with HIV/AIDS. The FITT principle of Ex R_x should be adjusted accordingly based on the individual's age and current health status.

Special Considerations

- There are no currently established guidelines regarding contraindications for exercise for individuals with HIV/AIDS.
- Supervised exercise, whether in the community or at home, is recommended for symptomatic individuals with HIV/AIDS or those with diagnosed comorbidities.
- In addition to supervised exercise sessions, individuals with HIV/AIDS require a higher level of health monitoring. This is especially important for those engaging in strenuous activity and/or interval training (*i.e.*, vigorous intensity aerobic exercise and/or resistance training).
- Individuals with HIV/AIDS should report increased general feelings of fatigue or perceived effort during activity, lower gastrointestinal distress, and shortness of breath if they occur.
- Minor increases in feelings of fatigue should not preclude participation, but dizziness, swollen joints, or vomiting should.
- The high (but more recently reducing) incidence of peripheral neuropathy may require adjustment of exercise type, intensity, and ROM.
- Regularly monitoring the health/fitness benefits related to PA and CVD risk factors is critical for clinical management and continued exercise participation.

ONLINE RESOURCES

Centers for Disease Control and Prevention:
http://www.cdc.gov/hiv/

INTELLECTUAL DISABILITY AND DOWN SYNDROME

Intellectual disability (ID) (older medical terminology referred to ID as *mental retardation*) is the most common developmental disability that occurs before age 18 yr in the United States with an estimated prevalence of 2.3% of the total population (161). Persons with ID experience significant limitations in two main areas: (a) intellectual functioning (*i.e.*, two standard deviations below the mean or an IQ <70 for mild/moderate ID and <35 for severe/profound ID) and (b) adaptive behavior (the use of everyday social and practical skills) (5). The etiology is not known in up to 30%–50% of all cases, but genetic disorders (*i.e.*, Down syndrome [DS], fragile X syndrome, phenylketonuria or PKU), birth trauma (*i.e.*, asphyxia), infectious disease (*i.e.*, toxoplasmosis, rubella, meningitis), maternal factors (*i.e.*, alcohol, smoking, and cocaine use), prematurity/low birth weight, and poverty/cultural deprivation (*i.e.*, malnutrition, maternal/child insufficient health care, inadequate educational support) are the major causes of ID (5).

Although there are many subpopulations of individuals with ID with their own unique attributes (*e.g.*, fragile X syndrome, PKU), the existing literature has focused on two main subpopulations—those with and without DS. The vast majority of adults with ID, with and without DS, are classified with *mild* ID (*i.e.*, >85% have an IQ between 50 and 70), and most of these individuals live in the community either at home or in group homes. Life expectancy for persons with mild ID without DS is now approaching that of the general population (22). Life expectancy of those with DS has seen a significant increase from a median age 13.5 yr in 1970 to 53 yr in the present day (232). With increasing life expectancy of persons with ID, causes of morbidity and mortality due to cardiovascular complications, obesity, and physical inactivity are reflecting that of the general population (137). Thus, it is becoming more likely that exercise professionals will encounter individuals with ID in need of both exercise testing and training.

Exercise Testing

Exercise responses in individuals with DS are unique and clearly different from individuals without DS. Thus, concerns and considerations for exercise testing and Ex R$_x$ are often different for individuals with and without DS. Exercise testing in general appears to be fairly safe in individuals with ID, and safety related to cardiovascular complications may not differ from the general population (80). However, although reports of exercise complications are rare or nonexistent, there is no scientific evidence for or against the safety of exercise testing in individuals with ID. Concerns have been raised regarding validity and reliability of exercise testing in this population, but individualized treadmill laboratory tests are reliable and valid, as are testing using the Schwinn Airdyne (*Box 11.2*) (80). However, only a few field tests are valid for estimating CRF in this population (80). It is recommended individuals with ID receive a full health-related physical fitness assessment including CRF, muscle strength and endurance, and body composition prior to beginning an exercise training program (78).

The following general points should be considered in order to ensure appropriate and valid test outcomes (80,83):

- Exercise preparticipation health screening should follow the general *ACSM Guidelines*, with the exception of individuals with DS. Because up to 50% of individuals with DS also have congenital heart disease (35) and up to 30% of individuals with DS may have significant atlantoaxial instability (*i.e.*, excessive movement of the joint between C1 and C2 usually caused by ligament laxity) (175), a careful medical history and physical evaluation of these individuals is needed. In addition, physician supervision of exercise tests may also be recommended for persons with DS.

Box 11.2	**Fitness Tests Recommendations for Individuals with Intellectual Disability (77)**	
	Recommended	**Not Recommended**
Cardiorespiratory fitness	■ Walking treadmill protocols with individualized walking speeds ■ Schwinn Airdyne using both arms and legs with 25-W stages ■ 20-m shuttle run ■ Rockport 1-mi walk	■ Treadmill running protocols ■ Cycle ergometry ■ Arm ergometry ■ 1–1.5-mi runs
Muscular strength and endurance	■ 1-RM using weight machines ■ Isokinetic testing ■ Isometric maximal voluntary contraction	■ 1-RM using free weights ■ Push-ups ■ Flexed arm hang
Anthropometrics and body composition	■ Body mass index ■ Waist circumference ■ Skinfolds ■ Air plethysmography ■ DEXA	
Flexibility	■ Sit and reach ■ Joint-specific goniometry	

DEXA, dual energy X-ray absorptiometry; 1-RM, one repetition maximum.

■ Familiarization with test procedures and personnel is required. Test validity and reliability have only been demonstrated following appropriate familiarization (81,241). The amount of familiarization will depend on the level of understanding and motivation of the individual being tested. Demonstration and practice should be performed; thus, several visits to the testing facility may be required prior to completion of the "actual" test. In particular, special care should be taken during familiarization for individuals with DS to ensure that all equipment fit their stature, which is generally small, including appropriate-sized mouthpiece or face mask for gas exchange measurements.

■ Provide an environment in which the participant feels valued and like a participating member. Give simple, one-step instructions and reinforce them verbally, visually, and regularly. Provide safety features to ensure participants do not fall or have fear of falling. Consider having two to three staff members on hand to monitor both the equipment (*e.g.*, BP, ECG, gas exchange) and participants balance.

■ Select appropriate tests (see *Box 11.2*) and individualize test protocols as needed. Only some tests of CRF have been shown to be valid and reliable in individuals with ID, whereas others have shown to be of poor value because of poor reliability or questionable validity (78). Apply the populations-specific formulas in *Table 11.5* when using CRF field tests.

■ CRF field tests are reliable but not valid for individual prediction of aerobic capacity in individuals with DS.

TABLE 11.5

Formulas for Predicting $\dot{V}O_{2max}$ from Field Test Performance in Individuals with Intellectual Disability

20-m shuttle run (82):
$\dot{V}O_{2max}$ (mL $\cdot$ kg^{-1} $\cdot$ min^{-1}) = 0.35 (number of 20-m laps) $-$ 0.59 (BMI) $-$ 4.5 (gender: 1 = boys, 2 = girls) + 50.8

600-yd run/walk (82):
$\dot{V}O_{2max}$ (mL $\cdot$ kg^{-1} $\cdot$ min^{-1}) = -5.24 (600-yd run time in min) $-$ 0.37 (BMI) $-$ 4.61 (gender: 1 = boys, 2 = girls) + 73.64

1-mi Rockport Walk Fitness test (287):
$\dot{V}O_{2max}$ (L $\cdot$ min^{-1}) = -0.18 (walk time in min) + 0.03 (body weight in kg) + 2.90

BMI, body mass index; $\dot{V}O_{2max}$, maximal oxygen consumption.

- In general, cycle ergometry protocols (no arm involvement) should not be used due to poor motor coordination in creating consistent forward pedal movement.
- Because HR$_{max}$ is altered in those with DS (80), the standard formula of 220 $-$ age to predict HR$_{max}$ should not be used. It is recommended that the following population-specific formula be used as a guide during exercise testing but should not be used for Ex R$_x$ (79): HR$_{max}$ = 210 $-$ 56 (age) $-$ 15.5 (DS status); insert 1 for DS not present and 2 for DS present.
- Individuals with ID, but without DS, may not differ from their peers without disabilities in aerobic capacity and overweight/obesity status. However, muscle strength is usually low in this population (77). Individuals with DS exhibit low levels of aerobic capacity and muscle strength and are often overweight and obese (13,55,310).
- The use of balance testing is an important consideration for this population. There are several techniques currently available to assess balance that range from functional measures (*e.g.*, timed up and go) (227) and the functional reach test (71) to more advanced technological measurements, such as pressure platforms (211).

Exercise Prescription

The general principles of exercise programming for healthy individuals apply to programs for persons with ID. However, because PA levels are low and body weight is often elevated into the overweight and obese range, especially in persons with DS, a focus on daily PA and caloric expenditure is desirable (80). The aerobic exercise training recommendations that follow are consistent with achieving an EE of $\geq$2,000 kcal $\cdot$ wk^{-1}. However, it is likely that several months of participation is needed before this EE can be achieved. Persons with ID who cannot meet these recommendations should be as active as their abilities allow. Exercise training programs improve aerobic and muscular fitness as well as balance in persons with ID (211).

FITT RECOMMENDATIONS FOR INDIVIDUALS WITH INTELLECTUAL DISABILITY AND DOWN SYNDROME (78)

FITT		Aerobic	Resistance	Flexibility
	Frequency	3–7 d · wk^{-1} to maximize caloric expenditure; includes 3–4 d · wk^{-1} of moderate-to-vigorous intensity exercise and light intensity PA on remaining days	2–3 d · wk^{-1}	At least 2–3 d · wk^{-1} but preferably daily with consideration for atlantoaxial instability in the neck
	Intensity	40%–80% $\dot{V}O_2R$ or HRR; RPE may not be an appropriate indicator of intensity in this population.	Begin with 12 repetitions using 60%–70% 1-RM for 1–2 wk. Progress to 75%–80% of 1-RM.	Stretch to the point of tightness or slight discomfort.
	Time	30–60 min · day^{-1}; intermittent exercise bouts of 10–15 min may be used	2–3 sets for major muscle groups	Hold static stretch for 10–30 s; 2–4 repetitions of each exercise
	Type	Primary activity is walking with progression to running using intermittent runs; swimming; combined arm and leg ergometry.	For safety purposes, machines are preferable to free weights.	Static stretching

1-RM, one repetition maximum; HRR, heart rate reserve; PA, physical activity; RPE, rating of perceived exertion; $\dot{V}O_2R$, oxygen uptake reserve.

Exercise Training Considerations

- Muscle strength and endurance is low in persons with ID and may limit the extent to which they can perform aerobic activities; thus, a focus on muscle strength is desirable (80).
- Yoga should be considered in that it not only impacts flexibility and strengthens joints but also facilitates social interaction when conducted in groups. However, caution is needed when prescribing yoga to persons with DS because of their joint laxity, especially when instability in the atlantoaxial and atlantooccipital areas is present.

Special Considerations

- Persons with ID may require additional encouragement during both exercise testing and training than persons without ID.
- Persons with ID may be on various medications including antidepressants, anticonvulsants, hypnotics, neuroleptics, and thyroid replacement.
- Many persons with ID have problems with motor control, coordination, balance, and gait and are at high risk for falls (132). Therefore, exercise professionals should consider incorporating neuromotor exercise training.
- Because of attention difficulties in this population, simple one-step instructions and demonstrations should always be used.
- Appropriate familiarization and practice time along with careful supervision is required for aerobic and muscle fitness training programs.
- Diverse activities are recommended to maximize enjoyment and adherence. Consider using music and simple games to promote exercise enjoyment and adherence. Also consider encouraging participants in sports programs such as those offered by Special Olympics.
- Group activities should be designed in ways that accommodate individuals, offering opportunities to reach appropriate exercise intensities.

Special Considerations for Individuals with Down Syndrome

- Individuals with DS typically have very low levels of aerobic capacity and muscle strength, often at levels approximately 50% of the level of expected based age and sex. Individuals with DS are often obese, and severe obesity is common.
- Almost all individuals with DS have low HR_{max} likely caused by a dampened catecholamine response to exercise (80).
- Many persons with DS have atlantoaxial instability, and thus, activities involving hyperflexion and hyperextension of the neck are contraindicated.
- Skeletal muscle hypotonia coupled with excessive joint laxity is commonly seen in this population (226). Increasing muscle strength, especially around major joints (*e.g.*, knee) is a priority. Also, caution should be used regarding involvement in contact sports.
- Exercise performance may be negatively affected by some physical characteristics which include short stature and limbs, malformation of feet and toes, and small mouth and nasal cavities.
- Some evidence suggests that the ACSM formula for estimating EE during walking may underestimate the oxygen uptake of a given speed in person with DS (1).
- Ear pathologies are common among individuals with DS (225). Physician clearance may be needed prior to participation in aquatic exercise.

ONLINE RESOURCES

Inclusive Fitness Coalition:
   http://incfit.org/node/83
American Association on Intellectual and Developmental Disabilities:
   http://www.aaidd.org
National Association for Down Syndrome:
   http://www.nads.org
National Center on Health, Physical Activity and Disability:
   http://www.nchpad.org
National Down Syndrome Society:
   http://www.ndss.org

KIDNEY DISEASE

Individuals are diagnosed with chronic kidney disease (CKD) if they have either kidney damage evidenced by microalbuminuria or reduced kidney function as indicated by a glomerular filtration rate (GFR) <60 mL $\cdot$ min^{-1} $\cdot$ 1.73 m^{-2} for $\geq$3 mo (156). CKD can be categorized into five stages based on the estimated GFR and the amount of albumin present in the urine and used to identify the risk of disease progression and poor outcome (*Table 11.6*) (156). Those in stage 1 (normal GFR and low albumin) are considered without CKD, and those in stage 5 (*i.e.*, GFR <15 mL $\cdot$ min^{-1} $\cdot$ 1.73 m^{-2}) are approaching the need for renal replacement therapy such as dialysis or transplantation. The symptoms and complications of late-stage CKD dictate the timing of initiation of renal replacement therapy. Most recent estimates

TABLE 11.6

Glomerular Filtration Rate (GFR) Categories in Chronic Kidney Disease (156)

GFR Category	GFR (mL $\cdot$ min^{-1} $\cdot$ 1.73 m^{-2})	Terms
G1	$\geq$90	Normal or high
G2	60–89	Mildly decreased[a]
G3a	45–59	Mildly to moderately decreased
G3b	30–44	Moderately to severely decreased
G4	15–29	Severely decreased
G5	<15	Kidney failure

NOTE: In the absence of kidney damage, neither GFR category G1 nor G2 fulfill the criteria for chronic kidney disease.
[a]Relative to young adult level.

indicate that more than 20 million adults in the United States (*i.e.*, ~10% of the adult population) have CKD (43), and the incidence is expected to increase due to the increasing prevalence of DM and obesity. Hypertension, diabetes mellitus, and CVD are very common in the CKD population with the prevalence of these comorbidities rising incrementally from stage 1 to stage 5 CKD (294).

Exercise Testing

Those who have not participated in regular exercise training in the previous 3 mo should be referred for medical clearance prior to beginning exercise (see *Chapter 2*). Because CVD is the major cause of death in individuals with CKD, when symptoms are present or CVD is diagnosed, exercise testing may be indicated as part of the medical clearance process prior to beginning an exercise program of moderate to vigorous intensity (139). In some cases, exercise testing may also be included in the workup for possible kidney transplantation or in those with CKD presenting with chest pain (168). However, some suggest that exercise testing for patients with end-stage renal disease (ESRD) (*i.e.*, stage 5 CKD), as well as those who are frail, is not warranted because their performance may be affected by muscle fatigue, and such testing may act as an unnecessary barrier to their participation in a training program (3). If performed, exercise testing of individuals with CKD should use standard test termination criteria and test termination methods (see *Chapter 5*).

Most research on patients with CKD has been done on individuals classified with category 5 CKD. These individuals have low functional capacities with values that are approximately 50%–80% of those seen in healthy age- and sex-matched controls (140). $\dot{V}O_{2peak}$ ranges between 15 and 25 mL $\cdot$ kg^{-1} $\cdot$ min^{-1} (140). $\dot{V}O_{2peak}$ values can increase with training by approximately 17%–23% but in general will never reach the values achieved by age- and sex-matched controls (140). This reduced functional capacity is thought to be related to several factors including a sedentary lifestyle, cardiac dysfunction, anemia, and musculoskeletal dysfunction. In those referred for exercise testing, the following considerations should be noted:

- Medical clearance should be obtained.
- Individuals with CKD are likely to be on multiple medications including those that are commonly used in the treatment of hypertension, dyslipidemia, and DM (see *Appendix A*).
- When performing an exercise test on individuals with category 1–4 CKD, standard procedures should be followed (see *Chapter 5*). However, in patients receiving maintenance hemodialysis, testing should be scheduled for nondialysis days, and BP should be monitored in the arm that does not contain the arteriovenous fistula (214).
- For comfort purposes, patients receiving continuous ambulatory peritoneal dialysis should be tested with little dialysate fluid in their abdomen (214).
- Standard procedures are used to test patients who are transplant recipients.
- Both treadmill and cycle leg ergometry protocols can be used to test individuals with kidney diseases. Because of the low functional capacity in this population,

more conservative treadmill protocols such as the modified Balke or Naughton are appropriate (213) (see *Chapter 5*). If cycle leg ergometry is used, initial warm-up work rates should be 20–25 W with the work rate increased by 10- to 30-W increments every 1–3 min (52,307).

■ In patients receiving maintenance hemodialysis, the peak heart rate (HR_{peak}) is often attenuated and may not surpass 75% of age-predicted maximum (215). Because HR may not always be a reliable indicator of exercise intensity in patients with CKD, RPE should always be monitored (see *Chapter 4*).

■ As a result of the very low functional capacity of individuals with CKD, traditional exercise tests may not always yield the most valuable information for Ex R_x and the assessment of exercise training adaptations (216). Consequently, a variety of physical performance tests that have been used in other populations (*e.g.*, older adults) can be used (see *Chapter 7*). Tests can be chosen to assess CRF, muscular strength, balance, and flexibility (212,216).

■ Isotonic strength testing should be done using a 3-RM or higher load (*e.g.*, 10–12-RM) because 1-RM testing is generally thought to be contraindicated in patients with CKD because of the fear of spontaneous avulsion fractures (20,138,214,250). There are equations to predict the 1-RM from a multiple-RM test (9,34). The estimated 1-RM value can be used to develop the resistance training Ex R_x.

■ Muscular strength and endurance can be safely assessed using isokinetic dynamometers employing angular velocities ranging from 60 degrees to 180 degrees $\cdot$ s^{-1} (68,119,213).

■ Muscle power should be assessed using a computerized dynamometer because power appears to be more related to functional ability than either muscular strength or endurance (216). To assess power, individuals should be asked to perform a repetition at a specific percentage of their estimated maximum as quickly as possible (14).

Exercise Prescription

Exercise training in those with CKD leads to BP reductions and improvements in aerobic capacity, HR variability, muscular function, and quality of life (120). The ideal FITT principle of Ex R_x for individuals with CKD has not been fully developed, but based on the research that has been done, programs for these patients should consist of a combination of aerobic and resistance training (120,138). The Kidney Diseases: Improving Global Outcomes (KDIGO) clinical practice guidelines recommend that those with CKD aim for PA of an aerobic nature 5 d $\cdot$ wk^{-1} for at least 30 min but do not provide more specific guidance regarding the Ex R_x (156). The National Kidney Foundation encourages patients with CKD to be active and provides some general recommendations that are in keeping with those given to the healthy adult population (195). Because the ideal FITT has not been developed for patients with CKD, it is prudent to modify the recommendations for the general population, initially using light-to-moderate intensities and gradually progressing over time based on individual tolerance. Medically cleared recipients

■ **FITT RECOMMENDATIONS FOR INDIVIDUALS WITH KIDNEY DISEASE** (140)

	Aerobic	Resistance	Flexibility
Frequency	3–5 d · wk^{-1}	2–3 d · wk^{-1}	2–3 d · wk^{-1}
Intensity	Moderate intensity (40%–59% $\dot{V}O_2R$, RPE 12–13 on a scale of 6–20)	65%–75 % 1-RM. Performance of 1-RM is not recommended; estimate 1-RM from a ≥3-RM test.	Static: stretch to the point of tightness or slight discomfort; PNF: 20%–75% of maximum voluntary contraction
Time	20–60 min of continuous activity; however, if this cannot be tolerated, use 3–5 min bouts of intermittent exercise aiming to accumulate 20–60 min · d^{-1}.	A minimum of 1 set of 10–15 repetitions, with a goal in most patients to achieve multiple sets. Choose 8–10 different exercises targeting the major muscle groups.	60 s per joint for static (10–30 s hold per stretch); 3–6 s contraction followed by 10–30 s assisted stretch for PNF
Type	Prolonged, rhythmic activities using large muscle groups (*e.g.*, walking, cycling, swimming)	Machines, free weights, or bands	Static or PNF

1-RM, one repetition maximum; PNF, proprioceptive neuromuscular facilitation; $\dot{V}O_2R$, oxygen uptake reserve.

of kidney transplants can initiate exercise training soon after the transplant operation (182,212).

Exercise Training Considerations

■ Some individuals with CKD are unable to do continuous exercise and therefore should perform intermittent exercise with intervals as short as 3 min interspersed with 3 min of rest (*i.e.*, 1:1 work-to-rest ratio). As the individual adapts to training, the duration of the work interval can be gradually increased, whereas the rest interval can be decreased. Initially, a total exercise time of 15 min can be used, and this can be increased within tolerance to achieve up to 20–60 min of continuous activity.
■ The clinical status of the individual is important to consider. The progression may need to be slowed if the individual has a medical setback.

- Individuals with CKD, including individuals with ESRD, should be gradually progressed to a greater exercise volume over time. Depending on the clinical status and functional capacity of the individual, the initial intensity selected for training should be light (*i.e.*, 30%–39% $\dot{V}O_2R$) and for as little as 10–15 min of continuous activity or whatever amount the individual can tolerate. The duration of PA should be increased by 3–5 min increments weekly until the individual can complete 30 min of continuous activity before increasing the intensity.

Special Considerations

- Hemodialysis
  - Exercise should ideally be performed on nondialysis days.
  - Performing exercise immediately postdialysis may increase the risk of a hypotensive response.
  - During any aerobic exercise, it may be beneficial to use RPE to guide exercise intensity because HR can be unreliable. Aim to achieve an RPE in the light (9–11) to moderate (12–13) intensity range.
  - Patients may exercise the arm with permanent arteriovenous access. They should always avoid placing weight or pressure on the access device (138).
  - Measure BP in the arm that does not contain the fistula.
  - If exercise is performed during dialysis, it should typically be done during the first half of the treatment to avoid hypotensive episodes, although some individuals may use late dialysis exercise to counteract a hypotensive response. Exercise modes typically used during dialysis are pedaling and stepping devices which can be used while seated in a dialysis chair. During dialysis, patients should not exercise the arm with permanent arteriovenous access.
- Peritoneal dialysis
  - Patients on continuous ambulatory peritoneal dialysis may attempt exercising with fluid in their abdomen; however, if this produces discomfort, then they should be encouraged to drain the fluid before exercising (138).
- Recipients of kidney transplants
  - During periods of rejection, the intensity of exercise should be reduced, but exercise can still be continued (212).

ONLINE RESOURCES

National Institute of Diabetes and Digestive and Kidney Diseases:
   http://www2.niddk.nih.gov/
National Kidney Foundation:
   http://www.kidney.org/
United States Renal Data System:
   http://www.usrds.org/atlas.htm
Kidney Disease: Improving Global Outcomes:
   http://kdigo.org/home/

MULTIPLE SCLEROSIS

Multiple sclerosis (MS) is a chronic, inflammatory autoimmune disease of the central nervous system (CNS) that currently affects an estimated 400,000 individuals in the United States and 2–3 million individuals worldwide (197). Although the exact cause of MS is still unknown, most researchers believe it involves an abnormal immune-mediated response that may be influenced by a combination of environmental, infectious, and genetic factors. MS is characterized by nerve demyelination due to an attack from activated T cells that cross the blood–brain barrier. Following the initial inflammatory response, damaged myelin form scar-like plaques (scleroses) in the brain and spinal cord that can impair nerve conduction and transmission (300). This can lead to a wide variety of signs and symptoms, which include visual disturbances, weakness, fatigue, and sensory loss. Initial symptoms often include transient neurological deficits such as numbness or weakness, blurred or double vision, cognitive dysfunction, and balance problems. *Box 11.3* lists the common signs and symptoms in persons diagnosed with MS.

The onset of MS usually occurs between the ages of 20 and 50 yr and affects women at a rate two to three times more than men. The disease course of MS is highly variable from individual to individual and within a given individual over time. However, four distinct disease courses are now recognized (*Table 11.7*). Of the individuals with MS, 85% are diagnosed with *relapsing-remitting MS* (RRMS), 10% with *primary progressive MS* (PPMS), and 5% with *progressive-relapsing MS* (PRMS) (170). Fifty percent of individuals initially diagnosed with RRMS will transition to a steady, progressive form of MS within 10 yr (*i.e., secondary progressive MS* [SPMS]), and 90% will transition to SPMS within 25 yr (197).

Box 11.3	Common Signs and Symptoms of Multiple Sclerosis

Symptoms

Muscle weakness	Bowel dysfunction
Symptomatic fatigue	Cognitive dysfunction
Numbness	Dizziness and vertigo
Visual disturbances	Depression
Walking, balance, and	Emotional changes
coordination problems	Sexual dysfunction
Bladder dysfunction	Pain

Signs

Optic neuritis	Paresthesia
Nystagmus	Spasticity

Reprinted with permission from (50).

TABLE 11.7	
Disease Courses of Multiple Sclerosis	
Type	**Characteristic**
Relapsing-remitting	Periodic exacerbations followed by full or partial recovery of deficits
Primary progressive	Continuous disease progression from onset with little or no plateaus or improvements
Secondary progressive	Slow and steady disease progression that transitioned from the relapsing-remitting type
Progressive-relapsing	Progression from onset with distinct relapses superimposed on the steady progression with or without full recovery

Table 11.8 is a summary of the Kurtzke Expanded Disability Status Scale (EDSS; range 0–10) that is commonly used to indicate the level of disability related to the progression of MS (160).

Persons with MS generally report lower exercise tolerance and higher perceived fatigue compared to age-matched persons without MS (93). Deconditioning (76), lower rates of PA (203), and higher energy cost of walking (89,207) may explain some of the exercise intolerance and fatigue that persons with MS experience as their condition progresses. Individuals with MS generally have a low maximal aerobic capacity (*i.e.*, <60% of predicted $\dot{V}O_{2peak}$) (153,246), and peak aerobic capacity continues to decrease with increasing levels of disability (153,231). HR and BP responses in persons with MS have been shown to be blunted during exercise (220) and may be a result of autonomic dysfunction (278) and/or a reduced skeletal intramuscular metabolic response (202).

In persons with MS who are mild-to-moderately disabled, aerobic exercise training studies have demonstrated improvements in $\dot{V}O_{2peak}$ (220,235), increased fatigue tolerance (282), increased walking capacity (235,298), improved overall quality of life (220), and a reduction in the risk factors associated with CVD (*e.g.*, waist circumference, blood triglycerides levels, glucose levels) (274). A recent study

TABLE 11.8	
Summary of Kurtzke Expanded Disability Status Scale (EDSS)	
Rating	**Disability**
0–2.5	None to minimal disability
3–5.5	Moderate disability but still ambulatory without assistive device
6–7	Severe disability but still ambulatory with assistive device
7.5–9	Essentially wheelchair-bound or bedbound
10	Death attributable to multiple sclerosis

examining 10 sessions of upper body endurance training (*i.e.*, six 3-min intervals at target HR corresponding to 65%–75% $\dot{V}O_{2peak}$) in persons with progressive MS who are severely disabled (EDSS of 6.5–8.0) demonstrated modest improvements in $\dot{V}O_{2peak}$ (272), suggesting that individuals who are severely disabled may still be capable of performing at a sufficient intensity to obtain cardiovascular benefits.

Decreased muscle performance is also commonly observed in MS. Persons with MS have lower isometric strength (202–204,262) and dynamic power production (41,50,230) compared with individuals without MS. Skeletal muscle weakness in MS may be due to changes in central (*e.g.*, lower central activation [204,238], lower motor unit discharge rates [70,238]) and peripheral (*e.g.*, alterations in contractile function) [204], decreased oxidative capacity [151] factors, and smaller muscle size [150,204]) as well as factors associated with force production. However, some of these physiological changes may be a secondary effect of lower PA levels in persons with MS (203). Several studies have demonstrated increases in isometric strength (158,179,312) and power (61,285) following a resistance training program in persons with MS. In addition, gains in functional capacity (61,158,246), greater muscular endurance (287), increased balance (118,133), improved gait kinematics (104), and reduction in symptomatic fatigue (104,312) have been observed after resistance training.

Exercise Testing

Exercise testing is useful in determining the fitness level, the physiological response to a given bout of exercise, and the effectiveness of exercise training in persons with MS. Prior to exercise testing, it is highly recommended to review an individual's medical history and list of medications as well as to conduct a functional assessment. The 6-min walk test (endurance), timed 5-repetition sit-to-stand (strength), timed 25-ft walk (gait speed), Berg Balance Scale (balance) (18), and Dynamic Gait Index (dynamic balance) (122) are commonly used functional tests.

- Avoid testing during an acute exacerbation of MS symptoms.
- Closely monitor for any signs of paresis, fatigue, overheating, or general worsening of symptoms as exercise intensity increases.
- Perform exercise testing earlier in the day because fatigue generally worsens throughout the day in individuals with MS.
- Conduct exercise testing in a climate-controlled room (72° to 74° F [22.2° to 24.4° C], low humidity)
- Use RPE in addition to HR to evaluate exercise intensity. HR and BP responses may be blunted because of autonomic dysfunction; therefore, HR may not be a valid indicator of exercise intensity.
- In most patients with MS, a cycle ergometer is the recommended method of testing aerobic fitness because this modality requires less balance and coordination compared with walking on a treadmill (297). Individuals with balance and coordination problems may require the use of an upright or recumbent cycle leg ergometer with foot straps.
- In select patients, a recumbent stepping ergometer or dual action stationary cycle (*e.g.*, NuStep or Schwinn Airdyne) that allows for the use of upper and

lower extremities may be advantageous because it distributes work to all extremities, thus minimizing the potential influence of local muscle fatigue or weakness in one limb on maximal exercise testing.

- Persons who are nonambulatory with sufficient upper body function can be assessed using an arm ergometer.
- Before starting an exercise test, a low-level warm-up of 1–2 min should be implemented.
- Depending on the disability and physical fitness level of the individual, the use of a continuous or discontinuous protocol of 3–5 min stages increasing work rate for each stage from 12 to 25 W for leg ergometry and 8 to 12 W for arm ergometry is recommended.
- In general, muscle strength and endurance can be determined using standard protocols in persons with MS. Each large muscle group and all limbs should be tested because weakness may present itself in a particular muscle group or limb due to the heterogeneity of lesion location and impact in MS. Isokinetic dynamometry can be used to evaluate muscle performance; however, in a clinical or community setting, an 8- to 10-RM or functional testing (*e.g.*, 30-s sit-to-stand test) can be used to measure muscular strength and endurance.
- Assessment of flexibility is important because increased muscle tone and spasticity may be evident in those with poor flexibility and can lead to contracture formation in persons with MS. Joint ROM can be measured using a goniometer.

Exercise Prescription

For individuals with minimal disability (EDSS 0–2.5), the FITT principle of Ex R_x is generally consistent with those outlined in *Chapter 6* for healthy adults. As MS symptoms and level of disability increase, the following modifications outlined may be required.

Exercise Training Considerations

- Whenever possible, incorporate functional activities (*e.g.*, stairs, sit-to-stand) into the exercise program.
- With individuals who have significant paresis, consider assessing RPE of the extremities separately using the 0–10 OMNI scale (*Figure 11.3*) (243) to evaluate effects of local muscle fatigue on exercise tolerance.
- During an acute exacerbation of MS symptoms, decrease the FITT of the Ex R_x to the level of tolerance. If the exacerbation is severe, focus on maintaining functional mobility and/or focus on aerobic exercise and flexibility. Recognize that in times of severe relapse, any exercise may be too difficult to perform.
- When strengthening weaker muscle groups or working with easily fatigued individuals, increase rest time (*e.g.*, 2–5 min) between sets and exercises as needed to allow for full muscle recovery. Focus on large postural muscle groups and minimize total number of exercises performed.
- Stretching is most effective when muscles are "warmed up" via exercise. Caution should be used if moist heat packs are used to warm a muscle due to the possibility of a reduced ability to thermoregulate body temperature due to MS.

■ **FITT RECOMMENDATIONS FOR INDIVIDUALS WITH MULTIPLE SCLEROSIS** (162)

	Aerobic	Resistance	Flexibility
Frequency	2–5 d · wk^{-1}	2 d · wk^{-1}	5–7 d · wk^{-1}, 1–2 times · d^{-1}
Intensity	40%–70% $\dot{V}O_2R$ or HRR; RPE 12–15	60%–80% 1-RM	Stretch to the point of feeling tightness or mild discomfort.
Time	Increase time initially to a minimum of 10 min before increasing intensity. Progress to 30–60 min as tolerated.	Begin with 1 and gradually work up to 2 sets of 10–15 repetitions.	Hold 30–60 s, 2–4 repetitions.
Type	Prolonged, rhythmic activities using large muscle groups (*e.g.*, walking, cycling, swimming)	Multijoint and single-joint exercises using machines, free weights, resistance bands, or body weight	Static stretching

1-RM, one repetition maximum; HRR, heart rate reserve; RPE, rating of perceived exertion; $\dot{V}O_2R$, oxygen uptake reserve.

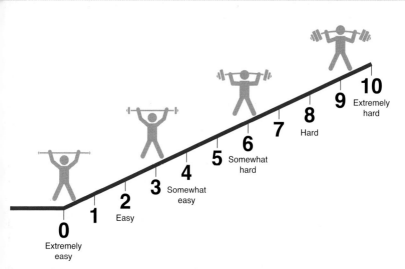

Figure 11.3 OMNI-Resistance Exercise Scale of perceived exertion. Used with permission from (243).

- Slow and gentle passive ROM exercise should be performed while seated or lying down to eliminate balance concerns.
- In spastic muscles, increase the frequency and time of flexibility exercises. Muscles and joints with significant tightness or contracture may require longer duration (several minutes to several hours) and lower load positional stretching to achieve lasting improvements. Very low-intensity, low-speed, or no-load cycling may be beneficial in those with frequent spasticity.

Special Considerations

- Commonly used disease-modifying medications such as Avonex, Betaseron, Rebif, and Copaxone can have transient side effects such as flu-like symptoms and localized irritation at the injection site. Take medication side effects into consideration with exercise testing and scheduling.
- Systemic fatigue is common in MS but tends to improve with increased physical fitness. It is important to help the individual understand the difference between more general centrally mediated MS fatigue and temporary peripheral exercise-related fatigue. Tracking the effects of fatigue may be helpful using an instrument such as the Modified Fatigue Impact Scale (197).
- Some individuals may restrict their daily fluid intake because of bladder control problems. They should be counseled to increase fluid intake with increased PA levels to prevent dehydration.
- Many individuals with MS have some level of cognitive deficit that may affect their understanding of testing and training instructions. They may also have short-term memory loss that requires written instructions and frequent verbal cueing and reinforcement.
- Watch for signs and symptoms of the *Uhthoff phenomenon* which typically involves a transient (<24 h) worsening of neurological symptoms, most commonly, visual impairment associated with exercise and elevation of body temperature. Symptoms can be minimized by using cooling strategies and adjusting exercise time and intensity.
- Use electric fans or cold neck packs and provide fluid replacement to minimize risk of hyperthermia and symptomatic fatigue during exercise, especially in individuals with MS with heat sensitivity.

ONLINE RESOURCES

National Center on Health, Physical Activity and Disability:
http://www.nchpad.org/156/1192/Multiple~Sclerosis~~Designing~an~Exercise~Program
National Institute for Neurological Disorders and Stroke:
http://www.ninds.nih.gov/multiple_sclerosis/multiple_sclerosis.htm
National Multiple Sclerosis Society:
http://www.nationalmssociety.org

OSTEOPOROSIS

Osteoporosis is a skeletal disease that is characterized by low BMD and changes in the microarchitecture of bone that increase susceptibility to fracture. The burden of osteoporosis on society and the individual is significant. Osteoporosis affects almost one out of every two women at some point in their lives. Although osteoporosis is thought of primarily as a disease of women, prevalence rates in men can be as high as 15% (147). More than 54 million individuals in the United States have osteoporosis or low bone density (198). Hip fractures, in particular, are associated with increased risk of disability and death. There is an estimated fivefold increase in all-cause mortality in the 3 mo following a hip fracture in older adults (107).

The official position of the International Society of Clinical Densitometry defines osteoporosis in postmenopausal women and in men ≥50 yr as a BMD T-score of the lumbar spine, total hip, or femoral neck of ≤−2.5 (261). The National Bone Health Alliance Working Group proposes additional diagnostic criteria for osteoporosis to include those with diagnosed osteopenia who have sustained a low-trauma vertebral, proximal humerus, pelvis, or distal forearm fracture or who have an elevated fracture risk per the World Health Organization's Fracture Risk Algorithm (FRAX) (270). It is important to recognize that osteoporotic fractures can occur in individuals with higher BMD levels, particularly in the elderly.

Recent evidence indicates that exercise can delay the onset of osteoporosis and reduce fracture risk (26,148,228). The benefits of exercise on bone health occur in both children and adults and are due primarily to increases in bone density, volume, and strength and to a parallel increase in muscle strength (6,26,148,228). Exercise also improves balance in both young and older populations, which can reduce falls and subsequent osteoporotic fracture risk (40,141). Thus, exercise can generally be regarded as the primary nonpharmacological treatment for prevention of osteoporosis. Nevertheless, many studies have concluded that large randomized controlled trials are still needed in both women and men to determine optimal Ex R_x for preventing both osteoporosis and fracture (26,148,228).

Exercise Testing

In general, when an exercise test is clinically indicated for those with osteoporosis, normal testing procedures should be followed (see *Chapter 5*). However, when exercise tests are performed in individuals with osteoporosis, the following issues should be considered:

- Use of cycle leg ergometry as an alternative to treadmill exercise testing to assess cardiorespiratory function may be indicated in patients with severe vertebral osteoporosis for whom walking is painful or risky.
- Multiple vertebral compression fractures leading to a loss of height and spinal deformation can compromise ventilatory capacity and result in a forward shift in the center of gravity. The latter may affect balance during treadmill walking.

- Maximal muscle strength testing may be contraindicated in patients with severe osteoporosis, although there are no established guidelines for contraindications for maximal muscle strength testing.
- Balance testing or fall risk assessment should be considered in patients with osteoporosis or low bone density. Available balance assessments include the four-stage balance test (45) and the Falls Efficacy Scale (288).

Exercise Prescription

Currently, little evidence exists regarding the optimal exercise regime for individuals with or at risk for osteoporosis. In general, weight-bearing aerobic exercise in combination with some form of high-impact, high-velocity, high intensity resistance training is considered the best choice for either population (6,26,99,228).

■ FITT RECOMMENDATIONS FOR INDIVIDUALS WITH OSTEOPOROSIS (6,99)

FITT		**Aerobic**	**Resistance**	**Flexibility**
	Frequency	4–5 d · wk^{-1}	Start with 1–2 non-consecutive d · wk^{-1}; may progress to 2–3 d · wk^{-1}	5–7 d · wk^{-1}
	Intensity	Moderate intensity (40%–59% $\dot{V}O_2R$ or HRR). Use of the CR-10 scale (0–10) with ratings of 3–4 might be a more appropriate method of establishing intensity.	Adjust resistance so that last 2 repetitions are challenging to perform. High intensity training is beneficial in those who can tolerate it.	Stretch to the point of tightness or slight discomfort.
	Time	Begin with 20 min; gradually progress to a minimum of 30 min (with a maximum of 45–60 min).	Begin with 1 set of 8–12 repetitions; increase to 2 sets after ~2 wk; no more than 8–10 exercises per session	Hold static stretch for 10–30 s; 2–4 repetitions of each exercise
	Type	Walking, cycling, or other individually appropriate aerobic activity (weight bearing preferred)	Standard equipment can be used with adequate instruction and safety considerations.	Static stretching of all major joints

HRR, heart rate reserve; $\dot{V}O_2R$, oxygen uptake reserve.

Special Considerations

- It is difficult to quantify exercise intensity in terms of bone loading forces. However, the magnitude of bone loading force generally increases in parallel with exercise intensity quantified by conventional methods (*e.g.*, %HRR for aerobic training or %1-RM for resistance training). Weight-bearing aerobic and high-velocity resistance training modes are recommended. Proper form and alignment are more important than intensity especially for those with a history of fractures (99).

- There are currently no established guidelines regarding contraindications to exercise for individuals with osteoporosis. The general recommendation is to prescribe moderate intensity weight-bearing exercise that does not cause or exacerbate pain. Exercises that involve explosive movements or high-impact loading should be avoided. Specific exercises or portions of group-led routines (*e.g.*, yoga, Pilates) that require excessive twisting, bending, or compression of the spine should also be carefully assessed and those types of movements avoided, particularly in those with very low spinal BMD values.

- Falls in those with osteoporosis increase the likelihood of a bone fracture. For older women and men at increased risk for falls, the Ex R$_x$ should also include activities that improve balance (see *Chapter 7* and the relevant ACSM position stand [6]). Primary considerations should be exercises that strengthen the quadriceps, hamstrings, and gluteal and trunk muscles because these are the muscles primarily responsible for balance (40).

- In light of the rapid and profound effects of immobilization and bed rest on bone loss and poor prognosis for recovery of BMD after remobilization, even the frailest elderly should remain as physically active as his or her health permits because this will best preserve musculoskeletal integrity. Even short bouts of standing or walking are desirable during prolonged illnesses.

- The recommendations in this section are generalized for exercise in patients with, or at risk for, osteoporosis. Modifications based on clinical judgment may be necessary for some patients (99).

ONLINE RESOURCES

American College of Sports Medicine Position Stand on Osteoporosis:
 http://www.acsm.org
International Society of Clinical Densitometry:
 http://www.iscd.org/official-positions/
National Institutes of Health Osteoporosis and Related Bone Diseases:
 http://www.niams.nih.gov/Health_Info/Bone/default.asp
National Osteoporosis Foundation:
 http://www.nof.org

PARKINSON DISEASE

Parkinson disease (PD) is one of the most common neurodegenerative diseases. More than 1.5 million individuals in the United States are believed to have PD, and 70,000 new cases are diagnosed each year (112). It is estimated 6 million individuals worldwide are currently living with PD (291). PD is a chronic, progressive neurological disorder characterized clinically by symptoms consisting of resting tremor, bradykinesia, rigidity, postural instability, and gait abnormalities (*Box 11.4*). PD is the result of damage to the dopaminergic nigrostriatal pathway of the midbrain, which results in a reduction in the neurotransmitter dopamine. The cause of PD is unknown; however, genetics and the environment are thought to be factors. Aging, autoimmune responses, and mitochondrial dysfunction may also contribute to the disease process (24,66,87,233).

Once motor signs and symptoms are clinically present, referred to as the motor phase of PD, severity of the disease can be classified as (a) *early disease*, characterized by minor symptoms of tremor or stiffness; (b) *moderate disease*, characterized by mild-to-moderate tremor and limited movement; and (c) *advanced*

Box 11.4	Common Movement Disorders in Individuals with Parkinson Disease (187)
Bradykinesia	Reduced movement speed and amplitude; at the extreme, it is known as *hypokinesia*, which refers to "poverty" of movement.
Akinesia	Difficulty initiating movements
Episodes of freezing	Motor blocks/sudden inability to move during the execution of a movement sequence
Impaired balance and postural instability	Difficulty maintaining upright stance with narrow base of support in response to a perturbation to the center of mass or with eyes closed; difficulty maintaining stability in sitting or when transferring from one position to another; can manifest as frequent falling
Dyskinesia	Overreactivity of muscles; wriggling/writhing movements
Tremor	Rhythmic activity alternating in antagonistic muscles, resembling a pill-rolling movement; usually resting tremor
Rigidity	Muscular stiffness throughout the range of passive movement in both extensor and flexor muscle groups in a given limb
Adaptive responses	Reduced activity, muscle weakness, reduced muscle length, contractures, deformity, reduced aerobic capacity

TABLE 11.9
The Hoehn and Yahr Staging Scale of Parkinson Disease (127)
Stage 0.0 = no signs of disease
Stage 1.0 = unilateral disease
Stage 2.0 = bilateral disease, without impairment of balance
Stage 2.5 = mild bilateral disease, with recovery on pull test
Stage 3.0 = mild-to-moderate bilateral disease; some postural instability; physically independent
Stage 4.0 = severe disability; still able to walk or stand unassisted
Stage 5.0 = wheelchair bound or bedridden unless aided

disease, characterized by significant limitations in activity regardless of treatment or medication (233). The progression of symptoms is described more comprehensively by the Hoehn and Yahr (HY) scale (127) (*Table 11.9*).

The symptoms of PD affect movement, and individuals with moderate and severe PD may have difficulty performing ADL. Resting tremors are often evident but can be suppressed by voluntary activity, sleep, and complete relaxation of axial muscles. Stress and anxiety increase resting tremors. Rigidity makes movement difficult and may increase EE. This increases the individual's perception of effort on movement and may be related to feelings of fatigue, especially postexercise fatigue. Bradykinesia and akinesia are characterized by a reduction or inability to initiate and perform purposeful movements. Postural instability or impaired balance is a serious problem in PD that leads to increased episodes of falling and exposes individuals with PD to the serious consequences of falls. Generally, patients with PD demonstrate slowed, short-stepped, shuffling walk with decreased arm swing and forward-stooped posture and have poorer walking economy when compared to persons without PD (49,94). Difficulty and slowness in performing turning, getting up, transfer, and ADL are common. Other problems including excessive salivation or drooling; soft, slurred speech; and small handwriting also impact quality of life. Individuals with PD also suffer from autonomic nervous system dysfunction including cardiovascular dysfunction, especially in advanced stages. Orthostatic hypotension, cardiac arrhythmias, sweating disturbances, and HR and BP disturbances can impact ADL, PA, and exercise.

Drug therapy is the primary intervention for the treatment of symptoms related to PD. Levodopa remains the mainstay of treatment and is the single most effective drug available to treat all cardinal features of PD. Despite its significant benefit, the effectiveness is limited to an average of approximately 10 yr. Long-term use is associated with motor complications including motor fluctuations and dyskinesias in about 50% of patients within 5 yr (223,279). Other side effects include nausea, sedation, orthostatic hypotension, and psychiatric symptoms (especially hallucinations). Levodopa is now always combined with Carbidopa to prevent systemic adverse effects (237). Other adjunctive drug groups are catechol-O-methyltransferase inhibitors, monoamine oxidase B inhibitors, amantadine, anticholinergics, and dopamine agonists. These drugs are used as a monotherapy or adjunct therapy to provide symptomatic relief in PD and may have side effects that are important when prescribing exercise to those with PD. For this reason, the exercise professional is advised to become familiar with these medications.

Individuals with severe PD may undergo surgical treatment. *Deep brain stimulation* (DBS) is an electrical stimulation of the deep brain nuclei, with the internal globus pallidus and subthalamic nucleus as the two main stimulation targets. DBS is the surgical intervention of choice when motor complications are inadequately managed with the medications. Improvement in motor function after either stimulation target is similar (86). DBS is more effective than medical therapy in advanced PD in improving dyskinesia, motor function, and quality of life (309).

Exercise is a crucial adjunct treatment in PD management. Regular exercise will decrease or delay secondary sequelae affecting musculoskeletal and cardiorespiratory systems that occur as a result of reduced PA. Because PD is a chronic progressive disease, sustained exercise is necessary to maintain benefits. Evidence demonstrates exercise improves gait performance, quality of life and aerobic capacity and reduces disease severity in individuals with PD (19,121,252,256,266). Exercise might also play a neuroprotective role in individuals with PD; however, the evidence is mostly limited to animal models (318).

Exercise Testing

Most individuals with PD have impaired mobility and problems with gait, balance, and functional ability, which vary from individual to individual. These impairments are often accompanied by low levels of physical fitness (*e.g.*, CRF, muscular strength and endurance, flexibility). The following are special considerations in performing exercise testing for individuals with PD:

- Because many individuals with PD are older and have reduced PA levels, assessment of cardiovascular risk may be warranted prior to beginning an exercise test.
- Tests of balance, gait, general mobility, ROM, flexibility, and muscular strength are recommended before exercise testing is performed. Results of the tests can guide how to safely exercise test the individual with PD.
- Static and dynamic balance evaluation and physical limitations of the individual should be used in making decisions regarding testing modes for test validity and safety. Clinical balance tests include the Functional Reach test (71), tandem stance (218), single limb stance (275), and pull tests (189,218,275). The Timed Up and Go (TUG) test (171,227) and chair sit-to-stand test (265) can be used to measure functional mobility.
- Gait observation can be done during the 10-m walk test at a comfortable walking speed (155,255).
- Manual muscle testing, arm curl tests, RM assessment using weight machines, dynamometers, and chair rise tests (100) can be used for strength evaluation;

goniometry, the sit-and-reach test, and the back scratch test can be used to evaluate flexibility (239); and the 6-min walk test can be used to assess CRF (73).

- Decisions regarding exercise testing protocols may be influenced by the severity of PD (see *Table 11.9*) or physical limitations of the individual. Use of a cycle leg ergometer alone or combined with arm ergometry may be more suitable for individuals with severe gait and balance impairment or with a history of falls (233). However, use of leg/arm ergometers may preclude individuals with PD from achieving a maximum cardiorespiratory response because of early muscular fatigue before the maximal cardiorespiratory levels are attained (311). Treadmill protocols can be used safely in individuals with a mild stage of PD (Hoehn and Yahr Stage 1–2) (311). Submaximal tests may be most appropriate in advanced cases (HY stage ≥3) or with severe mobility impairment.

- Autonomic nervous system dysfunction can occur in individuals with PD (317), increasing their risk of developing BP abnormalities (105), which can be further affected by medications (234).

- Individuals with very advanced PD (HY stage ≥4) and those unable to perform a GXT for various reasons, such as inability to stand without falling, severe stooped posture, and deconditioning, may require a radionuclide stress test or stress echocardiography.

- For an individual who is deconditioned, demonstrates lower extremity weakness, or has a history of falling, care and precautions should be taken, especially at the final stages of the treadmill protocol when fatigue occurs and the individual's walking may deteriorate. A gait belt should be worn, and a technician should stand by close to the subject to guard during the treadmill test.

- Use of symptom-limited exercise testing is strongly recommended. Symptoms include fatigue, shortness of breath, abnormal BP responses, and deteriorations in general appearance. Monitoring physical exertion levels during testing by using a scale such as the RPE scale (27) is recommended.

- Individuals with PD may experience orthostatic hypotension because of the severity of PD and medications (277). Antiparkinsonian medication intake should be noted prior to performing the exercise test.

- Issues to consider when conducting a GXT in individuals with PD include conducting the test during peak medication effect when an individual has optimal mobility, providing practice walking on a treadmill prior to testing, and using the modified Bruce protocol (see *Chapter 5*). These factors allow individuals with PD the opportunity to achieve maximal exercise (311). Although the Bruce protocol is the most commonly used protocol for exercise testing on a treadmill (146), it may be too strenuous for individuals with PD (311).

- For individuals with DBS, the signal from the DBS pulse generator interferes with the ECG recording. It is possible to perform the test when the DBS is deactivated; however, without the stimulation, the patient will be at a compromised mobile state and will not be able to achieve maximal tolerance. Potential risks when the DBS is deactivated are physical discomfort, tremor, cramping, and emotional symptoms (*e.g.*, nervousness, anxiety, pain). Clinicians should consult with a neurologist prior to performing the exercise test in these patients.

Deactivation of the DBS should be done by a trained clinician or neurologist. HR monitoring can be used when DBS is not activated. RPE should be used to monitor during exercise testing.

- In addition to the aforementioned concerns, standard procedures, contraindications to exercise testing, recommended monitoring intervals, and standard termination criteria are used to exercise test individuals with PD (see *Chapter 5*).
- There have been no known serious adverse effects exacerbated by the interaction of PD medications and exercise. A few episodes of systolic blood pressure (SBP) drops of >20 mm Hg during treadmill training sessions have been reported (271). However, no association between medication usage and drop in SBP during exercise was found.

Exercise Prescription

The main goal of exercise is to delay disability, prevent secondary complications, and improve quality of life as PD progresses. The FITT principle of Ex R_x should address CRF, muscle strength, flexibility, neuromotor training, and motor control. Because PD is a chronic and progressive disorder, an exercise program should be prescribed early when the individual is first diagnosed and continue on a regular, long-term basis. The Ex R_x should be reviewed and revised as PD progresses because different physical problems occur at different stages of the disease.

Four key health outcomes of an exercise program designed for individuals with PD are improved (a) gait, (b) transfers, (c) balance, and (d) joint mobility and muscle power to improve functional capacity (154). Because the FITT principle of Ex R_x recommendations for individuals with PD are based on limited literature, the FITT Ex R_x for healthy adults generally applies to those with PD (95); however, the limitations imposed by the disease process should be assessed, and the Ex R_x should be tailored accordingly.

It is important to note that the FITT principle of Ex R_x recommendations for resistance training in individuals with PD is based on a very limited literature. In general, resistance training increases strength in individuals with PD, but the majority of interventions tested were conservative (74). After a resistance training program, strength improvements are similar in individuals with PD compared to neurologically normal controls (53,253). Therefore, recommendations for resistance exercise in neurologically healthy, older adults may be applied to individuals with PD (253). General aerobic training at a moderate intensity may improve aerobic fitness, fatigue, mood, and quality of life in those with mild-to-moderate PD (292).

Exercise Training Considerations

- The selection of the exercise type is dependent on the individual's clinical presentation of PD severity. A stationary cycle, recumbent cycle, or arm ergometer are safer modes for individuals with more advanced PD.
- During resistance training, emphasize extensor muscles of the trunk and hip to prevent faulty posture. Train all major muscles of lower extremities to maintain mobility.

FITT RECOMMENDATIONS FOR INDIVIDUALS WITH PARKINSON DISEASE (252,292)

	Aerobic	Resistance	Flexibility
Frequency	3 d · wk^{-1}	2–3 d · wk^{-1}	≥2–3 d · wk^{-1} with daily being most effective
Intensity	Moderate intensity (40%–59% $\dot{V}O_2R$ or HRR; RPE of 12–13 on a scale of 6–20)	40%–50% of 1-RM for individuals beginning to improve strength; 60%–70% 1-RM for more advanced exercisers	Full extension, flexion, rotation, or stretch to the point of slight discomfort
Time	30 min of continuous or accumulated exercise	≥1 set of 8–12 repetitions; 10–15 repetitions in adults starting an exercise program	Hold static stretch for 10–30 s; 2–4 repetitions of each exercise
Type	Prolonged, rhythmic activities using large muscle groups (*e.g.*, walking, cycling, swimming, dancing)	For safety, avoid free weights; focus on weight machines and other resistance devices (*e.g.*, bands, body weight).	Slow static stretches for all major muscle groups

1-RM, one repetition maximum; HRR, heart rate reserve; RPE, rating of perceived exertion; $\dot{V}O_2R$, oxygen uptake reserve.

Recommendations for Neuromotor Exercise for Individuals with Parkinson Disease

Balance impairment and falls are major problems in individuals with PD. Balance training is a crucial exercise in all individuals with PD. A recent systemic review reported PA and exercise improved postural instability and balance performance in individuals with mild-to-moderate PD (67). Static, dynamic, and balance training during functional activities should be included. Clinicians should take steps to ensure the individual's safety (*e.g.*, using a gait belt and nearby rails or parallel bars and removing clutter on the floor) when using physical activities that challenge balance. Training programs may include a variety of challenging physical activities (*e.g.*, stepping in all directions, step up and down, reaching forward and sideways, obstacles, turning around, walking with suitable step length, standing up and sitting down) (159,187). Tai chi, tango, and waltz are other forms of exercise to improve balance in PD (72,106,166).

- Flexibility and ROM exercises should be emphasized for the upper extremities and trunk. All major joints of the body should be emphasized in all stages of PD (233).
- Spinal mobility and axial rotation exercises are recommended for all severity stages (255).
- Neck flexibility exercises should be emphasized because neck rigidity is correlated with posture, gait, balance, and functional mobility (92).
- Incorporate functional exercises such as the sit-to-stand, step-ups, turning over, and getting out of bed as tolerated to improve neuromotor control, balance, and maintenance of ADL.

Special Considerations

- Some medications used to treat PD further impair autonomic nervous system functions (105). Levodopa/Carbidopa may produce exercise bradycardia and transient peak dose tachycardia and dyskinesia. Caution should be used in testing and training an individual who has had a recent change in medications because the response may be unpredictable (233). Several nonmotor symptoms may burden exercise performance (47,229) (*Box 11.5*).
- The outcome of exercise training varies significantly among individuals with PD because of the complexity and progressive nature of the disease (233).
- Cognitive decline and dementia are common nonmotor symptoms in PD and burden the training and progression (277).

Box 11.5	Nonmotor Symptoms in Parkinson Disease (47)
Domains	**Symptoms**
Cardiovascular	Symptomatic orthostasis, fainting, light-headedness
Sleep/fatigue	Sleep disorders, excessive daytime sleepiness, insomnia, fatigue, lack of energy, restless legs
Mood/cognition	Apathy, depression, loss of motivation, loss of interest, anxiety syndromes and panic attacks, cognitive decline
Perceptual problems/ hallucinations	Hallucinations, delusion, double vision
Attention/memory	Difficulty in concentration, forgetfulness, memory loss
Gastrointestinal	Drooling, swallowing, choking, constipation
Urinary	Incontinence, excessive urination at night, increased frequency of urination
Sexual function	Altered interest in sex, problems having sex
Miscellaneous	Pain, loss of smell/taste and appetite/weight, excessive sweating, fluctuating response to medication

- Incorporate and emphasize fall prevention/reduction and education into the exercise program. Instruction on how to break falls should be given and practiced to prevent serious injuries. Most falls in PD occur during multiple tasks or long and complex movement (186,188).
- Balance training should be emphasized in all individuals with PD (103).
- Avoid using dual tasking or multitasking with novice exercisers. Individuals with PD have difficulty in paying full attention to all tasks. One activity should be completed before commencing of the next activity (155). Multitasking may better prepare an individual with PD for responding to a balance perturbation (268) and can be incorporated into training when they perform well in a single task.
- Although no reports exist suggesting resistive exercise may exacerbate symptoms of PD, considerable attention must be paid to the development and management of fatigue (96).
- Fall history should also be recorded. Patients with PD with more than one fall in the previous year are likely to fall again within the next 3 mo (154).
- Visual and auditory cueing can be used to improve gait in persons with PD during exercise (283).

ONLINE RESOURCES

American Parkinson Disease Association:
   http://www.apdaparkinson.org/userND/index.asp
Davis Phinney Foundation:
   http://www.davisphinneyfoundation.org/site/c.mvKWLaMOIqG/b.5109589
   /k.BFE6/Home.htm
Michael J. Fox Foundation for Parkinson's Research:
   http://www.michaeljfox.org
National Institute of Neurological Disorders and Stroke:
   http://www.ninds.nih.gov/parkinsons_disease/parkinsons_disease.htm
National Parkinson Foundation:
   http://www.parkinson.org/
Parkinson's Disease Foundation:
   http:// www.pdf.org
The Parkinson Alliance:
   http://www.parkinsonalliance.org/
Parkinson's Action Network:
   http://parkinsonsaction.org/
European Parkinson's Disease Association:
   http://www.epda.eu.com

SPINAL CORD INJURY

Spinal cord injury (SCI) results in a loss of somatic, sensory, and autonomic functions below the lesion level. Lesions in the cervical (C) region typically result in tetraplegia or tetraparesis (respectively, complete or incomplete loss of function below the C level of lesion), whereas lesions in the thoracic (T), lumbar (L), and sacral (S) regions lead to paraplegia or paraparesis (respectively, complete or incomplete loss of function below the T, L, or S level of lesion). Approximately 60% of persons with SCI have an incomplete injury (199) in which some functions controlled by spinal cord segments below the lesion level are intact. Approximately half of those with SCI have a C lesion, with the balance having T, L, or S lesions, and 80% of those with an SCI are male (199). SCI of traumatic origin often occurs at an early age. Individuals with SCI have a high risk for the development of secondary conditions (*e.g.*, shoulder pain, urinary tract infections, skin pressure ulcers, osteopenia, chronic pain, problematic spasticity, joint contractures, depression, obesity, T2DM, and CVD).

The SCI level and completeness have direct impacts on physical function and metabolic and cardiorespiratory responses to exercise. It is crucial to take into account the SCI lesion level when exercise testing and prescribing exercise for those with complete SCI. Those with complete SCI lesions from

- L2–S2 lack voluntary control of the bladder, bowels, and sexual function; however, the upper extremities and trunk usually have normal function.
- T6–L2 have respiratory and motor control that depends on the functional capacity of the abdominal muscles (*i.e.*, minimal at T6 to maximal at L2).
- T1–T6 can experience poor thermoregulation, orthostatic/exercise hypotension, and autonomic dysreflexia (*i.e.*, an unregulated, spinally mediated reflex response called the *mass reflex* that can be a life-threatening medical emergency with sudden hypertension, bradycardia, pounding headache, piloerection, flushing, gooseflesh, shivering, sweating above the level of injury, nasal congestion, and blotching of the skin). When there is no sympathetic innervation to the heart, resting HR may be bradycardic due to cardiac vagal dominance, and HR_{peak} is limited to ~115–130 beats · min^{-1}. Breathing capacity is further diminished by intercostal muscle paralysis; however, arm function is normal.
- C5–C8 are tetraplegic. Those with C8 lesions have voluntary control of the scapula, shoulder, elbow, and wrist but decreased hand function, whereas those with C5 lesions rely on the biceps brachii and shoulder muscles for self-care and mobility. Autonomic dysreflexia and orthostatic hypotension can occur.
- Above C4 requires ventilator support for breathing. Autonomic dysreflexia and orthostatic hypotension can occur.

Exercise Testing

When exercise testing individuals with SCI, consider the following issues:

- Initially, function should be assessed including ROM, strength, balance, transferability, wheelchair mobility, and upper and lower extremity motor involvement. This assessment will facilitate the choice of exercise testing equipment, protocols, and adaptations.
- Consider the purpose of the exercise test, the level and completeness of SCI, and the physical fitness level of the participant to optimize equipment and protocol selection.

- Choose an exercise mode that allows the person to engage the largest possible muscle mass. If substantial trunk and lower limb function is intact, consider combined voluntary arm and leg cycle ergometry or recumbent stepping. If complete or nearly complete, voluntary arm ergometry is the easiest to perform and is norm-referenced for the assessment of CRF (108). Other norm-referenced data exist for wheelchair exercise (269).

- If available, a stationary wheelchair roller system or motor-driven treadmill should be used with the participant's properly adjusted wheelchair. Motor-driven treadmill protocols allow for realistic simulation of external conditions such as slope and speed alterations (302).

- Incremental exercise tests for the assessment of CRF in the laboratory should begin at 0 W with incremental increases of 5–10 W per stage for persons with tetraplegia. Depending on function and fitness, individuals with paraplegia can use increments of 10–25 W per stage.

- For sport-specific indoor CRF assessments in the field, an incremental test adapted from the Léger and Boucher shuttle test around a predetermined rectangular court is recommended. Floor surface characteristics and wheelchair user interface should be standardized (164,302).

- After maximal-effort exercise in individuals with tetraplegia, it may be necessary to treat postexercise hypotension and exhaustion with rest, recumbency, leg elevation, and fluid ingestion.

- There are no special considerations for the assessment of muscular strength regarding the exercise testing mode beyond those for the general population with the exception of the lesion level, which will determine residual motor function, need for stabilization, and accessibility of testing equipment.

- Individuals with SCI requiring a wheelchair for mobility may develop joint contractures because of muscle spasticity, strength imbalance, and flexed joint position in the wheelchair (*i.e.*, hip flexion, hip adduction and knee flexion) and excessive wheelchair pushing and manual transfers (*i.e.*, anterior chest and shoulder). Therefore, intensive sport-specific training must be complemented with an upper extremity stretching of prime movers and strengthening antagonists program to promote muscular balance around the joints.

Exercise Prescription

The goals of exercise training include the prevention of deconditioning; improved wellness (*i.e.*, weight management, glucose homeostasis, lower cardiovascular risk); and improved muscular strength, muscular endurance, and flexibility for functional independence (wheelchair mobility, transfers, ADL), for prevention of falls and sports injuries, and for improved performance (safety and success in adaptive sports and recreational activities). Currently, there are no published consensus recommendations for developing an Ex R_x in the SCI population, and further research is warranted (25,124). Thus, the specific FITT principle of Ex R_x recommendations provided in the box is based from several systematic reviews and consensus documents as listed in the Ex R_x box.

■ FITT RECOMMENDATIONS FOR INDIVIDUALS WITH SPINAL CORD INJURY (101,219)

FITT		Aerobic	Resistance	Flexibility
	Frequency	Minimum of 2 d · wk^{-1}; progress to 3 d · wk^{-1}. Athletes can increase to 3–5 d · wk^{-1}.	Minimum of 2 d · wk^{-1}	Daily, especially in presence of joint contracture, spasticity, or frequent wheelchair propulsion and manual transfers
	Intensity	Beginners: moderate intensity (40%–59% HRR). Athletes: 75%–90% HRR	Initially, use 20-RM for each exercise.	Do not allow stretching discomfort >2 on the 0–10 pain scale.
	Time	Initially, bouts of 5–10 min alternating with 5-min active recovery periods. Gradually increase to at least 20 min per session and decrease or eliminate rest periods.	Initially, 1–2 sets of each exercise per session. Gradually progress to 3 sets of 8–10 repetitions.	Stretch each muscle group repeatedly for 3–4 min · d^{-1}, preferably after warm-up or following training/competition.
	Type	Engage the largest possible muscle mass: voluntary arm + leg ergometry or combined FES-LCE and voluntary arm ergometry or rowing, recumbent stepping, arm ergometry, wheelchair ergometry/rollers, or wheeling.	Accessible resistance exercise machines are convenient and safe. If not available, use dumbbells, cuff weights, or elastic bands/tubing.	Active stretching is preferred, but if this is not possible, low intensity passive stretching may be used by the individual or assistant.

20-RM, twenty repetition maximum; FES-LCE, functional electrical stimulation-leg cycle ergometry; HRR, heart rate reserve.

Exercise Training Considerations

- Include resistance exercises for all innervated muscle groups, typically involving the upper body but not ignoring paretic arm, trunk, or leg muscles.
- Resist overemphasis of "pushing" motions such as bench/chest press or rickshaw dips that develop the anterior shoulder/pectoral muscles, scapular protractors, and internal rotators (prime movers for functional skills such as wheelchair propulsion and transfers).
- Balance the "pushing" exercises with "pulling" exercises such as rowing and lat pulldowns that develop the scapular retractors and depressors, posterior deltoids, external rotator cuff muscles, and latissimus dorsi.
- If strength is the goal and arm overuse syndromes do not develop, increase resistance to 5- to 10-RM. As exercise tolerance increases and if arm overuse syndromes do not develop, increase volume to 3–4 sets per session.
- Advanced exercises for athletes may include ballistic medicine ball exercises, battling ropes training, and sport-specific skills requiring power and speed.
- Therapeutic exercises may be indicated for joints with muscle imbalance and spasticity. The primary goal is the prevention/correction of joint contractures and loss of ROM.
- All muscles should be stretched slowly, especially spastic muscles to minimize elicitation of stretch reflexes (spasticity) which can aggravate muscle imbalance and contracture. Emphasize prime mover muscles of the chest, anterior shoulders, and shoulder internal rotators. Adjacent joints must be stabilized to stretch the intended muscles/tendons.
- Stretch spastic muscles that may cause joint contractures (*e.g.*, elbow flexors, hip/knee flexors, hip adductors, and ankle plantar flexors). Passive/active standing can also stretch hip and plantar flexors.
- Progression (increased ROM) should be slow and based on pain tolerance, especially in advanced age, arthritis, permanent joint contracture, periodic immobilization (bed rest, hospitalizations), heterotopic ossification, and chronic overuse syndromes and pain.

Special Considerations

- Participants should empty their bowels and bladder or urinary bag before exercising because autonomic dysreflexia can be triggered by a full bladder or bowel distension.
- Skin pressure ulcers should be avoided at all costs, and potential risk areas should be checked on a regular basis.
- Individuals with complete SCIs above T6 may exhibit low cardiovascular performance, particularly among those with complete tetraplegia. They may reach their HR_{peak}, cardiac output ($\dot{Q}$), and oxygen consumption ($\dot{V}O_2$) at lower exercise levels than those with paraplegia with lesion levels below T5–T6 (131).
- During exercise, autonomic dysreflexia results in an increased release of catecholamines that increases HR, $\dot{V}O_2$, BP, and exercise capacity (257). BP may be elevated to excessively high levels (*i.e.*, SBP 250–300 mm Hg and/or diastolic

blood pressure [DBP] 200–220 mm Hg). In these situations, immediate emergency responses to decrease BP are needed (*i.e.*, stopping exercise; sitting upright; and identifying and removing the irritating stimulus such as an obstructed catheter/urinary collection device, tight clothing, or braces). Emergency medical attention should be sought immediately if the symptoms persist. In competition, athletes with a resting SBP ≥180 mm Hg should not be allowed to start the event.

- Novice unfit but healthy participants with SCI will probably experience muscular fatigue before achieving substantial central cardiovascular stimulus. Individuals with tetraplegia who have a very small active musculature will also experience muscular fatigue before exhausting central cardiorespiratory capacity.

- Those with SCI and limited or no recent standing history may be at an increased risk for fracture. Full weight-bearing activities should be limited to those individuals with a recent uncomplicated history of standing or for whom prior medical clearance for full weight bearing has been obtained.

- Individuals with higher SCI levels, especially those with tetraplegia, may benefit from use of lower body positive pressure by applying compressive antithromboembolic stockings, an elastic abdominal binder, electrical stimulation to leg muscles, and/or exercise in recumbent posture. Beneficial hemodynamic effects may include maintenance of BP, lower HR, and higher stroke volume during arm work to compensate for blood pooling below the lesion.

- Choose an exercise training mode that allows the person to engage the largest possible muscle mass. If the person's SCI is very incomplete, consider combined voluntary arm and leg cycle ergometry or recumbent stepping. If the SCI is complete or nearly complete, voluntary arm ergometry or wheelchair propulsion or ergometry may be the appropriate options.

- In persons with spastic paralysis above T12 who have substantial sensory loss and respond to the stimulation with sustainable static or dynamic contractions, hybrid exercise may provide higher intensity cardiovascular exercise than voluntary arm exercise alone. Hybrid exercise activates a larger muscle mass and elicits higher peak and submaximal training values of $\dot{V}O_2$, stroke volume, and ($\dot{Q}$) than either arm ergometry or functional electrical stimulation-leg cycle ergometry (FES-LCE) alone, especially for persons with tetraplegia (123,129). However, there is evidence that there may not be additional benefit of hybrid cycling versus handcycling in this population (10).

- Muscular strength training sessions from a seated position in the wheelchair should be complemented with nonwheelchair exercise bouts to involve all trunk stabilizing muscles. However, transfers (*e.g.*, from wheelchair to the exercise apparatus) should be limited because they increase the glenohumeral contact forces and the risk of repetitive strain injuries such as shoulder impingement syndrome and rotator cuff strain/tear, especially in individuals with tetraplegia (301). Special attention should be given to shoulder muscle imbalance and the prevention of repetitive strain injuries. The prime movers of wheelchair propulsion should be lengthened (*i.e.*, muscles of the anterior shoulder and chest), and antagonists should be strengthened (*i.e.*, muscles of the posterior shoulder, scapula, and upper back [84]).

- *Tenodesis* (*i.e.*, active wrist extensor driven finger flexion) allows functional grasp in individuals with tetraplegia who do not have use of the hand muscles. To retain the tenodesis effect, these individuals should never stretch the finger flexor muscles (*i.e.*, maximal and simultaneous extension of wrist and fingers).

- Individuals with SCI tend to endure higher core temperatures during endurance exercise than their able-bodied counterparts. Despite this enhanced thermoregulatory drive, they generally have lower sweat rates. The following factors reduce heat tolerance and should be avoided: lack of acclimatization, dehydration, glycogen depletion, sleep loss, alcohol, and infectious disease. During training and competition, the use of light clothing, ice vests, protective sunscreen cream, and mist spray are recommended (3,7).

ONLINE RESOURCES

National Center on Health, Physical Activity and Disability:
    http://www.nchpad.org/Articles/9/Exercise~and~Fitness
Spinal Cord Injury Rehabilitation Evidence:
    http://www.scireproject.com/rehabilitation-evidence/cardiovascular-health
    /exercise-rehabilitation-and-cardiovascular-fitness/fun
SCI Action Canada:
    http://sciactioncanada.ca/guidelines/
Peter Harrison Centre for Disability Sport:
    http://www.lboro.ac.uk/research/phc/educational-toolkit/
American Spinal Injury Association Learning Center:
    http://www.asia-spinalinjury.org/elearning/elearning.php

MULTIPLE CHRONIC DISEASES AND HEALTH CONDITIONS

Aging of current "baby boomers," improvements in the treatment of CVD and cancer, and the increased prevalence of overweight and obesity worldwide make it increasingly likely exercise professionals will be designing Ex R$_x$ for clients and patients with multiple chronic diseases and health conditions. For instance, a 2012 update from the Centers for Disease Control and Prevention estimated that half of the U.S. adult population (117 million) has at least one of the top 10 chronic disease conditions and that one in four has more than one of these conditions (308). *Chapters 9* through *11* present Ex R$_x$ guidelines for many chronic diseases and conditions. This section considers guidelines for individuals with more than one of these diseases or conditions. In general, the recommendations should follow the disease or condition with the most conservative guidelines. Exercise is generally safe for the majority of individuals with multiple diseases and chronic conditions who are medically stable and wish to participate in a light-to-moderate intensity exercise program (see *Chapters 1* and *2*). However, exercise professionals are encouraged to consult with their medical colleagues when there are questions about clients or patients with known disease and health conditions that may limit their participation in exercise programs.

Exercise Testing

Follow the preparticipation screening process in *Chapter 2* to determine if medical clearance is warranted for any single individual. If an exercise test is performed, refer to the information for the disease or condition that dictates the most conservative approach.

Exercise Prescription

In general, the FITT principle of Ex R_x for individuals with multiple diseases and health conditions will follow the recommendations for healthy adults (see *Chapter 6*) except when a disease or condition dictates a more conservative approach. Review the Ex R_x recommendations for each disease and condition to make this determination. The primary challenge is determining the specifics of the Ex R_x that should be recommended for the client or patient who presents with multiple chronic diseases because there is some variability in the exercise dose that most favorably impacts a particular disease, health condition, or CVD risk factor (*e.g.*, BP requires lower doses of exercise to improve than does high-density lipoprotein [HDL], abdominal adiposity, or bone density).

Special Considerations

- In those with multiple chronic diseases or conditions, it is important to make sure all are stable prior to initiating an exercise training program.
- In some instances, exercise training adaptations may allow exercise intensity increases to elicit symptoms of a disease. For instance, in the person with intermittent claudication, regular walking may allow an increase in exercise intensity that may subsequently uncover angina or dyspnea symptoms that were not present at lower intensity levels.
- A large body of scientific evidence supports the role of PA in delaying premature mortality and reducing the risks of many chronic diseases and health conditions. There is also clear evidence for a dose-response relationship between PA and health. Thus, any amount of PA should be encouraged even if the level is very low due to a chronic disease or condition.
- Begin with an Ex R_x for the single disease and health condition that confers the greatest risk and/or is the most limiting regarding ADL, quality of life, and/or starting or maintaining an exercise program. Also consider client and patient preference and goals.
- Alternatively, begin with the most conservative Ex R_x for the multiple diseases, health conditions, and/or CVD risk factors with which the client and patient presents.

■ Know the magnitude and time course of response of the various health outcome(s) that can be expected as a result of the Ex R_x that is prescribed in order to progress the client and patient safely and appropriately.

■ Frequently monitor signs and symptoms to ensure safety and proper adaptation and progression.

REFERENCES

1. Agiovlasitis S, Motl RW, Ranadive SM, et al. Prediction of oxygen uptake during over-ground walking in people with and without Down syndrome. *Eur J Appl Physiol*. 2011;111:1739–45.

2. Ahlborg L, Andersson C, Julin P. Whole-body vibration training compared with resistance training: effect on spasticity, muscle strength and motor performance in adults with cerebral palsy. *J Rehabil Med*. 2006;38(5):302–8.

3. American Association on Intellectual and Developmental Disabilities. *Intellectual Disability: Definition, Classification, and Systems of Support*. 11th ed. Washington (DC): American Association on Intellectual and Developmental Disabilities; 2010. 280 p.

4. American Cancer Society. *Cancer Facts and Figures* 2015 [Internet]. Atlanta (GA): American Cancer Society; [cited 2015 Jan 9]. Available from: http://www.cancer.org/research/cancerfactsstatistics/cancerfactsfigures2015/index

5. American College of Sports Medicine, Armstrong LE, Casa DJ, et al. American College of Sports Medicine position stand. Exertional heat illness during training and competition. *Med Sci Sports Exerc*. 2007;39(3):556–72.

6. American College of Sports Medicine, Chodzko-Zajko WJ, Proctor DN, et al. American College of Sports Medicine position stand. Exercise and physical activity for older adults. *Med Sci Sports Exerc*. 2009;41(7):1510–30.

7. American College of Sports Medicine, Sawka MN, Burke LM, et al. American College of Sports Medicine position stand. Exercise and fluid replacement. *Med Sci Sports Exerc*. 2007;39(2):377–90.

8. Anuurad E, Semrad A, Berglund L. Human immunodeficiency virus and highly active antiretroviral therapy-associated metabolic disorders and risk factors for cardiovascular disease. *Metab Syndr Relat Disord*. 2009;7(5):401–10.

9. Baechle TR, Earle RW, Wathen D. Resistance training. In: Baechle TR, Earle RW, editors. *Essentials of Strength Training and Conditioning*. 2nd ed. Champaign (IL): Human Kinetics; 2000. p. 395–425.

10. Bakkum AJ, de Groot S, Stolwijk-Swüste JM, et al. Effects of hybrid cycling versus handcycling on wheelchair-specific fitness and physical activity in people with long-term spinal cord injury: a 16-week randomized controlled trial. *Spinal Cord*. 2015;53(5):395–401.

11. Balemans AC, Van Wely L, De Heer SJ, et al. Maximal aerobic and anaerobic exercise responses in children with cerebral palsy. *Med Sci Sports Exerc*. 2013;45(3):561–8.

12. Bartels EM, Lund H, Hagen KB, Dagfinrud H, Christensen R, Danneskiold-Samsøe B. Aquatic exercise for the treatment of knee and hip osteoarthritis. *Cochrane Database Syst Rev*. 2007;(4):CD005523.

13. Baynard T, Pitetti KH, Guerra M, Unnithan VB, Fernhall B. Age-related changes in aerobic capacity in individuals with mental retardation: a 20-yr review. *Med Sci Sports Exerc*. 2008;40(11):1984–9.

14. Bean JF, Kiely DK, Herman S, et al. The relationship between leg power and physical performance in mobility-limited older people. *J Am Geriatr Soc*. 2002;50:461–7.

15. Bennett RM. Clinical manifestations and diagnosis of fibromyalgia. *Rheum Dis Clin North Am*. 2009;35:215–32.

16. Bennett RM, Friend R, Jones KD, Ward R, Han BK, Ross RL. The Revised Fibromyalgia Impact Questionnaire (FIQR): validation and psychometric properties. *Arthritis Res Ther*. 2009;11(4):R120.

17. Bennett RM, Friend R, Marcus D, et al. Criteria for the diagnosis of fibromyalgia: validation of the modified 2010 preliminary American College of Rheumatology criteria and the development of alternative criteria. *Arthritis Care Res*. 2014;66(9):1364–73.

18. Berg K, Wood-Dauphinee S, Williams JI, Gayton D. Measuring balance in the elderly: preliminary development of an instrument. *Physiotherapy Canada*. 1989;41(6):304–11.

19. Bergen JL, Toole T, Elliott RG III, Wallace B, Robinson K, Maitland CG. Aerobic exercise intervention improves aerobic capacity and movement initiation in Parkinson's disease patients. *NeuroRehabilitation*. 2002;17(2):161–8.

20. Bhole R, Flynn JC, Marbury TC. Quadriceps tendon ruptures in uremia. *Clin Orthop Relat Res*. 1985;(195):200–6.

21. Bidonde J, Busch AJ, Bath B, Milosavljevic S. Exercise for adults with fibromyalgia: an umbrella systematic review with synthesis of best evidence. *Curr Rheumatol Rev*. 2014;10(1):45–79.

22. Biftles AH, Petterson BA, Sullivan SG, Hussain R, Glasson EJ, Montgomery PD. The influence of intellectual disability on life expectancy. *J Gerontol A Biol Sci Med Sci*. 2002;57:M470–2.

23. Blanchard CM, Courneya KS, Stein K. Cancer survivors' adherence to lifestyle behavior recommendations and associations with health-related quality of life: results from the American Cancer Society's SCS-II. *J Clin Oncol*. 2008;26(13):2198–204.

24. Blandini F. Neural and immune mechanisms in the pathogenesis of Parkinson's disease. *J Neuroimmune Pharmacol*. 2013;8(1):189–201.

25. Bochkezanian V, Raymond J, de Oliveira CQ, Davis GM. Can combined aerobic and muscle strength training improve aerobic fitness, muscle strength, function and quality of life in people with spinal cord injury? A systematic review. *Spinal Cord*. 2015;53(6):418–31.

26. Bolam KA, van Uffelen JG, Taaffe DR. The effect of physical exercise on bone density in middle-aged and older men: a systematic review. *Osteoporos Int*. 2013;24:2749–62.

27. Borg GA. Psychophysical bases of perceived exertion. *Med Sci Sports Exerc*. 1982;14(5):377–81.

28. Borg GA. Scaling pain and related subjective somatic symptoms. In: Borg GA, editor. *Borg's Perceived Exertion and Pain Scales*. Champaign (IL): Human Kinetics; 1998. p. 63–7.

29. Branco JC, Bannwarth B, Failde I, et al. Prevalence of fibromyalgia: a survey in five European countries. *Semin Arthritis Rheum*. 2010;39(6):448–53.

30. Brehm MA, Balemans AC, Becher JG, Dallmeijer AJ. Reliability of a progressive maximal cycle ergometer test to assess peak oxygen uptake in children with mild to moderate cerebral palsy. *Phys Ther*. 2014;94(1):121–8.

31. Brosseau L, MacLeay L, Robinson V, Wells G, Tugwell P. Intensity of exercise for the treatment of osteoarthritis. *Cochrane Database Syst Rev*. 2003;(2):CD004259.

32. Brown JC, Huedo-Medina TB, Pescatello LS, Pescatello SM, Ferrer RA, Johnson BT. Efficacy of exercise interventions in modulating cancer-related fatigue among adult cancer survivors: a meta-analysis. *Cancer Epidemiol Biomarkers Prev*. 2011;20(1):123–33.

33. Brown JC, Schmitz KH. The prescription or proscription of exercise in colorectal cancer care. *Med Sci Sports Exerc*. 2014;46(12):2202–9.

34. Brzycki M. Strength testing — predicting a one-rep max from reps-to-fatigue. *J Physical Ed Rec Dance*. 1993;64:88–90.

35. Bull MJ. Health supervision for children with Down syndrome. *Pediatrics*. 2011;128:393–406.

36. Busch AJ, Barber KA, Overend TJ, Peloso PM, Schachter CL. Exercise for treating fibromyalgia syndrome. *Cochrane Database Syst Rev*. 2007;(4):CD003786.

37. Busch AJ, Webber SC, Brachaniec M, et al. Exercise therapy for fibromyalgia. *Curr Pain Headache Rep*. 2011;15(5):358–67.

38. Busch AJ, Webber SC, Richards RS, et al. Resistance exercise training for fibromyalgia. *Cochrane Database Syst Rev*. 2013;(12):CD010884.

39. Butler JM, Scianni A, Ada L. Effect of cardiorespiratory training on aerobic fitness and carryover to activity in children with cerebral palsy: a systematic review. *Int J Rehabil Res*. 2010;33(2):97–103.

40. Cadore EL, Rodríguez-Mañas L, Sinclair A, Izquierdo M. Effects of different exercise interventions on risk of falls, gait ability, and balance in physically frail older adults: a systematic review. *Rejuvenation Res*. 2013;16(2):105–14.

41. Carroll CC, Gallagher PM, Seidle ME, Trappe SW. Skeletal muscle characteristics of people with multiple sclerosis. *Arch Phys Med Rehabil*. 2005;86(2):224–9.

42. Centers for Disease Control and Prevention. National and state medical expenditures and lost earnings attributable to arthritis and other rheumatic conditions — United States, 2003. *MMWR Morb Mortal Wkly Rep*. 2007;56:4–7.

43. Centers for Disease Control and Prevention. *National Chronic Kidney Disease Fact Sheet: General Information and National Estimates on Chronic Kidney Disease in the United States*, 2014. Atlanta (GA): U.S. Department of Health and Human Services, Centers for Disease Control and Prevention; 2014. 4 p.

44. Centers for Disease Control and Prevention. Prevalence of doctor-diagnosed arthritis and arthritis-attributable activity limitation — United States, 2010–2012. *MMWR Morb Mortal Wkly Rep*. 2013;62:869–73.

45. Centers for Disease Control and Prevention. STEADI (Stopping Elderly Accidents, Deaths, and Injuries) Initiative for Health Care Providers. *Older Adults Falls Prevention* [Internet]. Atlanta (GA): Centers for Disease Control and Prevention; [cited 2014 Oct 21]. Available from: http://www.cdc.gov/steadi/materials.html

46. Cerebral Palsy International Sports and Recreation Association. *Classification and Sports Rules Manual*. 9th ed. Nottingham (United Kingdom): Cerebral Palsy International Sports & Recreation Association; 2006. 162 p.

47. Chaudhuri KR, Martinez-Martin P, Brown RG, et al. The metric properties of a novel non-motor symptoms scale for Parkinson's disease: results from an international pilot study. *Mov Disord*. 2007;22(13):1901–11.

48. Cheema BS, Kilbreath SL, Fahey PP, Delaney G, Atlantis E. Safety and efficacy of progressive resistance training in breast cancer: a systematic review and meta-analysis. *Breast Cancer Res Treat*. 2014;148:249–68.

49. Christiansen CL, Schenkman M, McFann K, Wolfe P, Kohrt WM. Walking economy in people with Parkinson's disease. *Mov Disord*. 2009;24(10):1481–7.

50. Chung LH, Remelius JG, van Emmerik RE, Kent-Braun JA. Leg power asymmetry and postural control in women with multiple sclerosis. *Med Sci Sports Exerc*. 2008;40(10):1717–24.

51. Clauw DJ. Fibromyalgia: an overview. *Am J Med*. 2009;122(12 Suppl):S3–13.

52. Clyne N, Jogestrand T, Lins LE, Pehrsson SK. Factors influencing physical working capacity in renal transplant patients. *Scand J Urol Nephrol*. 1989;23(2):145–50.

53. Corcos DM, Robichaud JA, David FJ, et al. A two-year randomized controlled trial of progressive resistance exercise for Parkinson's disease. *Mov Disord*. 2013;28(9):1230–40.

54. Courneya KS, Vardy J, Gill S, et al. Update on the Colon Health and Life-Long Exercise Change Trial: a phase III study of the impact of an exercise program on disease-free survival in colon cancer. *Curr Colorectal Cancer Rep*. 2014;10:321–8.

55. Cowley PM, Ploutz-Snyder LL, Baynard T, et al. Physical fitness predicts functional tasks in individuals with Down syndrome. *Med Sci Sports Exerc*. 2010;42(2):388–93.

56. Cramer L, Hildebrandt B, Kung T, et al. Cardiovascular function and predictors of exercise capacity in patients with colorectal cancer. *J Am Coll Cardiol*. 2014;64(13):1310–9.

57. Dadabhoy D, Clauw D. The fibromyalgia syndrome. In: Klippel JH, Stone JH, Crofford LJ, White PH, editors. *Primer on the Rheumatic Diseases*. 13th ed. New York (NY): Springer; 2008. p. 87–93.

58. Dagfinrud H, Kvien TK, Hagen KB. Physiotherapy interventions for ankylosing spondylitis. *Cochrane Database Syst Rev*. 2008;(1):CD002822.

59. Damiano DL. Activity, activity, activity: rethinking our physical therapy approach to cerebral palsy. *Phys Ther*. 2006;86(11):1534–40.

60. Darrah J, Wessel J, Nearingburg P, O'Connor M. Evaluation of a community fitness program for adolescents with cerebral palsy. *Ped Phys Ther*. 1999;11(1):18–23.

61. DeBolt LS, McCubbin JA. The effects of home-based resistance exercise on balance, power, and mobility in adults with multiple sclerosis. *Arch Phys Med Rehabil*. 2004;85(2):290–7.

62. De Groot S, Dallmeijer AJ, Bessems PJ, Lamberts ML, van der Woude LH, Janssen TW. Comparison of muscle strength, sprint power and aerobic capacity in adults with and without cerebral palsy. *J Rehabil Med*. 2012;44(11):932–8.

63. Deighton C, O'Mahony R, Tosh J, Turner C, Rudolf M. Management of rheumatoid arthritis: summary of NICE guidance. *BMJ*. 2009;338:b702.

64. De Jong Z, Munneke M, Kroon HM, et al. Long-term follow-up of a high intensity exercise program in patients with rheumatoid arthritis. *Clin Rheumatol*. 2009;28:663–71.

65. De Jong Z, Munneke M, Zwinderman AH, et al. Is a long-term high-intensity exercise program effective and safe in patients with rheumatoid arthritis? Results of a randomized controlled trial. *Arthritis Rheum*. 2003;48(9):2415–24.

66. Dias V, Junn E, Mouradian MM. The role of oxidative stress in Parkinson's disease. *J Parkinsons Dis*. 2013;3(4):461–91.

67. Dibble LE, Addison O, Papa E. The effects of exercise on balance in persons with Parkinson's disease: a systematic review across the disability spectrum. *J Neurol Phys Ther*. 2009;33(1):14–26.

68. Diesel W, Noakes TD, Swanepoel C, Lambert M. Isokinetic muscle strength predicts maximum exercise tolerance in renal patients on chronic hemodialysis. *Am J Kidney Dis*. 1990;16(2):109–14.

69. Dodd KJ, Taylor NF, Damiano DL. A systematic review of the effectiveness of strength-training programs for people with cerebral palsy. *Arch Phys Med Rehabil*. 2002;83(8):1157–64.

70. Dorfman LJ, Howard JE, McGill KC. Motor unit firing rates and firing rate variability in the detection of neuromuscular disorders. *Electroencephalogr Clin Neurophysiol*. 1989;73(3):215–24.

71. Duncan PW, Weiner DK, Chandler J, Studenski S. Functional reach: a new clinical measure of balance. *J Gerontol*. 1990;45(6):M192–7.

72. Earhart GM. Dance as therapy for individuals with Parkinson disease. *Eur J Phys Rehabil Med*. 2009;45(2):231–8.

73. Falvo MJ, Earhart GM. Six-minute walk distance in persons with Parkinson disease: a hierarchical regression model. *Arch Phys Med Rehabil*. 2009;90(6):1004–8.

74. Falvo MJ, Schilling BK, Earhart GM. Parkinson's disease and resistive exercise: rationale, review, and recommendations. *Mov Disord*. 2008;23(1):1–11.

75. Fang CT, Chang YY, Hsu HM, et al. Life expectancy of patients with newly-diagnosed HIV infection in the era of highly active antiretroviral therapy. *QJM*. 2007;100(2):97–105.

76. Feltham MG, Collett J, Izadi H, et al. Cardiovascular adaptation in people with multiple sclerosis following a twelve week exercise programme suggest deconditioning rather than autonomic dysfunction caused by the disease. Results from a randomized controlled trial. *Eur J Phys Rehabil Med*. 2013;49(6):765–74.

77. Fernhall B. The young athlete with a mental disability. In: Hebestreit H, Bar-Or O, editors. *The Young Athlete*. Malden (MA): Blackwell; 2008. p. 403–14.

78. Fernhall B, Baynard T. Intellectual disability. In: Ehrman JK, Gordon PM, Visich PS, Keteyian SJ, editors. *Clinical Exercise Physiology*. 3rd ed. Champaign (IL): Human Kinetics; 2013. p. 617–31.

79. Fernhall B, McCubbin JA, Pitetti KH, et al. Prediction of maximal heart rate in individuals with mental retardation. *Med Sci Sports Exerc*. 2001;33(10):1655–60.

80. Fernhall B, Mendonca G, Baynard T. Reduced work capacity in individuals with Down syndrome: a consequence of autonomic dysfunction? *Exerc Sport Sci Rev*. 2013;41:138–47.

81. Fernhall B, Pitetti KH, Rimmer JH, et al. Cardiorespiratory capacity of individuals with mental retardation including Down syndrome. *Med Sci Sports Exerc*. 1996;28(3):366–71.

82. Fernhall B, Pitetti KH, Vukovich MD, et al. Validation of cardiovascular fitness field tests in children with mental retardation. *Am J Ment Retard*. 1998;102(6):602–12.

83. Fernhall B, Tymeson G. Graded exercise testing of mentally retarded adults: a study of feasibility. *Arch Phys Med Rehabil*. 1987;68(6):363–5.

84. Figoni SF. Overuse shoulder problems after spinal cord injury: a conceptual model of risk and protective factors. *Clin Kinesiol*. 2009;63(2):12–22.

85. Fisher NM. Osteoarthritis, rheumatoid arthritis, and fibromyalgia. In: Myers J, Nieman DC, editors. *ACSM's Resources for Clinical Exercise Physiology: Musculoskeletal, Neuromuscular, Neoplastic, Immunologic, and Hematologic Conditions*. 2nd ed. Baltimore (MD): Lippincott Williams & Wilkins; 2010. p. 132–47.

86. Follett KA, Weaver FM, Stern M, et al. Pallidal versus subthalamic deep-brain stimulation for Parkinson's disease. *N Engl J Med*. 2010;362(22):2077–91.

87. Foltynie T, Kahan J. Parkinson's disease: an update on pathogenesis and treatment. *J Neurol*. 2013;260(5):1433–40.

88. Fowler EG, Knutson LM, Demuth SK, et al. Pediatric endurance and limb strengthening (PEDALS) for children with cerebral palsy using stationary cycling: a randomized controlled trial. *Phys Ther*. 2010;90(3):367–81.

89. Franceschini M, Rampello A, Bovolenta F, Aiello M, Tzani P, Chetta A. Cost of walking, exertional dyspnoea and fatigue in individuals with multiple sclerosis not requiring assistive devices. *J Rehabil Med*. 2010;42(8):719–23.

90. Fransen M, McConnell S. Exercise for osteoarthritis of the knee. *Cochrane Database Syst Rev*. 2008;(4):CD004376.

91. Fransen M, McConnell S, Hernandez-Molina G, Reichenbach S. Exercise for osteoarthritis of the hip. *Cochrane Database Syst Rev.* 2009;(3):CD007912.
92. Franzén E, Paquette C, Gurfinkel VS, Cordo PJ, Nutt JG, Horak FB. Reduced performance in balance, walking and turning tasks is associated with increased neck tone in Parkinson's disease. *Exp Neurol.* 2009;219(2):430–8.
93. Freal JE, Kraft GH, Coryell JK. Symptomatic fatigue in multiple sclerosis. *Arch Phys Med Rehabil.* 1984;65(3):135–8.
94. Gallo PM, McIsaac TL, Garber CE. Walking economy during cued versus non-cued treadmill walking in persons with Parkinson's disease. *J Parkinsons Dis.* 2013;3(4):609–19.
95. Garber CE, Blissmer B, Deschenes MR, et al. American College of Sports Medicine position stand. Quantity and quality of exercise for developing and maintaining cardiorespiratory, musculoskeletal, and neuromotor fitness in apparently healthy adults: guidance for prescribing exercise. *Med Sci Sports Exerc.* 2011;43(7):1334–59.
96. Garber CE, Friedman J. Effects of fatigue on physical activity and function in patients with Parkinson's disease. *Neurology.* 2003;60(7):1119–24.
97. Garcia A, Fraga GA, Vieira RC Jr, et al. Effects of combined exercise training on immunological, physical and biochemical parameters in individuals with HIV/AIDS. *J Sports Sci.* 2014;32(8):785–92.
98. Gavi MB, Vassalo DV, Amaral FT, et al. Strengthening exercises improve symptoms and quality of life but do not change autonomic modulation in fibromyalgia: a randomized clinical trial. *PLoS One.* 2014;9(3):e90767.
99. Giangregorio LM, McGill S, Wark JD, et al. Too fit to fracture: outcomes of a Delphi consensus process on physical activity and exercise recommendations for adults with osteoporosis with or without vertebral fractures. *Osteoporos Int.* 2015;26:891–910.
100. Gill TM, Williams CS, Tinetti ME. Assessing risk for the onset of functional dependence among older adults: the role of physical performance. *J Am Geriatr Soc.* 1995;43(6):603–9.
101. Ginis KA, Hicks AL, Latimer AE, et al. The development of evidence-informed physical activity guidelines for adults with spinal cord injury. *Spinal Cord.* 2011;49(11):1088–96.
102. Gomes Neto M, Ogalha C, Andrade AM, Brites C. A systematic review of effects of concurrent strength and endurance training on the health-related quality of life and cardiopulmonary status in patients with HIV/AIDS. *Biomed Res Int.* 2013;2013:319524.
103. Goodwin VA, Richards SH, Henley W, Ewings P, Taylor AH, Campbell JL. An exercise intervention to prevent falls in people with Parkinson's disease: a pragmatic randomised controlled trial. *J Neurol Neurosurg Psychiatry.* 2011;82(11):1232–8.
104. Gutierrez GM, Chow JW, Tillman MD, McCoy SC, Castellano V, White LJ. Resistance training improves gait kinematics in persons with multiple sclerosis. *Arch Phys Med Rehabil.* 2005;86(9):1824–9.
105. Haapaniemi TH, Kallio MA, Korpelainen JT, et al. Levodopa, bromocriptine and selegiline modify cardiovascular responses in Parkinson's disease. *J Neurol.* 2000;247(11):868–74.
106. Hackney ME, Earhart G. Effects of dance on gait and balance in Parkinson's disease: a comparison of partnered and nonpartnered dance movement. *Neurorehabil Neural Repair.* 2010;24(4):384–92.
107. Haentjens P, Magaziner J, Colón-Emeric CS, et al. Meta-analysis: excess mortality after hip fracture among older women and men. *Ann Intern Med.* 2010;152(6):380–90.
108. Haisma JA, van der Woude LH, Stam HJ, Bergen MP, Sluis TA, Bussmann JB. Physical capacity in wheelchair-dependent persons with a spinal cord injury: a critical review of the literature. *Spinal Cord.* 2006;44(11):642–52.
109. Häkkinen A. Effectiveness and safety of strength training in rheumatoid arthritis. *Curr Opinion Rheumatol.* 2004;16:132–7.
110. Häkkinen A, Häkkinen K, Hannonen P, Alen M. Strength training induced adaptations in neuromuscular function of premenopausal women with fibromyalgia: comparison with healthy women. *Ann Rheum Dis.* 2001;60(1):21–6.
111. Häkkinen A, Sokka T, Kotaniemi A, Hannonen P. A randomized two-year study of the effects of dynamic strength training on muscle strength, disease activity, functional capacity, and bone mineral density in early rheumatoid arthritis. *Arthritis Rheum.* 2001;44:515–22.
112. Hampton T. Parkinson disease registry launched. *JAMA.* 2005;293(2):149.

113. Hand GA, Jaggers JR, Lyerly GW, Dudgeon WD. Physical activity for CVD prevention in patients with HIV/AIDS. *Curr Cardiovasc Risk Rep*. 2009;3(4):288–95.

114. Hand GA, Lyerly GW, Jaggers JR, Dudgeon WD. Impact of aerobic and resistance exercise on the health of HIV-infected persons. *Am J Lifestyle Med*. 2009;3(6):489–99.

115. Hand GA, Phillips KD, Dudgeon WD, et al. Moderate intensity exercise training reverses functional aerobic impairment in HIV-infected individuals. *AIDS Care*. 2008;20(9):1066–74.

116. Haskell WL, Lee IM, Pate RR, et al. Physical activity and public health: updated recommendation for adults from the American College of Sports Medicine and the American Heart Association. *Med Sci Sports Exerc*. 2007;39(8):1423–34.

117. Häuser W, Klose P, Langhorst J, et al. Efficacy of different types of aerobic exercise in fibromyalgia syndrome: a systematic review and meta-analysis of randomised controlled trials. *Arthritis Res Ther*. 2010;12(3):R79.

118. Hayes HA, Gappmaier E, LaStayo PC. Effects of high-intensity resistance training on strength, mobility, balance, and fatigue in individuals with multiple sclerosis: a randomized controlled trial. *J Neurol Phys Ther*. 2011;35(1):2–10.

119. Headley S, Germain M, Mailloux P, et al. Resistance training improves strength and functional measures in patients with end-stage renal disease. *Am J Kidney Dis*. 2002;40(2):355–64.

120. Heiwe S, Jacobson S. Exercise training in adults with CKD: a systematic review and meta-analysis. *Am J Kidney Dis*. 2014;64(3):383–93.

121. Herman T, Giladi N, Gruendlinger L, Hausdorff JM. Six weeks of intensive treadmill training improves gait and quality of life in patients with Parkinson's disease: a pilot study. *Arch Phys Med Rehabil*. 2007;88(9):1154–8.

122. Herman T, Inbar-Borovsky N, Brozgol M, Giladi N, Hausdorff JM. The Dynamic Gait Index in healthy older adults: the role of stair climbing, fear of falling and gender. *Gait Posture*. 2009;29(2):237–41.

123. Hettinga DM, Andrews B. Oxygen consumption during functional electrical stimulation-assisted exercise in persons with spinal cord injury: implications for fitness and health. *Sports Med*. 2008;38(10):825–38.

124. Hicks AL, Martin Ginis KA, Pelletier CA, Ditor DS, Foulon B, Wolfe DL. The effects of exercise training on physical capacity, strength, body composition and functional performance among adults with spinal cord injury: a systematic review. *Spinal Cord*. 2011;49(11):1103–27.

125. Hochberg MC, Altman RD, April KT, et al. American College of Rheumatology 2012 recommendations for the use of nonpharmacologic and pharmacologic therapies in osteoarthritis of the hand, hip, and knee. *Arthritis Care Res*. 2012;64(4):465–74.

126. Hoeger Bement MK, Weyer A, Hartley S, Drewek B, Harkins AL, Hunter SK. Pain perception after isometric exercise in women with fibromyalgia. *Arch Phys Med Rehabil*. 2011;92(1):89–95.

127. Hoehn MM, Yahr M. Parkinsonism: onset, progression and mortality. *Neurology*. 1967;17 (5):427–42.

128. Hombergen SP, Huisstede BM, Streur MF, et al. Impact of cerebral palsy on health-related physical fitness in adults: systematic review. *Arch Phys Med Rehabil*. 2012;93(5):871–81.

129. Hooker SP, Figoni SF, Rodgers MM, et al. Metabolic and hemodynamic responses to concurrent voluntary arm crank and electrical stimulation leg cycle exercise in quadriplegics. *J Rehabil Res Dev*. 1992;29(3):1–11.

130. Hootman JM, Helmick C. Projections of US prevalence of arthritis and associated activity limitations. *Arthritis Rheum*. 2006;54(1):226–9.

131. Hopman MT, Oeseburg B, Binkhorst RA. Cardiovascular responses in persons with paraplegia to prolonged arm exercise and thermal stress. *Med Sci Sports Exerc*. 1993;25(5):577–83.

132. Hsieh K, Rimmer J, Heller T. Prevalence of falls and risk factors in adults with intellectual disability. *Am J Intellect Dev Disabil*. 2012;117(6):442–54.

133. Huisinga JM, Filipi ML, Stergiou N. Supervised resistance training results in changes in postural control in patients with multiple sclerosis. *Motor Control*. 2012;16(1):50–63.

134. Hurkmans E, van der Giesen FJ, Vliet Vlieland TP, Schoones J, van den Ende EC. Dynamic exercise programs (aerobic capacity and/or muscle strength training) in patients with rheumatoid arthritis. *Cochrane Database Syst Rev*. 2009;(7):CD006853.

135. Jaggers JR, Hand GA, Dudgeon WD, et al. Aerobic and resistance training improves mood state among adults living with HIV. *Int J Sports Med*. 2015;36(2):175–81.

136. Jaggers JR, Prasad VK, Dudgeon WD, et al. Associations between physical activity and sedentary time on components of metabolic syndrome among adults with HIV. *AIDS Care*. 2014;26(11):1387–92.

137. Janicki MP, Dalton AJ, Henderson CM, Davidson PW. Mortality and morbidity among older adults with intellectual disability: health services considerations. *Disabil Rehabil*. 1999;21 (5–6):284–94.

138. Johansen KL. Exercise and chronic kidney disease: current recommendations. *Sports Med*. 2005;35(6):485–99.

139. Johansen KL. Exercise in end-stage renal disease population. *J Am Soc Nephrol*. 2007;18(6): 1845–54.

140. Johansen KL, Painter P. Exercise in individuals with CKD. *Am J Kidney Dis*. 2012;59(1):126–34.

141. Johnson BA, Salzberg CL, Stevenson DA. A systematic review: plyometric training programs for young children. *J Strength Cond Res*. 2011;25(9):2623–33.

142. Jones CJ, Rakovski C, Rutledge D, Gutierrez A. A comparison of women with fibromyalgia syndrome to criterion fitness standards: a pilot study. *J Aging Phys Act*. 2015;23(1):103–11.

143. Jones KD, Burckhardt CS, Clark SR, Bennett RM, Potempa KM. A randomized controlled trial of muscle strengthening versus flexibility training in fibromyalgia. *J Rheumatol*. 2002;29(5):1041–8.

144. Jones KD, Clark SR, Bennett RM. Prescribing exercise for people with fibromyalgia. *AACN Clin Issues*. 2002;13(2):277–93.

145. Jones LW, Courneya KS, Mackey JR, et al. Cardiopulmonary function and age-related decline across the breast cancer survivorship continuum. *J Clin Oncol*. 2012;30:2530–7.

146. Kaminsky LA, American College of Sports Medicine. *ACSM's Resource Manual for Guidelines for Exercise Testing and Prescription*. 5th ed. Baltimore (MD): Lippincott Williams & Wilkins; 2005. 749 p.

147. Kanis JA, Bianchi G, Bilezikian JP, et al. Towards a diagnostic and therapeutic consensus in male osteoporosis. *Osteoporos Int*. 2011;22(11):2789–98.

148. Kemmler W, Häberle L, von Stengel S. Effects of exercise on fracture reduction in older adults: a systematic review and meta-analysis. *Osteoporos Int*. 2013;24:1937–50.

149. Kendrick AH, Johns DP, Leeming JP. Infection control of lung function equipment: a practical approach. *Respir Med*. 2003;97(11):1163–79.

150. Kent-Braun JA, Ng AV, Castro M, et al. Strength, skeletal muscle composition, and enzyme activity in multiple sclerosis. *J Appl Physiol*. 1997;83(6):1998–2004.

151. Kent-Braun JA, Sharma KR, Weiner MW, Miller RG. Effects of exercise on muscle activation and metabolism in multiple sclerosis. *Muscle Nerve*. 1994;17(10):1162–9.

152. Kenyon LK, Sleeper MD, Tovin MM. Sport-specific fitness testing and intervention for an adolescent with cerebral palsy: a case report. *Pediatr Phys Ther*. 2010;22(2):234–40.

153. Kerling A, Keweloh K, Tegtbur U, et al. Physical capacity and quality of life in patients with multiple sclerosis. *NeuroRehabilitation*. 2014;35(1):97–104.

154. Keus SH, Bloem BR, Hendriks EJ, Bredero-Cohen AB, Munneke M, Practice Recommendations Development Group. Evidence-based analysis of physical therapy in Parkinson's disease with recommendations for practice and research. *Mov Disord*. 2007;22(4):451–60.

155. Keus SHJ, Hendriks HJM, Bloem BR, et al. KNGF guidelines for physical therapy in Parkinson's disease. *Ned Tijdschr Fysiother*. 2004;114(Suppl 3):5–86.

156. Kidney Disease: Improving Global Outcomes. KDIGO 2012 Clinical Practice Guideline for the Evaluation and Management of Chronic Kidney Disease. *Kidney International Supplements*. 2013;3:134–5.

157. Kingsley JD, McMillan V, Figueroa A. The effects of 12 weeks of resistance exercise training on disease severity and autonomic modulation at rest and after acute leg resistance exercise in women with fibromyalgia. *Arch Phys Med Rehabil*. 2010;91(10):1551–7.

158. Kjølhede T, Vissing K, de Place L, et al. Neuromuscular adaptations to long-term progressive resistance training translates to improved functional capacity for people with multiple sclerosis and is maintained at follow-up. *Mult Scler*. 2014;21(5):599–611.

159. Kloos AD, Heiss D. Exercise for impaired balance. In: Kisner C, Colby LA, editors. *Therapeutic Exercise: Foundations and Techniques*. 5th ed. Philadelphia: Davis; 2007. p. 251–72.

160. Kurtzke JF. Rating neurologic impairment in multiple sclerosis: an expanded disability status scale (EDSS). *Neurology*. 1983;33(11):1444–52.

161. Larson SA, Lakin C, Anderson L, Kwak N, Lee JH, Anderson D. Prevalence of mental retardation and developmental disabilities: estimates from the 1994/1995 National Health Interview Survey Disability Supplements. *Am J Mental Retard*. 2001;106(3):231–52.

162. Latimer-Cheung AE, Martin Ginis KA, Hicks AL, et al. Development of evidence-informed physical activity guidelines for adults with multiple sclerosis. *Arch Phys Med Rehabil*. 2013; 94:1829–36.

163. Lawrence RC, Felson DT, Helmick CG, et al. Estimates of the prevalence of arthritis and other rheumatic conditions in the United States. Part II. *Arthritis Rheum*. 2008;58(1):26–35.

164. Léger L, Boucher R. An indirect continuous running multistage field test: the Université de Montréal track test. *Can J Appl Sport Sci*. 1980;5(2):77–84.

165. Lemmey AB, Marcora SM, Chester K, Wilson S, Casanova F, Maddison PJ. Effects of high-intensity resistance training in patients with rheumatoid arthritis: a randomized controlled trial. *Arthritis Rheum*. 2009;61(12):1726–34.

166. Li F, Harmer P, Fitzgerald K, et al. Tai chi and postural stability in patients with Parkinson's disease. *N Engl J Med*. 2012;366(6):511–9.

167. Ligibel JA, Denlinger C. New NCCN guidelines for survivorship care. *J Natl Compr Canc Netw*. 2013;11(5 Suppl):640–4.

168. Lin K, Stewart D, Cooper S, Davis CL. Pre-transplant cardiac testing for kidney-pancreas transplant candidates and association with cardiac outcomes. *Clin Transplant*. 2001;15(4): 269–75.

169. Lockette KF, Keyes AM. *Conditioning with Physical Disabilities*. Champaign (IL): Human Kinetics; 1994. 288 p.

170. Lublin FD, Reingold SC, National Multiple Sclerosis Society (USA) Advisory Committee on Clinical Trials of New Agents in Multiple Sclerosis. Defining the clinical course of multiple sclerosis: results of an international survey. *Neurology*. 1996;46(4):907–11.

171. Mak MK, Pang M. Balance confidence and functional mobility are independently associated with falls in people with Parkinson's disease. *J Neurol*. 2009;256(5):742–9.

172. Maltais DB, Robitaille NM, Dumas F, Boucher N, Richards CL. Measuring steady-state oxygen uptake during the 6-min walk test in adults with cerebral palsy: feasibility and construct validity. *Int J Rehabil Res*. 2012;35(2):181–3.

173. Mannerkorpi K, Iversen MD. Physical exercise in fibromyalgia and related syndromes. *Best Pract Res Clin Rheumatol*. 2003;17(4):629–47.

174. Mannerkorpi K, Nordeman L, Ericsson A, Arndorw M, GAU Study Group. Pool exercise for patients with fibromyalgia or chronic widespread pain: a randomized controlled trial and subgroup analyses. *J Rehabil Med*. 2009;41(9):751–60.

175. McKay SD, Al-Omari A, Tomlinson LA, Dormans JP. Review of cervical spine anomalies in genetic syndromes. *Spine*. 2012;37:E269–77.

176. McNeely ML, Courneya K. Exercise programs for cancer-related fatigue: evidence and clinical guidelines. *J Natl Compr Canc Netw*. 2010;8(8):945–53.

177. McNeely ML, Peddle C, Parliament M, Courneya KS. Cancer rehabilitation: recommendations for integrating exercise programming in the clinical practice setting. *Curr Cancer Ther Rev*. 2006;2(4):351–60.

178. The medical and psychological concerns of cancer survivors after treatment. In: Hewitt M, Greenfield S, Stovall E, editors. *From Cancer Patient to Cancer Survivor: Lost in Transition*. Washington (DC): National Academies Press; 2006. p. 66–186.

179. Medina-Perez C, de Souza-Teixeira F, Fernandez-Gonzalo R, de Paz-Fernandez JA. Effects of a resistance training program and subsequent detraining on muscle strength and muscle power in multiple sclerosis patients. *NeuroRehabilitation*. 2014;34(3):523–30.

180. Messier SP. Arthritic diseases and conditions. In: Kaminsky LA, editor. *ACSM's Resource Manual for Guidelines for Exercise Testing and Prescription*. 5th ed. Baltimore (MD): Lippincott Williams & Wilkins; 2006. p. 500–13.

181. Metsios G, Stavropoulos-Kalinoglou A, et al. Rheumatoid arthritis, cardiovascular disease and physical exercise: a systematic review. *Rheumatology*. 2008;47:239–48.

182. Miller TD, Squires RW, Gau GT, Ilstrup DM, Frohnert PP, Sterioff S. Graded exercise testing and training after renal transplantation: a preliminary study. *Mayo Clin Proc*. 1987;62(9):773–7.

183. Minor MA, Kay D. Arthritis. In: Larry Durstine J, Moore GE, editors. *ACSM's Exercise Management for Persons with Chronic Diseases and Disabilities*. 2nd ed. Champaign (IL): Human Kinetics; 2003. p. 210–6.

184. Mockford M, Caulton J. Systematic review of progressive strength training in children and adolescents with cerebral palsy who are ambulatory. *Pediatr Phys Ther*. 2008;20(4):318–33.

185. Morgan P, McGinley J. Gait function and decline in adults with cerebral palsy: a systematic review. *Disabil Rehabil*. 2014;36(1):1–9.

186. Morris ME. Locomotor training in people with Parkinson disease. *Phys Ther*. 2006;86(10): 1426–35.

187. Morris ME. Movement disorders in people with Parkinson disease: a model for physical therapy. *Phys Ther*. 2000;80(6):578–97.

188. Morris ME, Martin CL, Schenkman ML. Striding out with Parkinson disease: evidence-based physical therapy for gait disorders. *Phys Ther*. 2010;90(2):280–8.

189. Munhoz RP, Li JY, Kurtinecz M, et al. Evaluation of the pull test technique in assessing postural instability in Parkinson's disease. *Neurology*. 2004;62(1):125–7.

190. Munneke M, de Jong Z, Zwinderman AH, et al. High intensity exercise or conventional exercise for patients with rheumatoid arthritis? Outcome expectations of patients, rheumatologists, and physiotherapists. *Ann Rheum Dis*. 2004;63:804–8.

191. Murray CJ, Vos T, Lozano R, et al. Disability-adjusted life years (DALYs) for 291 diseases and injuries in 21 regions, 1990-2010: a systematic analysis for the Global Burden of Disease Study 2010. *Lancet*. 2012;380:2197–223.

192. Nakagawa F, Lodwick RK, Smith CJ, et al. Projected life expectancy of people with HIV according to timing of diagnosis. *AIDS*. 2012;26(3):335–43.

193. National Coalition for Cancer Survivorship Web site [Internet]. Silver Spring (MD): National Coalition for Cancer Survivorship; [cited 2015 Feb 19]. Available from: http://www.canceradvocacy.org/about-us/our-history

194. National Comprehensive Cancer Network. *NCCN Guidelines Survivorship Version 2.2014*. Fort Washington (PA): National Comprehensive Cancer Network; 2014. 72 p.

195. National Kidney Foundation. *Staying Fit with Kidney Disease* [Internet]. New York (NY): National Kidney Foundation; [cited 2015 Feb 19]. Available from: http://www.kidney.org/atoz/content/stayfit

196. National Lymphedema Network Medical Advisory Committee. *Position Statement of the National Lymphedema Network. Topic: Exercise* [Internet]. Berkeley (CA): National Lymphedema Network; [cited 2015 Feb 19]. Available from: http://www.lymphnet.org

197. National Multiple Sclerosis Society Web site [Internet]. New York (NY): National Multiple Sclerosis Society; [cited 2014 Nov 9]. Available from: http://www.nationalmssociety.org/About-the-Society/MS-Prevalence

198. National Osteoporosis Foundation. *What Is Osteoporosis* [Internet]. Arlington (VA): National Osteoporosis Foundation; [cited 2014 Nov 19]. Available from: http://nof.org/articles/7

199. National Spinal Cord Injury Statistical Center. *Spinal Cord Injury Facts and Figures at a Glance. March 2013* [Internet]. Birmingham (AL): University of Alabama at Birmingham; [cited 2014 Oct 22]. Available from: https://www.nscisc.uab.edu/PublicDocuments/fact_figures_docs/Facts%202013.pdf

200. Needle RH, Trotter RT II, Singer M, et al. Rapid assessment of the HIV/AIDS crisis in racial and ethnic minority communities: an approach for timely community interventions. *Am J Public Health*. 2003;93(6):970–9.

201. Ness KK, Wall MM, Oakes JM, Robison LL, Gurney JG. Physical performance limitations and participation restrictions among cancer survivors: a population-based study. *Ann Epidemiol*. 2006;16(3):197–205.

202. Ng AV, Dao HT, Miller RG, Gelinas DF, Kent-Braun JA. Blunted pressor and intramuscular metabolic responses to voluntary isometric exercise in multiple sclerosis. *J Appl Physiol*. 2000;88(3):871–80.

203. Ng AV, Kent-Braun J. Quantitation of lower physical activity in persons with multiple sclerosis. *Med Sci Sports Exerc*. 1997;29:517–23.

204. Ng AV, Miller RG, Gelinas D, Kent-Braun JA. Functional relationships of central and peripheral muscle alterations in multiple sclerosis. *Muscle Nerve*. 2004;29(6):843–52.

205. Nicassio PM, Moxham EG, Schuman CE, Gevirtz RN. The contribution of pain, reported sleep quality, and depressive symptoms to fatigue in fibromyalgia. *Pain.* 2002;100(3):271–9.

206. Nsenga Leunkeu A, Shephard RJ, Ahmaidi S. Six-minute walk test in children with cerebral palsy gross motor function classification system levels I and II: reproducibility, validity, and training effects. *Arch Phys Med Rehabil.* 2012;93(12):2333–9.

207. Olgiati R, Burgunder JM, Mumenthaler M. Increased energy cost of walking in multiple sclerosis: effect of spasticity, ataxia, and weakness. *Arch Phys Med Rehabil.* 1988;69(10):846–9.

208. Ortiz A, Ramirez-Marrero F, Rosario M, Venegas-Rios HL. Long-term participation in a community-based fitness program for Hispanic adults living with HIV influences health-related outcomes. *J Physical Ther Health Prom.* 2014;2(1):1–7.

209. Oursler KK, Katzel LI, Smith BA, Scott WB, Russ DW, Sorkin JD. Prediction of cardiorespiratory fitness in older men infected with the human immunodeficiency virus: clinical factors and value of the six-minute walk distance. *J Am Geriatr Soc.* 2009;57(11):2055–61.

210. Oursler KK, Sorkin JD, Smith BA, Katzel LI. Reduced aerobic capacity and physical functioning in older HIV-infected men. *AIDS Res Hum Retroviruses.* 2006;22(11):1113–21.

211. Oviedo GR, Guerra-Balic M, Baynard T, Javierre C. Effects of aerobic, resistance and balance training in adults with intellectual disabilities. *Res Dev Disabil.* 2014;35:2624–34.

212. Painter PL. Exercise after renal transplantation. *Adv Ren Replace Ther.* 1999;6:159–64.

213. Painter PL. Physical functioning in end-stage renal disease patients: update 2005. *Hemodial Int.* 2005;9(3):218–35.

214. Painter PL, Hector L, Ray K, et al. A randomized trial of exercise training after renal transplantation. *Transplantation.* 2002;74(1):42–8.

215. Painter PL, Krasnoff JB. End-stage metabolic disease: renal failure and liver failure. In: Durstine JL, Moore GE, editors. *ACSM's Exercise Management for Persons with Chronic Diseases and Disabilities.* 2nd ed. Champaign (IL): Human Kinetics; 2003. p. 126–32.

216. Painter PL, Marcus R. Assessing physical function and physical activity in patients with CKD. *Clin J Am Soc Nephrol.* 2013(8):861–72.

217. Palisano RJ, Snider LM, Orlin MN. Recent advances in physical and occupational therapy for children with cerebral palsy. *Semin Pediatr Neurol.* 2004;11(1):66–77.

218. Pastor MA, Day BL, Marsden CD. Vestibular induced postural responses in Parkinson's disease. *Brain.* 1993;116(Pt 5):1177–90.

219. Pelletier CA, Totosy de Zepetnek JO, MacDonald MJ, Hicks AL. A 16-week randomized controlled trial evaluating the physical activity guidelines for adults with spinal cord injury. *Spinal Cord.* 2015;53(5):363–7.

220. Petajan JH, Gappmaier E, White AT, Spencer MK, Mino L, Hicks RW. Impact of aerobic training on fitness and quality of life in multiple sclerosis. *Ann Neurol.* 1996;39(4):432–41.

221. Peterson MD, Lukasik L, Muth T, et al. Recumbent cross-training is a feasible and safe mode of physical activity for significantly motor-impaired adults with cerebral palsy. *Arch Phys Med Rehabil.* 2013;94(2):401–7.

222. Petrick JL, Reeve BB, Kucharska-Newton AM, et al. Functional status declines among cancer survivors: trajectory and contributing factors. *J Geriatr Oncol.* 2014;5(4):359–67.

223. Pezzoli G, Zini M. Levodopa in Parkinson's disease: from the past to the future. *Expert Opin Pharmacother.* 2010;11(4):627–35.

224. Physical Activity Guidelines Advisory Committee. *Physical Activity Guidelines Advisory Committee Report 2008,* [Internet]. Washington (DC): U.S. Department of Health and Human Services; [cited 2011 Jan 6]. 683 p. Available from: http://www.health.gov/paguidelines/Report/pdf/CommitteeReport.pdf

225. Pikora TJ, Bourke J, Bathgate K, Foley KR, Lennox N, Leonard H. Health conditions and their impact among adolescents and young adults with Down syndrome. *PLoS One.* 2014;9(5):e96868.

226. Pitetti K, Miller RA, Beets MW. Measuring joint hypermobility using the Beighton scale in children with intellectual disability. *Pediatr Phys Ther.* 2015;27:143–50.

227. Podsiadlo D, Richardson S. The timed "Up & Go": a test of basic functional mobility for frail elderly persons. *J Am Geriatr Soc.* 1991;39(2):142–8.

228. Polidoulis I, Beyene J, Cheung AM. The effect of exercise on pQCT parameters of bone structure and strength in postmenopausal women — a systematic review and meta-analysis of randomized controlled trials. *Osteoporos Int.* 2012;23:39–51.

229. Politis M, Wu K, Molloy S, G Bain P, Chaudhuri KR, Piccini P. Parkinson's disease symptoms: the patient's perspective. *Mov Disord.* 2010;25(11):1646–51.

230. Ponichtera JA, Rodgers MM, Glaser RM, Mathews TA, Camaione DN. Concentric and eccentric isokinetic lower extremity strength in persons with multiple sclerosis. *J Orthop Sports Phys Ther.* 1992;16:114–22.

231. Ponichtera-Mulcare JA, Mathews T, Barrett PJ, Gupta SC. Change in aerobic fitness of patients with multiple sclerosis during a 6-month training program. *Sports Med Train Rehabil.* 1997;7(3):265–72.

232. Presson AP, Partyka G, Jensen KM, et al. Current estimate of Down syndrome population prevalence in the United States. *J Pediatr.* 2013;163:1163–8.

233. Protas EJ, Stanley R. Parkinson's disease. In: Myers J, Nieman DC, editors. *ACSM's Resources for Clinical Exercise Physiology: Musculoskeletal, Neuromuscular, Neoplastic, Immunologic, and Hematologic Conditions.* 2nd ed. Baltimore (MD): Lippincott Williams & Wilkins; 2010. p. 44–57.

234. Pursiainen V, Korpelainen JT, Haapaniemi TH, Sotaniemi KA, Myllylä VV. Blood pressure and heart rate in Parkinsonian patients with and without wearing off. *Eur J Neurol.* 2007;14(4):373–8.

235. Rampello A, Franceschini M, Piepoli M, et al. Effect of aerobic training on walking capacity and maximal exercise tolerance in patients with multiple sclerosis: a randomized crossover controlled study. *Phys Ther.* 2007;87(5):545–55.

236. Reid S, Hamer P, Alderson J, Lloyd D. Neuromuscular adaptations to eccentric strength training in children and adolescents with cerebral palsy. *Dev Med Child Neurol.* 2010;52(4):358–63.

237. Rezak M. Current pharmacotherapeutic treatment options in Parkinson's disease. *Dis Mon.* 2007;53(4):214–22.

238. Rice CL, Vollmer TL, Bigland-Ritchie B. Neuromuscular responses of patients with multiple sclerosis. *Muscle Nerve.* 1992;15(10):1123–32.

239. Rikli RE, Jones C. *Senior Fitness Test Manual.* Champaign (IL): Human Kinetics; 2001. 176 p.

240. Rimaud D, Calmels P, Devillard X. Training programs in spinal cord injury. *Ann Readapt Med Phys.* 2005;48(5):259–69.

241. Rintala P, McCubbin JA, Dunn JM. Familiarization process in cardiorespiratory fitness testing for persons with mental retardation. *Sports Med Training Rehab.* 1995;6:15–27.

242. Ritter PL, González VM, Laurent DD, Lorig KR. Measurement of pain using the visual numeric scale. *J Rheumatol.* 2006;33(3):574–80.

243. Robertson RJ, Goss FL, Rutkowski J, et al. Concurrent validation of the OMNI perceived exertion scale for resistance exercise. *Med Sci Sports Exerc.* 2003;35(2):333–41.

244. Rock CL, Doyle C, Demark-Wahnefried W, et al. Nutrition and physical activity guidelines for cancer survivors. *CA Cancer J Clin.* 2012;62(4):243–74.

245. Rogers A, Furler BL, Brinks S, Darrah J. A systematic review of the effectiveness of aerobic exercise interventions for children with cerebral palsy: an AACPDM evidence report. *Dev Med Child Neurol.* 2008;50(11):808–14.

246. Romberg A, Virtanen A, Ruutiainen J, et al. Effects of a 6-month exercise program on patients with multiple sclerosis: a randomized study. *Neurology.* 2004;63(11):2034–8.

247. Rooks DS. Fibromyalgia treatment update. *Curr Opin Rheumatol.* 2007;19(2):111–7.

248. Rooks DS. Talking to patients with fibromyalgia about physical activity and exercise. *Curr Opin Rheumatol.* 2008;20(2):208–12.

249. Runciman P, Derman W, Ferreira S, Albertus-Kajee Y, Tucker R. A descriptive comparison of sprint cycling performance and neuromuscular characteristics in able-bodied athletes and paralympic athletes with cerebral palsy. *Am J Phys Med Rehabil.* 2014;94(1):28–37.

250. Ryuzaki M, Konishi K, Kasuga A, et al. Spontaneous rupture of the quadriceps tendon in patients on maintenance hemodialysis — report of three cases with clinicopathological observations. *Clin Nephrol.* 1989;32(3):144–8.

251. Satonaka A, Suzuki N, Kawamura M. Validity of submaximal exercise testing in adults with athetospastic cerebral palsy. *Arch Phys Med Rehabil.* 2012;93(3):485–9.

252. Scandalis TA, Bosak A, Berliner JC, Helman LL, Wells MR. Resistance training and gait function in patients with Parkinson's disease. *Am J Phys Med Rehabil.* 2001;80(1):38–43.

253. Schachter CL, Busch AJ, Peloso PM, Sheppard MS. Effects of short versus long bouts of aerobic exercise in sedentary women with fibromyalgia: a randomized controlled trial. *Phys Ther.* 2003;83(4):340–58.

254. Scharhag-Rosenberger F, Kuehl R, Klassen O, et al. Exercise training intensity prescription in breast cancer survivors: validity of current practice and specific recommendations. *J Cancer Surviv.* 2015;9(4):612–9.

255. Schenkman M, Cutson TM, Kuchibhatla M, et al. Exercise to improve spinal flexibility and function for people with Parkinson's disease: a randomized, controlled trial. *J Am Geriatr Soc.* 1998;46(10):1207–16.

256. Schenkman M, Hall DA, Barón AE, Schwartz RS, Mettler P, Kohrt WM. Exercise for people in early- or mid-stage Parkinson disease: a 16-month randomized controlled trial. *Phys Ther.* 2012;92:1395–410.

257. Schmid A, Schmidt-Trucksäss A, Huonker M, et al. Catecholamines response of high performance wheelchair athletes at rest and during exercise with autonomic dysreflexia. *Int J Sports Med.* 2001;22(1):2–7.

258. Schmitz KH, Courneya KS, Matthews C, et al. American College of Sports Medicine roundtable on exercise guidelines for cancer survivors. *Med Sci Sports Exerc.* 2010;42(7):1409–26.

259. Schneider CM, Dennehy CA, Roozeboom M, Carter SD. A model program: exercise intervention for cancer rehabilitation. *Integr Cancer Ther.* 2002;1(1):76–82.

260. Scholtes VA, Becher JG, Comuth A, Dekkers H, Van Dijk L, Dallmeijer AJ. Effectiveness of functional progressive resistance exercise strength training on muscle strength and mobility in children with cerebral palsy: a randomized controlled trial. *Dev Med Child Neurol.* 2010;52(6):e107–13.

261. Schousboe JT, Shepherd JA, Bilezikian JP, Baim S. Executive summary of the 2013 International Society for Clinical Densitometry Position Development Conference on bone densitometry. *J Clin Densitom.* 2013;16(4):455–66.

262. Schwid SR, Thornton CA, Pandya S, et al. Quantitative assessment of motor fatigue and strength in MS. *Neurology.* 1999;53(4):743–50.

263. Segura-Jiménez V, Romero-Zurita A, Carbonell-Baeza A, Aparicio VA, Ruiz JR, Delgado-Fernández M. Effectiveness of tai-chi for decreasing acute pain in fibromyalgia patients. *Int J Sports Med.* 2014;35(5):418–23.

264. Shih M, Hootman J, Kruger J, Helmick C. Physical activity in men and women with arthritis. *Am J Prev Med.* 2006;30(5):385–93.

265. Shrier I, Schur P. Flexibility versus stretching. *Br J Sports Med.* 2001;35(5):364.

266. Shulman LM, Katzel LI, Ivey FM, et al. Randomized clinical trial of 3 types of physical exercise for patients with Parkinson disease. *JAMA Neurol.* 2013;70(2):183–90.

267. Sidney S, Lewis CE, Hill JO, et al. Association of total and central adiposity measures with fasting insulin in a biracial population of young adults with normal glucose tolerance: the CARDIA study. *Obes Res.* 1999;7(3):265–72.

268. Silsupadol P, Shumway-Cook A, Lugade V, et al. Effects of single-task versus dual-task training on balance performance in older adults: a double-blind, randomized controlled trial. *Arch Phys Med Rehabil.* 2009;90(3):381–7.

269. Simmons OL, Kressler J, Nash MS. Reference fitness values in the untrained spinal cord injury population. *Arch Phys Med Rehabil.* 2014;95:2272–8.

270. Siris ES, Adler R, Bilezikian JP, et al. The clinical diagnosis of osteoporosis: a position statement from the National Bone Health Alliance Working Group. *Osteoporos Int.* 2014;25(5):1439–43.

271. Skidmore FM, Patterson SL, Shulman LM, Sorkin JD, Macko RF. Pilot safety and feasibility study of treadmill aerobic exercise in Parkinson disease with gait impairment. *J Rehabil Res Dev.* 2008;45(1):117–24.

272. Skjerbæk AG, Næsby M, Lützen K, et al. Endurance training is feasible in severely disabled patients with progressive multiple sclerosis. *Mult Scler.* 2014;20(5):627–30.

273. Slaman J, Dallmeijer A, Stam H, Russchen H, Roebroeck M, van den Berg-Emons R. The six-minute walk test cannot predict peak cardiopulmonary fitness in ambulatory adolescents and young adults with cerebral palsy. *Arch Phys Med Rehabil.* 2013;94(11):2227–33.

274. Slawta JN, McCubbin JA, Wilcox AR, Fox SD, Nalle DJ, Anderson G. Coronary heart disease risk between active and inactive women with multiple sclerosis. *Med Sci Sports Exerc.* 2002;34(6):905–12.

275. Smithson F, Morris ME, Iansek R. Performance on clinical tests of balance in Parkinson's disease. *Phys Ther.* 1998;78(6):577–92.

276. Somarriba G, Lopez-Mitnik G, Ludwig DA, et al. Physical fitness in children infected with the human immunodeficiency virus: associations with highly active antiretroviral therapy. *AIDS Res Hum Retroviruses.* 2013;29:112–20.

277. Stacy M. Medical treatment of Parkinson disease. *Neurol Clin.* 2009;27(3):605–31.

278. Sterman AB, Coyle PK, Panasci DJ, Grimson R. Disseminated abnormalities of cardiovascular autonomic functions in multiple sclerosis. *Neurology.* 1985;35(11):1665–8.

279. Stoessl AJ. Continuous dopaminergic therapy in Parkinson disease: time to stride back? *Ann Neurol.* 2010;68(1):3–5.

280. Stone PC, Minton O. Cancer-related fatigue. *Eur J Cancer.* 2008; 44(8):1097–1104.

281. Summer GD, Deighton CM, Rennie MJ, Booth AH. Rheumatoid cachexia: a clinical perspective. *Rheumatology.* 2008;47(8):1124–31.

282. Surakka J, Romberg A, Ruutiainen J, et al. Effects of aerobic and strength exercise on motor fatigue in men and women with multiple sclerosis: a randomized controlled trial. *Clin Rehabil.* 2004;18(7):737–46.

283. Suteerawattananon M, Morris GS, Etnyre BR, Jankovic J, Protas EJ. Effects of visual and auditory cues on gait in individuals with Parkinson's disease. *J Neurol Sci.* 2004;219(1–2):63–9.

284. Svien LR, Berg P, Stephenson C. Issues in aging with cerebral palsy. *Top Geriatr Rehabil.* 2008;25(1):26–40.

285. Taylor NF, Dodd KJ, Prasad D, Denisenko S. Progressive resistance exercise for people with multiple sclerosis. *Disabil Rehabil.* 2006;28(18):1119–26.

286. Teo-Koh SM, McCubbin JA. Relationship between peak VO_2 and 1-mile walk test performance of adolescent males with mental retardation. *Pediatr Exerc Sci.* 1999;11(2):144–57.

287. Thomas EN, Blotman F. Aerobic exercise in fibromyalgia: a practical review. *Rheumatol Int.* 2010;30(9):1143–50.

288. Tinetti ME, Richman D, Powell L. Falls efficacy as a measure of fear of falling. *J Gerontol.* 1990;45(6):239–43.

289. Tiozzo E, Jayaweera D, Rodriguez A, et al. Short-term combined exercise training improves the health of HIV-infected patients. *J AIDS HIV Res.* 2013;5:80–9.

290. Turk DC. The potential of treatment matching for subgroups of patients with chronic pain: lumping versus splitting. *Clin J Pain.* 2005;21(1):44–55.

291. Twelves D, Perkins KS, Counsell C. Systematic review of incidence studies of Parkinson's disease. *Mov Disord.* 2003;18(1):19–31.

292. Uc EY, Doerschug KC, Magnotta V, et al. Phase I/II randomized trial of aerobic exercise in Parkinson disease in a community setting. *Neurology.* 2014;83:413–25.

293. Unnithan VB, Clifford C, Bar-Or O. Evaluation by exercise testing of the child with cerebral palsy. *Sports Med.* 1998;26(4):239–51.

294. U.S. Renal Data System. *USRDS 2009 Annual Data Report: Atlas of Chronic Kidney Disease and End-Stage Renal Disease in the United States* [Internet]. Bethesda (MD): National Institutes of Health, National Institute of Diabetes and Digestive and Kidney Disease; [cited 2015 Jan 15]. Available from: http://www.usrds.org/atlas09.aspx

295. Valkeinen H, Alen M, Hannonen P, Häkkinen A, Airaksinen O, Häkkinen K. Changes in knee extension and flexion force, EMG and functional capacity during strength training in older females with fibromyalgia and healthy controls. *Rheumatology (Oxford).* 2004;43(2):225–8.

296. Valkeinen H, Häkkinen A, Hannonen P, Häkkinen K, Alén M. Acute heavy-resistance exercise-induced pain and neuromuscular fatigue in elderly women with fibromyalgia and in healthy controls: effects of strength training. *Arthritis Rheum.* 2006;54(4):1334–9.

297. van den Akker LE, Heine M, van der Veldt N, Dekker J, de Groot V, Beckerman H. Feasibility and safety of cardiopulmonary exercise testing in multiple sclerosis: a systematic review. *Arch Phys Med Rehabil.* 2015;96(11):2055–66.

298. van den Berg M, Dawes H, Wade DT, et al. Treadmill training for individuals with multiple sclerosis: a pilot randomised trial. *J Neurol Neurosurg Psychiatry.* 2006;77(4):531–3.

299. van den Ende CH, Hazes JM, le Cessie S, et al. Comparison of high and low intensity training in well controlled rheumatoid arthritis. Results of a randomised clinical trial. *Ann Rheum Dis.* 1996;55(11):798–805.

300. van der Kamp W, Maertens de Noordhout A, Thompson PD, Rothwell JC, Day BL, Marsden CD. Correlation of phasic muscle strength and corticomotoneuron conduction time in multiple sclerosis. *Ann Neurol.* 1991;29:6–12.

301. van Drongelen S, van der Woude LH, Janssen TW, Angenot EL, Chadwick EK, Veeger DH. Glenohumeral contact forces and muscle forces evaluated in wheelchair-related activities of daily living in able-bodied subjects versus subjects with paraplegia and tetraplegia. *Arch Phys Med Rehabil.* 2005;86(7):1434–40.

302. Vanlandewijck Y, Theisen D, Daly D. Wheelchair propulsion biomechanics: implications for wheelchair sports. *Sports Med.* 2001;31(5):339–67.

303. van Sighem A, Gras L, Reiss P, Brinkman K, de Wolf F. Life expectancy of recently diagnosed asymptomatic HIV-infected patients approaches that of uninfected individuals. *AIDS.* 2010;24(10):1527–35.

304. Verschuren O, Ketelaar M, Keefer D, et al. Identification of a core set of exercise tests for children and adolescents with cerebral palsy: a Delphi survey of researchers and clinicians. *Dev Med Child Neurol.* 2011;53(5):449–56.

305. Verschuren O, Takken T. Aerobic capacity in children and adolescents with cerebral palsy. *Res Dev Disabil.* 2010;31(6):1352–7.

306. Verschuren O, Zwinkels M, Obeid J, Kerkhof N, Ketelaar M, Takken T. Reliability and validity of short-term performance tests for wheelchair-using children and adolescents with cerebral palsy. *Dev Med Child Neurol.* 2013;55(12):1129–35.

307. Violan MA, Pomes T, Maldonado S, et al. Exercise capacity in hemodialysis and renal transplant patients. *Transplant Proc.* 2002;34(1):417–8.

308. Ward BW, Schiller JS, Goodman RA. Multiple chronic conditions among US adults: a 2012 update. *Prev Chronic Dis* [Internet]. 2014;11:130389. [cited 2015 Jan 6]. Available from: http://www.cdc.gov/pcd/issues/2014/pdf/13_0389.pdf. doi:10.5888/pcd11.130389.

309. Weaver FM, Follett K, Stern M, et al. Bilateral deep brain stimulation vs best medical therapy for patients with advanced Parkinson disease: a randomized controlled trial. *JAMA.* 2009;301(1):63–73.

310. Wee S, Pitetti KH, Goulopoulou S, Collier SR, Guerra M, Baynard T. Impact of obesity and Down syndrome on peak heart rate and aerobic capacity in youth and adults. *Res Dev Disabil.* 2014;36C:198–206.

311. Werner WG, DiFrancisco-Donoghue J, Lamberg EM. Cardiovascular response to treadmill testing in Parkinson disease. *J Neurol Phys Ther.* 2006;30(2):68–73.

312. White LJ, McCoy SC, Castellano V, et al. Resistance training improves strength and functional capacity in persons with multiple sclerosis. *Mult Scler.* 2004;10(6):668–74.

313. Wiart L, Darrah J, Kembhavi G. Stretching with children with cerebral palsy: what do we know and where are we going? *Pediatr Phys Ther.* 2008;20(2):173–8.

314. Wolfe F, Brähler E, Hinz A, Häuser W. Fibromyalgia prevalence, somatic symptom reporting, and the dimensionality of polysypmtomatic distress: results from a survey of the general population. *Arthritis Care Res.* 2013;65(5):777–85.

315. Wolfe F, Smythe HA, Yunus MB, et al. The American College of Rheumatology 1990 criteria for the classification of fibromyalgia: report of the multicenter criteria committee. *Arthritis Rheum.* 1990;33(2):160–72.

316. Yarasheski KE, Roubenoff R. Exercise treatment for HIV-associated metabolic and anthropomorphic complications. *Exerc Sport Sci Rev.* 2001;29(4):170–4.

317. Ziemssen T, Reichmann H. Cardiovascular autonomic dysfunction in Parkinson's disease. *J Neurol Sci.* 2010;289:74–80.

318. Zigmond MJ, Smeyne R. Exercise: is it a neuroprotective and if so, how does it work? *Parkinsonism Relat Disord.* 2014;20(Suppl 1):S123–7.

CHAPTER 12

Behavioral Theories and Strategies for Promoting Exercise

INTRODUCTION

The purpose of this chapter is to provide exercise and health care professionals a basic understanding of how to assist individuals to adopt and adhere to the exercise prescription (Ex R_x) recommendations that are made throughout the *Guidelines*. Chapter 1 of the *Guidelines* focuses on the public health recommendations for a physically active lifestyle, yet most of the public remains unaware of these recommendations (11). Furthermore, most adults in the United States do not engage in the recommended amounts of physical activity (PA) (99). Simply providing knowledge and promoting awareness of Ex R_x recommendations may be insufficient to produce behavior change (48); therefore, a better understanding of behavioral strategies that can be used to promote a physically active lifestyle is warranted.

Research has identified consistent correlates to engaging in regular exercise. Numerous demographic factors (*e.g.*, age, gender, socioeconomic status, education, ethnicity) are consistently related to the likelihood that an individual will exercise on a regular basis (10,57). Although these factors are not amenable to intervention, they do suggest who might benefit most from exercise intervention. This chapter focuses on (a) the role that modifiable factors have on the Ex R_x, (b) behavioral theories and models that have been applied to enhance exercise adoption and maintenance, (c) behavioral strategies and approaches that can be used to increase PA behaviors, and (d) unique considerations for special populations.

EXERCISE PRESCRIPTION

Given the flexibility in the *Frequency, Intensity, Time,* and *Type* (*FITT*) principle of Ex R_x for the targeted population, it is important to first understand what impact variations in the Ex R_x might have on adoption or maintenance of a habitually active lifestyle.

377

Frequency/Time

Ex R_x recommendations allow for flexibility in the different combinations of frequency and time to achieve them. A commonly held belief was that flexibility in terms of the time/duration and exercise volume recommended would allow individuals to overcome the most frequently reported barrier to regular exercise, that is, lack of time (71). However, the lack of any real change in PA levels in the United States from 1998 to 2008 suggests otherwise (17). Reviews of randomized trials have not identified differences in exercise adherence when different combinations of frequency and time are used to achieve the same total volume of PA (53,79). These results should be viewed with caution, however, because the included studies were randomized trials that *assigned* participants to different combinations. Allowing individuals to *self-select* frequency and time may positively influence adherence to exercise interventions.

Intensity

Although previous studies of the effects of exercise intensity on adherence suggest that individuals are more likely to adhere to lower intensity exercise programs (33,72), a more recent review suggests that this inverse relationship is not particularly strong and may be moderated by prior exercise behavior (79). There is evidence that individuals with more exercise experience fare better with higher intensity programs (65%–75% heart rate reserve [HRR]), whereas those adopting exercise for the first time may be better suited to, and self-select, moderate intensity programs (45%–55% HRR) (3).

Type

Although it is recommended that individuals participate in a variety of exercise types (*i.e.*, aerobic, resistance, neuromotor, and flexibility) (42), there have been few systematic tests of the effects of different exercise modalities on adoption and maintenance. Most of the research that has examined adherence has investigated aerobic activity, often with a focus on walking, yet there is no compelling evidence that exercise mode is related to adherence (79). To date, little is known about the characteristics of those who adopt and maintain resistance training and flexibility-exercise programs.

In the FITT principle of Ex R_x, "Type" universally refers to the mode or kind of exercise. However, in the area of health behavior, Type has an additional context, focusing more on program/delivery type (*i.e.*, home-based, supervised). Although the traditional approach in Ex R_x is to provide structured, supervised exercise programs, studies have shown comparable or greater adherence to home-based programs that include the provision of remotely delivered support (24,43). Interventions delivered entirely or predominantly via telephone have been shown to be effective in increasing PA in a range of populations (44), and technology-delivered interventions also hold promise for promoting PA with greater reach and lower cost (56). Although there are an abundance of commercially available apps that relate to PA and fitness, they generally lack the inclusion of evidence-based behavior change strategies, principles, and theories (62,86).

THEORETICAL FOUNDATIONS FOR UNDERSTANDING EXERCISE BEHAVIOR

Theories and models provide frameworks for understanding exercise participation and the factors that may facilitate or impede being physically active. Using appropriate theories can guide exercise and health professionals in determining appropriate strategies to assist individuals to adopt and maintain regular PA. The most widely used theories and models in the PA literature are described as follows. The purpose of this section is to provide a basic understanding of the theories and models. A later section describes the application of strategies that result from these theories and models.

Social Cognitive Theory

Social cognitive theory (SCT) is a comprehensive theoretical framework that has been extensively employed in understanding, describing, and changing exercise behavior. The theory and strategies derived from SCT have been successfully applied in exercise interventions across diverse populations (6,60,61). SCT is based on the principle of reciprocal determinism; that is, the individual (*e.g.*, emotion, personality, cognition, biology), behavior (*e.g.*, past and current achievement), and environment (*i.e.*, physical, social, and cultural) all interact to influence behavior (8). It is important to recognize that these are dynamic factors that influence each other differently over time. For example, an individual who begins an exercise program may feel a sense of accomplishment, encouraging even more exercise, which leads to making the environment more conducive to subsequent exercise (*e.g.*, buying home exercise equipment). Conversely, another individual may start an exercise program, work too hard and feel fatigued, lose motivation, and move the exercise equipment to the basement to make the environment less conducive to exercising. SCT posits that individuals learn from external reinforcements and punishments, by observing others, and through cognitive processes (9).

Central to SCT is the concept of *self-efficacy*, which refers to one's beliefs in his or her capability to successfully complete a course of action such as exercise (8). There are two salient types of self-efficacy when considering exercise behavior. Task self-efficacy refers to an individual's belief he or she can actually do the behavior in question, whereas barriers self-efficacy refers to whether an individual believes he or she can regularly exercise in the face of common barriers such as lack of time and poor weather. The higher the sense of efficacy, the greater the effort, persistence, and resilience an individual will exhibit, particularly when faced with barriers or challenges. Self-efficacy is one of the most consistently found correlates of PA in adults and youth (10). For example, an older adult who does not believe he or she can "lift weights" would not even consider enrolling in a program that included resistance training. This individual would have to work on increasing his or her confidence in his or her capability to perform resistance training. Strategies for enhancing self-efficacy are described later in this chapter.

Outcome expectations and expectancies, key concepts of SCT, are anticipatory results of a behavior and the value placed on these results (105). If specific outcomes are seen as likely to occur and are valued, then behavior change is more likely to occur (105). For example, an overweight adult who wants to lose weight and believes that walking will help is more likely to start and maintain such a program. Conversely, a woman who believes that resistance training will lead to looking "muscular" or "masculine" will be unlikely to start a resistance training program if these traits are perceived as undesirable.

Another important concept in SCT is *self-regulation* or *self-control*. Self-regulation/self-control is a person's ability to set goals, monitor progress toward those goals (or self-monitor), problem solve when faced with barriers, and engage in self-reward. A meta-analysis found that exercise interventions were most effective when self-monitoring was combined with at least one other technique within the self-regulation/self-control construct (61).

Transtheoretical Model

The transtheoretical model (TTM) was developed as a framework for understanding behavior change and is one of the most popular approaches for promoting exercise behavior (67,73,74). The popularity of the TTM stems from the intuitive appeal that individuals are at different stages of readiness to make behavioral changes and thus require tailored interventions. The TTM includes five stages of change: precontemplation (*i.e.*, no intention to be regularly active in the next 6 mo), contemplation (*i.e.*, intending to be regularly active in the next 6 mo), preparation (*i.e.*, intending to be regularly active in the next 30 d), action (*i.e.*, regularly active for <6 mo), and maintenance (*i.e.*, regularly active for ≥6 mo). As individuals attempt to change their behavior, they may move linearly through these stages, but repeated relapse and successful change after several unsuccessful attempts may also occur.

Associated with the five stages of change are the constructs of processes of change, decisional balance, and self-efficacy. The 10 processes of change illustrate the strategies used by individuals in attempting to advance through the five stages of change. Emphasizing experiential or cognitive processes of change (*e.g.*, understanding the risks of inactivity) is recommended in earlier, pre-action stages of change, whereas promoting behavioral processes of change (*e.g.*, rewarding oneself) is most helpful in later stages of change. Decisional balance involves weighing the pros and cons of changing exercise behavior. During pre-action stages of change, the cons typically outweigh the pros, whereas during action and maintenance, the pros typically outweigh the cons (74). Self-efficacy is lowest in the earliest stages of change and highest in the latest stages of change. There are specific processes of change and pattern in decisional balance and self-efficacy that have been shown to be most useful to facilitate progression through each of the stages of change for exercise (29,67) (*Figure 12.1*).

The TTM highlights different approaches to exercise adoption and maintenance that need to be taken with different individuals based on stage of change

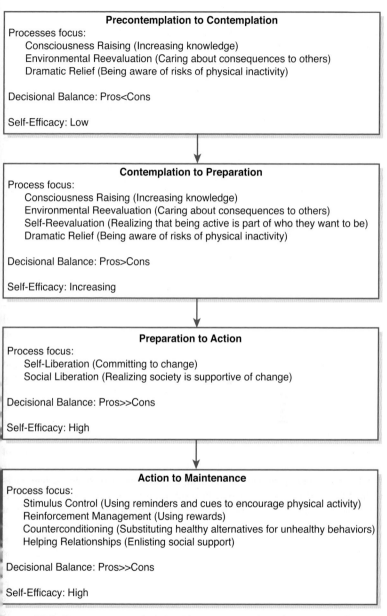

Precontemplation to Contemplation

Processes focus:
   Consciousness Raising (Increasing knowledge)
   Environmental Reevaluation (Caring about consequences to others)
   Dramatic Relief (Being aware of risks of physical inactivity)

Decisional Balance: Pros<Cons

Self-Efficacy: Low

Contemplation to Preparation

Process focus:
   Consciousness Raising (Increasing knowledge)
   Environmental Reevaluation (Caring about consequences to others)
   Self-Reevaluation (Realizing that being active is part of who they want to be)
   Dramatic Relief (Being aware of risks of physical inactivity)

Decisional Balance: Pros>Cons

Self-Efficacy: Increasing

Preparation to Action

Process focus:
   Self-Liberation (Committing to change)
   Social Liberation (Realizing society is supportive of change)

Decisional Balance: Pros>>Cons

Self-Efficacy: High

Action to Maintenance

Process focus:
   Stimulus Control (Using reminders and cues to encourage physical activity)
   Reinforcement Management (Using rewards)
   Counterconditioning (Substituting healthy alternatives for unhealthy behaviors)
   Helping Relationships (Enlisting social support)

Decisional Balance: Pros>>Cons

Self-Efficacy: High

Figure 12.1 Key processes and relationships to progress through the stages of change 58,67).

or readiness for behavior change. Stage-based interventions, across various groups and populations, have been effective in helping individuals make progress toward becoming regularly active (67,93). Strategies to facilitate transitioning through the stages of change are presented later in this chapter.

Health Belief Model

The health belief model (HBM) theorizes that an individual's beliefs about whether or not he or she is susceptible to disease, and his or her perceptions of the benefits of trying to avoid it, influence his or her readiness to act (82).

The theory is grounded in the notion that individuals are ready to act if they:

- Believe they are susceptible to the condition (*i.e.*, perceived susceptibility).
- Believe the condition has serious consequences (*i.e.*, perceived severity).
- Believe taking action reduces their susceptibility to the condition or its severity (*i.e.*, perceived benefits).
- Believe costs of taking action (*i.e.*, perceived barriers) are outweighed by the benefits.
- Are confident in their ability to successfully perform an action (*i.e.*, self-efficacy).
- Are exposed to factors that prompt action (*e.g.*, seeing their weight on the scale, a reminder from one's physician to exercise) (*i.e.*, cues to action).

Together, the six constructs of the HBM suggest strategies for motivating individuals to change their exercise behavior because of health issues (*Table 12.1*). For example, an individual would need to feel that he or she is at risk for having a heart attack (perceived susceptibility), feel that a heart attack would negatively impact his or her life (perceived severity), believe that starting an exercise program would reduce his or her risk (perceived benefits), feel that the amount of reduction in risk is worth the time and energy he or she would have to commit to exercise (perceived benefits outweigh perceived barriers), and believe he or she could exercise on a regular basis (self-efficacy). However, those factors alone are not enough for an individual to start exercising; he or she also needs some type of prompt (*e.g.*, a friend/relative having a heart attack) to actually begin to exercise (cue to action). Therefore, there is a need to prime individuals to be ready to change and also help devise ways to prompt them into taking action.

Given its obvious focus on health issues for understanding motivation, the HBM may be most suitable for understanding and intervening with populations that are motivated to be physically active primarily for health (39). Thus, the HBM has been applied to cardiac rehabilitation and diabetes mellitus (DM) prevention and management (64,92).

Self-Determination Theory

A theory that has recently received an increasing amount of attention related to exercise is self-determination theory (SDT) (25,40,96). The underlying assumption of SDT is individuals have three primary psychosocial needs that they are trying to satisfy: (a) self-determination or autonomy, (b) demonstration of competence or

TABLE **12.1**		
Health Belief Model Constructs and Strategies (82)		
Construct	**Exercise-Specific Definition**	**Change Strategy**
Perceived susceptibility	Beliefs about the chances of getting a disease/condition if do not exercise	■ Explain risk information based on current activity, family history, other behaviors, etc.
Perceived severity	Beliefs about the seriousness/ consequences of disease/ condition as a result of inactivity	■ Refer individual to medically valid information about disease. ■ Discuss different treatment options, outcomes, and costs.
Perceived benefits	Beliefs about the effectiveness of exercising to reduce susceptibility and/or severity	■ Provide information on benefits of exercise to preventing/treating condition or disease. ■ Provide information regarding all of the other potential benefits of exercise (*e.g.,* quality of life, mental health).
Perceived barriers	Beliefs about the direct and indirect costs associated with exercise	■ Discuss Ex R$_x$ options to minimize burden. ■ Provide information on different low-cost activity choices.
Cues to action	Factors that activate the change process and get someone to start exercising	■ Help individual look for potential cues. ■ Ask the individual what it would take for him or her to get started.
Self-efficacy	Confidence in ability to exercise	■ Assess level of confidence for different types of activity. ■ Use self-efficacy building techniques to enhance exercise confidence.

Ex R$_x$, exercise prescription.

mastery, and (c) relatedness or the ability to experience meaningful social interactions with others. The theory proposes that motivation exists on a continuum from amotivation to intrinsic motivation. Individuals with amotivation have the lowest levels of self-determination and have no desire to engage in exercise. Individuals with intrinsic motivation have the highest degree of self-determination and are interested in engaging in exercise simply for the satisfaction, challenge, or pleasure it brings. Between amotivation and intrinsic motivation lies extrinsic motivation; that is, when individuals engage in exercise for reasons that are external to the individual, such as being physically active to make oneself more attractive to others (40,96).

SDT suggests that the use of rewards to get individuals to start exercising may have limited effectiveness because they promote extrinsic motivation. Rather, programs should be designed to enhance autonomy by promoting choice and incorporating simple, easy exercises initially to enhance feelings of competence and enjoyment. Interventions that target strategies to increase autonomy have been effective at enhancing PA levels (19,89,90).

Theory of Planned Behavior

According to the theory of planned behavior (TPB), intention to perform a behavior is the primary determinant of actual behavior (1). Intentions reflect an individual's perceived probability or likelihood that he or she will exercise but do not always translate directly into behavior because of issues related to behavioral control (22). Intentions are determined by an individual's attitudes, subjective norms, and perceived behavioral control. Attitudes are influenced by behavioral beliefs that exercise will lead to certain outcomes (positive or negative) combined with the evaluation of those outcomes. Subjective norms are the social component and are influenced by individual's beliefs that others want him or her to be physically active (normative beliefs) combined with his or her motivation to comply with the desires of significant others. Finally, *perceived behavioral control* is influenced by the individual's belief about how easy or difficult performance of the behavior is likely to be (control beliefs) combined with the perceived power of the barrier or facilitator. Thus, an individual intends to be physically active if he or she believes exercise would lead to desire outcomes, is valued by someone whose opinion they value, and is within his or her control (*Figure 12.2*).

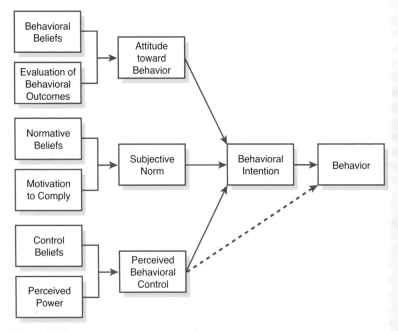

Figure 12.2 Theory of planned behavior (1).

Although intentions are the primary predictor of behavior, there is also a hypothesized direct link (dashed line in *Figure 12.2*) between perceived behavioral control and behavior. An individual's subjective norms may lead him or her toward healthier behavior, and he or she may also have a positive attitude, but powerful barriers outside of the person's control may act directly to limit exercise participation. For example, if an individual perceives low control over his or her ability to engage in exercise when the weather is poor, he or she is likely to skip an exercise session if it is raining.

In cross-sectional and prospective studies, the TPB consistently explains exercise intentions and behavior (14,32); however, there is less evidence that interventions based on the TPB are effective at increasing PA levels (49,101). This model has been applied most frequently to clinical populations, including patients with cancer (102), cardiac rehabilitation participants (13), and pregnant women (31).

Social Ecological Models

Social ecological models are important because they consider the impact of and connections between individuals and their environments. The explicit recognition of relations between individuals and their physical environments is a defining feature of ecological models (84,85). Ecological models posit that behavior results from influences at multiple levels, including intrapersonal factors (*e.g.*, biological, psychological), interpersonal/cultural factors (*e.g.*, family, friends, culture), organizational factors (*e.g.*, schools, worksites, churches), physical environments (*e.g.*, built, natural), and policies (*e.g.*, laws, regulations, codes) (*Table 12.2*). Importantly, environmental factors influence behavior not only directly but also indirectly through an individual's perceptions. A key belief is that interventions are most likely to be effective when they target multiple levels (84,85). For example, adding a walking path in a park is most likely to be effective in increasing PA when there is a campaign to promote awareness of the path perhaps combined with an intervention that targets individual beliefs and motivations about walking. Although research examining the impact of interventions based on ecological models is limited, results appear promising (85).

DECREASING BARRIERS TO PHYSICAL ACTIVITY

Individuals face a number of personal, social, and environmental-related barriers (*e.g.*, lack of time; inconvenience; lack of self-motivation; finding PA boring or not enjoyable; and lacking self-management skills, self-efficacy, social support, or places to be active) in both the adoption and maintenance of PA (16,66). *Table 12.3* outlines common challenges that individuals face in the adoption and maintenance of exercise that can be better understood and addressed through the application of different behavioral theories.

TABLE 12.2

Levels of Social Ecological Model and Potential Physical Activity Intervention Strategies

Social Ecological Level	Components	Potential Change Strategies
Intrapersonal factors	■ Knowledge, attitudes, behaviors, beliefs, perceived barriers, motivation, enjoyment ■ Skills and self-efficacy ■ Demographics (age, sex, education, and socioeconomic and employment status)	■ Focus on changing individual's knowledge, skills, and attitudes. ■ Use theories and approaches such as social cognitive theory, the transtheoretical model, theory of planned behavior, and self-determination theory. ■ Use demographic information to identify subgroups at risk or subgroups that require different approaches to intervention.
Interpersonal factors/social environment	■ Family, spouse, or partner ■ Peers ■ Coworkers ■ Access to social support ■ Influence of health professionals ■ Community norms ■ Cultural background	■ Use community education, support groups, and peer programs. ■ Social marketing campaigns may promote positive community attitudes and awareness toward participation in physical activity. ■ Use consistent, accurate, and encouraging messages to promote physical activity.
Organizational factors	■ Schools, workplaces, faith-based settings, and community organizations	■ Create opportunities for organizations, at both the individual and group level, to adopt or increase physical activity.
Physical environment	■ Natural factors such as weather or geography ■ Availability and access to exercise facilities ■ Aesthetics or perceived qualities of facilities or the natural environment ■ Safety such as crime rates and traffic ■ Community design ■ Public transportation options	■ Create walking trails or parks. ■ Enhance existing environments (*e.g.,* park/neighborhood cleanups). ■ Help individuals become more aware of opportunities for physical activity in their communities (*e.g.,* parks, trails, community centers).
Policy	■ Urban planning policies ■ Education policies such as physical education classes ■ Health policies ■ Environmental policies ■ Workplace and other organizational policies	■ Align physical activity participation with priorities such as reducing reliance on fossil fuels and the reduction of greenhouse gas emissions. ■ Emphasize the importance of regular physical education. ■ Require workplaces to provide support for physical activity.

TABLE 12.3

Most Common Exercise Barriers (16), Relevant Theories, and Potential Strategies

Common Problem	Percentage of Endorsing Barrier	Applicable Theories	Example Strategies
"I don't have enough time."	69%	SCT, TPB, SET	■ Discuss modifications to FITT principles ■ Examine priorities/goals ■ Brief counseling/motivational interviewing
"I don't have enough energy."	59%	SCT, HBM, SET, TPB	■ Discuss modifications to FITT principles ■ Brief counseling/motivational interviewing ■ Discuss affect regulation techniques for setting exercise intensity
"I'm just not motivated."	52%	SCT, HBM, TPB, TTM, SET, SDT	■ Discuss attitudes and outcome expectations ■ Determine stage of change and provide stage-tailored counseling ■ Examine perceived susceptibility and severity ■ Discuss potentially effective reinforcements
"It costs too much."	37%	HBM, TTM, SET	■ Examine exercise alternatives to meet goals ■ Evaluate exercise opportunities in the environment
"I'm sick or hurt."	36%	TTM	■ Discuss maintenance/relapse prevention ■ Discuss alternative exercises to keep progressing toward goals
"There's nowhere for me to exercise."	30%	SET	■ Evaluate exercise opportunities in the environment ■ Discuss different types of activities for which there are resources
"I feel awkward when I exercise."	29%	SCT, TPB	■ Examine self-efficacy ■ Examine alternative settings
"I don't know how to do it."	29%	SCT, HBM, TTM, TPB	■ Build task self-efficacy using appropriate strategies
"I might get hurt."	26%	SCT, HBM, TPB	■ Evaluate exercise prescription ■ Determine task-specific self-efficacy
"It's not safe."	24%	SCT, SET	■ Evaluate exercise opportunities in the environment

(continued)

TABLE 12.3			
Most Common Exercise Barriers (16), Relevant Theories, and Potential Strategies (Continued)			
Common Problem	**Percentage of Endorsing Barrier**	**Applicable Theories**	**Example Strategies**
"No one will watch my child if I exercised."	23%	SCT, SET	■ Develop social support structures ■ Examine opportunities for exercise in which childcare may be provided
"There is no one to exercise with me."	21%	SCT, TPB, TTM	■ Develop social support and exercise buddy system ■ Identify different types of activities one can do on his or her own

FITT, Frequency, Intensity, Time, and Type of exercise; HBM, health belief model; SCT, social cognitive theory; SDT, self-determination theory; SET, social ecological theory; TPB, theory of planned behavior; TTM, transtheoretical model.

COGNITIVE AND BEHAVIORAL STRATEGIES FOR INCREASING PHYSICAL ACTIVITY BEHAVIOR

Cognitive strategies are an essential component of interventions focused on exercise behavior change (6) and are especially effective at increasing PA levels (28). These strategies focus on changing the way individuals think, reason, and imagine about themselves in regard to exercise behavior. Behavioral strategies are also an important component of exercise interventions and refer to individual actions and reactions to various environmental stimuli. Because actions and reactions are thought to be learned, the behavioral approach to change posits that these actions and reactions can also be unlearned or modified. Evidenced-based cognitive and behavioral strategies that can be used to increase PA behavior are presented in *Table 12.4* and discussed in the following sections.

Enhancing Self-Efficacy

Self-efficacy, the confidence in one's ability to carry out actions necessary to perform certain behaviors (8), is a central component of most of the theories previously discussed (i.e., SCT, TTM, HBM, and TPB). Increased self-efficacy is related to PA behavior change (6). Individuals draw on various sources of efficacy information to increase exercise behavior, including mastery experience (e.g., experiencing success), which are the most powerful source, vicarious experience (e.g., observing others who are similar to them having positive experiences), verbal persuasion (e.g., encouragement from others), and physiological feedback

TABLE **12.4**	
Cognitive and Behavioral Strategies for Increasing Physical Activity	
Cognitive-Behavioral Strategy	**Description**
Enhancing self-efficacy	Increase individuals' confidence for increasing physical activity by ensuring their goals are realistic, watching others who are similar to them have positive experiences, offering encouragement, and helping them experience positive mood states.
Goal setting	Work with individuals to establish specific, measurable, action-oriented, realistic, timely, and self-determined (SMARTS) short and long term goals.
Reinforcement	Encourage individuals to reward themselves for meeting behavioral goals. Reinforcements can be external or internal.
Social support	Encourage individuals to enlist social support for physical activity from family, friends, and coworkers.
Self-monitoring	Encourage individuals to track their physical activity through a physical activity log, pedometer, smart watch, or other technology device.
Problem solving	Help individuals find ways to overcome barriers to physical activity.
Relapse prevention	Prepare individuals for lapses in physical activity and develop plans for overcoming them so that lapses do not become relapses.

(*e.g.*, enjoyment, positive mood states) (6). *Table 12.5* describes the sources of efficacy and outlines strategies that can be used to enhance an individual's sense of self-efficacy for exercise.

Goal Setting

Goal setting is a powerful tool for behavior change that leads to positive changes in exercise behavior (6). The exercise professional can work with the patients/clients to help develop, implement, measure, and revise goals on a consistent basis to provide direction to their efforts; enhance persistence; and learn new strategies. The SMARTS principle can be used to guide effective goal setting:

- **S**pecific: Goals should be precise.
- **M**easurable: Goals should be quantifiable.
- **A**ction-oriented: Goals should indicate what needs to be done.
- **R**ealistic: Goals should be achievable.
- **T**imely: Goals should have a specific and realistic time frame.
- **S**elf-determined: Goals should be developed primarily by the client/patient.

It is important for individuals to set both short- and long-term goals that allow for measurement and assessment on a regular basis. Individuals often focus on

TABLE 12.5		
Strategies for Enhancing Self-Efficacy		
Source of Self-Efficacy Information	**Description**	**Strategies**
Mastery experiences	Have person successfully perform the behavior.	■ Set realistic goals that can be achieved. ■ Progress gradually over time. ■ Provide proper instruction and demonstration. ■ Use physical activity logs to track progress.
Vicarious experiences	Have person watch others with similar background perform tasks.	■ Have appropriate group exercise leaders that individual can identify with. ■ Use videos to model behavior. ■ Discuss "success" stories of individuals with similar backgrounds and characteristics.
Verbal persuasion	Have others tell the person that he or she can be successful.	■ Give frequent feedback (*e.g.*, encouragement, compliments) and express confidence in the individual's abilities.
Physiological feedback	Communicate the meaning of symptoms associated with the behavior change.	■ Provide appropriate instruction and reassurance. ■ Discuss how physical activity makes the individual feel. ■ Provide education about the possible discomfort associated with physical activity. ■ Encourage using music, scenery, etc. to make physical activity pleasurable.

long-term goals; however, when attempting to initiate a new behavior, setting short-term achievable goals (*i.e.*, daily or weekly) is important for increasing self-efficacy (97). The exercise professional should regularly monitor progress, provide feedback, and discuss successes and struggles with the individual. Setting proper goals is an important part of numerous PA studies; however, because goal setting is incorporated into many theories and interventions, there is limited evidence on its sole contribution to changing exercise behavior (55,87,88).

Reinforcement

The use of positive reinforcement (*i.e.*, rewards) is emphasized in SCT, SDT, and TTM. Individuals should be encouraged to reward themselves for meeting behavioral goals. Extrinsic rewards include tangible, physical rewards such as money, a new pair of shoes, or a new book and are often used to initiate behavior change (68). Social reinforcement such as praise from an exercise professional or family member is also an extrinsic reinforcer. Intrinsic rewards are intangible rewards that come from within, such as a feeling of accomplishment, confidence, or enjoyment. Individuals are more likely to adhere to regular exercise over the long term if they are doing the activity for intrinsic reasons (83). It may be difficult to give intrinsic reinforcers to participants, but it may be possible to develop an environment that can promote intrinsic motivation. These environments focus on the autonomy of the participant and have been shown to lead to higher levels of PA (19). Environments promoting intrinsic motivation focus on (a) providing positive feedback to help the participant increase feelings of competence, (b) acknowledging participant difficulties within the program, and (c) enhancing sense of choice and self-initiation of activities to build feelings of autonomy.

Social Support

Social support is a powerful motivator to exercise for many individuals and important in SCT, TTM, TPB, and social ecological models and can come from an instructor, family members, workout partners, coworkers, neighbors, as well as exercise and other health professionals. Social support can be provided to clients/patients in various ways including (a) guidance (*i.e.*, advice and information), (b) reliable alliance (*i.e.*, assurance that others can be counted on in times of stress), (c) reassurance of worth (*i.e.*, recognition of one's competence that individuals in the exercise group or personal trainer believe in his or her abilities), (d) attachment (*i.e.*, emotional closeness with the personal trainer or at least one other individual in the exercise group), (e) social integration (*i.e.*, a sense of belonging and feeling comfortable in group exercise situations), and (f) opportunity for nurturance (*i.e.*, providing assistance to others in the exercise group) (103).

Providing social support in the form of guidance is most common when working with clients/patients. Individuals beginning an exercise program need to feel supported in times of stress or times when continuing to exercise is difficult (36,38). Moreover, individuals beginning an exercise program may have feelings of incompetence. Increasing one's confidence through mastery experiences, social modeling, and providing praise are practical ways to increase acknowledgment of one's competence (8).

Implementing ways to increase an individual's attachment and feelings of being part of a group is also important. The exerciser needs to feel comfortable. A method to make exercisers feel comfortable is to establish buddy groups. In group settings, exercisers can benefit from watching others complete their exercise routines and from instructors and fellow exercisers giving input on proper technique and execution. Creating supportive exercise groups within communities has been linked with greater levels of exercise behavior (48).

Self-Monitoring

Self-monitoring, an important component of SCT and TTM, involves observing and recording behavior and has been shown to be important in exercise behavior change (6,61). Self-monitoring of exercise can be in the form of a paper-and-pencil log, a heart rate monitor, pedometer, or "wearable" technology such as a smart watch. Technology devices can provide the individual with detailed feedback that includes minutes of exercise, exercise intensity, distance travelled, or step counts. Visual documentation (*e.g.*, workout log) can be useful for tracking progress toward goals, identifying barriers to changing behavior, and as a reminder to exercise.

Problem Solving

Individuals encounter a number of barriers that may impede efforts of becoming physically active (see *Table 12.3*). Problem solving can assist individuals in identifying strategies to reduce or eliminate barriers and includes four main steps: (a) identify the barrier, (b) brainstorm ways to overcome the barrier, (c) select a strategy generated in brainstorming viewed as most likely to be successful, and (d) analyze how well the plan worked and revise as necessary (12). Solutions to barriers should ideally be generated by the individual and not by the exercise professional. For example, if lack of time is a barrier to engaging in exercise, the individual, in conjunction with the exercise professional, can identify possible solutions for overcoming this barrier (*e.g.*, schedule exercise "appointments," incorporate PA into existing activities).

Relapse Prevention

Regularly active individuals will occasionally encounter situations that make sticking with their exercise program difficult or nearly impossible. Therefore, an important part of many theories and approaches is the development of strategies to help individuals overcome setbacks and maintain their PA levels (94). Although it is not unusual to have a lapse from an exercise program (*i.e.*, missing a few exercise sessions), preparing for situations which may result in a return to a sedentary lifestyle, or relapse, is most critical. Relapse prevention strategies include being aware of and anticipating high-risk situations (*e.g.*, travel, vacation, holidays, illness, competing family obligations, and poor weather) and having a plan to ensure that a lapse does not become a relapse (94). At times, missing planned exercise is unavoidable, yet good lapse and relapse strategies can help an individual to stay on track or to get back on track once the situation has passed. Finally, individuals should avoid "all-or-nothing" thinking and not get discouraged when they miss a session of planned exercise.

THEORETICAL STRATEGIES AND APPROACHES TO INCREASE EXERCISE ADOPTION AND ADHERENCE

Brief Counseling and Motivational Interviewing

A promising area for increasing exercise adoption is through the use of brief counseling, often conducted by health care professionals (4). These brief counseling approaches can be based on any of the theories previously discussed; however, it is imperative that they be more thorough than simply asking about PA levels and

Box 12.1	**Client-Centered Physical Activity Counseling (Five A's Model)**

Assess physical activity behavior, beliefs, knowledge, and readiness to change.
Advise client on the benefits of physical activity and the health risks of inactivity.
Agree collaboratively on physical activity goals based on client's interests, confidence, ability, and readiness to change.
Assist client to identify and overcome barriers using problem-solving techniques and social and environmental support and resources.
Arrange a specific plan for follow-up feedback, assessment, and support.

advising the patient to increase his or her exercise behavior. *Box 12.1* provides examples of established strategies and techniques that can be incorporated into counseling sessions. Numerous medical associations and Healthy People 2020 have adopted the position that primary care providers should make PA counseling a part of every routine patient visit (47), yet the U.S. Preventive Services Task Force concluded that the health benefit of behavioral counseling in the primary care setting to promote PA is small (65,95).

Motivational interviewing has evolved over the past two decades and can now be successfully applied to many health behaviors, including PA (59,69) and weight loss (5). Motivational interviewing is a person-centered method of communication where the professional and the client/patient work collaboratively for change. The professional's approach should be nonjudgmental, empathic, and encouraging. A major focus of motivational interviewing is to help the ambivalent individual realize the different intrinsic motivators that can lead to positive change. The approach respects client/patient autonomy and views the client as fully responsible for change. *Table 12.6* highlights some of the differences between traditional counseling and a motivational interviewing approach. Motivational interviewing can be adapted and used in combination with most existing theories to help motivate change and confidence among individuals who are seeking to adopt or maintain an exercise program. Because of theoretical similarities between motivational interviewing and SDT (*e.g.*, intrinsic motivation, autonomy), there is a growing interest to combine these in intervention development (78).

Principles of motivational interviewing can be applied in health care and public health settings, where time pressures are often great (81). In these settings, the primary goal is to help resolve ambivalence and increase motivation for change, which is also the initial phase of motivational interviewing, when "change talk" can occur. Change talk refers to an individual's mention or discussion of a desire or reason to change, making it more likely the change will occur (*Table 12.7*) (63). Several concrete and practical methods have been used in PA interventions (see [77]) and may be easily incorporated into these brief contact periods.

TABLE 12.6		
Comparison of Motivational Interviewing and Advice Giving		
	Motivational Interviewing	**Advice Giving**
Counseling aim	Explore why the individual isn't sure he or she wants to exercise and build his or her motivation to want to change.	Persuade the individual that he or she needs to change and start exercising by providing an Ex R$_x$.
Client	Help the individual explore why he or she is inactive, how and why he or she might begin exercising, and how exercising is consistent with personal values; use empathy	Explain that someone who is inactive may be at increased risk for disease (*e.g.*, diabetes mellitus, CVD)
Information presentation	Neutrally explain discrepancies between current activity level and recommended levels and allow client to react.	Give the evidence for why being inactive increases the risk of disease.
Questioning approach	Open-ended questioning to encourage exploration of thoughts and feelings regarding physical activity	Leading questions to have them "prove" to themselves the risks of their inactivity and why they should be active
Dealing with resistance	Use reflection to try to acknowledge their point; resistance is a sign that a new approach is needed; acknowledge that ambivalence to change is normal.	Have counterarguments ready and "correct" any misconceptions.
Summarizing	Use their language to summarize both the pros and cons of exercising.	Summarize the dangers of staying inactive and steps they should take to be active.

CVD, cardiovascular disease; Ex R$_x$, exercise prescription.

Stage of Change Tailored Counseling

The TTM is predicated on the notion of stages of change and that progression through the stages can be facilitated by the use of stage-specific strategies and processes of change that result in "tailoring" interventions. *Box 12.2* provides examples of how one might use specific strategies within each stage to tailor the intervention to an individual to help them progress to the next stage. Intervention studies have consistently found stage-tailored interventions that include all of the components of the TTM are appropriate for many different populations and are effective at enhancing PA levels (46,93).

Group Leader Interactions

Separate from attempts to implement individual behavior change is the concept of group interventions to improve exercise adoption and adherence

TABLE 12.7

Methods for Evoking Change Talk

Approach	Description	Examples
Ask evocative questions	Ask the person questions regarding: ■ Disadvantages of the status quo ■ Advantages of change ■ Optimism about change ■ Intention to change	"What do you think will happen if you don't change anything?" "What are some benefits of becoming more physically active?" "What changes would work best for you?" "What do you intend to do?"
Use the importance ruler	Ask simple questions to assess how important physical activity is to the person and what might make it more important.	"How important would you say it is for you to be physically active? (After response) "Why do you believe that?" "What would it take for you to increase the importance of exercise?"
Use the confidence rule	Ask simple questions to assess the person's confidence and what might increase his or her confidence.	"How confident are you that you can engage in regular physical activity? (After response) "What makes you feel that way?" "What would it take for you to feel more confident about this?"
Explore pros and cons	Encourage person to discuss the positive and negative aspects of his or her present behavior.	"Are there things that you like about being physically inactive?" "Are there disadvantages of being physically inactive?"
Elaborate	When health professional hears any arguments for change, encourage the person to elaborate to reinforce change talk.	"You said exercise might make you feel better. Can you tell me more about that?"
Query extremes	When the person has little desire for change, encourage him or her to consider extreme consequences of not changing and best consequences of changing.	"Suppose you continue on as you have, with no physical activity in your life. What do you imagine are the worse things that might happen to you?" "What might be the best results you could imagine if you make a change?"
Look back	Help the person remember a time in his or her life when he or she was physically active.	"You mentioned that you used to walk regularly. What was that like?"
Look forward	Help the person envision a changed future.	"If you don't like what you see in the future about yourself, how would you like things to be different?"
Explore values and goals	Ask the person to tell you what things are most important in his or her life and then ask if being inactive fits with this picture.	"What in life is most important to you?" (After a response) "Does being physically active or inactive matter to this?"

Adapted from (63,77).

Box 12.2	Example Strategies to Facilitate Stage Transitions

Precontemplation → Contemplation

- Provide information about the benefits of regular physical activity.
- Discuss how some of the barriers they perceive may be misconceived such as "It can be done in shorter and accumulated bouts if they don't have the time."
- Have them visualize what they would feel like if they were physically active with an emphasis on short-term, easily achievable benefits of activity such as sleeping better, reducing stress, and having more energy.
- Explore how their inactivity impacts individuals other than themselves such as their spouse and children.

Contemplation → Preparation

- Explore potential solutions to their physical activity barriers.
- Assess level of self-efficacy and begin techniques to build efficacy.
- Emphasize the importance of even small steps in progressing toward being regularly active.
- Encourage viewing oneself as a healthy, physically active person.

Preparation → Action

- Help develop an appropriate plan of activity to meet their physical activity goals and use a goal setting worksheet or contract to make it a formal commitment.
- Use reinforcement to reward steps toward being active.
- Teach self-monitoring techniques such as tracking time and distance.
- Continue discussion of how to overcome any obstacles they feel are in their way of being active.
- Encourage them to help create an environment that helps remind them to be active.
- Encourage ways to substitute sedentary behavior with activity.

Action → Maintenance

- Provide positive and contingent feedback on goal progress.
- Explore different types of activities they can do to avoid burnout.
- Encourage them to work with and even help others become more active.
- Discuss relapse prevention strategies.
- Discuss potential rewards that can be used to maintain motivation.

Adherence, social interaction, quality of life, physiological effectiveness, and functional effectiveness have all been studied in group settings and also compared to home-based programs, home-based programs involving some contact by health care professionals, and usual exercise classes. Exercising in a group, where the instructor purposefully creates group dynamics and goals, has consistently been shown superior to exercising in a usual exercise class (where each individual functions autonomously) or exercising at home with or without contact. These outcomes highlight the value of group-based PA interventions (15).

Exercise leaders have an influence on PA participation and the psychological benefits that occur as a result of PA (36). The exercise leader and group play significant roles in SCT and SDT. An exercise leader with a socially supportive leadership style is one that provides encouragement, verbal reinforcement, praise, and interest in the participant (38). Participants who have an exercise leader who has a socially supportive leadership style report greater self-efficacy, more energy, more enjoyment, stronger intentions to exercise, less fatigue, and less concern about embarrassment (41). In addition to the exercise leader, aspects of the exercise group may also influence PA participation. One such aspect is that of group cohesion, that is, a dynamic process reflected in the tendency of a group to stick together and remain united in the pursuit of its instrumental objectives and/or satisfaction of member affective needs. Five principles have been successfully used to improve cohesion and lower dropout rates among exercise groups (18,37):

- Distinctiveness — creating a group identity (*e.g.*, group name)
- Positions — giving members of the class responsibilities and roles for the group
- Group norms — adopt common goals for the group to achieve
- Sacrifice — individuals in the group giving up something for the greater good of the group
- Interaction and communication — the belief that the more social interactions that are made possible for the group, the greater the cohesion

SPECIAL POPULATIONS

An important area of exercise promotion is the proper tailoring of interventions to promote exercise behavior across diverse populations that present unique challenges. Proper tailoring requires an understanding of potential unique beliefs, values, environments, and obstacles within a population or individual. Although every individual is clearly unique, the following sections discuss behavioral considerations of some of the more common special groups with whom exercise professionals may work.

Cultural Diversity

In order to provide culturally competent care to exercisers, it is necessary to be exposed to and understand the cultural beliefs, values, and practices of the desired population. This includes but is not limited to housing, neighborhood characteristics, religion, access to resources, crime, race, ethnicity, age, ability level, and social class. For example, the higher levels of physical inactivity among African Americans compared to other racial/ethnic groups may be caused not only by environmental constraints but also by cultural beliefs (70). African American women have cited lack of PA exposure and thus lack of role models, family responsibilities (*i.e.*, need to be the caregiver), issues related to body size (*i.e.*, larger body sizes and curves tend to be appreciated, and thus, lower perceived need for PA), and hairstyles as barriers to PA (45). Including strategies that address these barriers may be essential in interventions focusing on this population.

Perhaps the most important characteristic of exercise interventions that target different racial/ethnic groups is being culturally sensitive and tailored. Culturally sensitive interventions should include surface structure and deep structure (76). Surface structure involves matching intervention materials and messages to observable, "superficial" characteristics of the target population. The people, places, language, music, food, locations, and clothing that are familiar to and preferred by the population should be used. For example, an intervention targeting African Americans should include pictures of African Americans in program materials. Deep structure involves incorporating the cultural, social, historical, environmental, and psychological forces that influence PA in the targeted population. For example, in Latino cultures, the family unit is very important. Thus, recommendations for increasing PA might incorporate methods to get all family members exercising together (*e.g.*, taking walks with the whole family). Including both dimensions within interventions can increase the receptivity and acceptance of the messages (surface structure) and saliency (deep structure) (76).

Older Adults

There are several challenges when working with promoting the adoption and adherence of exercise among older adults (see *Chapter 7*) (2,23). Older adults may lack knowledge about the benefits of PA or how to set up a safe and effective exercise program; therefore, the exercise professionals need to provide some initial education (106). Although typically viewed as beneficial, social support is not necessarily positive, especially in older adults (20). Family and friends may exert negative influences by telling them to "take it easy" and "let me do it." The implicit message is that they are too old or frail to be physically active (20).

Although older adults experience many of the commonly reported barriers to PA (*e.g.*, lack of time, motivation) (23,66), there are several barriers that may take on special significance, including lack of or indifferent social support; increased social isolation; fear of falling/safety; and physical ailments such as injury, chronic illness, and poor health (51,66). Quite possibly, the largest barrier to exercise participation in older adults is the fear that exercise will cause injury, pain, and discomfort or exacerbate existing conditions (66). In addition, older women in particular may have had little early-life exposure to PA due to social norms that were less accepting of this behavior in women. These unique barriers can be significant and require careful consideration when promoting PA and developing interventions for this population.

Youth

When working with children (see *Chapter 7*), it is important to recognize they are likely engaging in an exercise program because their parents wish them to.

implying an extrinsic motivation, and typically require tangible forms of social support (*e.g.*, transportation, payment of fees) (66). However, to help children maintain exercise behavior over their lifetime, they need help shifting toward a sense of autonomy (98) and to feel a sense of self-efficacy and behavioral control. Establishing a sense of autonomy and intrinsic motivation through the creation of a supportive environment, as discussed previously, should be a high priority when fostering PA among children and youth (19).

Schools are an appealing setting for implementing PA interventions, as they reach a majority of youth. Simple modifications to physical education classes (54,91), small changes during recess (80), and promoting structured PA within the classroom can increase PA (50). Although there is some concern that school-based PA programs will interfere with academic time and thus reduce academic performance, the data do not support this notion. With few exceptions, physical education, recess, and classroom-based PA interventions consistently show a positive or no association with academic achievement, academic behavior, and cognitive skills and attitudes (75).

Individuals with Obesity

PA decreases across body mass index categories, with individuals who are obese being the least active group (100). Although concerns about excess weight is the primary reason why many individuals with obesity adopt an exercise program (30), they may face additional, unique, weight-related barriers to engaging in PA such as feeling physically uncomfortable while exercising, being uncomfortable with their appearance, and not wanting to exercise in front of others (52). Individuals with obesity may have had negative mastery experiences with exercise in the past and will need to enhance their self-efficacy so they believe that they can successfully exercise (7,21). Furthermore, they may be quite deconditioned and perceive even moderate intensity exercise as challenging, so keeping activities fun and at a light intensity may be particularly important to promote positive perceptions of PA (34). Although goals should remain self-determined, individuals with obesity may need help setting realistic weight loss goals and identifying appropriate levels of PA to help them reach those goals (26).

Individuals with Chronic Diseases and Health Conditions

PA improves symptoms associated with a number of chronic diseases and health conditions. A concern when working with individuals with chronic diseases and health conditions is their ability to do the exercise both from a task self-efficacy perspective as well as in the face of the barriers specifically related to their condition (66). For example, individuals with arthritis report pain, fatigue, and mobility limitations as barriers to PA participation (27,104). Those with neurological conditions (*i.e.*, muscular dystrophy, multiple sclerosis, motor neuron disease, and Parkinson disease) cite fatigue, fear of falling or losing balance, and safety due to the progression of disease as barriers (35). Special consideration should be given to ensure activities are chosen to prevent, treat, or control the disease or health condition. Furthermore, being aware of the unique barriers and fears of individuals with chronic diseases and health conditions can help assure the physical activities chosen are appropriate.

ONLINE RESOURCES

National Physical Activity Plan:
  http://www.physicalactivityplan.org/
The Guide to Community Preventive Services, Behavioral and Social Approaches:
  http://www.thecommunityguide.org/pa/behavioral-social/index.html
National Cancer Institute Behavioral Research Program Theories Project:
  http://cancercontrol.cancer.gov/brp/research/theories_project/index.html
Exercise Is Medicine:
  http://exerciseismedicine.org

REFERENCES

1. Ajzen I. From intentions to actions: a theory of planned behavior. In: Kuhl J, Beckman J, editors. *Action Control: From Cognition to Behavior.* Heidelberg (Germany): Springer; 1985. p. 11–39.
2. American College of Sports Medicine, Chodzko-Zajko WJ, Proctor DN, et al. American College of Sports Medicine position stand. Exercise and physical activity for older adults. *Med Sci Sports Exerc.* 2009;41(7):1510–30.
3. Anton SD, Perri MG, Riley J III, et al. Differential predictors of adherence in exercise programs with moderate versus higher levels of intensity and frequency. *J Sport Exercise Psychol.* 2005;27:171–87.
4. Armit CM, Brown WJ, Marshall AL, Ritchie CB, Trost SG, Green A. Randomized trial of three strategies to promote physical activity in general practice. *Prev Med.* 2009;48(2):156–63.
5. Armstrong MJ, Mottershead TA, Ronksley PE, Sigal RJ, Campbell TS, Hemmelgarn BR. Motivational interviewing to improve weight loss in overweight and/or obese patients: a systematic review and meta-analysis of randomized controlled trials. *Obes Rev.* 2011;12(9):709–23.
6. Artinian NT, Fletcher GF, Mozaffarian D, et al. Interventions to promote physical activity and dietary lifestyle changes for cardiovascular risk factor reduction in adults: a scientific statement from the American Heart Association Jul 27. *Circulation.* 2010;122(4):406–41.
7. Baba R, Iwao N, Koketsu M, Nagashima M, Inasaka H. Risk of obesity enhanced by poor physical activity in high school students. *Pediatr Int.* 2006;48(3):268–73.
8. Bandura A. *Self-Efficacy: The Exercise of Control.* New York (NY): Freeman; 1997. 604 p.
9. Bandura A. *Social Foundations of Thought and Action: A Social-Cognitive Theory.* Englewood Cliffs (NJ): Prentice Hall; 1985. 544 p.
10. Bauman AE, Reis RS, Sallis JF, Wells JC, Loos RJ, Martin BW. Correlates of physical activity: why are some people physically active and others not? *Lancet.* 2012;380(9838):258–71.
11. Bennett GG, Wolin KY, Puleo EM, Masse LC, Atienza AA. Awareness of national physical activity recommendations for health promotion among US adults. *Med Sci Sports Exerc.* 2009;41(10):1849–55.
12. Blair SN, Dunn AL, Marcus BH, Carpenter RA, Jaret P. *Active Living Every Day.* 2nd ed. Champaign (IL): Human Kinetics; 2011. 174 p.
13. Blanchard CM, Courneya KS, Rodgers WM, et al. Is the theory of planned behavior a useful framework for understanding exercise adherence during phase II cardiac rehabilitation? *J Cardiopulm Rehabil.* 2003;23(1):29–39.

14. Blue CL. The predictive capacity of the theory of reasoned action and the theory of planned behavior in exercise research: an integrated literature review. *Res Nurs Health*. 1995;18(2):105–21.

15. Burke SM, Carron AV, Eys MA, Ntoumanis N, Estabrooks PA. Group versus individual approach? A meta-analysis of the effectiveness of interventions to promote physical activity. *Sport Exerc Psychol Rev*. 2006;2:19–35.

16. Canadian Fitness and Lifestyle Research Institute. *Progress in Prevention* [Internet]. Ottawa, Ontario (Canada): Canadian Fitness and Lifestyle Institute; [cited 2015 Aug 28]. Available from: http://www.cflri.ca/document/bulletin-04-barriers-physical-activity

17. Carlson SA, Fulton JE, Schoenborn CA, Loustalot F. Trend and prevalence estimates based on the 2008 Physical Activity Guidelines for Americans. *Am J Prev Med*. 2010;39(4):305–13.

18. Carron AV, Spink K. Team building in an exercise setting. *Sport Psychol*. 1993;7(1):8–18.

19. Chatzisarantis NL, Hagger M. Effects of an intervention based on self-determination theory on self-reported leisure-time physical activity participation. *Psychol Health*. 2009;24(1):29–48.

20. Chogahara M. A multidimensional scale for assessing positive and negative social influences on physical activity in older adults. *J Gerontol B Psychol Sci Soc Sci*. 1999;54(6):S356–67.

21. Conn VS, Minor MA, Burks KJ. Sedentary older women's limited experience with exercise. *J Community Health Nurs*. 2003;20(4):197–208.

22. Cooke R, Sheeran P. Moderation of cognition-intention and cognition-behaviour relations: a meta-analysis of properties of variables from the theory of planned behaviour. *Br J Soc Psychol*. 2004;43(Pt 2):159–86.

23. Cress ME, Buchner DM, Prohaska T, et al. Best practices for physical activity programs and behavior counseling in older adult populations. *J Aging Phys Act*. 2005;13(1):61–74.

24. Dalal HM, Zawada A, Jolly K, Moxham T, Taylor RS. Home based versus centre based cardiac rehabilitation: Cochrane systematic review and meta-analysis. *BMJ*. 2010;340:b5631.

25. Deci EL, Ryan R. *Intrinsic Motivation and Self-Determination in Human Behavior*. New York (NY): Plenum Publishing; 1985. 371 p.

26. Delahanty LM, Nathan D. Implications of the diabetes prevention program and Look AHEAD clinical trials for lifestyle interventions. *J Am Diet Assoc*. 2008;108(4 Suppl 1):S66–72.

27. Der Ananian C, Wilcox S, Saunders R, Watkins K, Evans A. Factors that influence exercise among adults with arthritis in three activity levels. *Prev Chronic Dis*. 2006;3(3):A81.

28. Dishman RK, Buckworth J. Increasing physical activity: a quantitative synthesis. *Med Sci Sports Exerc*. 1996;28(6):706–19.

29. Dishman RK, Vandenberg RJ, Motl RW, Nigg CR. Using constructs of the transtheoretical model to predict classes of change in regular physical activity: a multi-ethnic longitudinal cohort study. *Ann Behav Med*. 2010;40(2):150–63.

30. Donnelly JE, Blair SN, Jakicic JM, et al. American College of Sports Medicine position stand. Appropriate physical activity intervention strategies for weight loss and prevention of weight regain for adults. *Med Sci Sports Exerc*. 2009;41(2):459–71.

31. Downs DS, Hausenblas H. Exercising for two: examining pregnant women's second trimester exercise intention and behavior using the framework of the theory of planned behavior. *Womens Health Issues*. 2003;13(6):222–8.

32. Downs DS, Hausenblas H. The theories of reasoned action and planned behavior applied to exercise: a meta-analytic update. *J Phys Act Health*. 2005;2(1):76–97.

33. Duncan GE, Anton SD, Sydeman SJ, et al. Prescribing exercise at varied levels of intensity and frequency: a randomized trial. *Arch Intern Med*. 2005;165(20):2362–9.

34. Ekkekakis P, Lind E. Exercise does not feel the same when you are overweight: the impact of self-selected and imposed intensity on affect and exertion. *Int J Obes (Lond)*. 2006;30(4):652–60.

35. Elsworth C, Dawes H, Sackley C. A study of perceived facilitators to physical activity in neurological conditions. *Int J Ther Rehabil*. 2009;16(1):17–24.

36. Estabrooks PA. Sustaining exercise participation through group cohesion. *Exerc Sport Sci Rev*. 2000;28(2):63–7.

37. Estabrooks PA, Carron A. Group cohesion in older adult exercisers: prediction and intervention effects. *J Behav Med*. 1999;22(6):575–88.

38. Estabrooks PA, Munroe KJ, Fox EH, et al. Leadership in physical activity groups for older adults: a qualitative analysis. *J Aging Phys Act*. 2004;12(3):232–45.

39. Fitzpatrick SE, Reddy S, Lommel TS, et al. Physical activity and physical function improved following a community-based intervention in older adults in Georgia senior centers. *J Nutr Elder.* 2008;27(1–2):135–54.

40. Fortier MS, Duda JL, Guerin E, Teixeira PJ. Promoting physical activity: development and testing of self-determination theory-based interventions. *Int J Behav Nutr Phys Act.* 2012;9:20.

41. Fox LD, Rejeski WJ, Gauvin L. Effects of leadership style and group dynamics on enjoyment of physical activity. *Am J Health Promot.* 2000;14(5):277–83.

42. Garber CE, Blissmer B, Deschenes MR, et al. American College of Sports Medicine position stand. Quantity and quality of exercise for developing and maintaining cardiorespiratory, musculoskeletal, and neuromotor fitness in apparently healthy adults: guidance for prescribing exercise. *Med Sci Sports Exerc.* 2011;43(7):1334–559.

43. Geraedts H, Zijlstra A, Bulstra SK, Stevens M, Zijlstra W. Effects of remote feedback in home-based physical activity interventions for older adults: a systematic review. *Patient Educ Couns.* 2013;91(1):14–24.

44. Goode AD, Reeves MM, Eakin EG. Telephone-delivered interventions for physical activity and dietary behavior change: an updated systematic review. *Am J Prev Med.* 2012;42(1):81–8.

45. Harley AE, Odoms-Young A, Beard B, Katz ML, Heaney CA. African American social and cultural contexts and physical activity: strategies for navigating challenges to participation. *Women Health.* 2009;49:84–100.

46. Hutchison AJ, Breckon JD, Johnston LH. Physical activity behavior change interventions based on the transtheoretical model: a systematic review. *Health Educ Behav.* 2009;36(5):829–45.

47. Jacobson DM, Strohecker L, Compton MT, Katz DL. Physical activity counseling in the adult primary care setting: position statement of the American College of Preventive Medicine. *Am J Prev Med.* 2005;29(2):158–62.

48. Kahn EB, Ramsey LT, Brownson RC, et al. The effectiveness of interventions to increase physical activity. A systematic review. *Am J Prev Med.* 2002;22(4 Suppl):73–107.

49. Kelley K, Abraham C. RCT of a theory-based intervention promoting healthy eating and physical activity amongst out-patients older than 65 years. *Soc Sci Med.* 2004;59(4):787–97.

50. Kibbe DL, Hackett J, Hurley M, et al. Ten years of Take 10!®: integrating physical activity with academic concepts in elementary school classrooms. *Prev Med.* 2011;52:S43–50.

51. Lees FD, Clark PG, Nigg CR, Newman P. Barriers to exercise behavior among older adults: a focus-group study. *J Aging Phys Act.* 2005;13:23–33.

52. Leone LA, Ward D. A mixed methods comparison of perceived benefits and barriers to exercise between obese and nonobese women. *J Phys Act Health.* 2013;10:461–9.

53. Linke SE, Gallo LC, Norman GJ. Attrition and adherence rates of sustained vs. intermittent exercise interventions. *Ann Behav Med.* 2011;42(2):197–209.

54. Lonsdale C, Rosenkranz RR, Peralta LR, Bennie A, Fahey P, Lubans DR. A systematic review and meta-analysis of interventions designed to increase moderate-to-vigorous physical activity in school physical education lessons. *Prev Med.* 2013;56:152–61.

55. Lox CL, Martin Ginis KA, Petruzzello SJ. *The Psychology of Exercise: Integrating Theory and Practice.* 2nd ed. Scottsdale (AZ): Holcomb Hathaway Publishers; 2006. 450 p.

56. Lustria ML, Noar SM, Cortese J, Van Stee SK, Glueckauf RL, Lee J. A meta-analysis of web-delivered tailored health behavior change interventions. *J Health Commun.* 2013;18(9):1039–69.

57. Macera CA, Ham SA, Yore MM, et al. Prevalence of physical activity in the United States: Behavioral Risk Factor Surveillance System, 2001. *Prev Chronic Dis.* 2005;2(2):A17.

58. Marcus B, Forsyth L. *Motivating People to Be Physically Active.* Champaign (IL): Human Kinetics; 2003. 220 p.

59. Martins RK, McNeil D. Review of motivational interviewing in promoting health behaviors. *Clin Psychol Rev.* 2009;29(4):283–93.

60. McAuley E, Blissmer B. Self-efficacy determinants and consequences of physical activity. *Exerc Sport Sci Rev.* 2000;28(2):85–8.

61. Michie S, Abraham C, Whittington C, McAteer J, Gupta S. Effective techniques in healthy eating and physical activity interventions: a meta-regression. *Health Psychol.* 2009;28(6):690–701.

62. Middelweerd A, Mollee JS, van der Wal C, Brug J, Te Velde SJ. Apps to promote physical activity among adults: a review and content analysis. *Int J Behav Nutr Phys Act.* 2014;11(1):97.

63. Miller WR, Rollnick S. *Motivational Interviewing: Preparing People for Change.* 2nd ed. New York (NY): Guilford Press; 2002. 428 p.

64. Mirotznik J, Feldman L, Stein R. The health belief model and adherence with a community center-based, supervised coronary heart disease exercise program. *J Community Health.* 1995;20(3):233–47.

65. Moyer V, U.S. Preventive Services Task Force. Behavioral counseling interventions to promote a healthful diet and physical activity for cardiovascular disease prevention in adults: U.S. Preventive Services Task Force recommendation statement. *Ann Intern Med.* 2012;157:367–71.

66. Netz Y, Zeev A, Arnon M, Tenenbaum G. Reasons attributed to omitting exercising: a population-based study. *Int J Sport Exerc Psyc.* 2008;6:9–23.

67. Nigg CR, Geller KS, Motl RW, Horwath CC, Wertin KK, Dishman RK. A research agenda to examine the efficacy and relevance of the transtheoretical model for physical activity behavior. *Psychol Sport Exerc.* 2011;12(1):7–12.

68. Noland MP. The effects of self-monitoring and reinforcement on exercise adherence. *Res Q Exerc Sport.* 1989;60(3):216–24.

69. O'Halloran PD, Blackstock F, Shields N, et al. Motivational interviewing to increase physical activity in people with chronic health conditions: a systematic review and meta-analysis. *Clin Rehabil.* 2014;28(12):1159–71.

70. Pasick RJ, D'Onofrio CN, Otero-Sabogal R. Similarities and differences across cultures: questions to inform a third generation for health promotion research. *Health Educ Q.* 1996;23(Suppl):S142–61.

71. Pate RR, Pratt M, Blair SN, et al. Physical activity and public health. A recommendation from the Centers for Disease Control and Prevention and the American College of Sports Medicine. *JAMA.* 1995;273(5):402–7.

72. Perri MG, Anton SD, Durning PE, et al. Adherence to exercise prescriptions: effects of prescribing moderate versus higher levels of intensity and frequency. *Health Psychol.* 2002;21(5):452–8.

73. Prochaska JO, DiClemente CC, Norcross JC. In search of how people change. Applications to addictive behaviors. *Am Psychol.* 1992;47(9):1102–14.

74. Prochaska JO, Velicer W. The transtheoretical model of health behavior change. *Am J Health Promot.* 1997;12(1):38–48.

75. Rasberry CN, Lee SM, Robin L, et al. The association between school-based physical activity, including physical education, and academic performance: A systematic review of the literature. *Prev Med.* 2011;52:S10–20.

76. Resnicow K, Baranowski T, Ahluwalia JS, Braithwaite RL. Cultural sensitivity in public health: defined and demystified. *Ethn Dis.* 1999;9(1):10–21.

77. Resnicow K, Jackson A, Braithwaite R, et al. Healthy body/healthy spirit: a church-based nutrition and physical activity intervention. *Health Educ Res.* 2002;17(5):562–73.

78. Resnicow K, McMaster F. Motivational interviewing: moving from why to how with autonomy support. *Int J Behav Nutr Phys Act.* 2012;9:19.

79. Rhodes RE, Warburton DE, Murray H. Characteristics of physical activity guidelines and their effect on adherence: a review of randomized trials. *Sports Med.* 2009;39(5):355–75.

80. Ridges ND, Salmon J, Parrish A, Stanley RM, Okely AD. Physical activity during school recess: a systematic review. *Am J Prev Med.* 2012;43(3):320–8.

81. Rollnick S, Mason P, Butler C. *Health Behavior Change: A Guide for Practitioners.* Edinburgh (United Kingdom): Churchill Livingstone; 1999. 240 p.

82. Rosenstock IM, Strecher VJ, Becker MH. Social learning theory and the health belief model. *Health Educ Q.* 1988;15(2):175–83.

83. Ryan RM, Frederick CM, Lepes D, Rubio N, Sheldon KM. Intrinsic motivation and exercise adherence. *Int J Sport Psychol.* 1997;28:335–54.

84. Sallis JF, Cervero RB, Ascher W, Henderson KA, Kraft MK, Kerr J. An ecological approach to creating active living communities. *Annu Rev Public Health.* 2006;27:297–322.

85. Sallis JF, Floyd MF, Rodríguez DA, Saelens BE. Role of built environments in physical activity, obesity, and cardiovascular disease. *Circulation.* 2012;125(5):729–37.

86. Schoffman DE, Turner-McGrievy G, Jones SJ, Wilcox S. Mobile apps for pediatric obesity prevention and treatment, healthy eating, and physical activity promotion: just fun and games? *Transl Behav Med.* 2013;3(3):320–5.

87. Shilts MK, Horowitz M, Townsend MS. Goal setting as a strategy for dietary and physical activity behavior change: a review of the literature. *Am J Health Promot*. 2004;19(2):81–93.

88. Shilts MK, Horowitz M, Townsend MS. Guided goal setting: effectiveness in a dietary and physical activity intervention with low-income adolescents. *Int J Adolesc Med Health*. 2009;21(1): 111–22.

89. Silva MN, Markland D, Carraça EV, et al. Exercise autonomous motivation predicts 3-yr weight loss in women. *Med Sci Sports Exerc*. 2011;43(4):728–37.

90. Silva MN, Vieira PN, Coutinho SR, et al. Using self-determination theory to promote physical activity and weight control: a randomized controlled trial in women. *J Behav Med*. 2010;33(2): 110–22.

91. Slingerland M, Borghouts L. Direct and indirect influence of physical education-based interventions on physical activity: a review. *J Phys Act Health*. 2011;8:866–78.

92. Speer EM, Reddy S, Lommel TS, et al. Diabetes self-management behaviors and A1c improved following a community-based intervention in older adults in Georgia senior centers. *J Nutr Elder*. 2008;27(1–2):179–200.

93. Spencer L, Adams TB, Malone S, Roy L, Yost E. Applying the transtheoretical model to exercise: a systematic and comprehensive review of the literature. *Health Promot Pract*. 2006;7(4):428–43.

94. Stetson BA, Beacham AO, Frommelt SJ, et al. Exercise slips in high-risk situations and activity patterns in long-term exercisers: an application of the relapse prevention model. *Ann Behav Med*. 2005;30(1):25–35.

95. Task Force on Community Preventive Services. Recommendations to increase physical activity in communities. *Am J Prev Med*. 2002;22(4 Suppl):67–72.

96. Teixeira PJ, Carraça EV, Markland D, Silva MN, Ryan RM. Exercise, physical activity, and self-determination theory: a systematic review. *Int J Behav Nutr Phys Act*. 2012;9:78.

97. Thatcher J, Day M, Rahman R. *Sport and Exercise Psychology*. Exeter (United Kingdom): Sage Learning Matters Ltd; 2011. 240 p.

98. Thøgersen-Ntoumani C, Ntoumanis N. The role of self-determined motivation in the understanding of exercise-related behaviours, cognitions and physical self-evaluations. *J Sports Sci*. 2006;24(4):393–404.

99. Tucker JM, Welk GJ, Beyler NK. Physical activity in US adults: compliance with the Physical Activity Guidelines for Americans. *Am J Prev Med*. 2011;40(4):454–61.

100. Tudor-Locke C, Brashear MM, Johnson WD, Katzmarzyk PT. Accelerometer profiles of physical activity and inactivity in normal weight, overweight, and obese U.S. men and women. *Int J Behav Nutr Phys Act*. 2010;7:60.

101. Vallance JK, Courneya KS, Plotnikoff RC, Mackey JR. Analyzing theoretical mechanisms of physical activity behavior change in breast cancer survivors: results from the activity promotion (ACTION) trial. *Ann Behav Med*. 2008;35(2):150–8.

102. Vallance JK, Lavallee C, Culos-Reed NS, Trudeau MG. Predictors of physical activity among rural and small town breast cancer survivors: an application of the theory of planned behavior. *Psychol Health Med*. 2012;17(6):685–97.

103. Weiss RS. The provisions of social relationships. In: Rubin Z, editor. *Doing unto Others*. Englewood Cliffs (NJ): Prentice Hall; 1974. p. 17–26.

104. Wilcox S, Der Ananian C, Abbott J, et al. Perceived exercise barriers, enablers, and benefits among exercising and nonexercising adults with arthritis: results from a qualitative study. *Arthritis Rheum*. 2006;55(4):616–27.

105. Williams DM, Anderson ES, Winett RA. A review of the outcome expectancy construct in physical activity research. *Ann Behav Med*. 2005;29(1):70–9.

106. Winett RA, Williams DM, Davy BM. Initiating and maintaining resistance training in older adults: a social cognitive theory-based approach. *Br J Sports Med*. 2009;43(2):114–9.

Common
Medications

LIST OF COMMON MEDICATIONS

The first section of *Appendix A* is a listing of common medications that exercise and health care professionals are likely to encounter among their clients/patients that are soon to be, or are, physically active. This section includes the name of each drug, the brand name(s), and indications for drug use. This listing is not intended to be exhaustive nor all-inclusive and is not designed for the determination of pharmacotherapy/medication prescription for patients by clinicians/physicians. Rather, this listing should be viewed as a resource to further clarify the medical histories of research study participants, patients, and clients encountered by exercise professionals nationally and internationally. To this end, some brand names, although recently discontinued (*i.e.*, generic formulations only available) or no longer marketed in the United States, are included for reference. For a more detailed informational listing, the reader is referred to the American Hospital Formulary Service (AHFS) Drug Information (2) or the U.S. Food and Drug Administration, U.S. Department of Health and Human Services Web site from which the following listings were obtained.

Cardiovascular

β-Blockers

Indications: hypertension (HTN), angina, arrhythmias including supraventricular tachycardia, atrial fibrillation rate control, acute myocardial infarction (MI), migraine headaches, anxiety, essential tremor, and heart failure (HF) because of systolic dysfunction

Cardioselective		Noncardioselective	
Drug Name	Brand Name	Drug Name	Brand Name
Acebutolol[a]	Sectral	Carvedilol[b]	Coreg, Coreg CR
Atenolol	Tenormin	Labetalol[b]	Trandate
Betaxolol	Kerlone	Nadolol	Corgard
Bisoprolol	Zebeta	Pindolol[a]	Visken
Esmolol	Brevibloc	Propranolol	Inderal, Inderal LA
Metoprolol succinate	Toprol XL	Sotalol	Betapace
Metoprolol tartrate	Lopressor, Lopressor SR	Timolol	Blocadren
Nebivolol	Bystolic		

[a]β-Blockers with intrinsic sympathomimetic activity.
[b]Combined α- and β-blocker.

Angiotensin-Converting Enzyme Inhibitors (ACE-I)

Indications: HTN, coronary artery disease, HF caused by systolic dysfunction, diabetes nephropathy, chronic kidney disease, and cerebrovascular disease

Drug Name	Brand Name	Combination ACE-I + HCTZ[a]	ACE-I + CCB[b]
Benazepril	Lotensin	Lotensin HCT	Lotrel (+ amlodipine)
Captopril	Capoten	Capozide	
Enalapril	Vasotec	Vaseretic	Lexxel (+ felodipine)
Fosinopril	Monopril	Monopril HCT	
Lisinopril	Zestril, Prinivil	Prinzide, Zestoretic	
Moexipril	Univasc	Uniretic	
Perindopril	Aceon		Prestalia (+ amlodipine)
Quinapril	Accupril	Accuretic	
Ramipril	Altace		
Trandolapril	Mavik		Tarka (+ verapamil)

[a]HCTZ, hydrochlorothiazide, a thiazide diuretic.
[b]CCB, calcium channel blocker.

Angiotensin II Receptor Blockers (ARBs)

Indications: HTN, diabetic nephropathy, and HF

Drug Name	Brand Name	Combination ARB + Diuretic (HCTZ[a] or Chlorthalidone[b])	Combination ARB + HCTZ + CCB[c]	Combination ARB + CCB[d]
Azilsartan	Edarbi	Edarbyclor[b]		
Candesartan	Atacand	Atacand HCT[a]		
Eprosartan	Teveten	Teveten HCT[a]		
Irbesartan	Avapro	Avalide[a]		
Losartan	Cozaar	Hyzaar[a]		
Olmesartan	Benicar	Benicar HCT[a]	Tribenzor	Azor
Telmisartan	Micardis	Micardis HCT[a]		Twynsta
Valsartan	Diovan	Diovan HCT[a]	Exforge HCT	Exforge

[a]ARB + HCTZ for use in HTN and HF.
[b]ARB + chlorthalidone for use in HTN.
[c]ARB + HCTZ + CCB for use in HTN.
[d]ARB + CCB for use in HTN.

Direct Renin Inhibitor (DRI)

Indications: HTN

Drug Name	Brand Name	Combination DRI + HCTZ[a]
Aliskiren	Tekturna	Tekturna HCT

[a]DRI + HCTZ for use in HTN.

Calcium Channel Blockers (CCBs)

Dihydropyridines

Indications: HTN, isolated systolic HTN, angina pectoris, vasospastic angina, and ischemic heart disease

Drug Name	Brand Name
Amlodipine	Norvasc
Clevidipine (IV formulation only)	Cleviprex
Felodipine	Plendil
Isradipine	DynaCirc, DynaCirc CR
Nicardipine	Cardene, Cardene SR
Nifedipine	Adalat CC[a], Afeditab CR[a], Procardia[b], Procardia XL[a]
Nimodipine	Nymalize
Nisoldipine	Sular

[a]Long-acting.
[b]Short-acting.

Nondihydropyridines

Indications: angina, HTN, paroxysmal supraventricular tachycardia, and arrhythmia

Drug Name	Brand Name
Diltiazem	Cardizem
Diltiazem, extended-release	Cardizem CD or LA, Cartia XT, Dilt CD or XR, Diltia XT, Diltzac, Taztia XT, Tiazac
Verapamil	Calan, Verelan, Covera HS, Isoptin
Verapamil, controlled- and extended-release	Calan SR, Covera-HS, Verelan, Verelan PM
Verapamil + trandolapril	Tarka

Diuretics

Indications: edema, HTN, HF, and certain kidney disorders

Drug Name	Brand Name	Combined with HCTZ
Thiazides		
Bendroflumethiazide	(+ Nadolol) Corzide	
Chlorothiazide	Diuril	
Hydrochlorothiazide (HCTZ)	Microzide, Oretic	
Methyclothiazide	None	
Polythiazide	Renese	
Thiazide-like		
Chlorthalidone	Thalitone; (+ atenolol) Tenoretic	
Indapamide	Lozol	
Metolazone	Zaroxolyn	
Loop Diuretics		
Bumetanide	Bumex	
Ethacrynic acid	Edecrin	
Furosemide	Lasix	
Torsemide	Demadex	
Potassium-Sparing Diuretics		**Combined with HCTZ**
Amiloride	Midamor	Moduretic, Hydro-ride
Triamterene	Dyrenium	Dyazide, Maxzide
Mineralocorticoid (Aldosterone) Receptor Blockers		**Combined with HCTZ**
Eplerenone	Inspra	
Spironolactone	Aldactone	Aldactazide

Vasodilating Agents

Nitrates and Nitrites

Indications: angina, acute MI, HF, low cardiac output syndromes, and HTN

Drug Name	Brand Name
Amyl nitrite (inhaled)	Amyl Nitrite
Isosorbide mononitrate	Monoket
Isosorbide dinitrate	Dilatrate SR, Isordil
Isosorbide dinitrate + hydralazine HCl	BiDil
Nitric oxide (inhaled)	INOmax
Nitroglycerin capsules ER	Nitro-Time, Nitroglycerin Slocaps
Nitroglycerin lingual (spray)	Nitrolingual Pumpspray, NitroMist
Nitroglycerin sublingual	Nitrostat
Nitroglycerin topical ointment	Nitro-Bid
Nitroglycerin transdermal	Minitran, Nitro-Dur, Nitrek, Deponit
Nitroglycerin transmucosal (buccal)	Nitrogard

α-Blockers

Indications: HTN and benign prostatic hyperplasia

Drug Name	Brand Name
Doxazosin	Cardura, Cardura XL
Prazosin	Minipress
Tamsulosin	Flomax
Terazosin	Hytrin

Central α-Agonists

Indication: HTN

Drug Name	Brand Name
Clonidine	Catapres, Catapres-TTS (patch), Duraclon (injection form), Kapvay
Guanabenz	Wytensin
Guanfacine	Intuniv, Tenex
Methyldopa	Aldoril

Direct Vasodilators

Indications: HTN, hair loss, and HF

Drug Name	Brand Name
Hydralazine	(+ HCTZ) Hydra-Zide; (+ isosorbide dinitrate) BiDil
Minoxidil	Loniten
	Topical: Rogaine, Theroxidil
Sodium nitroprusside	Nipride, Nitropress

Peripheral Adrenergic Inhibitors

Indications: HTN and psychotic disorder

Drug Name	Brand Name
Reserpine	Raudixin, Serpalan, Serpasil

Others

Cardiac Glycosides

Indications: acute, decompensated HF in the setting of dilated cardiomyopathy and need to increase atrioventricular (AV) block to slow ventricular response with atrial fibrillation

Drug Name	Brand Name
Amrinone (inamrinone)	Inocor
Digoxin	Lanoxin, Lanoxicaps, Digitek
Milrinone	Primacor

Cardiotonic Agent

Indications: symptomatic management of stable angina pectoris in HF; specifically for heart rate reduction in patients with systolic dysfunction when in sinus rhythm with a resting heart rate ≥ 70 beats $\cdot$ min^{-1} and currently prescribed either with a maximally tolerated dose of β-blockers or with a contraindication to β-blocker use

Drug Name	Brand Name
Ivabradine	Corlanor, Procoralan

Antiarrhythmic Agents

Indications: specific for individual drugs but generally includes suppression of atrial fibrillation and maintenance of normal sinus rhythm, serious ventricular arrhythmias in certain clinical settings, and increase in AV nodal block to slow ventricular response in atrial fibrillation

Drug Name	Brand Name
Class I	
IA	
Disopyramide	Norpace (CR)
Procainamide	Procanbid
Quinidine	Quinora, Quinidex, Quinaglute, Quinalan, Cardioquin
IB	
Lidocaine	Xylocaine
Mexiletine	Mexitil
Phenytoin	Dilantin, Phenytek
IC	
Flecainide	Tambocor
Propafenone	Rythmol (SR)
Class II	
β-Blockers	
Atenolol	Tenormin
Bisoprolol	Zebeta
Esmolol	Brevibloc
Metoprolol	Lopressor, Lopressor SR, Toprol XL
Propranolol	Inderal, Inderal LA
Timolol	Blocadren
Class III	
Amiodarone	Cordarone, Nexterone (IV), Pacerone
Dofetilide	Tikosyn
Dronedarone	Multaq
Ibutilide	Corvert (IV)
Sotalol	Betapace, Betapace AF, Sorine
Class IV	
Diltiazem	Cardizem CD or LA, Cartia XT, Dilacor XR, Dilt CD or XR, Diltia XT, Diltzac, Tiazac, Taztia XT
Verapamil	Calan, Calan SR, Covera-HS, Verelan, Verelan PM

Antianginal Agents

Indications: adjunctive therapy in the management of chronic stable angina pectoris; may be used in combination with β-blockers, CCBs, nitrates, ACE-I, ARBs, and/or lipid-lowering therapy

Drug Name	Brand Name
Ranolazine	Ranexa

Antilipemic Agents

Indications: elevated total blood cholesterol, low-density lipoproteins (LDL), and triglycerides; low high-density lipoproteins (HDL); and metabolic syndrome

Drug Name	Brand Name
Bile Acid Sequestrants	
Cholestyramine	Prevalite
Colesevelam	Welchol
Colestipol	Colestid
Fibric Acid Sequestrants	
Fenofibrate	Antara, Fenoglide, Lipofen, Lofibra, Tricor, Triglide, Trilipix
Gemfibrozil	Lopid
HMG-CoA Reductase Inhibitors (Statins)	
Atorvastatin	Lipitor
Fluvastatin	Lescol (XL)
Lovastatin	Mevacor, Altoprev
Lovastatin + niacin	Advicor
Pitavastatin	Livalo
Pravastatin	Pravachol
Rosuvastatin	Crestor
Simvastatin	Zocor
Simvastatin + niacin	Simcor
Statin + CCB	
Atorvastatin + amlodipine	Caduet
Nicotinic Acid	
Niacin (vitamin B_3)	Niaspan, Nicobid, Slo-Niacin
Omega-3 Fatty Acid Ethyl Esters	
Omega-3-carboxylic acids (EPA and DHA)	Epanova
Icosapent ethyl (EPA)	Vascepa
Omega-3 fatty acid ethyl esters (EPA and DHA)	Lovaza
Cholesterol Absorption Inhibitor	
Ezetimibe	Zetia; (+ simvastatin) Vytorin

DHA, docosahexaenoic acid; EPA, eicosapentaenoic acid ; HMG-CoA, 3-hydroxy-3-methylglutaryl-coenzyme A.

Blood Modifiers

Anticoagulants

Indications: treatment and prophylaxis of thromboembolic disorders; to prevent blood clots, heart attack, stroke, and intermittent claudication or vascular death in patients with established nonvalvular atrial fibrillation, deep venous thrombosis, pulmonary embolism, heparin-induced thrombocytopenia, peripheral arterial disease, or acute ST-segment elevation with MI

Drug Name	Brand Name
Apixaban (selective inhibitor of factor Xa)	Eliquis
Argatroban (direct thrombin inhibitor)	Acova
Bivalirudin (direct thrombin inhibitor)	Angiomax
Dabigatran (direct thrombin inhibitor)	Pradaxa
Edoxaban (selective inhibitor of factor Xa)	Savaysa
Dalteparin (LMWH)	Fragmin
Enoxaparin (LMWH)	Lovenox
Fondaparinux (LMWH)	Arixtra
Rivaroxaban (selective inhibitor of factor Xa)	Xarelto
Warfarin (vitamin K antagonist)	Coumadin, Jantoven

factor Xa, serine endopeptidase also known as prothrombinase, thrombokinase, or thromboplastin; LMWH, low-molecular-weight heparin.

Antiplatelet Agents

Indications: Antiplatelet drugs reduce platelet aggregation and are used to prevent further thromboembolic events in patients who have suffered MI, ischemic stroke, transient ischemic attacks, or unstable angina and for primary prevention for patients at risk for a thromboembolic event. Some are also used for the prevention of reocclusion or restenosis following percutaneous coronary interventions and bypass procedures.

Drug Name	Brand Name
Aspirin (COX inhibitor)	None
Cilostazol (PDE inhibitor)	Pletal
Clopidogrel (ADP-R inhibitor)	Plavix
Dipyridamole (adenosine reuptake inhibitor)	Persantine; (+ aspirin) Aggrenox
Pentoxifylline	Trental
Prasugrel (ADP-R inhibitor)	Effient
Ticagrelor (ADP-R inhibitor)	Brilinta
Ticlopidine (ADP-R inhibitor)	Ticlid
Vorapaxar	Zontivity

ADP-R, adenosine diphosphate-ribose; COX, cyclooxygenase inhibitor; PDE, phosphodiesterase.

Respiratory

Inhaled Corticosteroids

Indications: asthma, nasal polyp, and rhinitis

Drug Name	Brand Name
Beclomethasone	Beclovent, Qvar, Vanceril
Budesonide	Pulmicort
Ciclesonide	Alvesco
Flunisolide	AeroBid
Fluticasone	Flovent
Mometasone furoate	Asmanex
Triamcinolone	Azmacort

Bronchodilators

Anticholinergics (Acetylcholine Receptor Antagonist)

Indications: Anticholinergic or antimuscarinic medications are used for the management of obstructive pulmonary disease and acute asthma exacerbations. They prevent wheezing, shortness of breath, and troubled breathing caused by asthma, chronic bronchitis, emphysema, and other lung diseases.

Drug Name	Brand Name	Combined with Sympathomimetic (β_2-Receptor Agonists)
Glycopyrrolate	Robinul	
Ipratropium	Atrovent	(+ Albuterol) Combivent
Tiotropium	Spiriva	

Sympathomimetics (β2-Receptor Agonists)

Indications: Relief of asthma symptoms and in the management of chronic obstructive pulmonary disease. They prevent wheezing, shortness of breath, and trouble breathing caused by asthma, chronic bronchitis, emphysema, and other lung diseases.

Drug Name	Brand Name	Combined with Steroid
Albuterol	ProAir, Proventil, Ventolin	
Formoterol (LA)	Foradil	(+ Budesonide) Symbicort (+ mometasone) Dulera
Indacaterol	Arcapta	
Levalbuterol	Xopenex	
Metaproterenol	Alupent, Metaprel	
Pirbuterol	Maxair	
Salmeterol (LA)	Serevent	(+ Fluticasone) Advair
Terbutaline	Brethine, Brethaire, Bricanyl	

Xanthine Derivatives

Indications: combination therapy in asthma and chronic obstructive pulmonary disease

Drug Name	Brand Name
Aminophylline	Phyllocontin, Truphylline
Caffeine	None
Theophylline	Theo-24, Uniphyl

Leukotriene Inhibitors and Antagonists

Indications: asthma, exercise-induced asthma, and rhinitis

Drug Name	Brand Name
Montelukast	Singulair
Zafirlukast	Accolate
Zileuton	Zyflo (CR)

Mast Cell Stabilizers

Indications: to prevent wheezing, shortness of breath, and troubled breathing caused by asthma, chronic bronchitis, emphysema, and other lung diseases

Drug Name	Brand Name
Cromolyn (inhaled)	Intal

Cough/Cold Products

Antihistamines

First Generation

Indications: allergy, anaphylaxis (adjunctive), insomnia, motion sickness, pruritus of skin, rhinitis, sedation, and urticaria (hives)

Drug Name	Brand Name
Brompheniramine (Brompheniramine maleate)	Lodrane, Bidhist; combinations available with pseudoephedrine and phenylephrine
Carbinoxamine (Carbinoxamine maleate)	Arbinoxa, Palgic
Chlorpheniramine	Aller-Chlor, Chlor-Trimeton; combinations available with pseudoephedrine and phenylephrine
Clemastine	Dayhist, Tavist
Cyproheptadine	Periactin
Diphenhydramine	Benadryl, Nytol; combinations available with acetaminophen (APAP), pseudoephedrine, and phenylephrine
Doxylamine	Aldex, Unisom SleepTabs, GoodSense Sleep Aid
Promethazine	Phenergan; Promethazine VC Syrup (with pseudoephedrine)
Triprolidine	Zymine, Zymine-D (with pseudoephedrine), Allerfrim (with pseudoephedrine), Aprodine (with pseudoephedrine)

Second Generation

Indications: allergic rhinitis and urticaria (hives)

Drug Name	Brand Name
Acrivastine	Semprex-D (with pseudoephedrine)
Cetirizine	Zyrtec, Zyrtec-D (with pseudoephedrine)
Desloratadine	Clarinex, Clarinex-D (with pseudoephedrine)
Fexofenadine	Allegra, Allegra-D (with pseudoephedrine)
Levocetirizine	Xyzal
Loratadine	Claritin, Claritin-D (with pseudoephedrine), Alavert, Alavert-D (with pseudoephedrine)

Sympathomimetic/Adrenergic Agonists

Indications: allergic rhinitis and nasal congestion

Drug Name	Brand Name
Phenylephrine	Sudafed PE
Pseudoephedrine	Sudafed; many combinations

Expectorant

Indication: abnormal sputum (thin secretions/mucus)

Drug Name	Brand Name
Guaifenesin	Robitussin, Guiatuss, Mucinex (many combinations), DayQuil Mucus Control

Antitussives

Indications: cough and pain

Drug Name	Brand Name
Benzonatate	Tessalon
Codeine	Codeine; many combinations
Dextromethorphan	Robitussin CoughGels, Robitussin Pediatric Cough Suppressant; many combinations
Hydrocodone	Many combinations

Hormonal

Human Growth Hormone

Indications: cachexia associated with acquired immunodeficiency syndrome (AIDS), growth hormone deficiency, and short bowel syndrome

Drug Name	Brand Name
Somatropin	Genotropin, Norditropin, Nutropin, Humatrope, Omnitrope
Mecasermin (IV)	Increlex
Tesamorelin (IV)	Egrifta

Adrenals — Corticosteroids

Indications: adrenocortical insufficiency, adrenogenital syndrome, hypercalcemia, thyroiditis, rheumatic disorders, collagen diseases, dermatologic diseases, allergic conditions, ocular disorders, respiratory diseases (*e.g.*, asthma, chronic obstructive pulmonary disorders), hematologic disorders, gastrointestinal diseases (*e.g.*, ulcerative colitis, Crohn disease), and liver disease among others

Drug Name	Brand Name
Beclomethasone	QVAR, Beclovent
Betamethasone	Celestone, Celestone Soluspan (injectable)
Budesonide	Entocort EC, Pulmicort
Ciclesonide	Alvesco
Cortisone	Cortisone
Dexamethasone	Decadron
Fludrocortisone	Florinef
Flunisolide	Aerospan, Nasalide, Nasarel
Fluticasone	Flovent; with salmeterol: Advair
Hydrocortisone	Cortef, Hydrocortone
Methylprednisolone	Medrol, Meprolone, Solu-Medrol, Depo-Medrol, A-Methapred
Mometasone	Asmanex
Prednisolone	Orapred, Orapred ODT, Prelone, Pediapred
Prednisone	Sterapred, Prednisone Intensol
Triamcinolone	Aristospan, Aristocort, Kenalog, Azmacort

Androgenic-Anabolic

Indications: hypogonadism in males, catabolic and wasting disorders, endometriosis, hereditary angioedema, fibrocystic breast disease, and precocious puberty

Drug Name	Brand Name
Danazol	Danocrine
Fluoxymesterone	Halotestin, Androxy
Methyltestosterone	Android, Testred, Virilon
Oxandrolone	Oxandrin
Testosterone	Striant, AndroGel, Androderm, Natesto, Testim, Delatestryl (injectable)

Estrogens

Indications: menopause and perimenopause in women, osteoporosis, moderate to severe vasomotor symptoms, corticosteroid-induced hypogonadism, metastatic breast carcinoma, prostate carcinoma, Alzheimer disease

Drug Name	Brand Name	Combinations
Estradiol	Elestrin, EstroGel, Evamist, Menostar, Alora, Climara, Vivelle, Vivelle-Dot, Estraderm, Estrace, Estrasorb	(+ Norgestimate) Prefest; (+ norethindrone acetate) Activella; (+ drospirenone) Angeliq
Estradiol (acetate)	Femtrace	
Estradiol (cypionate)	Depo-Estradiol	(+ Testosterone) Depo-Testadiol
Estradiol (valerate)	Delestrogen	
Estradiol (ethinyl)		(+ Norethindrone) Femhrt
Estrogens (conjugated)	Premarin, Cenestin (synthetic), Enjuvia (synthetic)	(+ Medroxyprogesterone) Prempro, Premphase
Estrogens (esterified)	Ogen, Ortho-Est, Menest	(+ Methyltestosterone) Covaryx

Contraceptives

Drug Name	Brand Name
Estrogen–progestin combinations	Oral: Beyaz, Yaz, Alesse, Lybrel, Lessina, Aviane, LoSeasonique, Loestrin, Yasmin, Microgestin, Sprintec, Ortho-Cyclen, Ortho Tri-Cyclen
Transdermal	Ortho Evra
Vaginal ring	NuvaRing
Intrauterine	Mirena
Progestins: etonogestrel	Parenteral implant: Implanon, Nexplanon
Progestins: levonorgestrel	Oral: Next Choice, Plan B One-Step
Progestins: norethindrone	Oral: Micronor, Nor-QD

Thyroid Agents

Indications: hypothyroidism and pituitary thyroid-stimulating hormone suppression

Drug Name	Brand Name
Levothyroxine	Levothroid, Synthroid, Levoxyl, Unithroid
Liothyronine	Cytomel
Liotrix	Thyrolar
Thyroid	Armour

Antidiabetic

Indication: management of Type 2 diabetes mellitus

Class: α-Glucosidase Inhibitors (Slow Absorption of Carbohydrates in the Gastrointestinal Tract)

Drug Name	Brand Name
Acarbose	Precose
Miglitol	Glyset

Class: Amylin Analogue (Mimics Amylin, a Hormone Secreted with Insulin to Inhibit Glucose, for Postprandial Glycemic Control)

Drug Name	Brand Name
Pramlintide	Symlin

Class: Biguanides (Decrease Sugar Production by Liver and Decreases Insulin Resistance)

Drug Name	Brand Name	Combination
Metformin	Glucophage, Fortamet, Glumetza	(+ Glipizide) Metaglip; (+ glyburide) Glucovance

Class: Sodium-Glucose Co-Transporter 2 (SGLT2) Inhibitor

Drug Name	Brand Name	Combination
Canagliflozin	Invokana	(+ Metformin) Invokamet
Dapagliflozin	Farxiga	(+ Metformin) Xigduo XR
Empagliflozin	Jardiance	

Class: Dipeptidylpeptidase-4 Inhibitors (Enhance Insulin Release by Preventing Breakdown of Glucagon-like Peptide 1 [GLP-1] that is a Potent Antihyperglycemic Hormone)

Drug Name	Brand Name	Combination
Alogliptin	Nesina	(+ Metformin) Kazano; (+ pioglitazone) Oseni
Linagliptin	Tradjenta	
Saxagliptin	Onglyza	(+ Metformin) Kombiglyze
Sitagliptin	Januvia	(+ Metformin) Janumet

Class: Glucagon-like Peptide 1 Receptor Agonists (Activate GLP-1 that is a Potent Antihyperglycemic Hormone that Stimulates Insulin Release)

Drug Name	Brand Name
Exenatide	Byetta
Liraglutide	Victoza

Class: Meglitinides (Short-Acting Stimulation of β Cells to Produce More Insulin)

Drug Name	Brand Name	Combination
Nateglinide	Starlix	
Repaglinide	Prandin	(+ Metformin) PrandiMet

Class: Sulfonylureas (Stimulate β Cells to Produce More Insulin)

Drug Name	Brand Name	Combination
Chlorpropamide — first generation	Diabinese	
Glimepiride	Amaryl	(+ Pioglitazone) Duetact; (+ rosiglitazone) Avandaryl
Glipizide	Glucotrol	(+ Metformin) Metaglip
Glyburide	DiaBeta, Glynase, Micronase	(+ Metformin) Glucovance
Tolazamide — first generation	Tolinase	
Tolbutamide — first generation	Orinase	

Class: Thiazolidinediones (Improve Sensitivity of Insulin Receptors in Muscle, Liver, and Fat Cells)

Drug Name	Brand Name	Combination
Pioglitazone	Actos	(+ Metformin) Actoplus Met (XR); (+ glimepiride) Duetac
Rosiglitazone	Avandia	(+ Metformin) Avandamet; (+ glimepiride) Avandaryl

Class: Insulin

Rapid-Acting	Intermediate-Acting	Intermediate- and Rapid-Acting Combination	Long-Acting
Humalog	Humulin L	Humalog Mix	Humulin U
Humulin R	Humulin N	Humalog 50/50	Lantus injection
NovoLog	Novolin L	Humalog 75/25	Levemir
Novolin R	Novolin N	Novolin 70/30	
Iletin II R		NovoLog 70/30	
Apidra			

Central Nervous System

Antidepressants

Indication: depression

Drug Name	Brand Name
Amitriptyline (TCA)	Elavil; (+ chlordiazepoxide) Limbitrol, Limbitrol DS
Amoxapine (TCA)	Asendin
Bupropion	Wellbutrin (SR and XL), Zyban
Citalopram (SSRI)	Celexa
Clomipramine (TCA)	Anafranil
Desipramine (TCA)	Norpramin
Desvenlafaxine (SNRI)	Pristiq
Doxepin (TCA)	Adapin, Sinequan
Duloxetine (SNRI)	Cymbalta
Escitalopram (SSRI)	Lexapro
Fluoxetine (SSRI)	Prozac, Sarafem; (+ olanzapine) Symbyax
Fluvoxamine (SSRI)	Luvox (CR)
Imipramine (TCA)	Tofranil, Tofranil-PM
Isocarboxazid (MAO-I)	Marplan
Levomilnacipran (SNRI)	Fetzima
Maprotiline (TeCA)	Ludiomil
Milnacipran (SNRI)	Savella
Mirtazapine (TeCA)	Remeron
Nefazodone	Serzone (brand d/c 2004)
Nortriptyline (TCA)	Pamelor
Paroxetine (SSRI)	Paxil (CR), Pexeva
Phenelzine (MAO-I)	Nardil
Protriptyline (TCA)	Vivactil
Selegiline (MAO-I)	Emsam
Sertraline (SSRI)	Zoloft
Tranylcypromine (MAO-I)	Parnate
Trazodone (SARI)	Desyrel Dividose, Oleptro
Trimipramine (TCA)	Surmontil
Venlafaxine (SNRI)	Effexor (XR)
Vilazodone (SARI)	Viibryd

MAO-I, monoamine oxidase inhibitor; SARI, serotonin antagonist reuptake inhibitor; SNRI, serotonin-norepinephrine reuptake inhibitor; SSRI, selective serotonin reuptake inhibitor; TCA, tricyclic antidepressant; TeCA, tetracyclic antidepressant.

Antipsychotics

Indications: behavioral syndrome, bipolar disorder, Gilles de la Tourette syndrome, hyperactive behavior, psychotic disorder, and schizophrenia

Drug Name	Brand Name
Aripiprazole (atypical)	Abilify
Asenapine (atypical)	Saphris
Chlorpromazine (typical)	Thorazine
Clozapine (atypical)	Clozaril, FazaClo
Fluphenazine (typical)	Permitil, Prolixin
Haloperidol (typical)	Haldol
Iloperidone (atypical)	Fanapt
Lithium	Eskalith (CR), Lithobid
Loxapine (typical)	Adasuve, Loxitane
Lurasidone (atypical)	Latuda
Mesoridazine (phenothiazine)	Serentil
Molindone (typical)	Moban
Olanzapine (atypical)	Zyprexa; (+ fluoxetine) Symbyax
Paliperidone (atypical)	Invega
Perphenazine (typical)	Perphenazine, Trilafon
Prochlorperazine (typical)	Compazine
Pimozide	Orap
Promazine	Sparine
Quetiapine (atypical)	Seroquel
Risperidone (atypical)	Risperdal
Thioridazine (typical)	Mellaril
Thiothixene (typical)	Navane
Triflupromazine	Vesprin
Valproic acid	Depakote (ER), Depakene
Ziprasidone (atypical)	Geodon

Antianxiety

Indications: anxiety and panic disorder

Drug Name	Brand Name
Alprazolam	Xanax (XR), Niravam
Buspirone	Buspar
Chlordiazepoxide	Limbitrol (DS), Librium; (+ clidinium) Librax
Clonazepam	Klonopin
Clorazepate	Tranxene
Diazepam	Valium
Lorazepam	Ativan
Meprobamate	Equanil, Miltown, Meprospan
Oxazepam	Serax

Sedative-Hypnotics

Indications: general anesthesia, insomnia, and sedation

Drug Name	Brand Name
Amobarbital	Amytal
Butabarbital	Butisol
Chloral hydrate	Somnote, Aquachloral Supprettes
Dexmedetomidine	Precedex
Estazolam	ProSom
Eszopiclone	Lunesta
Flurazepam	Dalmane
Fospropofol	Lusedra
Mephobarbital	Mebaral
Promethazine	Phenergan, Phenadoz, Prometh
Propofol	Diprivan
Quazepam	Doral, Dormalin
Ramelteon	Rozerem
Secobarbital	Seconal
Temazepam	Restoril
Triazolam	Halcion
Zaleplon	Sonata
Zolpidem	Ambien (CR), Intermezzo, Edluar

Stimulants

Indications: attention deficit hyperactivity disorder, narcolepsy, obstructive sleep apnea, and shift work sleep disorder

Drug Name	Brand Name
Amphetamine salts	Adderall (XR)
Armodafinil	Nuvigil
Caffeine	NoDoz, Vivarin
Dexmethylphenidate	Focalin (XR)
Dextroamphetamine	Dexedrine, Dextrostat
Lisdexamfetamine	Vyvanse
Methamphetamine	Desoxyn
Methylphenidate	Concerta, Metadate (CD or ER), Ritalin (LA, SR), Methylin (ER)
Modafinil	Provigil

Nicotine Replacement Therapy

Indication: smoking cessation assistance

Drug Name	Brand Name
Nicotine	Solution: Nicotrol NS
	Inhalant: Nicotrol Inhaler
	Transdermal: Nicotrol Step 1, 2, 3; NicoDerm CQ Step 1, 2, 3
Nicotine polacrilex	Lozenges: Commit
	Chewing gum: Nicorette, Nicorette DS

Nonsteroidal Anti-inflammatory Drugs (NSAIDs)

Indications: fever, headache, juvenile rheumatoid arthritis, migraine, osteoarthritis, pain, primary dysmenorrhea, and rheumatoid arthritis

Drug Name	Brand Name
Celecoxib	Celebrex
Diclofenac	Arthrotec, Cataflam, Voltaren
Diflunisal	Dolobid
Etodolac	Lodine
Fenoprofen	Nalfon
Flurbiprofen	Ansaid
Ibuprofen	Advil, Ibu-Tab, Menadol, Midol, Motrin, Nuprin, Genpril, Haltran
Indomethacin	Indocin
Ketoprofen	Actron, Orudis, Oruvail
Ketorolac	Toradol
Meclofenamate	Meclomen
Mefenamic acid	Ponstel
Meloxicam	Mobic
Nabumetone	Relafen
Naproxen	Aleve, Anaprox, Naprelan, Naprosyn
Oxaprozin	Daypro, Daypro Alta
Piroxicam	Feldene
Sulindac	Clinoril
Tolmetin	Tolectin

Opioids
Opiate Agonists

Indications: pain, chronic nonmalignant pain, MI, delirium, acute pulmonary edema, preoperative sedation, cough, and opiate dependence

Drug Name	Brand Name
Codeine	Codeine; (+ acetaminophen [APAP], pseudoephedrine, and phenylephrine Tylenol with Codeine no. 3 and no. 4
Fentanyl	Actiq, Fentora; Duragesic (topical)
Hydrocodone	(+ APAP) Bancap HC, Ceta-Plus, Lorcet, Hydrocet, Lortab, Vicodin, Anexsia Co-Gesic, Zydone; (+ ibuprofen) Vicoprofen, Reprexain
Hydromorphone	Dilaudid, Exalgo
Levorphanol	Levo-Dromoran
Meperidine	Demerol
Methadone	Dolophine, Intensol, Methadose
Morphine	Avinza, MS Contin, Oramorph SR, Kadian
Opium	None
Oxycodone	OxyIR, OxyContin, Endocodone, Percolone, Roxicodone; (+ APAP) Percocet Tylox, Endocet, Roxicet; (+ aspirin [ASA]) Percodan, Endodan, Roxiprin
Oxymorphone	Opana (ER)
Remifentanil	Ultiva (IV)
Sufentanil	Sufenta (IV)
Tapentadol	Nucynta
Tramadol	Ultram (ER); (+ APAP) Ultracet

Opiate Partial Agonists (Pain and Opiate Dependence)

Indications: general anesthesia (adjunctive) and pain

Drug Name	Brand Name
Buprenorphine	Butrans (topical), Suboxone (sublingual strip), Subutex (sublingual tablet), Buprenex (injectable)
Butorphanol	Stadol (injectable), Stadol NS (nasal spray)
Nalbuphine	Nubain (injectable)
Pentazocine	(+ Naloxone) Talwin Nx; (+ acetaminophen) Talacen; Talwin (injectable)

Analgesics and Antipyretics

Indications: dysmenorrhea, fever, headache, and pain

Drug Name	Brand Name
Acetaminophen	Tylenol, many combinations

Unclassified

Antigout

Indication: to treat or prevent gout or treat hyperuricemia (excess uric acid in the blood)

Drug Name	Brand Name
Allopurinol	Zyloprim
Colchicine	Colcrys
Febuxostat	Uloric
Probenecid	(+ Colchicine) Col-Probenecid
Sulfinpyrazone	Anturane

THE EFFECT OF COMMON MEDICATIONS ON THE RESPONSE TO EXERCISE

The second section of *Appendix A* contains *Table A.1* that lists the common medications with available published data regarding their influence on the response to exercise, specifically hemodynamics; the electrocardiogram (ECG); and exercise capacity. Exercise data are presented by drug category and then by specific drug when information is available. The influence of common medications during rest and/or exercise is presented with the directional relationships when specified in the literature. *Exercise capacity* is a generic term that often was used and not defined by a specific measure in the literature. In instances in which measures of exercise capacity were reported, they are listed, that is, maximal volume of oxygen consumed per unit time ($\dot{V}O_{2max}$), endurance, performance, and tolerance, often times with no clear distinctions among them provided by the author.

TABLE A.1

Effects of Medications on Hemodynamics, the Electrocardiogram (ECG), and Exercise Capacity

Medications	Cardiac Output Q̇	Heart Rate (HR)	Blood Pressure (BP)	ECG Changes	Exercise Capacity
I. Cardiovascular Medications					
β-Blockers (BB)	↓ or ↔ Exercise (5)	↓ Rest and exercise ↓ Rest less by intrinsic sympathomimetic activity (ISA) + BB ↓ Exercise less by cardioselective BB (5)	↓ Rest and exercise	↓ Rest ↓ Ischemia during exercise	↓V̇O₂ₘₐₓ acute administration and ↑ chronic administration (5)
Angiotensin-converting enzyme inhibitors (ACE-I)	↔ Exercise (5)	↔ Exercise (5)	↓ Rest and exercise (5)		↔ Performance (5); ↑ tolerance patients with congestive heart failure (CHF) (7)
Captopril		↔ Exercise	↓ Rest and exercise		
Angiotensin II receptor blockers (ARBs)		↓ or ↔ Rest and exercise	↓ Rest and exercise		↔
Calcium channel blockers (CCB)					
Nondihydropyridines (non-DHP)			↓ Exercise (5)		↔ Performance and endurance; responses can be variable (5)
Diltiazem	↔ Exercise (5)	↓ Exercise patients with hypertension (5)			
Verapamil		↓ Exercise patients with hypertension (5)			

Dihydropyridine	↔ Exercise (5)	↓ Exercise (greater vs. non-DHP) (5)		↔ Performance and endurance; responses can be variable (5)
Nifedipine	↔ Exercise (5) ↓ Stroke volume (5)	↔ Exercise (5)		
II. Vasodilating Agents				
Nitrates	↑ Rest ↑ or ↔ Exercise	↓ Rest ↓ or ↔ Exercise	↑ Rest HR ↑ or ↔ Exercise HR ↓ Exercise ischemia	↑ Patients with angina (7) ↔ Patients without angina ↑ or ↔ Patients with CHF
α-Blockers	↔ Exercise (5)	↓ Exercise systolic BP (SBP) (not diastolic BP [DBP]) (5)	↓ Exercise ischemia	↔ Performance (5)
Prazosin	↔ Exercise (5)	↑ Exercise acute administration ↔ Exercise chronic administration (5)		
Doxazosin	↑ Exercise at 50% $\dot{V}O_{2max}$	↑ Exercise at 75% $\dot{V}O_{2max}$ ↔ Exercise up to 50% $\dot{V}O_{2max}$ (5)		
Central α-agonist	↔ Exercise (5)	↓ Exercise (5)		
Clonidine	↔	↓ BP regular exercisers (5) ↔ During exercise SBP		Blunts the sympathetic response to exercise; consider avoiding if exercising (5)
Guanabenz	↔ Exercise			

(continued)

TABLE A.1

Effects of Medications on Hemodynamics, the Electrocardiogram (ECG), and Exercise Capacity (Continued)

Medications	Cardiac Output Q̇	Heart Rate (HR)	Blood Pressure (BP)	ECG Changes	Exercise Capacity
III. Others					
Cardiac glycosides					
Digitalis		↓ Patients with atrial fibrillation and possibly CHF Not significantly altered in patients with sinus rhythm	↔ Rest and exercise	Rest may produce nonspecific ST-T wave changes During exercise, may produce ST-segment depression	↑ Patients with atrial fibrillation or CHF
Antiarrhythmic agents		All antiarrhythmic agents may cause new or worsened arrhythmias (i.e., proarrhythmic effect).			
Class I					
Quinidine		↑ or ↔ Rest and exercise	↓ or ↔ Rest	↑ or ↔ Rest HR Exercise may result in false negative test results.	↔
Disopyramide			↔ Exercise	Rest may prolong QRS and QT intervals.	
Procainamide		↔ Rest and exercise	↔ Rest and exercise	Rest may prolong QRS and QT intervals. Exercise may result in false positive test results.	↔

Medication				
Tocainide	↔ Rest and exercise	↔ Rest and exercise	↔ Rest and exercise	↔
Moricizine	↔ Rest and exercise	↔ Rest and exercise	Rest may prolong QRS and QT intervals. ↔ Exercise	↔
Propafenone	↓ Rest ↓ or ↔ Exercise	↔ Rest and exercise	↓ Rest HR ↓ or ↔ Exercise HR	↔
Class II				
β-Blockers (see Class I)				
Class III				
Amiodarone	↓ Rest and exercise (7)	↔ Rest ↑ Exercise	↓ Rest HR	↔ or ↑ (7)
Sotalol	↔ (7)		↔ Exercise	
Class IV				
CCB (see Class III)				
IV. Antilipemic Agents				↔ Performance (5)
V. Blood Modifiers				
Anticoagulants	↔ Rest and exercise	↔ Rest and exercise	↔ Rest and exercise	↔
Antiplatelet	↔ Rest and exercise	↔ Rest and exercise	↔ Rest and exercise	↔
VI. Respiratory Inhaled corticosteroids	↔ Rest and exercise (5)	↔ Exercise (5)	↔ Exercise (5)	↔

(continued)

TABLE A.1

Effects of Medications on Hemodynamics, the Electrocardiogram (ECG), and Exercise Capacity (Continued)

Medications	Cardiac Output Q̇	Heart Rate (HR)	Blood Pressure (BP)	ECG Changes	Exercise Capacity
Bronchodilators		↔ Rest and exercise	↔ Rest and exercise	↔ Rest and exercise	↔ V̇O$_{2max}$; ↑ or ↔ in patients with chronic obstructive pulmonary disease (COPD) (1,3,6)
Anticholinergics		↔ Rest and exercise	↔	↑ or ↔ HR	↑ or ↔ in patients with COPD (1,3,6)
Sympathomimetics (β$_2$-receptor agonists)		↔ Rest and exercise (5)	↔		↔ Performance or V̇O$_{2max}$ (5); ↑ or ↔ in patients with COPD (1,3,6)
— Albuterol		May ↑ exercise (5)			↔ Performance and V̇O$_{2max}$ (5)
Pseudoephedrine		↔ Rest and exercise May ↑ exercise (5)	↔ Exercise May ↑ exercise SBP (5)	May produce premature ventricular contractions (PVC) (5)	↔ Performance (5)
Xanthine derivatives				Rest and exercise may produce PVCs.	
— Theophylline		↑ Rest ↔ Exercise (5)			↔ Performance and V̇O$_{2max}$ (5)
— Caffeine	↔ (5)	↑ Resting ↑ or ↔ Exercise (5)	↑ Exercise (5)		↑ Endurance (5)
Mast cell stabilizers		↔ Rest and exercise	↔	↔	↔ V̇O$_{2max}$ (5)
Antihistamines		↑ Rest ↔ Exercise (5)			↔ Performance and endurance (5)

Medications	Heart Rate	Blood Pressure	ECG	Exercise Capacity
VII. Hormonal				
Human growth hormone	↔ Rest and exercise	↔	↔	↑ Performance and $\dot{V}O_{2max}$ (5)
Androgenic-anabolic	↔ or Rest and exercise (5)	↑ DBP (5)	↔	↔ or ↑ Performance and $\dot{V}O_{2max}$ (5)
Thyroid agents	↑ Rest and exercise	↑ Rest and exercise	↑ HR May provoke arrhythmias	↔ Unless angina worsens during exercise
Levothyroxine				↑ Cardiopulmonary reserve ↔ Recovery and performance (4)
VIII. Central Nervous System				
Antidepressants	↑ or ↔ Rest and exercise	↓ or ↔ Rest and exercise	Variable rest	
Antipsychotics				
— Lithium	↔ Rest and exercise	↔ Rest and exercise		
Antianxiety	↑ or ↔ Rest and exercise	↓ or ↔ Rest and exercise	Variable rest	
Stimulants	↑ (5)	↑ (5)		↑ or ↔ Endurance and performance
Nicotine replacement therapy	↑	↑		↔ or ↓
Nonsteroidal anti-inflammatory drugs (NSAIDs)				↔ or ↑ Performance dose related (5)

(continued)

TABLE A.1

Effects of Medications on Hemodynamics, the Electrocardiogram (ECG), and Exercise Capacity (Continued)

Medications	Cardiac Output Q̇	Heart Rate (HR)	Blood Pressure (BP)	ECG Changes	Exercise Capacity
Opioids					↔
Analgesics and antipyretics					↔ Performance (5)
IX. Unclassified					
Antigout		↔ Rest and exercise	↔ Rest and exercise	↔ Rest and exercise	↔
Alcohol		↔ Rest and exercise	Rest and exercise Chronic use may have role in ↑ BP. ↑ BP after acute ingestion (5)	Rest and exercise may provoke arrhythmias.	↓ Performance and V̇O$_{2max}$ (5)
Marijuana					→

, increased; ↓, decreased; ↔, not changed; V̇O$_{2max}$, maximal volume of oxygen consumed per unit time.

Table A.1 is not intended to be inclusive because that would require an evidence-based meta-analysis of the literature that is beyond the scope of the *Guidelines*. Thus, *Table A.1* serves as a reference guide for exercise and other health care professionals. It is important to note exercise may impact the pharmacokinetic (*i.e.*, what the body does to the medication) and pharmacodynamic (*i.e.*, what the medication does to the body) properties of a medication, necessitating a change in (a) dose, (b) dosing interval, (c) length of time the patient or client takes the medication, and/or (d) the exercise prescription.

The primary sources used to extract the information in *Table A.1* were *Pharmacology in Exercise and Sports* (7) and *Sport and Exercise Pharmacology* (5). In addition, a literature search by generic drug name or class and exercise response and/or capacity was performed using MEDLINE and Google Scholar on or before December 31, 2014.

ONLINE RESOURCES

The American Hospital Formulary Service Drug Information:
    http://www.ahfsdruginformation.com
U.S. Food and Drug Administration, U.S. Department of Health and Human Services:
    http://www.accessdata.fda.gov/scripts/cder/drugsatfda/index
    .cfm?fuseaction=Search.Search_Drug_Name
MICROMEDEX 2.0 (unbiased, referenced information about medications):
    http://www.micromedex.com/

REFERENCES

1. Aguilaniu B. Impact of bronchodilator therapy on exercise tolerance on COPD. *Int J Chron Obstruct Pulmon Dis*. 2010;5:57–71.
2. American Society of Health-System Pharmacists. *AHFS Drug Information 2014*. Bethesda (MD): American Society of Health-System Pharmacists; 2014. 3840 p.
3. Liesker JJ, Wijkstra PJ, Ten Hacken NH, Koëter GH, Postma DS, Kerstjens HA. A systematic review of the effects of bronchodilators on exercise capacity in patients with COPD. *Chest*. 2002;121: 597–608.
4. Mainenti MR, Teixeira PF, Oliveira FP, Vaisman M. Effect of hormone replacement on exercise cardiopulmonary reserve and recovery performance in subclinical hypothyroidism. *Braz J Med Biol Res*. 2010;43(11):1095–101.
5. Reents S. *Sport and Exercise Pharmacology*. Champaign (IL): Human Kinetics; 2000. 360 p.
6. Scuarcialupi MEA, Berton DC, Cordoni PK, Squassoni SD, Fiss E, Neder JA. Can bronchodilators improve exercise tolerance in COPD patients without dynamic hyperinflation? *J Bras Pneumol*. 2014;40(2):111–8.
7. Somani SM. *Pharmacology in Exercise and Sports*. Boca Raton (FL): CRC Press; 1996. 384 p.

Emergency Risk Management

INTRODUCTION

Having a well-thought-out emergency response system in place at all types of exercise settings is critical to providing a safe environment for participants and represents a fundamental practice in risk management. Emergency policies, procedures, and practices for health/fitness facilities and clinical exercise testing laboratories have been previously described in detail in recommendations published by the American College of Sports Medicine (ACSM) and American Heart Association (AHA) (2,3,4,8) (*Box B.1*). The types of settings in which exercise takes place vary markedly from rooms that are essentially hotel amenities to medically supervised clinical exercise centers. Such facilities often serve different purposes and clientele; may or may not have organized program offerings; and may or may not have exercise professionals trained in emergency preparedness. *Appendix B* provides an overview of emergency risk management for exercise settings typically overseen by qualified exercise or health care professionals trained in emergency preparedness.

The following ACSM standards on emergency response risk management are highlighted (2):

■ Facilities offering exercise services must have written emergency response system policies and procedures that are reviewed and rehearsed regularly and include documentation of these activities. These policies enable staff to handle basic first-aid situations and emergency cardiac events.

  ■ The emergency response system must be fully documented (*e.g.*, staff training, emergency instructions) and the documents kept in an area that can be easily accessed by the staff.

  ■ The emergency response system should identify a local coordinator (*e.g.*, a staff person that is responsible for the overall level of emergency readiness).

  ■ Exercise facilities should use local health care or medical personnel to help them develop their emergency response program.

  ■ The emergency response system must address the major emergency situations that might occur. Among those situations are medical emergencies

Box B.1	American College of Sports Medicine (ACSM) and American Heart Association (AHA) Emergency Risk Management Comprehensive Resources

The fourth edition of the *ACSM's Health/Fitness Facility Standards and Guidelines* (2) provides the most comprehensive information published to date on developing an emergency response system for the nonclinical or health/fitness exercise setting, and the reader is referred to this textbook for more detailed information regarding these types of settings. Additional information on matters of preparing emergency policies, procedures, and practices specific to clinical, research, health/fitness, or other exercise settings can be found in the contents of the joint ACSM/AHA publications (3,4). Emergency procedures specific to the clinical exercise testing setting have been described by the AHA (8).

that are reasonably foreseeable with the onset of moderate or more intense exercise such as hypoglycemia, sudden cardiac arrest (SCA), myocardial infarction, stroke, heat illness, and common orthopedic injuries. The response system must also address other foreseeable emergencies not necessarily associated with physical activity such as fires, chemical accidents, or severe weather.

- The emergency response system must provide a contingency plan that describes basic steps and instructions for each type of emergency situation and the roles each staff member or responder plays in an emergency. In addition, the emergency response system needs to provide locations for all emergency equipment, the location for all emergency exits, and accessible telephones for calling 911 as well as other contact information and steps necessary for contacting the local emergency medical services (EMS).
- The emergency response system must be physically reviewed and rehearsed at least two times per year with notations maintained in a logbook that indicate when the rehearsals were performed and who participated.
- The emergency response system must address the availability of first-aid kits and other medical equipment within the facility.

◀ Exercise facilities in the health/fitness or community setting must have as part of their written emergency response system a public access defibrillation program.

- Every site with automated external defibrillators (AEDs) should strive to get the response time from collapse caused by cardiac arrest to defibrillation to ≤3 min (*e.g.*, AEDs located throughout the facility so that the walk to retrieve an AED is ≤1.5 min).
- A skills and practice session with the AED is recommended every 3–6 mo for most exercise settings.
- The AED should be monitored and maintained according to the manufacturer's specifications on a daily, weekly, and monthly basis, and all related

information should be carefully documented and maintained as part of the facility's emergency response system records.

■ Exercise facilities must have in place a written system for sharing information with users and employees or independent contractors regarding the handling of potentially hazardous materials including the handling of bodily fluids by the facility's staff in accordance with the standards of the Occupational Safety and Health Administration (OSHA). These standards include the following:

  ▪ Provide appropriate training for staff on the handling of bodily fluids.
  ▪ Store all chemicals and agents in proper locations. Ensure these materials are stored off the floor and in an area that is off-limits to users. These areas should also have locks to prevent accidental or inappropriate entry.
  ▪ Provide regular training to workers in the handling of hazardous materials.
  ▪ Post the appropriate signage to warn users that they may be exposed to these hazardous agents.

Other key points regarding medical emergency plans and special circumstances such as clinical exercise testing or participation are as follows:

■ All personnel involved with exercise testing and supervision in a clinical exercise setting should be certified in basic cardiopulmonary resuscitation (CPR) and preferably advanced cardiac life support (ACLS).

■ There should be a physician immediately available at all times when maximal sign or symptom-limited exercise testing is performed on high-risk individuals.

■ Telephone numbers for emergency assistance should be posted clearly on or near all telephones. Emergency communication devices must be readily available and working properly.

■ Designated personnel should be assigned to the regular maintenance (*i.e.*, monthly and/or as determined by hospital and/or facility protocol) of the emergency equipment and regular surveillance of all pharmacological substances.

■ Incident reports should be clearly documented including the event time and date, witnesses present, and a detailed report of the medical emergency care provided. Copies of all documentation should be preserved on site maintaining the injured personnel's confidentiality, and a corresponding follow-up postincident report is highly recommended.

■ If a medical emergency occurs during exercise testing and/or training in the clinical exercise setting, the nearest available physician and/or other trained CPR provider should be solicited along with the medical emergency response team and/or paramedic (*i.e.*, if exercise is conducted outside of the hospital setting). In the medical exercise setting, the physician or lead medical responder should decide whether to evacuate the patient to the emergency department based on whether the medical emergency is life-threatening or not. If a physician is not available and there is any likelihood of decompensation, then transportation to the emergency department should be made immediately.

SPECIAL CIRCUMSTANCES: EMERGENCY EQUIPMENT AND DRUGS

Records should be kept documenting proper functioning of medical emergency equipment such as a manual defibrillator, AED, oxygen supply, and suction (*i.e.*, daily for all days of operations). All malfunctioning medical emergency equipment should be locked or removed immediately with operations suspended until repaired and/or replaced. In addition, expiration dates for pharmacological agents and other supportive supplies (*e.g.*, intravenous equipment, intravenous fluids) should be kept on file and readily available for review.

Emergency equipment and drugs should be available in any area where maximal exercise testing is performed on high-risk individuals such as in hospital-based exercise programs. Only personnel authorized by law and policy to use certain medical emergency equipment (*e.g.*, defibrillators, syringes, needles) and dispense drugs can lawfully do so. It is expected that such personnel be immediately available during maximal exercise testing of individuals with known cardiovascular disease in the clinical exercise setting. For more details, the reader is referred to guidelines on clinical exercise laboratories published by the AHA (8).

ADDITIONAL INFORMATION ON AUTOMATED EXTERNAL DEFIBRILLATORS

AEDs are computerized, sophisticated devices that provide voice and visual cues to guide lay and health care providers to safely defibrillate pulseless ventricular tachycardia/fibrillation (VF) SCA. Early defibrillation plays a critical role for successful survival of SCA for the following reasons:

- VF is the most frequent SCA witnessed.
- Electrical defibrillation is the treatment for VF.
- With delayed electrical defibrillation, the probability of success diminishes rapidly.
- VF deteriorates to asystole within minutes.

According to the 2010 AHA Guidelines for CPR and Emergency Cardiovascular Care, "rescuers must be able to rapidly integrate CPR with use of the AED" (7). Three key components must occur within the initial moments of a cardiac arrest and include the following:

1. Activation of the EMS
2. CPR
3. Operation of an AED

Automated External Defibrillator Implementation Guidelines

Because delays in CPR or defibrillation reduces SCA survival, the AHA urges the placement and use of AEDs in medical and nonmedical settings (*e.g.*, airports, airplanes, casinos, health/fitness facilities) (7). In hospital settings, CPR and an AED should be used immediately for cardiac arrest incidents. For out-of-hospital events when an AED is available, the AED should be used as soon as possible. Survival rate is improved when AED use is preceded by CPR (7).

For more detailed explanations on the expanding role of AEDs and management of various cardiovascular emergencies, refer to the 2010 AHA Guidelines for Cardiopulmonary Resuscitation and Emergency Cardiovascular Care (7) or any AHA subsequent updates. Important elements for implementing an AED program as previously described by the AHA are highlighted in *Table B.1* (1).

TABLE B.1	
American Heart Association Recommendations for Implementing an Automated External Defibrillator (AED) Program	
Get medical oversight	The U.S. Food and Drug Administration (FDA) may require a physician's prescription to purchase an AED. Other roles of the physician may include reviewing or making recommendations on policies and procedures, developing training plans, and helping assess each use of an AED. A designated individual should be responsible for day-to-day program implementation.
Work with local EMS	Most states require coordinating a public or community AED program with local EMS and providing follow-up data to EMS after any use of the AED.
Choose an AED	There are several suitable AEDs on the market. Select one that is easy to use and has adequate technical support from the manufacturer.
Make sure program support is available	Some AED manufacturers provide help with program planning, implementation, and ongoing support. They can assist with placement, medical authorization, registration, training, and supplies.
Place AEDs in visible and accessible locations	Effective AED programs are designed to deliver a shock to a victim within 3 min after the person collapses. Use a 3-min response time as a guideline to determine how many AEDs are needed and where to place them.
Develop a training plan	AED users should be certified in CPR and the use of an AED. The training should be done with enough regularity that the emergency plan and AED are familiar if needed.
Raise awareness of the AED program	Provide information to all stakeholders within an organization or company about the AED program. This information should include location of the device(s).
Implement an ongoing maintenance routine	Visually inspect the AED on a weekly or monthly basis to ensure they are in working order. Use a written checklist to assess the readiness of the AEDs and supplies.

CPR, cardiopulmonary resuscitation; EMS, emergency medical services.
Adapted from (1).

LEGAL ISSUES

According to the AHA, all 50 states and the District of Columbia now include using an AED as part of their Good Samaritan laws (1). In addition, the Cardiac Arrest Survival Act of 2000 provides limited immunity to rescuers using AEDs (6). The AHA encourages those involved with risk management to review its state's Good Samaritan Act and laws on AEDs (11). Several states have also passed laws requiring fitness facilities to have an AED (2). Because the requirements and immunity provisions vary from state to state, it is necessary to seek legal consultation on the interpretation and application of these laws.

Litigation cases involving sudden cardiac death and AEDs in the exercise setting vary widely and have included (a) not having an AED on premises, (b) not deploying an AED that existed on premises, (c) deploying but not utilizing a properly functioning AED within a reasonable response time, and (d) deploying an improperly functioning AED (11). Although the outcomes of such legal cases vary, it is the position of the ACSM that a professional standard of care exists for all exercise facilities in the public or community setting to have and properly deploy an AED when needed as part of their emergency response system. This recommendation (guideline) was introduced by the ACSM as early as 2002 in its joint publication with the AHA (4) and became a requirement (standard) in the third edition of *ACSM's Health/Fitness Facility Standards and Guidelines* published in 2007.

To minimize liability following an incident, exercise facilities should have post-emergency procedures in place including the completion of an incident report, taking photographs of conditions where the event occurred, and inspecting equipment that was involved in the emergency (5).

ONLINE RESOURCES

The following links provide additional information on emergency risk management. The reader will find sample plans for medical incidents/nonemergency situations and use of AEDs in the exercise setting; however, specific plans must be customized according to individual program needs and local standards. The ACSM recommends particular attention to local, state, and federal laws governing emergency risk management policies and procedures.

Automated External Defibrillator Implementation Guide (1):
http://www.heart.org/idc/groups/heart-public/@wcm/@ecc/documents
/downloadable/ucm_455415.pdf
State Laws on Cardiac Arrest and Defibrillators (11):
http://www.ncsl.org/research/health/laws-on-cardiac-arrest-and
-defibrillators-aeds.aspx
Occupational Safety and Health Administration: Emergency Action Plans (9):
http://www.osha.gov/pls/oshaweb/owadisp.show_document?p_id=9726&p
_table=STANDARDS
Public Access Defibrillator Guidelines (10):
http://www.foh.dhhs.gov/whatwedo/AED/HHSAED.ASP

REFERENCES

1. *AED Implementation Guide* [Internet]. Dallas (TX): American Heart Association; 2012 [cited 2015 Jan 11]. Available from: http://www.heart.org/idc/groups/heart-public/@wcm/@ecc/documents/downloadable/ucm_455415.pdf

2. American College of Sports Medicine. *ACSM's Health/Fitness Facility Standards and Guidelines.* 4th ed. Champaign (IL): Human Kinetics; 2012. 256 p.

3. Balady GJ, Chaitman B, Driscoll D, et al. Recommendations for cardiovascular screening, staffing, and emergency policies at health/fitness facilities. *Circulation.* 1998;97(22):2283–93.

4. Balady GJ, Chaitman B, Foster C, et al. Automated external defibrillators in health/fitness facilities: supplement to the AHA/ACSM Recommendations for Cardiovascular Screening, Staffing, and Emergency Policies at Health/Fitness Facilities. *Circulation.* 2002;105(9):1147–50.

5. Eickhoff-Shemek J, Herbert D, Connaughton DP. Risk Management for Health/Fitness Professionals. Baltimore (MD): Lippincott Williams and Wilkins; 2009. 407 p.

6. *Federal Cardiac Arrest Survival Act* [Internet]. Newtown (PA): HeartSine; [cited 2015 Aug 25]. Available from: http://heartsine.com/pdf/PDF-other/Cardiac_Arrest_Survival_Act_Text.pdf

7. Field JM, Hazinski MF, Sayre MR, et al. Part 1: executive summary: 2010 American Heart Association Guidelines for Cardiopulmonary Resuscitation and Emergency Cardiovascular Care. *Circulation.* 2010;122(18 Suppl 3):S640–56.

8. Myers J, Arena R, Franklin B, et al. Recommendations for clinical exercise laboratories: a scientific statement from the American Heart Association. *Circulation.* 2009;119(24):3144–61.

9. Occupational Safety and Health Administration. *Emergency Action Plans* [Internet]. Washington (DC): U.S. Department of Labor; [cited 2015 Aug 25]. Available from: http://www.osha.gov/pls/oshaweb/owadisp.show_document?p_id=9726&p_table=STANDARDS

10. *Public Access Defibrillation Guidelines* [Internet]. Washington (DC): U.S. Department of Health and Human Services; 2001 [cited 2015 Aug 25]. Available from: http://www.foh.dhhs.gov/whatwedo/AED/HHSAED.ASP

11. *State Laws on Cardiac Arrest and Defibrillators* [Internet]. Washington (DC): National Conference of State Legislatures; [cited 2015 Aug 25]. Available from: http://www.ncsl.org/research/health/laws-on-cardiac-arrest-and-defibrillators-aeds.aspx

Electrocardiogram Interpretation

The tables in *Appendix C* provide a quick reference source for electrocardiogram (ECG) recording and interpretation. Each of these tables should be used as part of the overall clinical profile when making diagnostic decisions about an individual.

TABLE C.1

Limb and Augmented Lead Electrode Placement[a]

Lead	Electrode Location and Polarity	Heart Surface Viewed
Lead I	Left arm (+), right arm (−)	Lateral
Lead II	Left leg (+), right arm (−)	Inferior
Lead III	Left leg (+), left arm (−)	Inferior
aVR	Right arm (+)	None
aVL	Left arm (+)	Lateral
aVF	Left leg (+)	Inferior

Exercise modifications: The limb leads are positioned over the left and right infraclavicular region for the arm leads and over the left and right lower quadrants of the abdomen for the leg leads. This ECG configuration minimizes motion artifacts during exercise. However, torso-placed limb leads should be noted for all ECG tracings to avoid misdiagnosis of an ECG tracing. The most common changes observed are produced by right axis deviation and standing that may obscure or produce Q waves inferiorly or anteriorly and T wave or frontal QRS axis changes even in normal people (5,7).

TABLE C.2

Precordial (Chest Lead) Electrode Placement

Lead	Electrode Placement	Heart Surface Viewed
V_1	Fourth intercostal space just to the right of the sternal border	Septum
V_2	Fourth intercostal space just to the left of the sternal border	Septum
V_3	At the midpoint of a straight line between V_2 and V_4	Anterior
V_4	On the midclavicular line in the fifth intercostal space	Anterior
V_5	On the anterior axillary line and on a horizontal plane through V_4	Lateral
V_6	On the midaxillary line and on a horizontal plane through V_4 and V_5	Lateral

Adapted from (6).

TABLE C.3

Electrocardiogram Interpretation Steps

1. Check for correct calibration (1 mV = 10 mm) and paper speed (25 mm · s^{-1}).
2. Verify the heart rate and determine the heart rhythm.
3. Measure intervals (PR, QRS, QT).
4. Determine the mean QRS axis and mean T-wave axis in the limb leads.
5. Look for morphologic abnormalities of the P wave, QRS complex, ST segment, T wave, and U wave (*e.g.*, chamber enlargement, conduction delays, infarction, repolarization changes).
6. Interpret the present ECG.
7. Compare the present ECG with previous available ECGs.
8. Offer conclusion, clinical correlation, and recommendations.

TABLE **C.4**			
Resting Electrocardiogram: Normal Limits (3,8,9,11)			
Parameter	**Normal Limits**	**Abnormal if:**	**Possible Interpretation(s)**[a]
Heart rate	60–100 beats · min^{-1}	<60 beats · min^{-1}	Bradycardia
		>100 beats · min^{-1}	Tachycardia
P wave	<0.12 s	Broad and notched (>0.12 s) in leads I, II, aVL, and V_4–V_6 and inverted in V_1	Left atrial hypertrophy
	<2.5 mm tall	Peaked (>2.5 mm tall) in leads II, III, and aVF and upright in V_1	Right atrial hypertrophy or enlargement
		Peaked and broad in leads I, II, III, aVL, aVF, and V_4–V_6 and biphasic in V_1	Combined atrial hypertrophy
PR interval	0.12–0.20 s	<0.12 s	Preexcitation (i.e., W-P-W or L-G-L)
		>0.20 s	First-degree AV block
QRS duration	0.06–0.10 s	If ≥0.11 s	Conduction abnormality (i.e., incomplete or complete bundle branch block, W-P-W, IVCD, or electronic pacer)
QT interval	Rate dependent	QTc long	Drug effects, electrolyte abnormalities, or ischemia
	Normal QT = $K \sqrt{RR}$, where K = 0.37 for men and children and 0.40 for women	QTc short	Digitalis effect, hypercalcemia, or hypermagnesia
QRS axis	−30 to +110 degrees	<−30 degrees	Left axis deviation (i.e., chamber enlargement, hemiblock, or myocardial infarction)
		>+110 degrees	Right axis deviation (i.e., RVH, pulmonary disease, or myocardial infarction)
		Indeterminate	All limb leads transitional
T wave	Upright in leads I, II, and V_3–V_6; inverted in aVR; flat, inverted, or biphasic in III and V_1–V_2	Upright, inverted, flattened, or biphasic alone or with ST-segment changes	Can be a normal variant; ischemia, LVH, or caused by physiologic conditions (posture changes, respiration, drugs)

(continued)

TABLE C.4

Resting Electrocardiogram: Normal Limits (3,8,9,11) (Continued)

Parameter	Normal Limits	Abnormal if:	Possible Interpretation(s)[a]
T axis	Generally same direction as QRS axis	The T axis (vector) is typically deviated away from the area of "mischief" (i.e., ischemia, bundle branch block, or hypertrophy).	Chamber enlargement, ischemia, drug effects, or electrolyte disturbances
ST segment	Generally at isoelectric line (PR segment) or within 1 mm	Elevation of ST segment	Normal variant (early repolarization), injury, ischemia, pericarditis, or electrolyte abnormality
	The ST segment may be elevated up to 1–2 mm in leads V_1–V_4.	Depression of ST segment 80 ms after the J-point	Injury, ischemia, electrolyte abnormality, drug effects, or normal variant
Q wave	<0.04 s and <25% of R wave amplitude (exceptions lead III and V_1)	>0.04 s and/or >25% of R wave amplitude except lead III and V_1	Myocardial infarction or pseudoinfarction (as from chamber enlargement, conduction abnormalities, W-P-W, COPD, or cardiomyopathy)
Transition zone	Usually between V_2–V_4	Before V_2	Counterclockwise rotation (early transition)
		After V_4	Clockwise rotation (late transition)

[a]If supported by other electrocardiograms and related clinical criteria.
AV, atrioventricular; COPD, chronic obstructive pulmonary disease; IVCD, intraventricular conduction delay; L-G-L, Lown-Ganong-Levine syndrome; LVH, left ventricular hypertrophy; QTc, QT corrected for heart rate; RVH, right ventricular hypertrophy; W-P-W, Wolff-Parkinson-White syndrome.

TABLE C.5

Romhilt-Estes Electrocardiogram Criteria for the Screening of Left Ventricular Enlargement

	Points
1. Any of the following	
R or S in limb lead ≥20 mm	
S wave in V_1, V_2, V_3 ≥25 mm	
R wave in V_4, V_5, V_6 ≥25 mm	3
2. Any ST shift	3
Typical strain ST-T changes	1
3. LAD >15 degrees	2
4. QRS interval >0.09 s	1
5. Intrinsicoid deflection >0.04 s	1
6. P-terminal force V_1 >0.04	3
Total (LVH >5 points, probable LVH >4 points)	13

NOTE: The Romhilt-Estes point score system for screening left ventricular hypertrophy via electrocardiogram is associated with a median specificity of 95% (2).
LAD, left axis deviation; LVH, left ventricular hypertrophy.
Adapted with permission from (10).

TABLE C.6

Localization of Transmural Infarcts[a] (Location of Diagnostic Q Wave)

Typical ECG Leads	Infarct Location
V_1–V_3	Anteroseptal
V_3–V_4	Localized anterior
V_4–V_6, I, aVL	Anterolateral
V_1–V_6	Extensive anterior
I, aVL	High lateral
II, III, aVF	Inferior
V_1–V_2	Septal or true posterior (R/S >1)
V_1, V_{3R}, V_{4R}	Right ventricular

When diagnostic Q waves are present in the inferior leads and the R wave is greater than the S wave in V_1 or V_2, this can reflect the presence of posterior extension of the inferior myocardial infarction.
$_R$, V_{4R}, right precordial leads.

TABLE C.7

Supraventricular versus Ventricular Ectopic Beats[a]

Parameter		Supraventricular (Normal Conduction)	Supraventricular (Aberrant Conduction)	Ventricular
QRS complex	Duration	Up to 0.10 s	≥0.11 s	≥0.11 s
	Configuration	Normal	Widened QRS usually with unchanged initial vector	Widened QRS often with abnormal initial vector
			P wave precedes QRS	QRS usually not preceded by a P wave
P wave		Present or absent but with relationship to QRS	Present or absent but with relationship to QRS	Present or absent but without relationship to QRS
Rhythm		Usually less than compensatory pause	Usually less than compensatory pause	Usually compensatory pause

[a]Numerous ECG criteria exist to try to distinguish premature ventricular contractions (PVCs) from aberrant conduction (1,4). A major clinical problem is the patient with a wide QRS tachycardia. Such tachycardias can be ventricular or supraventricular with aberrant conduction. Typically, ventricular tachycardia is characterized by a significant shift in frontal plane axis. In contrast, a wide QRS (supraventricular tachycardia) maintains proximity to the axis in absence of this arrhythmia. A good rule of thumb is that any wide QRS tachycardia in a patient with heart disease or a history of heart failure is likely to be ventricular tachycardia, especially if atrioventricular (AV) dissociation is identified.

TABLE C.8

Atrioventricular Block

Interpretation	P Wave Relationship to QRS	PR Interval	R–R Interval
First-degree atrioventricular (AV) block	1:1	>0.20 s	Regular or follows P–P interval
Second-degree AV block: Mobitz I (Wenckebach)	>1:1	Progressively lengthens until a P wave fails to conduct	Progressively shortens; pause less than two other cycles
Second-degree AV block: Mobitz II	>1:1	Constant but with sudden dropping of QRS	Regular except for pause, which usually equals two other cycles
Third-degree AV block	None	Variable but P–P interval constant	Usually regular (escape rhythm)

TABLE C.9

Atrioventricular (AV) Dissociation[a]

Type of AV Dissociation	Electrophysiology	Example	Significance	Comment
AV dissociation resulting from complete AV block	AV block	Sinus rhythm with complete AV block	Pathologic	Unrelated P wave and QRS complexes P–P interval is shorter than R–R interval
AV dissociation by default causing interference	Slowing of the primary or dominant pacemaker with escape of a subsidiary pacemaker	Sinus bradycardia with junctional escape rhythm	Physiologic	Unrelated P wave and QRS complexes P–P interval is longer than R–R interval
AV dissociation by usurpation	Acceleration of a subsidiary pacemaker usurping control of the ventricles	Sinus rhythm with either AV junctional or ventricular tachycardia	Physiologic	Unrelated P wave and QRS complexes P–P interval is longer than R–R interval
Combination	AV block and interference	Atrial fibrillation with accelerated AV junctional pacemaker and block below this pacemaker	Pathologic	Unrelated P wave and QRS complexes

[a]What is meant by AV dissociation? When the atria and ventricles beat independently, their contractions are "dissociated," and AV dissociation exists. Thus, P waves and QRS complexes in the ECG are unrelated. AV dissociation may be complete or incomplete, transient or permanent. The causes of AV dissociation are block and interference, and both may be present in the same ECG. Block is associated with a pathologic state of refractoriness, preventing the primary pacemaker's impulse from reaching the lower chamber. An example of this is sinus rhythm with complete AV block. Interference results from slowing of the primary pacemaker or acceleration of a subsidiary pacemaker. The lower chamber's impulse "interferes" with conduction by producing physiologic refractoriness, and AV dissociation results. An example of this is sinus rhythm with AV junctional or ventricular tachycardia and no retrograde conduction into the atria. A clear distinction must be made between block and interference. Table C.9 describes the four types of AV dissociation.

REFERENCES

1. American College of Sports Medicine. *ACSM's Resource Manual for Guidelines for Exercise Testing and Prescription.* 7th ed. Baltimore (MD): Lippincott Williams & Wilkins; 2014. 896 p.

2. Bauml MA, Underwood D. Left ventricular hypertrophy: an overlooked cardiovascular risk factor. *Cleve Clin J Med.* 2010;77(6):381–7.

3. Chou T-C. *Electrocardiography in Clinical Practice: Adult and Pediatric.* 4th ed. Philadelphia (PA): Saunders; 1996. 717 p.

4. Dubin D. *Rapid Interpretation of EKG's.* 6th ed. Tampa (FL): Cover; 2000. 368 p.

5. Gamble P, McManus H, Jensen D, Froelicher V. A comparison of the standard 12-lead electrocardiogram to exercise electrode placements. *Chest.* 1984;85:616–22.

6. Goldberger AL. *Clinical Electrocardiography: A Simplified Approach.* 7th ed. Philadelphia (PA): Mosby Elsevier; 2006. 352 p.

7. Jowett NI, Turner AM, Cole A, Jones PA. Modified electrode placement must be recorded when performing 12-lead electrocardiograms. *Postgrad Med J.* 2005;81(952):122–5.

8. Levine S, Coyne BJ, Colvin LC. *Clinical Exercise Electrocardiography.* Burlington (MA): Jones and Barlett; 2016. 384 p.

9. Menown IB, Mackenzie G, Adgey AA. Optimizing the initial 12-lead electrocardiographic diagnosis of acute myocardial infarction. *Eur Heart J.* 2000;21:275–83.

10. Wagner GS. *Marriott's Practical Electrocardiography.* 9th ed. Baltimore (MD): Williams & Wilkins; 1994. 352 p.

11. Whyte G, Sharma S. *Practical ECG for Exercise Science and Sports Medicine.* Champaign, (IL): Human Kinetics; 2010. 176 p.

American College of Sports Medicine Certifications

INTRODUCTION

Exercise practitioners are becoming increasingly aware of the advantages of maintaining professional credentials. In efforts to ensure quality, reduce liability, and remain competitive, more and more employers are requiring professional certification of their exercise staff. Additionally, in efforts to improve public safety, mandates for certification by state and/or regulatory agencies (*e.g.*, licensure) as well as third-party payers now exist. The American College of Sports Medicine (ACSM) offers five primary and five specialty certifications for exercise professionals.

ACSM Primary and Specialty Certifications

Primary Certifications

- ACSM Certified Group Exercise Instructor^{SM} (GEI)
- ACSM Certified Personal Trainer^{SM} (CPT)
- ACSM Certified Exercise Physiologist^{SM} (EP-C)
- ACSM Certified Clinical Exercise Physiologist® (CEP)
- ACSM Registered Clinical Exercise Physiologist® (RCEP)

Specialty Certifications and Credentials

- Exercise is Medicine Credential®
- ACSM/NCHPAD Certified Inclusive Fitness Trainer^{SM}
- ACSM/ACS Certified Cancer Exercise Trainer^{SM}
- ACSM/NPAS Physical Activity in Public Health Specialist^{SM}
- ARP/ACSM Certified Ringside Physician®

ACS, American Cancer Society; ARP, Association for Ringside Physicians; NCHPAD, National Center on Health, Physical Activity and Disability; NPAS, National Physical Activity Society

JOB DEFINITIONS AND SCOPE OF PRACTICE

ACSM Certified Group Exercise Instructor^{SM}: The GEI (a) possesses a minimum of a high school diploma and (b) works in a group exercise setting with apparently healthy individuals and those with health challenges who are able to exercise independently to enhance quality of life, improve health-related physical fitness, manage health risk, and promote lasting health behavior change. The GEI leads safe and effective exercise programs using a variety of leadership techniques to foster group camaraderie, support, and motivation to enhance muscular strength and endurance, flexibility, cardiorespiratory fitness, body composition, and any of the motor skills related to the domains of health-related physical fitness.

ACSM Certified Personal Trainer^{SM}: The CPT (a) possesses a minimum of a high school diploma and (b) works with apparently healthy individuals and those with health challenges who are able to exercise independently to enhance quality of life, improve health-related physical fitness, performance, manage health risk, and promote lasting health behavior change. The CPT conducts basic preparticipation health screening assessments; submaximal aerobic exercise tests; and muscular strength/endurance, flexibility, and body composition tests. The CPT facilitates motivation and adherence as well as develops and administers programs designed to enhance muscular strength/endurance, flexibility, cardiorespiratory fitness, body composition, and/or any of the motor skill–related components of physical fitness (*i.e.*, balance, coordination, power, agility, speed, and reaction time).

ACSM Certified Exercise Physiologist^{SM}: The EP-C is a health fitness professional with a minimum of a bachelor's degree in exercise science. The EP-C performs preparticipation health screenings, conducts physical fitness assessments, interprets results, develops exercise prescriptions, and applies behavioral and motivational strategies to apparently healthy individuals and individuals with medically controlled diseases and health conditions to support clients in adopting and maintaining healthy lifestyle behaviors. The academic preparation of the EP-C also includes fitness management, administration, and supervision. The EP-C is typically employed or self-employed in commercial, community, studio, corporate, university, and hospital settings.

ACSM Certified Clinical Exercise Physiologist® The CEP is an allied health professional with a minimum of a bachelor's degree in exercise science. The CEP works with patients and clients challenged with cardiovascular, pulmonary, and metabolic diseases and disorders as well as with apparently healthy populations in cooperation with other health care professionals to enhance quality of life, manage health risk, and promote lasting health behavior change. The CEP conducts preparticipation health screening and maximal and submaximal graded exercise tests and performs strength, flexibility, and body composition tests. The CEP develops and administers programs designed to enhance cardiorespiratory fitness, muscular strength and endurance, balance, and range of motion. The CEP educates his or her clients about testing, exercise program components, and clinical and lifestyle self-care for control of chronic disease and health conditions.

ACSM Registered Clinical Exercise Physiologist®: The RCEP (a) is an allied health professional with a minimum of a master's degree in exercise science and (b) works the application of physical activity and behavioral interventions for those with clinic diseases and health conditions that have been shown to provide therapeutic and/or functional benefit. Persons whom RCEP services are appropriate for may include, but are not limited to, individuals with cardiovascular, pulmonary, metabolic, orthopedic, musculoskeletal, neuromuscular, neoplastic, immunologic, and hematologic disease. The RCEP provides primary and secondary prevention and rehabilitative strategies designed to improve physical fitness and health in populations ranging across the lifespan. The RCEP provides exercise screening, exercise and physical fitness testing, exercise prescriptions, exercise and physical activity counseling, exercise supervision, exercise and health education/promotion, and measurement and evaluation of exercise and physical activity–related outcome measures. The RCEP works individually or as part of an interdisciplinary team in a clinical, community, or public health setting. The practice and supervision of the RCEP is guided by published professional guidelines, standards, and applicable state and federal laws and regulations.

ACSM CERTIFICATION DEVELOPMENT

The process of developing a certification examination begins with a job task analysis (JTA) (1). The purpose of the JTA is to (a) define the major areas of professional practice (*i.e.*, domains), (b) delineate the tasks performed "on the job," and (c) identify the knowledge and skills (KSs) required for safe and competent practice. The domains are subsequently weighted according to the importance and frequency of performance of their respective tasks. The number of examination test items is then determined based on the domain weight. Each examination reflects the content and weights defined by the JTA. By linking the content of the examination to the JTA (*e.g.*, what professionals do), it is possible to ensure that the examination is practice related.

Examination development continues with question writing. Content experts representing academia and practice are selected and trained on examination item writing. This examination writing team is charged with the task of creating test items that are representative of and consistent with the JTA. Each test item is evaluated psychometrically, undergoing extensive testing, editing, and retesting before being included as a scored item on the examination. Finally, passing scores are determined using a criterion-referenced methodology. Passing scores for each examination are associated with a minimum level of mastery necessary for safe and competent practice. Setting passing scores in this manner ensures that qualified candidates will become certified regardless of how other candidates perform on the examination.

The eligibility criteria, competencies, and primary populations served by ACSM's primary certifications are listed in *Table D.1*.

Certification **domains**, **complete job tasks**, and **KSs statements** for each certification for all five primary ACSM certifications, ACSM/NCPAD Certified Inclusive Fitness Trainer^{SM}, ACSM/ACS Certified Cancer Exercise Trainer^{SM}, and ACSM/NPAS Physical Activity in Public Health Specialist^{SM} can be found online at http://certification.acsm.org/outlines. Because every question on each of the certification examinations must refer to a specific knowledge or skill statement within the associated JTA, these documents provide a resource to guide exam preparation.

TABLE D.1

American College of Sports Medicine's Certifications at a Glance

Certification	Primary Population Served	Eligibility Criteria	Competencies
ACSM Certified Group Exercise Instructor^SM	Apparently healthy individuals and those with health challenges who are able to exercise independently	■ ≥18 yr ■ High school diploma or equivalent ■ Current CPR and AED certifications (must contain a live skills component) — AED not required for those practicing outside of the United States and Canada	■ Develops and implements a variety of exercises in group settings and modifies exercise according to need ■ Leads safe and effective exercise using a variety of leadership techniques to enhance the motor skills related to the domains of physical fitness
ACSM Certified Personal Trainer^SM	Apparently healthy individuals and those with health challenges who are able to exercise independently	■ ≥18 yr ■ High school diploma or equivalent ■ Current CPR and AED certifications (must contain a live skills component such as the American Heart Association [AHA] or the American Red Cross) — AED not required for those practicing outside of the United States and Canada	■ Identifies health risk factors, performs fitness appraisals and preparticipation health screenings, and develops exercise programs that promote lasting behavior change ■ Incorporates suitable and innovative activities to improve functional capacity and manages health risk to promote lasting behavior change

Certification	Population	Requirements	Job tasks
...SM Certified Exercise Physiologist^SM	Apparently healthy individuals and those with medically controlled diseases	■ Bachelor's degree in an exercise science, exercise physiology, kinesiology, or exercise science–based degree (one is eligible to sit for the examination if the candidate is in the last term of his or her degree program) ■ Current CPR and AED certifications (must contain a live skills component such as the AHA or the American Red Cross) — AED not required for those practicing outside of the United States and Canada	■ Applies knowledge of exercise science including kinesiology, functional anatomy, exercise physiology, nutrition, program administration, psychology, and injury prevention in the health/fitness setting ■ Performs preparticipation health screenings and fitness assessments ■ Interprets assessment results and develops exercise prescriptions ■ Performs duties related to fitness management, administration, and program supervision ■ Incorporates suitable physical activities to improve functional capacity ■ Applies appropriate behavioral change techniques to effectively educate and counsel on lifestyle modification
ACSM Certified Clinical Exercise Physiologist®	Apparently healthy individuals and those with cardiovascular, pulmonary, and metabolic disease	■ Bachelor's degree in an exercise science, exercise physiology, kinesiology, or exercise science–based degree (one is eligible to sit for the exam if the candidate is in the last term of his or her degree program) ■ Minimum of 400 h of clinical experience for graduates from a CAAHEP-accredited program or 500 h of clinical experience for graduates from a non-CAAHEP-accredited program ■ Current certification for the AHA BLS for Healthcare Provider or American Red Cross CPR/AED for the Professional Rescuer or equivalent (must contain live skills component) — AED not required for those practicing outside of the United States and Canada	■ Applies extensive knowledge of functional anatomy, exercise physiology, pathophysiology, electrocardiography, human behavior/ psychology, gerontology, and graded exercise testing in the clinical setting ■ Provides exercise supervision/leadership and counsels patients on lifestyle modification ■ Conducts emergency procedures in exercise testing and training settings

(continued)

TABLE D.1

American College of Sports Medicine's Certifications at a Glance (Continued)

Certification	Primary Population Served	Eligibility Criteria	Competencies
ACSM Registered Clinical Exercise Physiologist®	Apparently healthy individuals and those with cardiovascular, pulmonary, metabolic, orthopedic/musculoskeletal, neuromuscular, neoplastic, immunologic, and hematologic disorders	■ Graduate degree in clinical exercise physiology with coursework in clinical assessment, exercise testing, exercise prescription, and exercise training (one is eligible to sit for the exam if the candidate is in the last term of his or her degree program) ■ Minimum of 600 h of clinical experience (external to classroom/laboratory) working with individuals with chronic disease ■ Current certification for the AHA BLS for Healthcare Provider or American Red Cross CPR/AED for the Professional Rescuer or equivalent (must contain live skills component) — AED not required for those practicing outside of the United States and Canada	■ Performs exercise screening and exercise and fitness testing ■ Develops exercise prescriptions and supervises exercise programs ■ Conducts exercise and physical activity education counseling ■ Conducts measurement and evaluation of exercise and physical activity–related outcomes

AED, automated external defibrillators; BLS, basic life support; CAAHEP, Commission on Accreditation of Allied Health Education Programs; CPR, cardiopulmonary resuscitation

ONLINE RESOURCES

American College of Sports Medicine Certifications:
http://certification.acsm.org/get-certified
American College of Sports Medicine Certifications Job Task Analysis:
http://certification.acsm.org/exam-content-outlines
American College of Sports Medicine Code of Ethics for Certified and
Registered Professionals:
http://certification.acsm.org/faq28-codeofethics
Clinical Exercise Physiology Association:
http://www.acsm-cepa.org

REFERENCE

1. Paternostro-Bayles M. The role of a job task analysis in the development of professional certifications. *ACSM Health Fitness J.* 2010;14(4):41–2.

Accreditation of Exercise Science Programs

Advances in the exercise profession have been substantial over the past decade. Specific conditions that are considered essential for a formalized profession to exist are now in place (1). These include

- A standardized system to develop skills
- A standardized system to validate skills

The Committee on Accreditation for the Exercise Sciences (CoAES) under the auspices of the Commission on Accreditation of Allied Health Education Programs (CAAHEP) now validates and accredits university curriculum in the exercise sciences (*i.e.*, standardized skills development). The National Commission for Certifying Agencies (NCCA) provides a standardized, independent, and objective third-party evaluation of examination design, development, and performance to ensure certification integrity (*i.e.*, skills validation).

An increase in the number of accredited graduate and undergraduate programs will help to further establish exercise science as a profession. Accreditation assures that an appropriate curriculum is being provided and that students are graduating with the competencies necessary to be an exercise physiologist or clinical exercise physiologist. The primary role of the CoAES is to establish standards and guidelines for academic programs that facilitate the preparation of students seeking employment in the preventive and clinical exercise field. The secondary role of the CoAES is to establish and implement a process of self-study, review, and recommendation for all programs seeking CAAHEP accreditation (http://www.coaes.org). A number of organizations participate in CoAES including American College of Sports Medicine (ACSM), American Council on Exercise (ACE), The Cooper Institute, National Academy of Sports Medicine (NASM), and National Council on Strength and Fitness (NCSF).

Accreditation of exercise science programs also serves a very important public interest. Along with certification and licensure, accreditation is a tool intended to help assure a well-prepared and qualified workforce providing health care services (CAAHEP: http://www.caahep.org).

ONLINE RESOURCES

Commission on Accreditation of Allied Health Education Programs:
http://www.caahep.org

Committee on Accreditation for the Exercise Sciences:
http://www.coaes.org

The National Commission for Certifying Agencies under the National Organization for Competency Assurance:
http://www.credentialingexcellence.org

REFERENCE

1. Costanzo DG. ACSM certification: The evolution of the exercise professional. *ACSM Health Fitness J*. 2006;10(4):38–9.

Contributing Authors to the Previous Two Editions

CONTRIBUTORS TO THE NINTH EDITION

Kelli Allen, PhD
VA Medical Center
Durham, North Carolina

Mark Anderson, PT, PhD
University of Oklahoma Health
  Sciences Center
Oklahoma City, Oklahoma

Gary Balady, MD
Boston University School of Medicine
Boston, Massachusetts

Michael Berry, PhD
Wake Forest University
Winston-Salem, North Carolina

Bryan Blissmer, PhD
University of Rhode Island
Kingston, Rhode Island

Kim Bonzheim, MSA, FACSM
Genesys Regional Medical Center
Grand Blanc, Michigan

Barry Braun, PhD, FACSM
University of Massachusetts
Amherst, Massachusetts

Monthaporn S. Bryant, PT, PhD
Michael E. DeBakey VA Medical Center
Houston, Texas

Thomas Buckley, MPH, RPh
University of Connecticut
Storrs, Connecticut

John Castellani, PhD
United States Army Research Institute
  of Environmental Medicine
Natick, Massachusetts

**Dino Costanzo, MA, FACSM,
ACSM-RCEP, ACSM-PD,
ACSM-ETT**
The Hospital of Central Connecticut
New Britain, Connecticut

Michael Deschenes, PhD, FACSM
The College of William and Mary
Williamsburg, Virginia

Joseph E. Donnelly, EdD, FACSM
University of Kansas Medical Center
Kansas City, Kansas

Bo Fernhall, PhD, FACSM
University of Illinois at Chicago
Chicago, Illinois

Stephen F. Figoni, PhD, FACSM
VA West Los Angeles Healthcare
  Center
Los Angeles, California

Nadine Fisher, EdD
University of Buffalo
Buffalo, New York

Charles Fulco, ScD
United States Army Research Institute
of Environmental Medicine
Natick, Massachusetts

**Carol Ewing Garber, PhD, FACSM,
ACSM-RCEP, ACSM-HFS,
ACSM-PD**
Columbia University
New York, New York

Andrew Gardner, PhD
University of Oklahoma Health
Sciences Center
Oklahoma City, Oklahoma

**Neil Gordon, MD, PhD, MPH,
FACSM**
Intervent International
Savannah, Georgia

Eric Hall, PhD, FACSM
Elon University
Elon, North Carolina

Gregory Hand, PhD, MPH, FACSM
University of South Carolina
Columbia, South Carolina

**Samuel Headley, PhD, FACSM,
ACSM-RCEP**
Springfield College
Springfield, Massachusetts

Kurt Jackson, PT, PhD
University of Dayton
Dayton, Ohio

Robert Kenefick, PhD, FACSM
United States Army Research Institute
of Environmental Medicine
Natick, Massachusetts

Christine Kohn, PharmD
University of Connecticut School of
Pharmacy
Storrs, Connecticut

Wendy Kohrt, PhD, FACSM
University of Colorado—Anschutz
Medical Campus
Aurora, Colorado

I-Min Lee, MBBS, MD, ScD
Brigham and Women's Hospital,
Harvard Medical School
Boston, Massachusetts

David X. Marquez, PhD, FACSM
University of Illinois at Chicago
Chicago, Illinois

Kyle McInnis, ScD, FACSM
Merrimack College
North Andover, Massachusetts

Miriam Morey, PhD, FACSM
VA and Duke Medical Centers
Durham, North Carolina

Michelle Mottola, PhD, FACSM
The University of Western Ontario
London, Ontario, Canada

Stephen Muza, PhD, FACSM
United States Army Research Institute
of Environmental Medicine
Natick, Massachusetts

Patricia Nixon, PhD
Wake Forest University
Winston-Salem, North Carolina

**Jennifer R. O'Neill, PhD, MPH,
ACSM-HFS**
University of South Carolina
Columbia, South Carolina

Russell Pate, PhD, FACSM
University of South Carolina
Columbia, South Carolina

Richard Preuss, PhD, PT
McGill University
Montreal, Quebec, Canada

Kathryn Schmitz, PhD, MPH, FACSM, ACSM-HFS
University of Pennsylvania
Philadelphia, Pennsylvania

Carrie Sharoff, PhD
Arizona State University
Tempe, Arizona

Maureen Simmonds, PhD, PT
University of Texas Health Science
 Center
San Antonio, Texas

Paul Thompson, MD, FACSM, FACC
Hartford Hospital
Hartford, Connecticut

CONTRIBUTORS TO THE EIGHTH EDITION

Kelli Allen, PhD
VA Medical Center
Durham, North Carolina

Lawrence E. Armstrong, PhD, FACSM
University of Connecticut
Storrs, Connecticut

Gary J. Balady, MD
Boston University School of Medicine
Boston, Massachusetts

Michael J. Berry, PhD, FACSM
Wake Forest University
Winston-Salem, North Carolina

Craig Broeder, PhD, FACSM
Benedictine University
Lisle, Illinois

John Castellani, PhD, FACSM
U.S. Army Research Institute of
 Environmental Medicine
Natick, Massachusetts

Bernard Clark, MD
St. Francis Hospital and Medical
 Center
Hartford, Connecticut

Dawn P. Coe, PhD
Grand Valley State University
Allendale, Michigan

Michael Deschenes, PhD, FACSM
College of William and Mary
Willamsburg, Virginia

J. Andrew Doyle, PhD
Georgia State University
Atlanta, Georgia

Barry Franklin, PhD, FACSM
William Beaumont Hospital
Royal Oak, Michigan

Charles S. Fulco, ScD
U.S. Army Research Institute of
 Environmental Medicine
Natick, Massachusetts

Carol Ewing Garber, PhD, FACSM
Columbia University
New York, New York

Paul M. Gordon, PhD, FACSM
University of Michigan
Ann Arbor, Michigan

Sam Headley, PhD, FACSM
Springfield College
Springfield, Massachusetts

John E. Hodgkin, MD
St. Helena Hospital
St. Helena, California

John M. Jakicic, PhD, FACSM
University of Pittsburgh
Pittsburgh, Pennsylvania

Wendy Kohrt, PhD, FACSM
University of Colorado—Denver
Aurora, Colorado

Timothy R. McConnell, PhD, FACSM
Bloomsburg University
Bloomsburg, Pennsylvania

Kyle McInnis, ScD, FACSM
University of Massachusetts
Boston, Massachusetts

Miriam C. Morey, PhD
VA and Duke Medical Centers
Durham, North Carolina

Stephen Muza, PhD
U.S. Army Research Institute of
    Environmental Medicine
Natick, Massachusetts

Jonathan Myers, PhD, FACSM
VA Palo Alto Health Care System/
    Stanford University
Palo Alto, California

Patricia A. Nixon, PhD, FACSM
Wake Forest University
Winston-Salem, North Carolina

Jeff Rupp, PhD
Georgia State University
Atlanta, Georgia

Ray Squires, PhD, FACSM
Mayo Clinic
Rochester, Minnesota

Clare Stevinson, PhD
University of Alberta
Edmonton, Canada

Scott Thomas, PhD
University of Toronto
Toronto, Canada

Yves Vanlandewijck, PhD
Katholieke Universiteit Leuven
Leuven, Belgium

Index

Note: Page numbers followed by *b*, *f*, or *t* indicate boxed, figures, or table material.